Merriman's Assessment of the Lower Limb

For Elsevier:

Commissioning Editor: Robert Edwards
Development Editor: Kim Benson
Project Manager: Andrew Palfreyman
Design: Charles Gray
Illustrations Manager: Kirsteen Wright
Illustrations: Joanna Cameron
DVD: CreationVideo

Merriman's Assessment of the Lower Limb

Edited by

Ben Yates MSc BSc (Hons) FCPodS DpodM
Consultant Podiatric Surgeon, Trauma and Orthopaedics,
Great Western Hospital, Swindon, UK

THIRD EDITION

CHURCHILL LIVINGSTONE

ELSEVIER

EDINBURGH LONDON NEW YORK OXFORD PHILADELPHIA ST LOUIS SYDNEY TORONTO 2008

CHURCHILL
LIVINGSTONE
ELSEVIER

First edition 1995
Second edition 2002
Reprinted 2005, 2006, 2007
Third edition 2009

ISBN: 978-0-08-045107-7

British Library Cataloguing in Publication Data
A catalogue record for this book is available from the British Library.

Library of Congress Cataloging in Publication Data
A catalog record for this book is available from the Library of Congress.

Note
Knowledge and best practice in this field are constantly changing. As new research and experience broaden our knowledge, changes in practice, treatment and drug therapy may become necessary or appropriate. Readers are advised to check the most current information provided (i) on procedures featured or (ii) by the manufacturer of each product to be administered, to verify the recommended dose or formula, the method and duration of administration, and contraindications. It is the responsibility of the practitioner, relying on their own experience and knowledge of the patient, to make diagnoses, to determine dosages and the best treatment for each individual patient, and to take all appropriate safety precautions. To the fullest extent of the law, neither the Publisher nor the Editor assumes any liability for any injury and/or damage to persons or property arising out or related to any use of the material contained in this book.

The Publisher

Printed in China

Contents

Contributors

A R Bird PhD BPod(Hons)
Lecturer, Department of Podiatry and the Musculoskeletal Research Centre
La Trobe University
Victoria
Australia

I Bristow MSc(Oxon) BSc(Hons) MChS FHEA
Lecturer, School of Health Professions and Rehabilitation Sciences
University of Southampton
UK

J Burns PhD
NHMRC Australian Clinical Research Fellow
Institute for Neuromuscular Research
The Children's Hospital at Westmead
New South Wales
Australia

M Hanley BSc(Hons) Psychology MSc PhD
Principal Lecturer, Postgraduate programmes
The University of Northampton
Northampton
UK

D Hocken
Consultant Vascular Surgeon
Great Western Hospital
Swindon
UK

K B Landorf PhD
Senior Lecturer and Research Coordinator
Department of Podiatry and Musculoskeletal Research Centre
La Trobe University
Bundoora
Australia

C McCarthy MBChB FRCR
Consultant Radiologist
Nuffield Orthopaedic Hospital
Oxford
UK

A McInnes BSc(Hons) DPodM
Senior Lecturer
Podiatry Division School of Health Professions
Eastbourne
UK

H B Menz BPod(Hons) PhD
Associate Professor and Reader
Musculoskeletal Research Centre
La Trobe University
Victoria
Australia

James RD Murray MA FRCS(Orth)
Consultant Orthopaedics and Trauma Surgeon
Avon Orthopaedic Centre and Frenchay Hospital
North Bristol NHS Trust
Bristol
UK

C B Payne DipPod(NZ) MPH
Lecturer, Department of Podiatry and the Musculoskeletal Research Centre
School of Human Biosciences
La Trobe University
Melbourne
Australia

A Percivall BSc MSc DPodM FCPodS
Senior Lecturer, School of Podiatry
University College Northampton
Northampton
UK

A Redmond PhD MSc DPodM FCPod
Arthritis Research Campaign Senior Lecturer
School of Medicine University of Leeds
Leeds Institute of Molecular Medicine
Section of Musculoskeletal Disease
Chapel Allerton Hospital
Leeds
UK

S Rees BSc MSc PhD FRSM
Senior Lecturer and Clinical Fellow
West Middlesex University Hospital
UK

I Reilly DPodM BSc FCPodS DMS
Consultant Podiatric Surgeon
Northamptonshire PCT
Northampton
UK

W J Ribbans BSc(Hons) MB BS MChOrth PhD FRCS FRCS(Ed) FRCSEd(Tr and Orth) FFSEM(UK)
Professor of Surgical Sciences
University of Northampton
Consultant Orthopaedic Surgeon
Northampton General Hospital
Northampton
UK

M C Spruce PhD
Lecturer, School of Health Professions and Rehabilitation Sciences
University of Southampton
Southampton
UK

P Thomson BSc MChS
Podiatry Centre Dunfermline
UK

R Turner MB ChB MRCP
Consultant Dermatologist
Oxford Radcliffe Hospitals
Oxford
UK

W Tyrrell MEd FHBA DPodM MChS FCPod Med
Principal Lecturer
Director of Enterprise
Cardiff School of Health Sciences
University of Wales Institute Cardiff
Cardiff
Wales

B Yates MSc BSc(Hons) FCPodS DpodM
Consultant Podiatric Surgeon
Trauma and Orthopaedics
Great Western Hospital
Swindon
UK

Preface

Many textbooks make reference to the assessment of the lower limb but very few are dedicated entirely to this purpose. Those that are tend to focus on only one of the components of the process, e.g. skin disorders or on a specific client group such as paediatrics. The purpose of this book is to produce a textbook which encompasses all aspects of lower limb assessment. Problems affecting the lower limb can lead to pain and morbidity through a reduction or loss of mobility and loss of time from work. Occasionally lower limb pathology can be life threatening. Effective and efficient management of these problems can only be based on a thorough assessment.

Throughout the book the term 'practitioner' is used in its broadest sense to denote any person who has an interest in the management of lower limb problems. Although the podiatrist has a natural claim to specialising in caring for the foot, the range of practitioners with an interest in the lower limb includes: general medical practitioners, nurses, occupational therapists, orthopaedic surgeons, orthotists, physiotherapists, bioengineers, diabetologists, rheumatologists and vascular surgeons.

This is the third edition of this textbook and, like its predecessors, it is divided into four parts: Approaching the patient, Systems examination, Laboratory and hospital investigations and Specific client groups. The textbook has been thoroughly revised with thirteen new chapter authors. Throughout the text there is a clear emphasis on evidence-based practice to underpin assessment techniques.

In Section one, Approaching the patient provides an introduction to the assessment process and covers in detail the assessment interview, the presenting problem and the reliability and validity of outcome measures used in the assessment of lower limb pathology. For the third edition these chapters have been updated and chapter four completely rewritten to cover the assessment of health outcome measures that can be used in both clinical practice and clinical research.

Systems examination covers the separate components of lower limb assessment: medical and social history, vascular, neurological, musculoskeletal, dermatological and footwear assessments. Details relating to anatomy and physiology have been discussed where relevant. Again, the chapters in this section have been revised as part of the third edition. The chapter on musculoskeletal assessment has been completely rewritten and divided in to two sections: orthopaedic assessment and functional assessment. The chapters have been written respectively by a professor of orthopaedics and a NIHR research lecturer in musculoskeletal medicine who is also a podiatrist. Although some areas are covered in both sections they are approached in different ways with different assessment aims. This gives the reader a more holistic overview of lower limb musculoskeletal assessment of both function and pathology.

Laboratory and hospital investigations focuses on those tests which may be performed to confirm, support or clarify the clinical examination: blood analysis, urine analysis, microbial identification and histopathology. The previous chapter on radiographic imaging has been completely rewritten as diagnostic imaging to incorporate the ever increasing use of more sophisticated imaging modalities such as MRI and ultrasound. The chapter on methods of analysing gait has been revised and updated and logically follows on from musculoskeletal assessment. Reliance on tests without the appropriate clinical examination is unwise, creates higher costs, may worry the patient unnecessarily and overworks support departments. It is intended that this part of the book demonstrates when and how these tests can be used to aid the assessment process.

The last part of the book focuses on Specific client groups, and the assessment of the lower limb in these patients. The sports, paediatric and older patient all require a different approach to assessment often based upon the unique characteristics associated with that client group. The presenting pathologies within theses groups are often different to others and their assessment is also covered in detail. Assessment of the surgical patient is designed to cover the specific issues related to this type of unique treatment, whether the surgery is being performed under local or general anaesthesia. Pain in the foot can arise due to a multitude of factors, affects all age groups and has a highly morbid effect on our lives; for this reason, it has been given a separate chapter which has been completely rewritten and covers the common causes of foot pain. The early diagnosis of the at-risk foot is recognised as a means of reducing morbidity, mortality and minimising the cost of in-hospital care for these patients. The at-risk foot chapter has been rewritten to cover these issues in detail.

The most obvious addition to the third edition is the incorporation of a DVD to support the text. There are many aspects of assessment where an image is worth a thousand words. The ability to visualise an assessment technique provides a tremendous learning opportunity for the viewer. The DVD is divided into sections incoporating vascular assessment; neurological assessment; assessment of the at-risk foot and musculoskeletal assessment which is further divided into the hip, the knee, and the foot and ankle. Assessment of the painful foot is divided into the rearfoot, the midfoot, the forefoot and there is also a section on the painful ankle. Diagnostic imaging relies on visual images to make a diagnosis and there is an extensive image library incorporated on the DVD to supplement the text in the chapter. Still images of a dynamic ultrasound assessment are hard to interpret and the DVD therefore includes video footage of patients undergoing ultrasound examination of common foot pathologies.

Case histories and comments support some of the chapters, particularly those in Systems examination and Specific client groups. These have been used to illustrate certain points and reflect real life experiences. Where appropriate, photographs, figures and tables have also been used to support and further illustrate points raised in the text. Sections of colour plates have been specifically used to support Chapters 8, 12 and 18. Each chapter has been thoroughly referenced and some indicate Further Reading.

Clearly there is more than one approach to undertaking an assessment. *Assessment of the Lower Limb* has been written to support good clinical practice for all professionals with an interest in the foot and lower limb. Whatever approach the practitioner adopts, it is hoped that this text will be a valuable asset.

Ben Yates

Acknowledgements

A big thank you to all the contributors for their time and effort in revising or rewriting the chapters. Particular thanks to Mr David Hocken (Consultant Vascular Surgeon), Mr James Murray (Consultant Orthopaedic Surgeon), Ms Catherine McCarthy (Consultant Radiologist), Dr Michelle Spruce (Podiatrist) for giving up their time to help make the DVD and to the team at Creation Video for its production. To all the staff at Elsevier, especially Robert, Kim and Veronika, who have helped and cajouled me and the contributors to produce the book on time.

Finally to my wife Elaine and children Katherine and Rory for their love, support and understanding.

Part 1

Approaching the patient

CHAPTER

1

Assessment

B Yates

Chapter contents

Introduction

Patients present with a range of signs and symptoms for which they are seeking relief and if possible a cure. However, before this can be achieved, it is essential to undertake a primary patient assessment. Ineffective and inappropriate treatment may result if the practitioner has not taken into account information obtained from the assessment. To avoid missing important information a flexible but systematic approach should be adopted for assessment. This chapter explores why it is necessary to undertake an assessment and considers specific aspects of the assessment process.

Why undertake a primary patient assessment?

Information from the assessment helps the practitioner to:

- arrive at a differential diagnosis or definitive diagnosis
- identify the likely cause of the problem (aetiology), e.g. trauma, pathogenic microorganism
- identify any factors that may influence the choice of treatment, e.g. poor blood supply, current drug regimen
- assess the extent of pathological changes so that a prognosis can be made
- establish a baseline in order to identify whether the condition is deteriorating or improving
- determine the need for further investigations (e.g. X-rays)
- assess whether a second opinion is necessary.

All the above information is essential if the practitioner is to provide effective treatment and care for the patient.

Table 1.1 Components of an assessment

Component	
Assessment interview	Presenting problem Personal details Medical history Family history Social history Current health status
Observation and clinical examination	Vascular Neurological Musculoskeletal Dermatological Footwear
Laboratory and hospital tests	Urinalysis Microbiology Blood tests History Gait analysis X-rays Other imaging techniques Electrocardiography (ECG) Nerve conduction studies

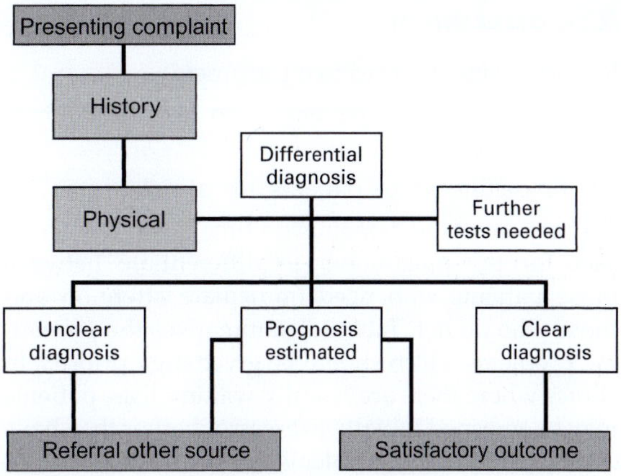

Figure 1.1 The stages of assessment.

The assessment process

Assessment comprises three elements: the interview, observation and tests (Table 1.1). Information from the interview and observation is used to formulate ideas about the likely diagnosis and cause. Further information may be sought via the interview and the use of clinical and specialist tests or investigations. The practitioner uses the data gained from the assessment to formulate a hypothesis(es) from which a diagnosis will be reached. This diagnosis will be used to inform the management plan (Fig. 1.1). Where possible, the cause (aetiology) of the problem should be identified, as part of the management plan would be to eradicate or reduce the effects of the cause.

What has been outlined above is the ideal. In reality, patients often present with ill-defined problems and it is not possible to reach a definitive diagnosis. In these instances the practitioner explores a range of likely possibilities and develops the management plan in relation to these possibilities. This approach focuses on symptom reduction and palliation.

To make a good assessment, a practitioner requires good interviewing (communication) and observational skills. It is also essential that the practitioner has effective listening skills and knows when and which questions to ask the patient (see Ch. 2). Research has shown that most diagnoses are based on observation and information volunteered by the patient (Lee et al 2006, Sandler 1979). For patients with complex pathology, it may not be appropriate to follow normal models of diagnostic practice as many conditions will not present in a typical 'textbook' fashion. This has led to the development of subspecialty models of clinical assessment such as the 'permeable brick wall' theory for neuromuscular assessment developed by Maitland et al (2001). This theory recommends that the clinician should treat a patient's presenting symptoms rather than follow a treatment programme based on an exact diagnosis, as this may not be possible because of the variable and mixed nature of neurological symptoms and conditions.

Clinical, laboratory and hospital-based tests provide additional data. Clinical tests include physical examination of the patient (e.g. assessing ranges of motion at joints, taking a pulse) as well as near-patient tests, e.g. assessing blood glucose levels with a glucometer. Most clinical tests are relatively quick and inexpensive to carry out and in most instances give fairly reliable and valid results. Technological advances mean that there is an increasing number of available clinical tests. Tests in laboratories and hospitals are more expensive and can be time-consuming. Such tests should only be used when it is necessary to confirm a suspected diagnosis, in cases of differential diagnosis or when the outcome of the test will have a positive influence on treatment.

Risk assessment

Risk assessment serves two purposes:

- Identification of patients who need immediate attention
- Predicting which patients are 'at risk'.

On account of the demands on time it is often necessary for the practitioner to differentiate between those patients who need immediate attention and those who do not. Table 1.2 summarises the presenting problems which should be given high priority. In clinics where there are lengthy waiting lists, patients may be screened initially to assess whether they have one or more of the problems listed in Table 1.2 and are then given immediate treatment.

The term 'at risk' usually denotes those patients at risk of developing ulceration and infection. Identifying those 'at risk' is a complex task. Currently, there is sparse research into risk factors related to lower limb problems, and thus it is difficult to produce risk-assessment methods that are robust and valid. Considerable research has been undertaken into the risk assessment of pressure ulcers (Lothian 1987, Sharp & McLaws 2006). In relation to the lower limb some work has been undertaken into developing methods of risk assessment to identify patients with diabetes who are at risk of developing foot ulcers (Zahra 1998, Boyko et al 2006). Risk assessment has also been applied to numerous other health problems such as falls in the older population (DeMott et al 2007), muscle flexibility and muscle injury (Witvrouw et al 2003), and deep vein thrombosis (McCaffrey et al 2007).

Table 1.2 Presenting problems which should be given high priority

Problem	*Features*
Pain	Constant, weightbearing and non-weightbearing Affects patient's usual daily activities
Infection	Raised temperature (pyrexia) Sign of acute inflammation Signs of spreading cellulitis Lymphangitis, lymphadenitis
Ulceration	Loss of skin May or may not be painful May expose underlying tissues
Acute swelling	Unrelieved pain Very noticeable swelling May have associated signs of inflammation
Abnormal skin changes	Distinct colour change Discharge may be malodorous Itching Bleeding

Making a diagnosis

Arriving at a diagnosis is a complex activity. Studies of clinical reasoning show that practitioners use one or more of the following approaches (Higgs & Jones 2000):

- Hypothetico-deductive reasoning
- Pattern recognition
- Interpretative model.

Hypothetico-deductive reasoning is based on generating hypotheses using clinical data and knowledge. These hypotheses are tested through further inquiry during the assessment. The evidence gained is evaluated in relation to existing knowledge and a conclusion reached on the basis of probability (Buckingham & Adams 2000, Gale 1982).

Pattern recognition is a process of recognising the similarity between a set of signs and symptoms. The important aspect of the use of categorisation in clinical reasoning is the link practitioners make between the pattern they are currently observing and previous cases showing the same or similar patterns.

The interpretative model is different from the other two models. This approach is based on the practitioner gaining a deep understanding of the patient's perspective and the influence of contextual factors. Protagonists of this approach believe that the meaning patients give to their problems, including their understanding of and their feelings about their problem, can significantly influence their levels of pain tolerance, disability and the eventual outcome (Ferurestein & Beattie 1995).

Studies have shown that with all these approaches there is an association between clinical reasoning and knowledge (De Bruin et al 2005, Higgs & Jones 2000). There is a symbiotic relationship between the knowledge base of practitioners and their clinical reasoning ability. It is not possible to develop problem-solving skills in the absence of cognitive knowledge related to the specific problem. The ability to diagnose a condition improves when the knowledge of basic science is combined with clinical knowledge (De Bruin et al 2005).

There are three partners in the assessment process: the practitioner, the patient and the wider environment. The ability of a practitioner to undertake an effective assessment and make a diagnosis is influenced by a range of factors:

- Personal values, beliefs and perceptions
- Knowledge base related to the problem(s)
- Reasoning skills (cognition and metacognition)
- Previous clinical experience
- Familiarity with similar cases.

There can be enormous differences between practitioners, both in their assessment findings and in their diagnoses. For example, Comroe & Botelho (1947) undertook a landmark study in which 22 doctors were asked to examine 20 patients and note whether cyanosis was present. Under controlled conditions the patient were also assessed for cyanosis with an oximeter. When the results of the clinical assessment were compared with the results with the oximeter, only 53% of the doctors diagnosed cyanosis in subjects with extremely low oxygen content, and 26% said cyanosis was present in subjects with normal oxygen content. Curran & Jagger (1997) found poor agreement between podiatrists when diagnosing common conditions of the leg and foot. Agreement improved when a patient expert system was used. Expert patient systems are increasingly being used, in particular in medicine (Adams et al 1986, Adlassnig 2001). These computer-based systems provide practitioners with a wealth of information and are used to guide and direct clinical decision making.

Unfortunately, making a diagnosis is not a precise science, and errors can and do occur. Practitioners should always keep an open mind when making a diagnosis, reflect on the process they have used, keep up to date with current literature and technology, and request a second opinion when they are unsure. If a diagnosis is not possible, the practitioner should focus on treating the patient's symptoms.

Sometimes a practitioner may generate more than one possible diagnosis; in these instances the practitioner has to undertake a differential diagnosis, i.e. decide which is the most likely diagnosis from several possibilities. When arriving at a differential diagnosis the practitioner should take into account the factors listed in Table 1.3. For example, many conditions affect specific age groups (e.g. the osteochondroses), whereas other conditions have specific presenting features (e.g. the sudden, acute, nocturnal pain associated with gout).

Table 1.3 Factors to be considered in differential diagnosis

Social history	Age Gender Race Social habits Occupation Leisure pursuits
Medical history	Family history Medication Previous treatment for the condition (self or medical)
Symptoms	Onset Type of pain Aggravated by/relieved by Seasonal variation
Signs	Site Appearance Symmetry
Specific tests	Imaging techniques Urinalysis Microbiology Blood analysis Biopsy Foot pressure analysis Electrical conductive studies

The patient is the key partner in the assessment process. Some patients want a greater role in decision making and their healthcare management. In addition, patients are increasingly being seen as consumers of healthcare. As such, they have expectations of the type and quality of the health services they receive.

Patients' perceptions, beliefs and expectations related to their lower limb problems can be influenced by the following factors:

- Home environment
- Work environment
- Culture
- Socioeconomic status
- Language skills
- General state of health.

The above factors can affect patients' needs, communication skills and, ultimately, the choices they make.

The wider health environment and context cannot be ignored in the assessment process. Healthcare is a political issue and changes in government policy can radically affect available services. Finance is another major influencing factor that may limit the range of clinical and laboratory tests that may be used. Conversely, technological advances have led to improved clinical and laboratory test equipment. Employing organisations can affect the assessment process in a variety of ways, e.g. use of specific frameworks of operation. Profession-specific frameworks and the status of knowledge within the profession can also be influencing factors.

Aetiology

Information from the assessment can enable the practitioner to identify the cause of the problem. A variety of aetiological factors can result in disorders of the lower limb. These can be divided into hereditary, congenital (present at birth) or acquired:

- **Hereditary conditions** may manifest immediately after birth, e.g. epidermolysis bullosa, or may not appear until some years after, e.g. Huntington's chorea.
- **Congenital conditions** include chromosomal abnormalities, e.g. Down's syndrome, developmental defects, e.g. spina bifida, or birth injuries such as cerebral palsy.
- **Acquired conditions** are those that arise after birth. Infection by a pathogenic organism resulting in sepsis is a common example of an acquired condition affecting the lower limb.

Many conditions occur as a result of more than one factor, i.e. they are multifactorial. Atherosclerosis is thought to be due to the interplay of a number of factors, including dietary intake, familial high cholesterol level, high blood pressure, sedentary lifestyle and stress. In many cases predisposing factors present in conjunction with an exciting factor before the condition manifests. An example is an infected ingrown toenail, where the nail may be naturally involuted, and poor nail-cutting technique, localised trauma, or poor hygiene may all be contributing factors.

If the cause of a condition can be identified (e.g. poor proprioception, contamination by a pathogen) then treatment can be aimed at eradicating or reducing its effects. Knowing what has caused a problem can assist in identifying the most appropriate treatment and help to produce an accurate prognosis. For example, if the cause of pain in the foot is chronic ischaemia due to atherosclerosis, the prognosis may be poor unless radical (bypass) surgery is performed. Conversely if the foot pain is due to acute ischaemia that has occurred as a result of hosiery constricting the peripheral circulation, the prognosis is good and advice may be all that is required. Unfortunately, it is not always possible to isolate the cause; for these cases the term *idiopathic* (unknown cause) is used.

Time management

The assessment process is fundamental to a satisfactory outcome for both patient and practitioner. However, practitioners often find themselves working within strict time constraints and may feel they have insufficient time in which to undertake a full primary patient assessment. It is important that the practitioner does not compromise the assessment process to save on time. Although such actions may save time in the short term, they may have unfortunate long-term effects. The practitioner who does not obtain important information or fails to recognise salient clinical findings may reach an incorrect diagnosis and/or implement treatment that puts the patient at considerable risk. In the long term, this will lead to avoidable patient suffering and extra time being spent in dealing with the complications arising from treatment.

To use time effectively, it is important to plan and prioritise activities. The time allotted to a primary assessment may be as little as 10 minutes if the condition is straightforward to diagnose and there are few aetiological factors. More complex conditions may require far more detailed assessment necessitating a longer appointment time or multiple appointments. With experience, practitioners should be able to undertake a routine assessment in approximately 10 minutes. This does not mean a diagnosis has always to be made within this time frame, but the practitioner should have determined the need for further assessment or investigation. Further time may be required if the problem is complex, if a definitive diagnosis cannot be reached or if laboratory or hospital tests are required. Table 1.4 summarises the essential components of any assessment.

Re-assessment

Assessment should not be something that is only undertaken on the patient's first visit. Every time the patient attends the clinic a mini-assessment should

Table 1.4 The essential components of an assessment that should be carried out with all patients. Further tests and examination should be used if indicated from the information obtained from the essential assessment

Observation	Gait as the patient walks into the room to detect abnormal function Facial features for signs of current health status
Interview	Presenting problem Personal details Medical history Family history Social history Current health status
Observation	Skin and nails to detect trophic changes and abnormal lesions Position of lower limb to note deformity, swelling, inflammation Footwear
Tests	Pulses, capillary filling time

be undertaken so that the following can be noted:

- Changes to the patient's general health status
- Changes to the status of the lower limb
- The patient's perception of previous treatment
- Effects of previous treatment
- Information about treatment from other practitioners.

The process of assessment, diagnosis and treatment should be an uninterrupted loop: at every subsequent consultation, the patient should be re-assessed and evaluated (Fig. 1.2).

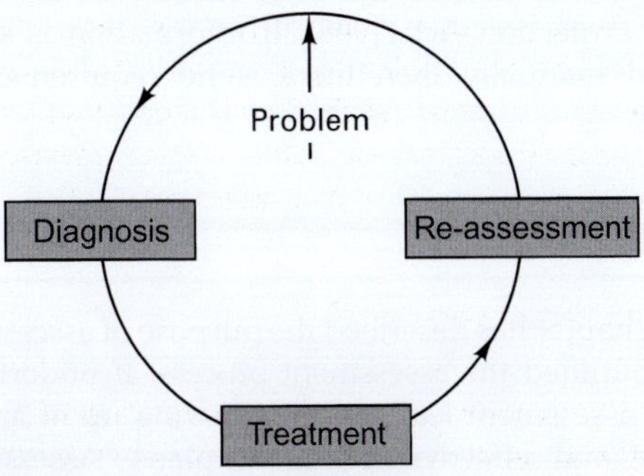

Figure 1.2 The assessment loop.

Recording assessment information

Information gained from the assessment should be accurately and clearly noted in the patient's record. This record is the storehouse of knowledge concerning the patient and his or her medical history. It should contain a summary of the main points from the assessment and sufficient data to justify the diagnosis. Ideally, whether in a hospital or primary care setting, healthcare practitioners should use the same patient record. This ensures that all practitioners involved with the care of the patient are aware of each other's assessments and interventions. Although this is good practice, the keeping of separate records by each healthcare professional, e.g. general practitioner, district (home) nurses, podiatrists, is still prevalent. This practice does not facilitate teamworking.

Two methods may be used to record the assessment information. In the first the practitioner records, in a logical sequence, assessment and diagnostic details on a blank sheet of paper. In the second method, a pro-forma is used; this may vary from a form with a few headings to a very detailed form with boxes in which to record specific details. Such pro-formas can be self-designed or purchased from specialist suppliers.

Whatever the method used, it is important that all details are recorded in such a way that practitioners not involved with the assessment can familiarise themselves with the salient details and any previous treatment. Records may be handwritten or word-processed. If records are handwritten, the handwriting must be legible and in ink (black). The use of software packages is already prevalent and it is likely that computers will eventually be the prime means of recording patient data. Many hospitals have now moved to a purely electronic 'paperless' system with all patient information being stored electronically. The main advantages for such a system is that information is not lost, it is legible, and can be accessed by all members of the healthcare team at multiple sites.

The record should be made at the time of the assessment. This is termed contemporaneous and is an important medicolegal issue. Any blank spaces in a paper assessment form should be scored through. The original record should not be altered or disguised. If it proves necessary to amend the record, the nature of the amendment should be clear and the amendment should be signed and dated by the practitioner making the alteration.

The use of abbreviations should be avoided (Bradshaw & Braid 1999). Profession-specific abbreviations can be particularly problematic in patient records that have been completed by more than one healthcare profession. However, the use of abbreviations in patient records is common. In a survey of podiatrists, Curran (1994) found that 97% used abbreviations in their patient records.

All entries should be dated and signed. In particular, details regarding the patient's medication should always be dated, as the medication may have been changed by the time the patient attends for the next appointment. The patient's name or the patient identifier should appear on every page, except the front cover where only the patient number should be used as an identifier. Records should always be written in such a way so as not to be offensive or contain subjective opinions. Under the Patient's Charter and Data Protection Act, patients have the right to view their medical notes.

Most professional bodies provide guidance on recording information in patient records. For example, the Society of Chiropodists and Podiatrists (2000) has produced guidelines on minimum standards in clinical practice, which contain specific information on record keeping. Bradshaw & Braid (1999) identified the following four reasons for poor record keeping:

- Illegible handwriting
- Incomplete information
- Inaccurate information
- Ambiguous abbreviations.

It is suggested that practitioners as part of their continuing professional development receive periodic reminders and refresher sessions related to record keeping (Bradshaw & Braid 1999). Regular audit of medical records improves record keeping (Donnelly 1995).

The information recorded from the assessment may be used for:

- ensuring contraindicated treatments are not used
- clinical and epidemiological research
- audit
- planning
- legal purposes.

Retrospective and prospective analyses of patient records are commonly used for clinical and epidemiological research, audit and planning. If well documented, they can provide a wealth of information. However, one of the problems with patient records is that there is no standardised manner in which information is collected. For example, the use of clinical terms can be ambiguous.

The International Statistical Classification of Diseases, Injuries and Causes of Death was established by the World Health Organization as a universal system for collecting data. The system was originally designed for mortality statistics but has evolved to cover a broad range of diseases. It is updated every 10 years to keep abreast of the constantly changing information base. This system can be used to record diseases for the purpose of clinical and epidemiological research and audit.

In an increasingly litigious society it is important that high standards of record keeping are maintained. The St Paul International Insurance Company (1991) states that 35–40% of all malpractice claims in the USA cannot be defended because of 'documentation problems'. The Society of Chiropodists and Podiatrists (1998) found that inadequate patient records were the main reason why legal claims against chiropodists and podiatrists succeeded.

Confidentiality

The information volunteered by the patient and recorded in the patient's notes should be treated as confidential and not divulged to any other party without the consent of the patient. However, the information can be made available to all those involved with the care of that patient.

Patient records, whether in manual or electronic format, are subject to the Data Protection Act 1998, which became effective from March 2000. This means that patients have the right of access, for a preset fee, to information stored about them. The act gives rights to individuals in respect of personal data held about them by others. Where information about a patient is stored electronically it is a legal requirement that practitioners (or their employing organisation) comply with the notification requirements of the Data Protection Act (1998). If information is solely stored manually then there is no requirement to notify.

Summary

This chapter has described the purpose of assessment and outlined the assessment process. If undertaken well, assessment leads to the drawing up of appropriate and effective treatment plans. Assessment should be seen as pivotal to good patient–

practitioner interaction. Assessment also involves continuous evaluation throughout the patient journey to ensure that treatment is delivered in the most effective manner possible.

References

Adams I D, Chan M, Clifford P 1986 Computer aided diagnosis of abdominal pain: a multi centre study. British Medical Journal 293:80–84

Adlassnig K 2001 The section on medical expert and knowledge based systems at the department of medical computer sciences of the university of Vienna medical school. Artificial Intelligence in Medicine 21(1–3):139–146

Boyko E, Ahroni J, Cohen V et al 2006 Prediction of diabetic foot ulcer occurrence using commonly available clinical information: the Seattle diabetic foot study. Diabetes Care 29:1202–1207

Bradshaw T, Braid S 1999 The practice of recording clinical treatment and audit of practice – an overview for podiatrists. British Journal of Podiatry 2:8–12

Buckingham C, Adams A 2000 Classifying clinical decision making: interpreting nursing intuition, heuristics, and medical diagnosis. Journal of Advance Nursing 32:990–998

Comroe J H, Botelho S 1947 The unreliability of cyanosis in the recognition of arterial anoxemia. American Journal of the Medical Sciences 214:1–6

Curran M 1994 Use of abbreviations in chiropody/podiatry. Journal of British Podiatric Medicine 49:71–72

Curran M, Jagger C 1997 Interobserver variability in the diagnosis of foot and leg disorders using a computer expert system. The Foot 7:7–10

Data Protection Act 1998 EC Data Protection Directive (95/46/EC)

De Bruin A, Schmidt H, Rikers M 2005 The role of basic science knowledge and clinical knowledge in diagnostic reasoning: a structural equation modelling approach. Academic Medicine 80:765–763

DeMott T, Richardson J, Thies S et al 2007 Falls and gait characteristics among older persons with peripheral neuropathy. American Journal of Physical Medicine and Rehabilitation 86:125–132

Donnelly A 1995 Improve your nurses' record collection. Nursing Management 2:18–19

Ferurestein M, Beattie P 1995 Biobehavioural factors affecting pain and disability in low back pain: mechanisms and assessment. Physical Therapy 75:267–280

Gale J 1982 Some cognitive components of the diagnostic thinking process. British Journal of Educational Psychology 52:64–72

Higgs J, Jones M 2000 Clinical reasoning in the health professions, 2nd edn. Butterworth-Heinemann, London

Lee J, Chan A, Phillips D 2006 Diagnostic practice in nursing: a critical review of the literature. Nursing Health Sciences 8:57–65

Lothian P 1987 The practical assessment of pressure sore risk. CARE Science and Practice 5:3–7

Maitland G, Hengeveld E, Banks K et al 2001 Maitland's vertebral manipulation, 6th edn. Butterworth-Heinemann, Oxford

McCaffrey R, Bishop M, Adonis-Rizzo M et al 2007 Development and testing of a DVT risk assessment tool: providing evidence of validity and reliability. Worldviews Evidence Based Nursing 4:14–20

Sandler G 1979 Costs of unnecessary tests. British Medical Journal i:1686–1688

Sharp C, McLaws M 2006 Estimating the risk of pressure ulcer development: Is it truly evidence based? International Wound Journal 3:344–353

Society of Chiropodists and Podiatrists 1998 Defensive practice (editorial). Podiatry Now 1:1

Society of Chiropodists and Podiatrists 2000 Guidelines on minimum standards of clinical practice, December

St Paul International Insurance Company 1991 Defensible documentation. St Paul House, 61–63 London Rd, Redhill, Surrey RH1 1NA (information leaflet for healthcare professionals)

Witvrouw E, Danneels L, Asselman P et al 2003 Muscle flexibility as a risk factor for developing muscle injuries in male professional soccer players. A prospective study. American Journal of Sports Medicine 31:41–46

Zahra J 1998 Can podiatrists predict diabetic foot ulcers using a risk assessment card? British Journal of Podiatry 1:79–88

CHAPTER 2

The assessment interview

M Hanley

Chapter contents

Introduction

The professional skill of being able to appropriately plan and conduct an assessment interview has long been recognised as a key factor in successful clinical assessment (Dickson et al 1997). Indeed, it has been argued that communication skills of healthcare professionals are at least as important as their clinical skills in fulfilling the professional role (Alexander 2001). The significance of successful communication in healthcare has also been reflected in government policy, with the need to improve such skills identified as a key area for education and training in *The NHS plan* (Department of Health 2000). A key part of communicating successfully in a healthcare setting is having the ability to conduct a satisfactory assessment interview. This chapter focuses on the purpose of the interview, the skills required to communicate effectively, explore how the interview should be structured and identify the pitfalls to avoid. It concludes by examining the features of a good assessment interview.

Is an interview different from a normal conversation?

An interview is based on a conversation between two or more people. As individuals we converse with a broad range of people, and our conversation serves many purposes. The conversation in an interview differs from an ordinary conversation in several ways:

- It is an opportunity for an exchange of information.
- It has a specific purpose, e.g. to solve a problem.
- It has an outcome, e.g. a course of treatment.
- It has less flexibility than an ordinary conversation.
- The interviewer has a perceived position of authority/power over the interviewee; it is important that this power is not abused. Every effort should be made to put the interviewee (the patient) at ease.
- A written record of the interview is usually kept.

Practitioners may also have other types of conversation with patients, requiring additional skills such as counselling, teaching and advising. These are discussed in the companion textbook, *Clinical skills in treating the foot* (2nd edition, Elsevier Churchill Livingstone, 2005).

Aims of the assessment interview

The assessment interview is a conversation with a purpose that takes place between the practitioner and the patient. Patients present with problems which may have physical, psychological and social dimensions. Patients often have their own ideas and concerns about the problems they present with, and about the medical care that they may or may not receive. Likewise, practitioners approach the interview with perceptions of their role, which will have been influenced by their training, past experiences, attitudes and beliefs. The availability of resources and facilities will contribute to the practitioner's response to the patient. It is essential that the practitioner and the patient develop common ground during the interview and that both are aware of each other's perspectives. If this cannot be achieved, the interview may be an unsatisfactory experience for both of them.

The prime purpose of the interview is to identify the cause of the patient's concerns and the appropriate actions to be taken. This is best achieved by the patient and the practitioner working in partnership to reduce or resolve these concerns. It is essential that practitioners provide ample opportunity for patients to convey their concerns and worries. In other words, the interview should be patient-centred. Research has shown that this is not always the case and despite the time afforded to clinical interviews, many are conducted rather poorly (Newell 1994).

Information gathered collectively from the interview and examination should facilitate the identification of the patient's health problem and, where appropriate, a diagnosis can be made. Besides aiding the diagnostic process, the interview serves other important purposes:

- The information gained may be of help when drawing up a treatment plan. For example, the interview can provide a picture of the patient's social circumstances, which may affect the manner of, or the actual, advice given.
- It provides an opportunity to gain the patient's trust and build confidence in the practitioner.
- It facilitates the development of a therapeutic relationship between the healthcare practitioner and the patient.

However, not all healthcare students are aware of how to communicate effectively and, as a result, communication skills training is becoming a common part of the curriculum of healthcare courses (Hargie et al 1998, Sleight 1995).

Communicating effectively

Since the interview has a particularly significant role in the assessment of the patient, it is important to ensure that the meeting is successful. In other words, good communication skills are essential if you are to achieve an effective assessment interview. What is meant by communication? In its simplest form it can be seen as the transmission of information from one person and the receiving of information by another. Unfortunately, the communication process is not that simple; if it was, there would not be communication breakdowns or misunderstandings between people about what was said.

Communication may be influenced by certain characteristics of:

- the sender (e.g. ability to express ideas clearly, verbal skills, attitude towards the patient)
- the receiver (e.g. the extent to which the receiver is paying attention, their ability to hear and understand the conversation, and their beliefs and expectations)
- the social environment in which the interview is being conducted (e.g. disruption due to background noise).

With so many opportunities for these forms of interference, it is not surprising that many attempts to communicate effectively fail. Consequently, healthcare professionals should develop their communication skills to make the best use of the interview.

A common question asked is: 'Are some people born with good communication skills or is it a skill you can learn?'. The answer has to be that it is a combination of the two. We can all think of people we consider to be good communicators; these people appear to have an inherent skill. For others, communication may not come so easily. It is particularly important for health practitioners to be aware of and develop effective communication skills because so much clinical information is gathered through the assessment interview. Research has shown that clinical communication and relationship skills can be developed strategically through education and training (Stein et al 2005), and that good communication can be an effective intervention in longer-term patient care (Trummer et al 2006).

A myriad of books are available on the subject of communication skills. However, just reading a book does not automatically mean you become a good communicator. Observing others, noting good and bad points, receiving feedback from others, role-play exercises, videotaping and audiotaping of interactions, and practising with friends are all helpful ways in which such skills can be developed. Being an effective communicator is a skill – and like any clinical skill it should be regularly practised and reviewed.

Although you may not be able to change the communication characteristics of the patient or the social environment, you can ensure that your contribution to the interview is as effective as possible. You can do this by sending clear and appropriate messages to the patient and by ensuring that you understand fully what the patient is trying to communicate to you. To achieve this, you need to pay careful attention to three key components of the communication process:

- Questioning skills
- Listening skills
- Non-verbal communication skills.

Each of these skills will be considered in turn below.

Questioning skills

The prime purpose of the assessment interview is to gain as much information as possible from the patient so that a diagnosis and treatment plan can be determined. To achieve this objective, the practitioner uses a range of questioning skills. There are three categories of question:

- Open
- Closed
- Leading.

Open questions

Open questions invite the patient to give answers consisting of more than one word. Patients are in a much better position to construct the response they wish to give. Examples of open questions are:

- What happened when you went into hospital?
- What do you look for when buying a pair of shoes?
- What do you think is causing the problem?

These kinds of question can elicit information from the patient that you may not have expected. Open questions are often preferable to closed questions such as 'When you were in hospital did they test your blood sugar or did you have an X-ray?'. The patient may legitimately answer 'no' to these direct questions and so fail to tell you that they did have a test – one you did not mention.

Closed questions

Although closed questions may serve a useful purpose during the assessment interview, but if used incorrectly they can limit the responses a patient may give. Closed questions may require:

- a yes/no response, e.g. do you have rheumatoid arthritis?
- the patient to select, e.g. is the pain worse in the morning or the afternoon?
- the patient to provide factual information, e.g. how long have you had diabetes?

Within the assessment interview closed questions can be useful as a quick means of gaining and verifying information. Patients often find this type of question easier to answer than the more open type of question. They can be used to focus the assessment interview in a particular direction. On the other hand, if used too much, they limit what the patient can say. As a result the patient may not volunteer important information.

Leading questions

Leading questions should be avoided where possible. In general, they give responses that a professional expects to receive and are of limited use in a therapeutic setting. Examples of leading questions are:

- You don't smoke, do you?
- That doesn't hurt, does it?
- You said you get the pain a lot; that must mean you get it every day?

Although you may get the answer you want or expect to hear, it does not necessarily mean it is true, as the patient may feel pressured into giving the answer the practitioner is looking for.

In addition to specific styles of question, the practitioner may also use a range of *interview techniques* to elaborate further on the issues raised. These techniques are often referred to as probes. Probing questions are a very useful adjunct to both open and closed questions. In general they aim at finding out more from the patient. In particular, they are useful in gaining indepth rather than superficial information. Examples include:

- Could you describe the type of pain you are experiencing?
- What makes you think it might be linked to your circulation?

You might also use silence as a probe to encourage the patient to expand on a given answer, or say 'yes', 'uh-hm' or simply nod, techniques that are particularly useful when you feel the patients may have more to say and are thinking about expanding their answer.

General pointers when questioning patients

The following points should be borne in mind when interviewing patients:

- Show empathy. Authier (1986) defined empathy as being 'attuned to the way another person is feeling and conveying that understanding in a language he/she understands'.
- Use language that is simple, direct and understandable. Avoid medical and technical terms. The 'fog index' can be used to assess the complexity of a piece of communication. It is primarily used in written communication but has also been used, although less frequently, to analyse the complexity of the spoken word. It involves a mathematical equation that produces a score. For example, tabloid newspapers have a fog index score between 3 and 6, whereas government policy documents can achieve a score of 20+. Applying the fog index to spoken communication or a health education leaflet will give an indication of the complexity of that particular communication. If it receives a high fog index score, the average patient may find it very difficult to understand.
- Avoid presenting the patient with a long list of conditions. This is especially important during medical history taking. It is unlikely that a patient has experienced more than one or two of the problems on a list. Patients may fall into the habit of replying 'no' to all the items on the list and fail to respond in the affirmative to ones they do suffer from. Strategies that can be used to avoid this situation include a pre-assessment questionnaire (see Ch. 5) or breaking up the list of closed questions with some open questions.
- Don't ask the patient more than one question at a time. For example, if asking a closed-type question do not say, 'Could you tell me when you first noticed the condition, when the pain is worse and what makes it better?'. By the end of the question the patient will have forgotten the first part.
- Attempt to get the patient to give you an honest answer using his or her own words. Avoid putting words into the patient's mouth.
- Clarify inconsistencies in what the patient tells you.
- Get the patient to explain what he means by using certain terms, e.g. 'nagging pain'. Your interpretation of this term may differ from the patient's.
- Pauses are an integral part of any communication. They allow time for participants to take in and analyse what has been communicated and provide time for a response to be formulated. Allow the patient time to think how he wishes to answer your question. Avoid appearing as if you are undertaking an interrogation.
- In the early stages of the interview it is often better to use the term 'concern' rather than 'problem'. Asking patients what concerns them may elicit a very different response from asking them what the problem is. Some patients may feel they do not have a problem as such but are worried about some symptom or sign they have noticed. Asking them what concerns them may get them to reveal this rather than a denial that they have any problems.
- Asking personal and intimate questions can be very difficult. Do not start the interview with this type of question; wait until further into the interview when hopefully the patient is more at ease with you. Try to avoid showing any embarrassment when asking an intimate question as this may well make the patient feel uncomfortable.
- It is important that the patient understands why you are asking certain questions. Remember that the assessment interview is a two-way process: besides gathering information from the patient it can be used for giving information to him.
- Some patients, on account of a range of circumstances such as hearing difficulties, speech deficit or language difference, may not be able to communicate with the practitioner. In these instances it is important that the practitioner involves someone known to the patient to communicate on his behalf, e.g. relative, friend or carer.
- The patient may have difficulty listening and interpreting what you are saying through fear, anxiety, physical discomfort or cognitive impairment. Be aware of non-verbal and verbal messages that can give clues to the patient's emotional state.

Listening skills

Listening is an active and not a passive skill. Many people ask questions but do not listen to the response. A common example is the general introductory question: 'How are you?'. Most responses tend to be in the affirmative: 'Fine', 'OK'. Occasionally, someone responds by saying they have not been too well, only to get the response from the supposed listener: 'Great; pleased to hear everything is fine'. Similarly, do not limit your attention to what you want to hear or expect to hear. Listen to all that is being said and watch the patient's non-verbal behaviour. The average rate of speech is 100–200 words a minute; however, we can assimilate the spoken word at around 400 words per minute. As a result the listener has 'extra time' to understand and interpret what is being said. If you have asked a question you should listen to *all* of the answer. Often when trying to understand the clinical nature of a patient's problem, there is a great temptation to listen to the first part of an answer and then to immediately use this information to try to make a diagnosis. This may mean that you are not paying careful attention to important clinical information that the patient may give at the end of their reply. Finally, it is important that you don't let your mind wander on to unrelated thoughts such as what you are going to do after the interview. Before you know it you will have missed a good chunk of what the patient has been telling you and have most probably missed important and relevant information.

To be a good listener you need to set aside your own personal problems and worries and give your full attention to the other person. It is inevitable that, at times, one's attention does wander. This may be due to lack of concentration, tiredness or because the patient has been allowed to wander off the point. In the case of the former do not be afraid to say to the patient, 'Sorry, could I ask you to go over that again?'. In the latter case, politely interrupt the patient and use your questioning skills to bring the conversation back to the subject in hand.

During the interview the techniques of paraphrasing, reflection and summarising can be used to aid listening and ensure you understand what the patient is trying to convey.

Paraphrasing

This technique is used to clarify what a person has just said to you to get them to confirm its accuracy or to encourage them to expand their response. It involves re-stating, using your own and the patient's words, what the patient has said.

Reflection

This technique is similar to prompting in that it is used to encourage the patient to continue talking about a particular issue that may involve feelings or concerns. It may be used when the patient appears to be reluctant to continue or is 'drying up'. It involves the practitioner repeating in the patient's own words what has just been said.

Summarising

This technique is used to identify what you consider to be the main points of what the patient is trying to tell you. It can also be a useful means of controlling the interview when a patient continues to talk at length about an issue. To summarise, the practitioner draws together the salient points from the whole conversation. At the end of the summary the patient may agree with, add to or make corrections to what the practitioner has said. Summarising serves a useful purpose in checking the validity, clarity and understanding of old information; it does not aim to develop new information.

The basic skills of a good listener are highlighted in Box 2.1.

Non-verbal communication skills

Non-verbal communication involves all forms of communication apart from the purely spoken (verbal) message. It is through this medium that we create first impressions of people and, similarly, people make initial judgements about us. Once made, first impressions are often difficult to change, yet research has shown they are not always reliable. Therefore, it is particularly important that we consider non-verbal communication here since it affects not only how we are perceived when we communicate but also how we make judgements about patients.

Box 2.1 Skills of a good listener

- Looking at the patient when they start to talk
- Using body language such as nodding, leaning forwards to demonstrate to the speaker that you are interested in what is being said
- Not constantly looking at the time
- Adopting a relaxed posture
- Using paraphrasing, reflecting and summarising to show the patient that you are listening to and understanding what they are saying

Non-verbal behaviour includes behaviours such as posture, touch, personal space, physical appearance, facial expressions, gestures and paralanguage (i.e. the vocalisations associated with verbal messages, such as tone, pitch, volume, speed of speech). It is said that we primarily communicate non-verbally. Remember the old adage 'a picture says a thousand words'. Your body language and paralanguage will send an array of messages to your patient even before you say anything. Non-verbal communication serves many useful purposes. It can be used to (Dickson et al 1997, Hargie et al 1994):

- replace, support or complement speech
- regulate the flow of verbal communication
- provide feedback to the person who is transmitting the message, e.g. looking interested
- communicate attitudes and emotions.

Non-verbal communication is the main mode of conveying our emotional state in most types of human interaction. In fact, in a typical practitioner–client interaction, only a small amount of the social meaning will be conveyed verbally, with a significant amount being communicated through non-verbal channels (Buller & Street 1992).

Due to the broad literature in this area the following section will focus on selected aspects of non-verbal behaviour and how they may influence the success of the assessment interview. For the interested reader, a wide range of books are available on non-verbal communication, many specialising in the clinical interaction (see recommended reading at the end of this chapter).

Eye contact

Eye-to-eye contact is frequently the first stage of interpersonal communication. It is the way we attract the other person's attention. Direct eye-to-eye contact creates trust between two people; hence, the innate distrust felt of someone who avoids eye contact. However, we do not keep constant eye-to-eye contact throughout a conversation. The receiver looks at the speaker for approximately 25–50% of the time, whereas the speaker looks at the other person for approximately half as long. So in other words, people tend to look more at the other person when they are listening compared with when they are speaking.

Too much eye contact is interpreted as staring and is seen as a hostile gesture. Too little is interpreted as a lack of interest, attention or trustworthiness. Interviewers cannot afford to look inattentive because patients may interpret this as meaning that they have said enough and as a result may stop talking. Conversely, withdrawing eye contact may be used as a legitimate way indicating to patients to stop talking.

Healthcare practitioners should be aware of the frequency and duration of eye contact they have with their patients. The use of eye contact is important for assessing a range of patient needs and providing feedback and support, and its use during the interview should be based on the professional judgement of the practitioner (Davidhizar 1992). Certainly eye-to-eye contact is recommended at the beginning of the interview, to gain rapport and trust, and at the end of the interview by way of closing the interview. However, you should always be aware of potential cultural and gender differences in appropriate level of eye contact. For example, Hall (1984) has reported that on average women tend to make more eye-to-eye contact compared with men, so adjust your non-verbal behaviour accordingly.

Facial expression

Facial expression is arguably the most important form of human communication next to speech itself (Hargie et al 1994). It is via our facial expression we communicate most about our emotional state, and the meaning of a wide range of facial expressions (e.g. happy or sad) have been shown in one classic study to be recognised universally (Ekman & Fresen 1975). Smiling, together with judicious eye-to-eye contact, signifies a receptive and friendly persona and inspires a feeling of confidence and friendliness. Facial expressions often carry even more weight in a social interaction than the spoken word. For example, if a practitioner is giving a very positive verbal message to the patient but, at the same time, the practitioner's facial expression communicates anxiety and doubt, then it is likely that the patient will pay more attention to the facial message. This is because verbal behaviour is much easier to control than non-verbal and, as a result, non-verbal communication is likely to be more honest! Therefore, it is important that practitioners are always aware of the message they are communicating using their facial expressions.

Posture and gestures

The manner in which we hold ourselves and the way in which we move says a lot about us as individuals. This area of non-verbal behaviour is often referred to as *kinesics* and includes all those movements of the body which complement the spoken word (e.g. gestures, limb movements, head nods, etc.). One particularly important aspect is posture. Four types of posture have been identified:

- *Approaching posture*, which conveys interest, curiosity and attention, e.g. sitting upright and slightly forward in a chair facing towards the person you are communicating with
- *Withdrawal posture*, which conveys negation, refusal and disgust, e.g. distance between the receiver and the communicator, shuffling, gestures indicating agitation
- *Expansion*, which conveys a sense of pride, conceit, mastery, self-esteem, e.g. expanded chest, hands behind head with shoulders in air, erect head and trunk
- *Contraction*, which conveys depression, dejection, e.g. sitting in a chair with head drooped, arms and legs crossed or head held in hands, avoiding eye contact.

Clearly, the posture adopted by the healthcare practitioner is important in developing a rapport and a working therapeutic relationship with the patient.

When we speak we also tend to use our arms and hands to reinforce and complement the verbal message. Self-directed gestures such as ring twisting, self-stroking and nail biting may indicate anxiety. Be aware of self-participation in these types of activities as you may convey a non-verbal message of anxiety to your patient when verbally you are trying to convey a confident approach. The healthcare professional should be sensitive to the non-verbal gestures used by the patient as these may reveal more about the patient's thoughts and feelings than they are able to communicate verbally (Harrigan & Taing 1997).

Touch

The extent to which touching is permissible or encouraged is related to culture (McDaniel & Andersen 1998). In general, Britain is not known as a nation of 'touchers'. During the assessment it may be necessary to touch patients to examine a part of the body. This type of touching, known as functional touching, is generally acceptable to most patients as part of the role of the practitioner and as such does not carry any connotation of a social relationship. However, people from certain cultures may find it difficult to accept, even in medical settings. Prior to functional touching of a patient, it is important that you inform the patient what you intend to do and the reasons for doing it.

During the interview you may wish to use touch as a means of reassuring the patient, to indicate warmth, show empathy or as a sign of care and concern (McCann & McKenna 1993). A hand lightly placed on a shoulder or holding a patient's hand are means of showing concern and giving reassurance. It is difficult to produce guidelines for when this type of touching should or should not be used. Practitioners must feel confident and happy in its use, and must also take into account a multitude of communication cues from the patient before deciding whether it is or is *not* appropriate (Davidhizar & Newman 1997).

Proxemics

All of us have a sense of our own personal territory. When someone invades that territory, depending on the situation, we can be fearful, disturbed or pleased and happy. As with touch, our sense of personal space is affected by culture. In some cultures individuals have a large personal space, whereas in others they have a very small personal space. Encroaching on someone else's personal space can be perceived as intimidation and, in the case of the assessment interview, may put patients on their guard. As a result the patient may become reluctant to disclose relevant information. Hall (1969) defined the four zones of personal space (Table 2.1).

The zone in which people interact is highly influenced by social status and people who have an equal status tend to interact at closer distances (Zahn 1991). The assessment interview usually takes place in the social/consultative and the personal zones. During the interview it may be necessary to enter the intimate zone. During the interview it may be necessary to enter the intimate zone to carry out an intervention or examination that requires closer contact. Before doing this, you should ask the patient's permission.

Table 2.1 Four zones of personal space (Hall 1969)

Zone	*Distance*	*Activities*
Intimate	0–0.5 m	Intimate relationships/close friends
Personal	0.5–1.2 m	What is usually termed 'personal space'
Social/consultative	1.2–3 m	Distance of day-to-day interactions
Public	+3 m	Distance from significant public figures

Social interactions are not only influenced by distance but also by bodily orientation. The angle at which you conduct the assessment interview may have a significant effect on the success of the interaction. There are four main ways in which you can position yourself to interact with the patient (Fig. 2.1): (i) conversation, (ii) cooperation, (iii) competition, and (iv) co-action. Research indicates that the conversation position is most appropriate for an assessment interview. When GPs sat at a 90° angle to their patients during a clinical interview, the amount of clinician–patient information exchanged increased by up to *six* times compared with when they interacted face-to-face (Pietroni 1976). Clearly, the healthcare professional needs to be aware of the physical position they adopt when assessing a patient as this will have a significant impact on the kind of relationship they are hoping to achieve (Worchel 1986).

Physical appearance

We use our clothing and accessories to make statements about ourselves to others. Clothing can be seen as an expression of conformity or self-expression, comfort, economy or status. Uniforms are used as intentional means of communicating a message to others; often the message is to do with status. Uniforms are also used in the healthcare professions for cover and protection. Whether one wears a uniform (white coat, coloured top and trousers) for the assessment interview is open for debate, but one should pay attention to issues of cleanliness and appearance

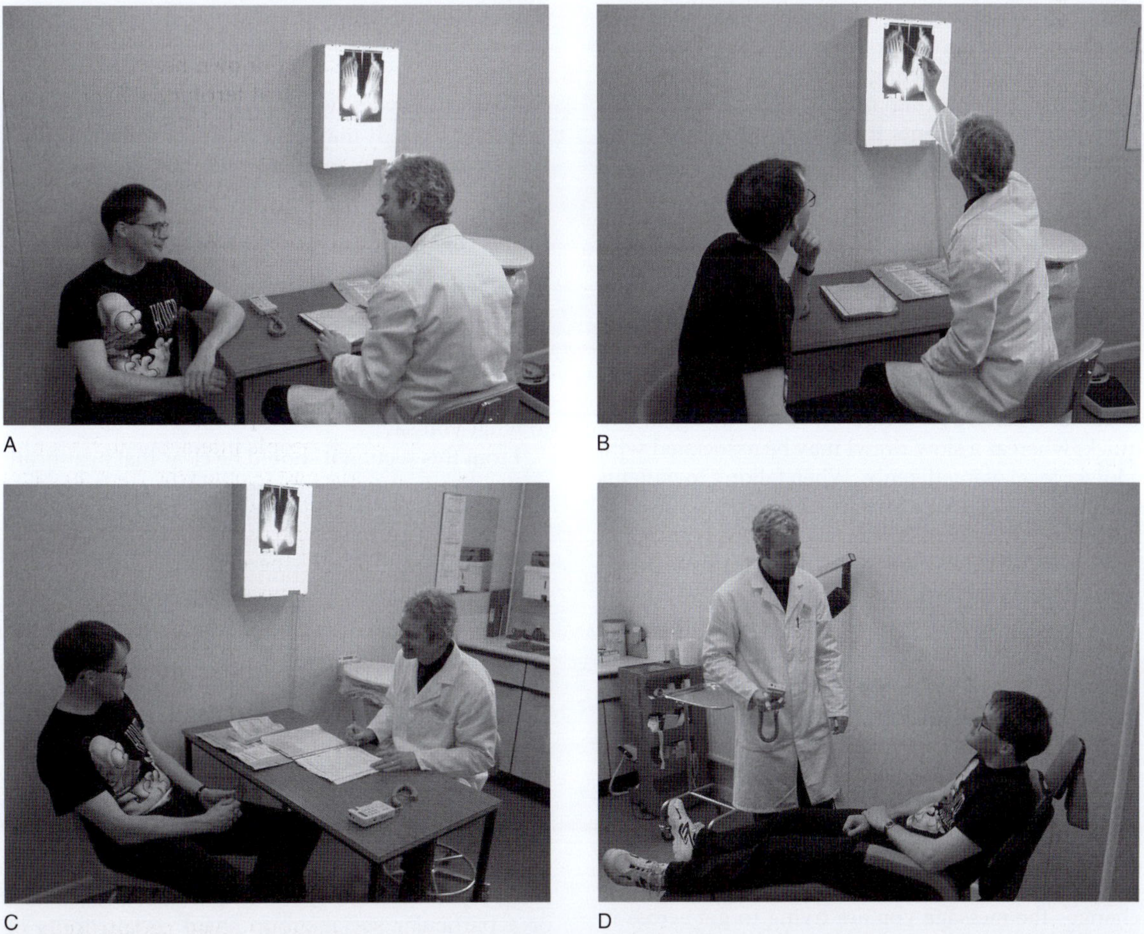

A B C D

Figure 2.1 Body orientation may influence the success of the interview. The four positions commonly encountered when two people interact are: **A** conversation, **B** cooperation **C** competition and **D** co-action. Which of these orientations do you think would be most appropriate for the assessment interview?

of dress, hair, hands, footwear and accessories such as jewellery – they all send messages to the patient. In addition to physical factors, which can be altered, you should also be aware of how 'non-changeable' physical characteristics may have a role in your interaction with the patient. For example, physically attractive and/or taller people are typically judged more favourably in general social interactions (Hensley & Cooper 1987, Melamed & Bozionelos 1992). Research has shown that within a healthcare environment, children make judgements about healthcare professionals on the basis of height. In general, taller health professionals are judged to be stronger and more dominant than their smaller colleagues, but they are not considered to be more intelligent or more empathetic (Montepare 1995).

Finally, healthcare practitioners should also be aware of the impact of their appearance on any health promotion message that they hope to communicate. For example, the patient will often pay attention to the footwear worn by the practitioner. Avoid giving conflicting verbal and non-verbal messages, e.g. wearing high-heeled slip-on shoes while advising patients that they should not wear this type of shoe.

Paralanguage

This involves the manner in which we speak. It includes everything from the speed at which we speak to the dialect we use. Paralanguage is the **bold**, underlining, *italics* and punctuation marks in our everyday speech. An individual who speaks fast is often considered by the receiver to be intelligent and quick, whereas a slow drawl may be associated with a lower level of intelligence. When talking to patients we should be careful not to speak too quickly as they will not understand what we say. Conversely, if speech is too slow, the patient may not have confidence in the practitioner.

When we speak we use pitch, intonation and volume to affect the message we transmit. Individuals who speak at a constant volume and do not use intonation and/or alter their pitch often come across as monotonous, dull and boring. Such speech is often difficult to listen to. Intonation and pitch should be used to highlight the important parts of your question and can be used to change the point you are trying to make. For example, in the following examples you can see how changing the point of emphasis changes the message you are trying to get across in this sentence:

- **You** must use the cream on your foot daily (i.e. treatment is the responsibility of the patient).
- You **must** use the cream on your foot daily (i.e. it is essential that the treatment is carried out).
- You must use the **cream** on your foot daily (i.e. it is important that the cream is used and not some other substance).
- You must use the cream on your **foot** daily (i.e. the cream should be used on the foot and not some other part of the body).
- You must use the cream on your foot **daily** (i.e. treatment needs to be on a regular basis).

The fluency with which we speak also tends to convey messages about mental and intellectual abilities. Repeated hesitations, repetitions, interjections of 'you know' or 'um' and false starts do not inspire confidence in the receiver (Christenfeld 1995). We all experience occasions when we are not as fluent as at other times. These occasions tend to occur when we are tired or under great stress. If possible, these times should be kept to a minimum during clinical assessment.

Dialect conveys which part of the country we originate from. It may also cause us to use vocabulary a person from another part of the country is not familiar with. Avoid using colloquial terms. Dialect, on the other hand, is not so easy to alter. The only time it should be considered is when patients cannot understand what the practitioner is saying. Finally, volume should not be changed too regularly. Shouting at the patient should be avoided. In the clinical setting, as in life in general, shouting certainly does not guarantee that the other person will listen more to what you say!

From this section it should be clear that healthcare professionals need to be sensitive to the kind of atmosphere they are creating through their non-verbal communication, and the role this may have in the subsequent interaction with the patient. The extent to which you establish a satisfactory rapport will depend heavily on your non-verbal skills and how you develop them in your clinical work (Grahe & Bernieri 1999).

Stereotyping

Healthcare practitioners should be aware of their own underlying psychological characteristics, which may have a profound effect on the interaction, i.e. stereotypes. A stereotype is a belief that all members of a particular social group share certain traits or characteristics (Baron & Byrne 2000). For example, you might hold particular ideas about the characteristics of patients who are alcoholic, elderly, from an upper social class group, from a minority ethnic group or female. You probably already hold a range of stereotypes about a wide group of patients whom you have never actually treated! While stereotypes are not always negative, they do share a common characteristic in that they reduce the ability of the healthcare worker to see the patient as an *individual*. Consequently, any information gathered from the patient during the assessment interview is likely to be interpreted in the light of such stereotypes (Price 1987). Ganong et al (1987) conducted a review of 38 studies, in which they examined stereotyping by nurses and nursing students. Their results indicated that nurses held stereotypes about patients on the basis of age, gender, diagnosis, social class, personality and family structure. However, the impact on actual patient care was harder to classify. What does seem to be the case is that patients were less likely to be seen as having unique concerns, health problems and social circumstances. Consequently, in addition to practising interviewing skills, it is important for healthcare practitioners to reflect on any belief systems they may hold regarding particular patient groups, and consider how such views may impair the overall success of the assessment interview.

The healthcare practitioner should also pay particular attention to the needs of patients for whom the traditional assessment interview format may present difficulties. This may include patients with speech or hearing difficulties, those with a learning disability or who have difficulty with the use of language, and also patients who come from a different cultural background. For example, research has shown that healthcare professionals differed significantly in how they were perceived when communicating with patients from a different cultural background. The most skilled communicators are generally considered to be more empathetic by patients, but they are also more likely to have had some previous experience of working across cultures (Gibson & Zhong 2005). This finding would again reinforce the importance of experience and practise in the development of good communication skills – particularly when working in challenging situations.

Finally, you should also carefully consider the design of the physical environment in which the interview takes place and ensure that this does not add to any communication difficulties a patient may have. This is particularly important if you work in a busy clinic where background noise in the environment may hinder communication with patients with hearing difficulties (Park & Song 2005).

Documenting the assessment interview

It is essential to make a permanent record of the findings of the interview either during or at the end of the assessment. This record acts as an aide-memoire for future reference when monitoring and evaluating the treatment plan and as a means of communicating your findings to another practitioner who may collaborate in treating the patient.

Despite recent discussions within the field of podiatry regarding changing to electronic data management systems, the majority of patient records are still stored on paper. However, the use of computerised records is on the increase, particularly in private practice. It may well be in the future that paper records are discarded completely, and replaced by computerised records. Whatever the future may hold, the need for clear, accurate recording of information will be the same. The recording of assessment findings, together with the recording of treatment provided, forms a legal document. Patient records would certainly be used if action was taken by a patient against a practitioner, or if certain agencies required detailed evidence of management and progress in the case of disability awards.

Patient records may take a variety of forms: at the simplest level a plain piece of paper may be used. If using plain paper it is essential to adopt an order to the presentation of your assessment findings: e.g. name, address, doctor, age, sex, weight, height, main complaint, medical history, etc. This is considered further in Chapter 5. A variety of patient record cards are used in the National Health Service (NHS) and private practice. Many practitioners and health agencies produce their own tailor-made record card. The Association of Chief Chiropody Officers (ACCO) produced a standard record in 1986 for charting foot conditions, diagnoses and treatment progress.

Handwritten recording of information requires the following:

- The writing is legible and in permanent ink, not pencil. If another practitioner cannot read your writing the information is of no use.
- The information is set in a clear and logical order. It is essential to use an accepted method.
- Location and size of lesions or deformities are recorded accurately. The use of prepared outlines of the feet are very good for indicating anatomical sites and save additional writing.
- Abbreviations are avoided where possible. What is obvious to you may not be so obvious to another practitioner.

- Entries are dated. Recording the medication a patient is taking is useless unless it is dated. Once dated the information can be updated as and when there is a change.
- Each entry should be signed and dated by the practitioner.

Structuring the assessment interview

Preparation

In order to achieve a good assessment interview it is essential you prepare yourself for the interview. The following should be taken into consideration.

Purpose

It is essential that the practitioner is clear about the purpose of the interview. In some instances the assessment interview may be used as a screening mechanism to identify patients for further assessment. It may be used to gain information from patients so that their needs can be prioritised and those judged to be urgent can be seen to first. On the other hand, the assessment interview may be aimed at undertaking a full assessment of the patient, with treatment provided at the end of the interview.

Letter of application

Was the patient referred or self-referred? If the patient was referred by another healthcare practitioner there should be an accompanying letter of referral. Read this carefully so you are fully informed of the reasons for referral. This information should be used as a starting point for the assessment. If patients have referred themselves directly (self-referred) they should complete any appropriate documentation prior to the interview. Information on application forms can be used to prioritise patients and ensure the most suitable practitioner sees them.

You may wish to give the patient a short health questionnaire to complete prior to the assessment. This questionnaire may be sent to the patient before they come for the interview or the patient may be asked to fill it in on arrival. These questionnaires provide the practitioner with important information before the start of the interview. Patients should be allowed adequate time to complete the questionnaire so that they can think about their responses. The advantage of such a questionnaire is that the practitioner does not have to ask the patient a series of routine questions during the interview. However, some patients may be reluctant to fill in a form without having met the practitioner or may be reluctant to disclose information in writing.

Prior to the interview, try to read all the information you have about the patient. You can then come across to patients someone who is well informed or someone who has taken an interest in him.

Patient expectations

Does the patient know what to expect from the assessment interview? Some new patients, prior to attending their assessment appointment, are sent an information sheet or booklet explaining the purpose of the assessment interview and what will happen during it. Such initiatives are helpful. The cause of a poor interview may be that the patient's expectations of what will happen are very different from what actually happens. For example, a patient who expected immediate treatment and had not envisaged any need for history taking may well say, 'Why are you asking me all these questions?'. Box 2.2 lists the information a patient information booklet should contain.

Waiting room

Patients can spend a lot of time in the waiting room, especially if they arrive too early or are kept waiting due to unavoidable circumstances. Try sitting in the

Box 2.2 Information booklet for patients to read before the interview

The booklet should contain the following information:

- The purpose of the assessment interview
- How long the interview should take
- What will happen during the interview
- Specific information the patient may be asked to provide, e.g. list of current medication
- Specific items the patient may be asked to bring, e.g. footwear
- Examples of questions patients are likely to be asked
- The possible outcomes of the assessment interview, e.g. whether the patient will receive treatment at the end of it.

The booklet may also contain a health questionnaire for the patient to complete and bring to the assessment interview.

waiting room in your clinic. Look around you: how welcoming is it? The waiting room sets the scene for the rest of the interview. Where possible, ensure that it is in good decorative order, clean, with magazines to read and informative, eye-catching posters or pictures on the wall. Make the most of a captive audience to put over important health education information. TV monitors showing health promotion videos may be useful method of reinforcing important information.

Displaying the name of the practitioner outside the clinic may be useful. Some clinics, like several high street banks, have a display of photographs with the names and titles of those who work in that department or centre.

Interview room

The assessment interview may be carried out in an office or in a clinic. Both have advantages and disadvantages. Using an office prevents the patient being put off by surrounding clinical equipment. It facilitates eye-to-eye contact by sitting in chairs, and provides a non-clinical environment. This is especially useful if treatment is not usually provided at the end of the assessment. On the other hand, using a clinic ensures that clinical equipment is readily to hand and the patient can be moved into different positions on the treatment couch/plinth.

During the interview you should ensure that you are not disturbed. If there is a phone in the room, redirect calls. Ensure the receptionist does not interrupt. While a patient is in the room, you should be giving them your full, undivided attention. Constant disturbances not only makes the assessment interview a protracted occasion but also can prompt the patient into feeling that their problem is not worthy of your attention.

The interview

When the patient enters the room, welcome them to the clinic, preferably by name. This personalises the occasion for the patient and at the same time ensures that you have the correct patient. If you have difficulty with the patient's name, ask politely how to pronounce it rather than doing so incorrectly. Introduce yourself. As part of the Patient's Charter you should be wearing a name badge but a personal introduction is usually preferable, especially if the patient's eyesight is poor. It is useful to shake the patient by the hand since touch is an important aspect of non-verbal behaviour (as discussed earlier), although this may be influenced by personal preference and religious protocol.

At this stage you may find it helpful to make one or two general conversation points about the weather, the time of year or some news item. This enables patients to see you as a fellow human. Remember that during the interview they are going to give a lot of themselves to you. It is important that patients feel you are someone they wish to disclose information to. Use the introduction as an opportunity to explain the purpose of the interview and what will happen.

The positioning of patient and practitioner can influence the success of the assessment interview. Ideally, you and the patient should be at the same level in order to facilitate eye-to-eye contact. Barriers such as desks are often used in medical interviews. They can be considered as means of making the interview formal. Standing over a patient who is sitting down or lying on a couch may be intimidating.

Data gathering

It is essential that the practitioner is clear as to what areas should be covered in the interview. A logical and ordered approach should be adopted. However, it is not always possible or desirable to stick to an ordered approach. Patients tend to talk around issues or elect to give information about a question that you asked earlier at the end of the interview. You must make allowances for this.

Effective and efficient use of time is paramount. Experienced practitioners combine the interview with the examination. This is achieved by, for example, feeling pulses and skin temperature while simultaneously asking questions about medical history. This technique is a matter of preference; some prefer to complete the interview before commencing the examination. After each assessment interview reflect on it. Ask yourself how you could improve your performance and how you could make better use of the time. This will help you to make the best use of the data-gathering stage of the interview. Peer appraisal is another mechanism that you may find helpful in aiding you to develop good data-gathering skills.

Closure

Bringing the assessment interview to a close is a difficult task. When do you know you have enough information? This is a difficult question to answer. Some presenting problems, together with information from the patient, can be easily diagnosed. Other problems are not so easy to resolve and may require further questioning and investigations.

General medical practitioners have been shown to give their patients, on average, six minutes of their time. Psychotherapists, on the other hand, spend an hour or more on each assessment. Unfortunately the demands on practitioners' time means they are often not in a position to give the patient as much time as they would like.

As a general rule of thumb the interview should be brought to a close when the practitioner feels the patient has been given an opportunity to talk about the problem. Body language can be used to convey the closing of the interview. Standing up from a sitting position, shuffling of papers, withdrawing eye-to-eye contact are all ways by which the end of the interview can be conveyed to the patient, together with a verbal message.

The patient should not leave the interview without fully understanding what is to happen next and without an opportunity to ask questions. A range of outcomes may result from the assessment interview (Box 2.3). Patients should know which outcome applies to them. They should always be given the opportunity to raise any queries or concerns they may have prior to leaving the assessment. This is one of the most important parts of the assessment and should not be hurried. The patient must leave the assessment fully understanding the findings of the assessment interview and what action, if any, is to be taken, and it is the responsibility of the healthcare professional to ensure that they have communicated such information clearly (Calkins et al 1997).

It is helpful to provide written instructions as a follow-up to the interview. For example, if the patient is to be offered a course of treatment write down what will the treatment involve, when will it be given, who will give it and any problems the patient may experience.

Box 2.3 Outcomes from the assessment interview

- Treatment is not required; the patient requires advice and reassurance
- The patient can look after the problem once appropriate self-help advice has been given
- A course of treatment is required; the patient should be informed as to whether treatment will commence straight after the assessment interview or at a later date
- The patient needs to be referred to another practitioner for treatment
- Further examination and investigations are required before a definitive diagnosis can be made
- A second opinion is required
- The urgency for treatment should be prioritised

Confidentiality

The information a patient divulges during the interview is confidential. It should not be disclosed to other people unless the patient has given consent. The Data Protection Act 1998 requires that all personal data held on computers should be 'secure from loss or unauthorised disclosure'. In the UK, the General Medical Council (2006) and the NHS (2003) have laid down guidelines on confidentiality. These guidelines can be accessed electronically at their respective websites (www.gmc-uk.org. and www.dh.gov.uk).

What makes a good assessment interview?

The prime purpose of the assessment interview is to draw out information, experiences and opinions from the patient. It is the duty of the interviewer to guide and keep the interview to the subject in hand. At the same time, it is equally important to encourage the patient to talk and to clear up any misunderstandings as you go along. Keeping the balance between these two competing aims is not an easy task. One way of checking on this is to ask yourself who is doing most of the talking. Is it you or the patient? If you are to achieve the aims of the assessment interview it should be the patient. However, if the interview is moving towards the closure phase or you are discussing treatment protocols then it is likely to be the practitioner doing most of the talking.

It is not essential that you like the patient you are interviewing. What is important is that you adopt a professional approach, demonstrate empathy and deal with the patient in a competent and courteous manner. It is essential that you do not make value judgements based on your own biases and prejudices: respect the patient and avoid stereotyping. Do not jump to conclusions before reaching the end of the interview.

As emphasised earlier, the assessment interview should be patient-centred; its prime purpose is to gain information from the patient. However, one sometimes comes across patients who cannot seem to stop talking. What can the practitioner do in these instances? The first question to ask is why the patient is talking so much. Is it because they are lonely and welcome the opportunity to talk, are they self-centred, overly anxious, avoiding telling you what the real concern is by talking about minor issues? The reason will influence the action you take. If you feel the patient wants to tell you something but is finding it difficult, try reflecting or summarise what you think has been said. Ask if there is anything else the patient would like to discuss. Encourage patients by telling them that you want to help them as much as you can; the more they tell you about their concerns the more you can help them.

On the other hand, if you feel you need to control a talkative patient you may find the following techniques helpful:

- Use eye contact and your body language to inform the patient that you are bringing a particular section of the interview to a close.
- Politely interrupt the patient, summarise what they have said and say what is to happen next.
- Ask questions that bring the patient back to the topic under discussion.

The opposite of talkative patients are those who are reluctant to disclose information about themselves. This may be because they do not see the purpose of the questions you are asking, or they are shy, cannot articulate their concerns, are fearful of what the outcomes may be or are too embarrassed to disclose certain information. Your response will depend on the cause of the reticence.

Explaining why you need to know certain information will be helpful if the patient is hesitant. For example, a patient may wonder why you need to know what medication they are taking when all they wants is to have a corn treated. If you feel the patient cannot articulate what they want to say, you may find that closed questions can help. This type of questioning limits responses but can be helpful for a patient who has difficulty putting concerns and problems into words. You need to use a range of closed questions and avoid leading questions if you are to ensure you reach an accurate diagnosis.

The shy or embarrassed person may find self-disclosure very difficult. It has been shown that people tend to disclose more about themselves as they get older. In general, females disclose more than males. When privacy is ensured and the interviewer shows empathy, friendliness and acceptance, patients have been shown to disclose more information. Reciprocal disclosure can also be helpful.

Feedback

In order to develop your interview technique it is important that you obtain feedback on your performance. Mention has already been made of self and peer assessment of the interview. This is a valuable process, which should be ongoing. Patient feedback is another valuable mechanism. Questionnaires (postal or self-administered) and structured or unstructured interviews are ways in which patient reactions to the interview can be obtained. Suggestions as to how to improve interviews should be welcomed.

Summary

The interview is the process of initiating an assessment of the lower limb. The relationship created between the practitioner and the patient during the interview will hopefully lead to an effective diagnosis. A good interview can provide the majority of the information required, without having to resort to tests, investigations and unnecessary examination. However, there is no one formula that can be applied to all assessment interviews. Each patient should be treated as an individual with specific needs. Practitioners should develop their interviewing skills so that the interview achieves a successful outcome for a patient and the practitioner during each step of the patient's journey.

References

Alexander J 2001 How much do we know about the giving and receiving of information? International Journal of Nursing Studies 38(5):495–496

Authier J 1986 Showing warmth and empathy. In: Hargie O (ed) A handbook of communication skills. Routledge, London

Baron R A, Byrne D 2000 Social psychology, 9th edn. Allyn & Bacon, Boston

Buller D, Street R 1992 Physician–patient relationships. In: Feldman R S (ed) Applications of nonverbal behavioural theories and research. Lawrence Erlbaum Associates, Hillsdale, New Jersey

Calkins D, Davis R, Reiley P et al 1997 Patient–physician communication at hospital discharge and patients' understanding of the postdischarge treatment plan. Archives of Internal Medicine 157:1026

Christenfeld N 1995 Does it hurt to say um. Journal of Nonverbal Behavior 19:171

Data Protection Act 1998 EC Data Protection Directive (95/46 EC)

Davidhizar R 1992 Interpersonal communication: a review of eye contact. Infection Control and Hospital Epidemiology 13:222

Davidhizar R, Newman J 1997 When touch is not the best approach. Journal of Clinical Nursing 6:203

Department of Health 2000 The NHS plan. Department of Health, London

Dickson D, Hargie O, Morrow N 1997 Communication skills training for health professionals, 2nd edn. Chapman & Hall, London

Ekman P, Fresen W V 1975 Unmasking the face. Prentice-Hall, Englewood Cliffs, New Jersey

Ganong L H, Bzdek V, Manderino M A 1987 Stereotyping by nurses and nursing students: a critical review of research. Research in Nursing and Health 10:49

General Medical Council 2006 Professional conduct and discipline: Fitness to practice. GMC, London

Gibson D, Zhong M 2005 Inner cultural communication competence in the healthcare context. International Journal of Cultural Relations 29(5):621–634

Grahe J, Bernieri F 1999 The importance of nonverbal cues in judging rapport. Journal of Nonverbal Behavior 23:253

Hall E T 1969 The hidden dimension. Doubleday, New York

Hall J A 1984 Nonverbal sex differences: communication accuracy and expressive style. Johns Hopkins University, Baltimore

Hargie O, Saunders C, Dickson D 1994 Social skills in interpersonal communication, 3rd edn. Routledge, London

Hargie O, Dickson D, Boohan M et al 1998 A survey of communication skills training in UK schools of medicine: present practices and prospective proposals. Medical Education 32:25

Harrigan J, Taing K 1997 Fooled by a smile: detecting anxiety in others. Journal of Nonverbal Behavior 21:203

Hensley W, Cooper R 1987 Height and occupational success: a review and critique. Psychological Reports 60:843

McCann K, McKenna H P 1993 An examination of touch between nurses and elderly patients in a continuing care setting in Northern Ireland. Journal of Advanced Nursing 18:38

McDaniel E, Andersen P 1998 International patterns of interpersonal tactile communication. Journal of Nonverbal Behavior 22:59

Melamed J, Bozionelos N 1992 Managerial promotion and height. Psychological Reports 71:587

Montepare J 1995 The impact of variations in height in young children's impressions of men and women. Journal of Nonverbal Behavior 19:31

National Health Service Circular No 2003 A code of practice on the confidentiality of personal health information. London

Newell, R 1994 Interviewing skills for nurses and other healthcare professionals. A structured approach. Routledge, London

Park E, Song M 2005 Communication barriers perceived by older patients and nurses. International Journal of Nursing Studies 42(2):159–166

Pietroni P 1976 Non-verbal communication in the GP surgery. In: Tanner B (ed) Language and communication in general practice. Hodder & Stoughton, London

Price B 1987 First impressions: paradigms for patient assessment. Journal of Advanced Nursing 12:699

Sleight P 1995 Teaching communication skills: part of medical education. Journal of Human Hypertension 9:67

Stein T, Frankel R, Krupat E 2005 Enhancing clinician communication skills in a large healthcare organisation: a longitudinal case study. Patient Education and Counseling 58(1):4–12

Trummer U, Mueller U, Nowak P et al 2006 Does physician-patient communication that aims at empowering patients improve clinical outcomes? A case study. Patient Education and Counseling 61(2):299–306

Worchel S 1986 The influence of contextual variables on interpersonal spacing. Journal of Nonverbal Behavior 10:230

Zahn G L 1991 Face-to-face communication in an office setting: the effects of position, proximity and exposure. Communication Research 18:737

Further reading

Davis C 1994 Patient practitioner interaction: an experiential manual for developing the art of healthcare, 2nd edn. Slack Inc, New Jersey

Hargie O 1997 The handbook of communication skills, 2nd edn. Routledge, London

CHAPTER

3

The presenting problem

B Yates

Chapter contents

Introduction

Most patients consult a practitioner because they have concerns about or problems with their lower limbs. Problems are usually quite specific and focused. Patients may have problems with painful feet, an ingrowing toe nail or difficulty accommodating a bunion in footwear. Concerns relate to when the patient is worried or anxious about something. This may be concerning a particular problem or pathology, e.g. they are worried about an ulcer that is taking a long time to heal. Conversely, a patient may have concerns but no specific problems or pathology, e.g. a patient may be concerned about the appearance of their feet, are they wearing the right type of running shoe?

The role of the practitioner is to discover what are the patient's concern(s) and problem(s) so that an effective management plan can be drawn up and implemented. This may involve just giving reassurance and advice to implementing a treatment plan aimed at resolving or reducing the effects of a specific problem or pathology.

During the assessment interview the patient should be given ample opportunity to express their concerns and talk about any problems they may have. This chapter concentrates on acquiring information about the patient's presenting problem(s). However, the practitioner should always remember it is also important to identify any concerns the patient may have.

The problem

What one person perceives as a problem may be accepted as being normal by another. A major concern for one person may be a minor issue for another. Defining what is normal and acceptable, and what is abnormal or unacceptable and therefore a problem, is fraught with difficulties.

When patients attend for their appointments they bring with them their own ideas of what is a problem and what is normal. A variety of factors can influence a patient's perception (Box 3.1). For example, if there has been media coverage emphasising a link between verrucae and cancer of the cervix this might result in many women, who had previously ignored their verrucae, to seek treatment. Having a friend who has developed a malignant melanoma may make people

Box 3.1 Factors that influence a patient's perceptions of what is normal and what is a problem

- Age
- Gender
- Culture
- Socioeconomic base
- Knowledge base
- Previous experiences
- Views of family and friends
- Media
- Socioeconomic background
- Life expectations

more vigilant for signs associated with this condition and prompt them to seek advice when previously they may have been oblivious to the situation.

People from socioeconomic groups 1 and 2 are more likely to seek medical assistance than those from socioeconomic groups 4 and 5 (Bygren 2001, Townsend & Davidson 1982). People who work are also less likely to seek medical attention, and there are also differences between ethnic groups. There is also growing evidence that white middle-class men are less likely to seek medical treatment for illness probably due to 'traditional masculine behaviour' and a belief that the problem will go away (Galdas et al 2005). Variation is also seen in the type of healthcare accessed. Delay in utilisation of emergency medicine is more common in people who infrequently see their general practitioner (GP) (Rucker et al 2001), whereas there is little if any difference in people seeking palliative care for cancer (Kessler et al 2005).

It is important that the practitioner allows the patient to describe the problem in their own words. This should enable the practitioner to determine the 'needs' of the patient and the significance of the concern or problem. The practitioner's perception of the problem is not always the same as that of the patient. For example, a mother may be concerned that her 3-year-old child has flat feet. The practitioner considers this to be normal for a child of that age. However, during the consultation, the practitioner notices a small verruca on the apex of the right second toe and suggests that it is treated. The mother accepts the treatment but leaves the clinic still concerned about her child's flat feet, as the practitioner failed to alleviate the mother's main concern. An effective solution would have consisted of advice and reassurance regarding the flat feet as well as treatment of the verruca.

Encouraging the patient to tell you about concerns and problems

How can you encourage patients to tell you why they have sought your help? A whole range of factors can make it difficult for the patient to articulate the problem in words. Some patients may be frightened or embarrassed, others may be concerned that they are wasting your time and yet others may be worried that you will think they are silly to be concerned about a minor problem. It is essential that patients are made to feel that they are not wasting your time and that you are genuinely interested in their concerns and problems.

Most patients present with discomfort or pain. For example, a patient may present with discomfort from a bunion rubbing on footwear. The patient may also be concerned about the appearance of the bunion and scared that she will develop a deformity similar to her grandmother's. A skilled practitioner will identify all the anxieties the patient is experiencing: the problems with the current discomfort, the difficulty in finding appropriate shoes to wear, the worry about the unsightly appearance of the bunion and the fear that it may get worse.

It is important that you consider how best to start the conversation. Asking the patient 'What are you complaining of?', 'What's the problem?' or 'What is it that's wrong with you?' are probably not the best ways to start. The last question may result in the patient responding 'That's what I've come here for you to find out'. 'How can I help you?' or 'Would you like to tell me about what concerns you?' may be preferable. Open questions should be used (see Ch. 2). The patient should not feel rushed; avoid interrupting and putting words into the patient's mouth. Record in the patient's own words what they are concerned about and what they see as a problem. Avoid medical jargon wherever possible.

Having obtained an idea of the patient's concerns, it may help to find out if they have any thoughts about the cause. Ask the reason for such conclusions as this may help determine the aetiology of the condition and could help guide management. The answers to these questions may also reveal whether the patient and practitioner share the same views.

When patients do reveal what is worrying them, avoid being judgemental and making comments such as 'Oh, that's nothing!' or 'I don't know why you are so worried!'. Remember it is a problem to the patient even if it is relatively innocuous matter for you. Patients may not reveal their real reason for coming to see you until they are just about to leave. This can be a source of annoyance to the busy practitioner. Do try to give the patient time even if it is at the end of the consultation. Patients may also not tell you the real reason for seeking treatment if they think it may affect your decision to offer treatment. An example of this is a foot deformity for which the patient would like surgical correction for cosmetic reasons rather than for any disability or pain the deformity may cause. Conversely, if a patient does not like the treatment offered, they may play down the significance of the problem.

Patients with special needs

Some patients may find it hard to tell you about their concerns and problems. This may be more than simply having poor powers of description. The patient may be deaf, dumb, have suffered a stroke, have a speech impediment, or have learning or language difficulties. It is important you give these patients extra time. Avoid jumping to too many conclusions. If the patient can write, ask them to write down the nature of the complaint. Friends, relatives, or carers may be able to provide valuable details and information or act as interpreters.

Why did the patient seek your help?

A variety of factors can influence why a patient has chosen to visit your practice. Box 3.2 gives the usual reasons for a patient choosing a particular practitioner. It is important to find out what made the patient choose you. For example, a patient who has been referred by a friend or relative may find it easy to disclose her concerns to you. The friend/relative might have been complimentary about your abilities. On the other hand, a patient who is seeking a second opinion may want you to give a different diagnosis from the one given by the previous practitioner. As a result they may not disclose all the salient features of the problem. It is important to remember that legal claims associated with a patient's problem may affect the patient's perspective.

Box 3.2 Reasons for a patient choosing a practitioner

- Applied for treatment at their local health service
- Found your name in the *Yellow Pages*
- Saw an advertisement
- Noticed your plate outside the practice
- Were advised by a friend or relative to seek your help
- Were referred by another health practitioner, e.g. their GP
- Are seeking a second opinion because they were unhappy with the response of the first practitioner

Assessment of the problem

Assessment of the problem involves acquiring information about the history of the problem. The history must be taken logically and systematically. An assessment of the current level of pain and discomfort should also be done.

History of the problem

History taking involves finding answers to a range of questions (Box 3.3). Many diseases can be identified by the pattern of symptoms they display. Research has shown that history taking can be more effective in diagnosing a problem than clinical tests alone (Sandler 1979), although in truth it is difficult to analyse them separately (Sapira 1989) as the history should dictate the clinical tests or investigations performed.

Where is the problem?

Locating the site of the patients problem is essential. Getting the patient to show you by pointing with one finger is the best way of trying to identify the site of pain. If the patient has difficulty reaching the area, you may find it helpful to present an outline picture of the lower limb and ask them to mark the area affected. For example, pain may start in one area but

Box 3.3 The history of the problem: questions to ask the patient

- Where is the problem?
- How did it start?
- What caused it?
- How long have you had the problem?
- When does it trouble you?
- What makes it worse?
- What makes it better?
- What treatments have you tried?
- Are you treating it at the moment?

then radiate to other areas. Some problems may have a precise location; others may be far more diffuse or have multiple sites. These variations may yield helpful clues about the diagnosis.

Isolating a localised area in the case of pain can be helpful in differentiating enthesopathy from the more general discomfort associated with instep plantar fasciitis. During the physical examination you may touch the area and attempt to elicit the symptoms in order to make sure you have isolated the area. Do not forget to tell the patient that this is what you are going to do. Palpation should use no more pressure than necessary to elicit symptoms and isolate the particular anatomy affected. It is essential that you record, either on a diagram or in words, the location of the problem and give an indication in the records whether it is localised or diffuse. For example, a patient with Morton's neuroma may not only complain of acute pain at one particular site, but may also describe a paraesthesia which radiates towards the apex of the toes. Diagrams may be preferable to written descriptions. Another practitioner treating the patient on a different occasion can see exactly where the problem lies. It is essential that dimensions of skin lesions or ulcers are recorded. This approach allows progress to be monitored for improvement or deterioration.

How did it start?

It is important to identify how the problem started. The problem may have had a sudden or an insidious onset. For example, rheumatoid arthritis may have an acute sudden onset accompanied by raised temperature and severe joint pains, or more commonly a slow insidious onset with general aches and pains, which gradually get worse and more regular. Besides trying to locate the start of the condition, it is also important to record the symptoms the patient initially experienced. For example, was there anything visible at the start, such as a rash, swelling or erythema? Were there any symptoms, e.g. the throbbing associated with acute inflammation? Initial symptoms may be different from the patient's current symptoms, especially if the condition had an acute onset but is now chronic or the patient has had some form of treatment already for the condition.

How long have you had the problem?

It may be necessary to jog the patient's memory, especially if the problem started some time ago. Using family occasions such as weddings or births, national events or the season of the year may help the patient to pinpoint which time of the year it started.

When does it trouble you?

Some conditions may give rise to constant symptoms. Others may occur especially at night or during the day. For example, one of the distinguishing features of gout is nocturnal pain. Chronic ischaemia is associated with pain in the calf muscle (intermittent claudication) after a period of walking and the maximum distance the patient can walk prior to experiencing pain gives an indication of the severity of the problem. Many musculoskeletal problems are worse first thing in the morning or after a period of rest. This is a classic feature of plantar fasciitis (sometimes referred to post-static dyskinesia).

What makes it worse and what makes it better?

Some conditions may improve on rest, others can deteriorate. Patients may discover all sorts of ways to alleviate their symptoms, e.g. wearing particular shoes, adopting a different walking pattern. Such information can provide valuable clues. In instances where patients alter their gait because of a problem affecting one part of their foot or leg they may develop secondary compensatory problems elsewhere. It is essential that the practitioner identifies the original problem, as treatment for the secondary problem will not be successful until the initial problem is identified. Seasonal variation is not uncommon in vascular and joint pathology, and information on seasonal changes in symptoms should always be sought in chronic conditions.

What treatments have you tried? Are you treating it at the moment?

It is important to find out if the patient has or is presently using any medications. This should include prescription-only medicines, over-the-counter remedies and alternative medicines. Sometimes treatments can mask or alter the clinical features of a problem and make diagnosis difficult. For example, using 1% hydrocortisone cream for a fungal infection of the skin may mask the inflammatory response and blur the distinctive border between infected and non-infected areas. If the patient has seen another healthcare practitioner for the same problem, record any diagnosis or treatment received. Such information can help your own diagnostic assessment of the problem and avoid unnecessary duplication of treatment.

It is important that you record the information the patient gives you in response to all these questions. All critical events should be dated.

Dimensions of pain

Pain is a subjective, multidimensional phenomenon that can be affected by social and psychological factors. In the same way as individuals differ over what they perceive as a problem, individuals also differ when it comes to the assessment of their pain. Pain caused by apparently similar conditions affects individuals in very different ways. Practitioners should avoid making assumptions about the severity of pain an individual is experiencing. Patients vary in their abilities to cope with pain. Some are more than willing to complain about mild discomfort, whereas others make no complaint despite being in considerable pain.

Tolerance and coping strategies are subjective concepts that are difficult to quantify. A patient's state of mind and personal circumstances may make their pain worse or demand that they ignore it. For example, it is well known that runners may continue to run in a race despite having sustained an injury. Patients living with the constant pain of a chronic condition such as rheumatoid arthritis may express little concern for a problem that others without such a condition would find intolerable.

The assessment of pain requires information about its character, distribution, severity, duration, frequency and periodicity. This information, coupled with the history of the problem and details of the patient's concerns, helps the practitioner to arrive at the correct diagnosis and draw up an effective treatment plan.

Character

Pain can be superficial or deep. Pain arising in the skin often gives rise to a pricking sensation if brief or burning if protracted. Deep pain is more nebulous and is often associated with a dull ache. Patients may use a variety of adjectives to describe their pain (Box 3.4).

Distribution

Pain may be localised, diffuse or radiating. Initially, a problem may give rise to localised pain but as it becomes chronic and the disease process spreads, the pain can be felt over a wider area. Radiating pain can result from the extent of the disease or from pain being referred from one site to another; for example, a trapped spinal nerve can lead to pains in the leg (radiculopathy). Usually, referred pain does not get worse when direct pressure is applied to the site affected. However, if the pain has a localised cause it usually worsens when direct pressure is applied.

Box 3.4 Descriptors used for pain

- Burning
- Deep
- Aching
- Throbbing
- Sharp
- Intermittent
- Stabbing
- Shooting
- Bursting
- On touching
- On weightbearing

Severity

Certain conditions give rise to severe pain, e.g. myocardial infarction. However, a patient's ability to tolerate and cope with pain differs so much that a description of the severity of the pain must be assessed alongside the other features.

Duration

Pain may be fleeting or may be persistent. Ascertaining the duration of the pain can provide valuable information. For example, pain due to intermittent claudication may last a few minutes to half an hour. The pain associated with deep vein thrombosis is persistent. These differences can be helpful in differential diagnosis.

Frequency and periodicity

Some conditions lead to pain occurring in a regular pattern; others result in a less predictable pain pattern. It may be that the pain recurs infrequently or regularly. Again this can help in the diagnosis and gauging the severity or stage of the condition.

Techniques for assessing pain

Weir et al (1998) in a survey of podiatrists found that 53% did not assess their patient's foot pain. This is of concern, as the accurate assessment of pain is critical for the identification of suitable and effective interventions.

A range of techniques can be used to provide more objective information about the dimensions of pain experienced by a patient and its effect on the patient's quality of life. These are covered in detail in Chapter 4.

Numerical pain rating scales

Different dimensions such as severity, frequency and duration can be assessed. For example, patients may be asked to score the frequency of their pain using a 1–5 scale, where 1 signifies persistent, present all the time, and 5 indicates infrequent, occurring fewer than two times a week.

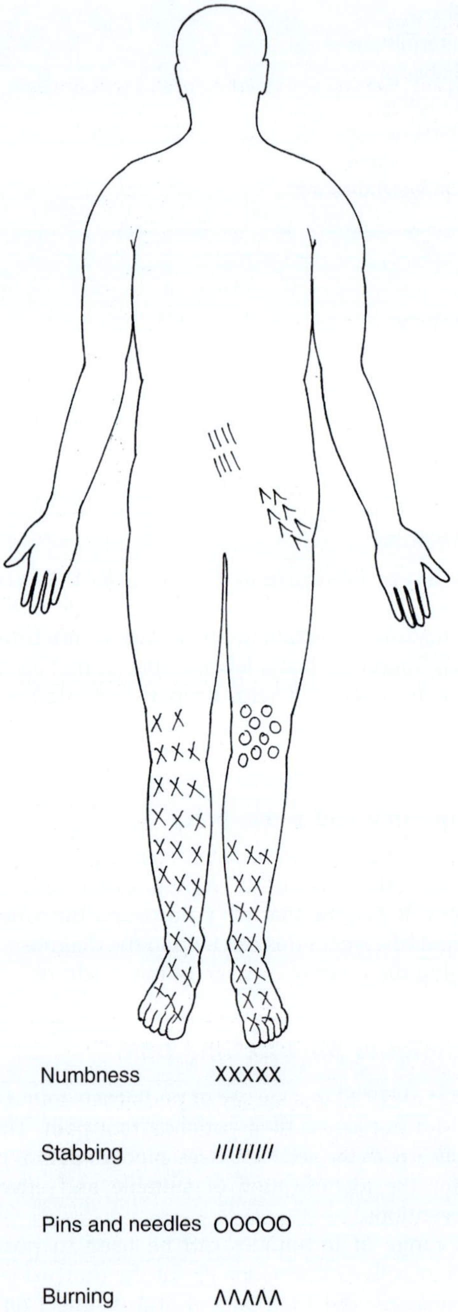

Figure 3.1 A pain chart.

Verbal descriptor scales

Descriptive scales can also be used. The following descriptors can assess severity: slight, quite a lot, very bad, agonising. Verbal descriptor scales (VDS) are reliant on the ability of patients to use words that best describe their pain. It is not possible to compare the descriptors used by individual patients.

Visual analogue scales

These scales can be used to assess the severity of pain. The technique involves asking the patient to indicate how severe their problem is and is more useful for acute than chronic conditions. It is a valuable method of determining before and after pain rates following an intervention.

Body-part questionnaires

These questionnaires usually relate to pain in a particular anatomical part, e.g. Boeckstyns (1987) developed a knee pain questionnaire.

Charts

Charts can be used for patients to indicate where the pain occurs and, by using different symbols, the type of pain that occurs (Fig. 3.1). Pain charts have been used as an aid to the psychological evaluation of patients with low back pain (Ransford et al 1976). This method should be used with great caution and with the assistance of a suitably qualified psychologist to prevent incorrect conclusions being reached.

Pain diary

It may be helpful, especially if a patient is not clear about the duration and frequency of the pain, to get them to keep a diary of the pain over a specific period of time. **Figure 3.2** illustrates a pain chart. The categories used in the chart were devised by the Pain Research Institute, Liverpool. While pain diaries can be helpful, they may lead patients to focus on their problem and could even exacerbate it.

The information gained from a patient presenting with a painful first metatarsophalangeal joint is shown in Table 3.1. The data used for this example suggest a diagnosis of gout. Laboratory tests and further assessments, i.e. medical and social history, may confirm this diagnosis.

Table 3.1 Information gained from assessment of a patient with a painful first metatarsophalangeal joint

The problem(s)	I've got a very painful big toe. I can't sleep at night for the pain.
The concern(s)	Do you think it is something serious? Will I have to have my foot off?
Where is the problem?	The big toe joint on my left foot.
How did it start?	The pain started one night. I woke up in a lot of pain. My toe was bright red and throbbing. The next day it was really swollen.
How long have you had the problem?	It started about a week ago.
When does it trouble you?	It hurts all the time, especially at night.
What makes it worse?	If I knock it at all and when I walk on it.
What makes it better?	The pain eases a bit when I take a painkiller but when the tablet wears off the pain is just as bad again.
What treatments have you tried? Are you treating it at the moment?	Just painkillers. I have been taking quite strong ones these last few days.

	Mon	Tues	Wed	Thur	Fri
6.00					
7.00					
8.00					
9.00					
10.00					
11.00					
12.00					
13.00					
14.00					
15.00					
16.00					
17.00					
18.00					
19.00					
20.00					
21.00					
22.00					

5 Excruciating

4 Very severe

3 Severe

2 Moderate

1 Just noticeable

0 No pain

S Sleeping

Figure 3.2 Pain diary.

Summary

It is essential that the practitioner acquires a clear and accurate understanding of the patient's concern(s) and problems in order to devise an effective management plan. These terms have been emphasised in different ways in this chapter, although 'problem' and 'concern' may be used synonymously elsewhere.

If the basic history part of the assessment concerning the presenting problem is inadequately dealt with or not undertaken the result of an inaccurate diagnosis occurring is all too clear to see. Some of these issues are emphasised in more detail in Chapter 5, which forms a prerequisite for systems analysis by functional enquiry and physical examination.

References

Boeckstyns M E H 1987 Development and construct validity of a knee pain questionnaire. Pain 31:47–52

Bygren L 2001 Egalitarian aspects of medical and social services. Journal of Public Health Policy 22(2):175–181

Galdas P, Cheater F, Marshall P 2005 Men and health seeking behaviour: literature review. Journal of Advance Nursing 49(6):616–623

Kessler D, Peters T, Lee L et al 2005 Social class and access to specialist palliative care services. Palliative Medicine 19(2):105–110

Ransford A O, Cairns D, Mooney V 1976 The pain drawing as an aid to the psychologic evaluation of patients with low-back pain. Spine 1(2:6):127–134

Rucker D, Brennan T, Burstin H 2001 Delay in seeking emergency care. Academic Emergency Medicine 8(2):163–169

Sandler G 1979 Costs of unnecessary tests. British Medical Journal 2:21–24

Sapira J 1989 Why perform a routine history and physical examination. Southern Medical Journal 82(3):364–365

Townsend P, Davidson N 1982 Inequalities in health: the Black Report. Penguin, Harmondsworth, 76–89

Weir E C, Burrow J G, Bell F 1998 Podiatrists and pain assessment – a cross sectional study. British Journal of Podiatry 1(4):128–133

CHAPTER 4

Health outcome assessment

K B Landorf, J Burns

Chapter contents

Introduction

Evaluation of the effect of treatment is an essential component of clinical practice. Such evaluations, or outcome assessments, range from simple measures like death (i.e. the patient is dead or alive) to more complex assessment relating to a broader, more holistic view of a person's life that includes physical, psychological and social issues. Assessments such as these allow clinicians to monitor the progress of a patient in response to advice or treatment. They also provide important objective information for the patient about whether their condition is improving or worsening. Equally important, however, is the role of outcome assessment in research evaluating health interventions (Spilker 1991) including clinical trials assessing treatments for musculoskeletal disorders (Keller et al 1993). Accordingly, health outcome assessment spans both clinical practice and clinical research, and is therefore an important issue about which both clinicians and researchers need to have a clear understanding.

Outcome measurement

Surrogate outcome measurement

Until relatively recently, clinician-based or laboratory measures (e.g. foot alignment or plantar pressure), referred to as *surrogate outcomes* (Guyatt & Rennie 2002), were often used to evaluate outcomes of treatment. Unfortunately, patients do not generally consider these surrogate measures important for understanding their health. Surrogate outcomes place little or no emphasis on an appraisal from the person being treated (Jenkinson & McGee 1998), whose only concern might be that they want their pain to reduce. Consequently, decisions regarding the effect of an intervention based on surrogate outcomes rely on the health professional's judgement, rather than on the patient's appraisal of their own health (Friedman et al 1998, Staquet et al 1999). Reasons for using surrogate outcomes include:

- they are usually easier to measure than a broader evaluation of an individual's health
- they often have the effect of decreasing sample size requirements in clinical trials.

To illustrate this issue further, a common example of a surrogate outcome from medicine is that of measuring tumour size as the primary outcome of success of a cancer treatment (Gebski et al 2002). Of course there would be a high likelihood that tumour size and progression of the disease are highly correlated. However, it is not necessarily the case that a decrease in tumour size correlates to a good therapeutic outcome from the patient's perspective. Indeed, adverse effects of treatment can have a negative impact on the individual's quality of life, both in the short and long term. This clinician-based focus is an historical problem in medicine and medical research where patient input had customarily been considered too subjective.

Bias towards clinician-based measures also exists in professions that care for foot and foot-related disorders, for example measuring arch height, frontal plane calcaneal position or plantar pressure distribution. Clearly, these surrogate outcomes have little meaning to the average patient who wants more relevant feedback about whether a prescribed treatment is working. Another key issue also needs to be considered when evaluating surrogate outcomes, particularly in relation to foot-related disorders. Because little is known about the actual relationship between these surrogate measures and a person's health status, it is unclear whether a change in, for example, foot alignment, correlates to an improvement in the patient's health status. Often, good-quality evidence that provides certainty about these links is not available. With this in mind, clinicians and researchers need to be careful when interpreting changes in these surrogate outcomes as being meaningful to the patient.

Due to the limitations of surrogate outcome measures, which tend to focus on disease, *health outcome* assessment has developed rapidly over the past two decades. Not surprisingly, health outcome assessment focuses more on the concept of what is important to the patient. The World Health Organization's definition of 'health' is that which is 'not merely the absence of disease or infirmity, but a state of complete physical, mental, and social well-being' (World Health Organization 1958). Clearly, this definition of health is more holistic and consumer-centred than clinician-based measures (Bowling 2005). However, in their early development, health outcome measures were created by clinicians, incorporating issues that they thought were important to patients. Whether these clinician-generated health outcome measures were, indeed, important to patients is an area of great conjecture. In the light of this, *health status* measurement has developed to include a broader account of 'health', which encompasses the patient's (or consumer's) perspective of their health (Jenkinson & McGee 1998). Put more simply, health status (and health-related quality of life) measurement attempts to evaluate what is important to patients, ideally from the patient's perspective.

Health status and quality-of-life measurement

With the aforementioned concerns about surrogate outcomes in mind, health status measurement has taken on increasing importance. Health status incorporates the notion of *health-related quality of life*, which is an important, and some would argue, fundamental measure of the impact of a disease or abnormality on an individual (Testa & Simonson 1996). Health-related quality of life characterises and measures what consumers experience as a result of healthcare (Staquet et al 1999). Emphasis is taken away from the disease process, while highlighting the broader appraisal of an individual's health by that individual (Muldoon et al 1998). Measurement of health-related quality of life is usually by self-report (i.e. self-reported questionnaire), although in paediatrics it can be acceptable to use a proxy (e.g. a parent/guardian). Health-related quality of life includes such areas as somatic sensation (e.g. pain), physical function, cognitive function and psychological well-being, social function and life satisfaction (Jenkinson & McGee 1998, Bowling 2005). A summary of health outcome terms used thus far in this chapter can be found in Table 4.1.

Measurement of health status and quality of life via self-reported questionnaire is a complex area that is developing rapidly (Scientific Advisory Committee of the Medical Outcomes Trust 2002). These questionnaires or instruments pose relevant questions relating to a person's quality of life. Each question or item is then scored individually or added together to produce a summary score. Scores can also be weighted to place more importance on certain sections of the instrument (Streiner & Norman 1995). In addition, many questionnaires group items together into like areas, known as *domains* or *subscales* (e.g. 'pain', 'function', 'vitality', etc.). Domains can also be scored individually or combined to give an overall numerical score of health and well-being, although this feature is not available for all instruments (McDowell 2006). Questionnaire development is a science of its own and rigorous methods should be employed to develop an instrument that will measure appropriately and accurately. Questions and their grouping into domains need to be developed using

Table 4.1 Terms used in health outcome assessment

Term	*Explanation*
Health outcome	A measurement that evaluates the health of an individual, in particular as a result of an intervention (Kane 1997). Can be a laboratory or clinician-generated measure, or one that is a subjective measure from the patient
Surrogate outcome	A proxy measurement that is generally known to be associated with a construct of interest (Herbert et al 2005). Tends to reflect 'disease', rather than 'ill-health' and its consequences (Bowling 2005). For example, a simple clinical or laboratory test may be used rather than a detailed assessment of subjective issues that are important to patients (e.g. health-related quality of life) (Guyatt & Rennie 2002)
Health status	A broad health construct that encompasses an individual's subjective perception of their health, including physical, psychological and social issues that impact on well-being (Jenkinson & McGee 1998, Bowling 2005). Sometimes used interchangeably with health-related quality of life. Provides a broader interpretation of an individual's health compared with a surrogate outcome
Health-related quality of life	A subjective measure of one's ability to perform usual tasks and their impact on one's everyday physical, emotional and social well-being (Fayers & Hays 2005, Jenkinson & McGee 1998). Sometimes used interchangeably with health status. Provides a broader interpretation of an individual's health compared with a surrogate outcome
Quality of life	A comprehensive measure of the quality of an individual's life. It incorporates, but is not limited to, health-related quality of life, and takes into account factors such as the environment that one lives in (Bowling 2005)

sound measurement principles, including item inclusion, psychometrics, validity and reliability testing (Streiner & Norman 1995). Appropriate development will ensure that instruments measure what they are supposed to measure and that they do so in a reproducible manner (Muldoon et al 1998).

Health status measures can be classified under two broad categories: (i) *generic* measures, which assess universal aspects of general health and well-being; and (ii) *specific* measures, which assess a specific medical condition or region of the body (Patrick & Deyo 1989). It is generally accepted that when measuring health status, both a generic and a specific measuring instrument should be used, as they measure distinct but complementary aspects of patients' health (Kantz et al 1992, Bombardier et al 1995, Hawker et al 1995). Generic instruments allow some commonality of measurement, and as such, comparison between different conditions (Patrick & Deyo 1989). However, due to their non-specific nature, they are generally less responsive to change compared with specific instruments (Patrick & Deyo 1989). Table 4.2 presents a summary of the categories discussed above.

Table 4.2 Categories of health status measures

Category	*Subcategory*	*What does it measure?*
Generic	None	Universal aspects of general health and well-being
Specific	Specific region of the body (e.g. foot) Specific medical condition (e.g. onychocryptosis) Specific population (e.g. with rheumatoid arthritis)	Health status relative to a region of the body or medical condition

Before discussing specific examples of health outcome measures in more detail, a brief look at the important issues of validity and reliability is needed.

Choosing an outcome measure: issues of validity and reliability

It is not the intention of this chapter to discuss in detail the concepts of validity and reliability. Readers are referred to many excellent texts if further detail is required (Bowling 2005, Bowling & Ebrahim 2005, McDowell 2006, Portney & Watkins 2008, Streiner & Norman 1995). However, some mention of the issues that relate to validity and reliability need to be covered – this is important when deciding whether to use an outcome measure in research or practice, or when evaluating the results of research that has used a particular outcome measure.

When measuring the outcome of an intervention, either for research purposes or in the clinical setting, it is necessary to ensure the outcome measure being used is appropriate (Boynton & Greenhalgh 2004). For health outcome measures, often self-reported questionnaires, to be 'appropriate' they need to be both valid and reliable. *Validity* refers to whether the outcome measure or the instrument measures what it is intended to measure (Portney & Watkins 2008). *Reliability* is the degree of consistency with which an outcome measure or an instrument measures a variable (Portney & Watkins 2008). When choosing an outcome measure the researcher or clinician should ensure it has been subjected to appropriate validity and reliability testing; that is, it has been proved through rigorous investigation to be both valid and reliable. Importantly, an instrument or questionnaire that has been shown to have good validity and reliability is confirmed to be of good quality and can be used with confidence (McDowell 2006).

Validity has a number of constructs, including: face validity, content validity, criterion validity and construct validity (Peat 2001). Briefly, *face validity* (also known as measurement validity) refers to the extent that an outcome measure measures what it is intended to measure. *Content validity* relates to the extent that the items included in an outcome measure cover the area being researched. *Criterion validity* refers to whether the outcome measure agrees with a gold standard (i.e. does it agree with another measure currently considered to be the best). *Construct validity* relates to whether the outcome measure agrees with other tests used for measuring the construct in question.

Reliability of an outcome measure refers to the consistency or repeatability of an instrument or questionnaire. That is, if the outcome measure was used multiple times on one patient would the same answer be arrived at, provided that the patient's health status did not change (Bowling 2005). Reliability encompasses both *test–retest reliability* (often measured via intraclass correlation coefficients (ICCs) and measurement error) as well as *internal consistency* (often measured via Cronbach's alpha) (Streiner & Norman 1995).

Issues relating to responsiveness to change (an instrument's ability to detect clinically important changes over time), floor and ceiling effects (where many patients achieve the lowest or highest score), and interpretability are also important (Terwee et al 2007). However, because of the complex nature of these issues they will not be covered in depth in this chapter, and the interested reader is referred to many excellent texts on this subject (Fayers & Hays 2005, McDowell 2006, Streiner & Norman 1995). Clearly, the aforementioned issues of validity and reliability are relatively complex, particular if one is new to the area of health outcome measurement. In such a case, the vast array of statistics associated with these issues can detract from a clinician or researcher wanting to take the plunge into health outcomes assessment. With this in mind, Suk and colleagues (Suk et al 2005) recommend the following checklist to assist in choosing (or even developing) an outcome measuring instrument for use in clinical practice or research:

1. Is the instrument internally consistent?
2. Is the instrument reproducible (reliable)?
3. Does the instrument demonstrate criterion validity?
4. Does the instrument demonstrate construct validity?
5. Does the instrument demonstrate content validity?
6. Does the instrument detect changes over time that matter to patients?
7. Will the instrument be deemed acceptable to patients?
8. Is this instrument feasible to administer clinically?

Ideally, an instrument should be able to satisfy each of the questions in the above checklist. In reality, some instruments will not satisfy this checklist, so if this is the case, then the most appropriate one should be chosen. If available instruments are simply not appropriate, or indeed none exist, development of a new instrument is warranted. However, many instruments already exist, so the indiscriminate development of a new instrument should be discouraged until it is absolutely clear that a new one is warranted.

In summary, it is important that outcome measures are appropriate and are of good quality. To achieve this, they need to be properly designed and validated. If an outcome measure has not been formerly validated, or alternatively, been found to be not valid, then it should not be used. Prior to applying an instrument in practice or research, detailed information should be gathered on the instrument's validity and reliability.

With the above in mind, this chapter will now return to discussion about the different categories of health outcome measures, including specific examples of commonly used instruments. First, the simple visual analogue scale, arguably the most commonly used outcome measure in clinical practice, will be reviewed. Second, clinician-based outcome measures will be briefly covered. Third, patient-reported outcome measures will be discussed in more detail. The focus of this section will be on foot-related outcome measures, although generic instruments will also be mentioned to provide a broader perspective of health status. Key resources for foot-related outcome measures will be provided to assist readers to further their knowledge if required.

Specific outcome measures

Visual analogue scale

Often clinicians and researchers want to assess a single (uni-dimensional) construct, such as pain, in as simple a manner as possible. One such method that is well accepted is the visual analogue scale (VAS). The VAS is a 100 mm straight line, which has at each end labels that define the extreme limits (i.e. range) of the sensation or response being measured (McDowell 2006). The line is most frequently presented horizontally on a page, but it can be presented vertically (Scott & Huskisson 1979b).

Although primarily used to measure pain, the VAS can be used to measure other constructs as well (e.g. anxiety, satisfaction, comfort). When used for the measurement of pain, the extreme left end of the scale (i.e. 0 mm) is labelled 'no pain' and the right end of the scale (i.e. 100 mm) is labelled 'pain as bad as it could be' (Huskisson 1974, Scott & Huskisson 1976). Alternatively, the labels 'worse pain imaginable' or 'agonising pain' can be used at the extreme right end of the scale (McDowell 2006). **Figure 4.1** shows a typical example of a VAS formatted for the measurement of pain.

The patient rates the degree of pain they are experiencing for the condition in question by marking a point on the 100 mm line that corresponds to their level of pain relative to the two extremes. The distance from the 0 mm point to the mark that the patient draws is then measured to determine the level of pain. VAS are relatively simple for clinicians to explain to patients and are easy for patients to use. In addition, they can be easily used by patients at home (i.e. away from the clinical setting) if ongoing assessment is required.

The VAS has been validated as a measure for the following types of pain: experimentally induced pain; pain intensity; unpleasantness of pain; and chronic clinical pain (Duncan et al 1989, Price et al 1983, Price & Harkins 1987). When used to measure pain, the VAS has also been shown to be reliable, with test–retest correlations ranging from 0.95 to 0.99 (Revill et al 1976). With respect to serial assessment of pain over longer periods of time (e.g. every month for a year), one study found that it is acceptable to show patients their initial scores (Scott & Huskisson 1979a). Caution is needed with non-literate patients where reliability, while still acceptable, is not as good as with literate patients (Ferraz et al 1990).

Clearly, the VAS has been extensively validated and been shown to be a reliable tool to measure pain, but how are the results obtained interpreted? For example, what scores on a VAS relate to mild, moderate or severe pain? One study pooled the findings of 11 randomised trials (1080 patients) that evaluated the effects of analgesia using VAS (Collins et al 1997). The results showed that patients who scored their pain as 'moderate' had a mean of 49 mm, with 85% of them scoring over 30 mm. Those reporting 'severe' pain had a mean of 75 mm, and 85% scored over 54 mm.

In addition, what amount of change in pain can be viewed as positive for the patient? Although this is a highly complex and contentious area, there has been some research on this issue. For example, one study found that a 33% decrease in postoperative pain represented a reasonable standard for determining a meaningful change from the patient's perspective (Jensen et al 2003). Another study established that

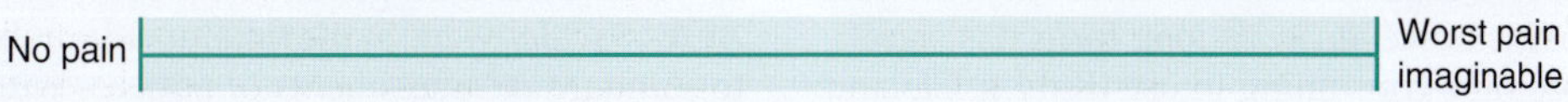

Figure 4.1 An example of a VAS used for measuring pain.

patients experiencing pain postoperatively of less than 40 mm on a VAS were 'adequately' satisfied, and the complete elimination of pain was not required for good patient satisfaction (Jensen et al 2005).

The issue of meaningful change has received some attention of late, with researchers attempting to determine what change in pain level is important to patients. More broadly, the amount of change required on any outcome measure – not just pain – to be considered important to a patient has been recently referred to as the 'minimal important difference' (Schunemann & Guyatt 2005), although it has also been referred to by many other terms including: minimal clinically important difference, clinically significant difference and meaningful change. Unfortunately, there are few examples of this type of research (i.e. calculation of the minimal important difference) in the foot and ankle literature. The literature on emergency medicine indicates the minimal important difference for the VAS ranges between 9 mm and 13 mm (Kelly 1998, Kelly 2001). That is, a change in pain of 9–13 mm on a VAS is, on average, considered important by patients. The minimal important difference is a valuable piece of information, not only when interpreting findings from instruments such as the VAS, but also for clinical trials, in which it can be used to assist in prospective sample size calculations.

Although the VAS is one of the most frequently used instruments to measure constructs such as pain, there are other methods such as the numerical rating scale, the verbal rating scale and the Oucher scale. The *numerical rating scale* is a simple mechanical device where the patient moves a slider and the numerical rating is read from the back of the device (McDowell 2006). Alternatively, the *verbal rating scale* can be used where the patient indicates their level of pain, for example, using the numbers 0–10. This simple and clinically useful method correlates well with the VAS (Murphy et al 1988). It has also been shown to have adequate validity and reliability (Jensen et al 1999). The *Oucher scale* is a pain scale that is specifically used for children between the ages of 3 and 12 years (Knott et al 1994). To indicate their level of pain, children can choose a face from a series of faces with varying expressions of pain.

Finally, more complex, multi-dimensional measures of pain have also been developed, and the McGill Pain Questionnaire (Melzack 1975) is one of the most well known. In contrast with the VAS, the McGill Pain Questionnaire measures beyond just pain intensity; however, in its long form it is significantly more time consuming to use (Kahl & Cleland 2005). Moreover, the newer health status measures also generally have a pain component embedded in them, making more complex pain measurements, such as the McGill Pain Questionnaire, somewhat redundant. If a specific component of pain is required to be measured in addition to the more generalised pain assessed in the newer health status measures, a simple VAS would probably be sufficient. For example, in a randomised trial evaluating low-Dye taping for plantar heel pain (Radford et al 2006), 'first step' pain – the pain experienced in the heel on first stepping out of bed in the morning – was measured using a VAS, as well as more generalised foot pain using a foot specific health status measure (the Foot Health Status Questionnaire, covered below).

In summary, the VAS is a highly useful and easy to use instrument to measure constructs such as pain. It has demonstrated good validity and reliability, and is a mainstay in clinical research where an assessment of pain is required. An easier method, the verbal rating scale is a satisfactory alternative in clinical practice. However, the VAS has some limitations, including its unidimensionality and the fact that it does not evaluate broader quality-of-life issues.

Clinician-based outcome measures

American Orthopaedic Foot and Ankle Society clinical rating scales

The American Orthopaedic Foot and Ankle Society (AOFAS) first reported on these scales in the medical literature in 1994 (Kitaoka et al 1994). Since this time, they have been widely adopted in orthopaedic foot and ankle research. The scales, or 'clinical rating systems', were generated by clinicians (i.e. members of the AOFAS) and hence, are clinician-based outcome measures. Four rating systems were originally developed: the Ankle-Hindfoot Scale; the Midfoot Scale; the Hallux Metatarsophalangeal-Interphalangeal Scale; and the Lesser Toe Metatarsophalangeal-Interphalangeal Scale.

Each scale contains a series of items, some of which are subjective (e.g. level of pain) and some objective (e.g. range of joint motion). Clearly, the 'objective' components of these scales are surrogate in nature. Points are given to each response for each of the items. For example, in the pain section: 40 points is given to no pain; 30 points to mild, occasional pain; 20 points to moderate, daily pain; and 0 points to severe, almost always present pain. Points are then added to generate a score of 0–100. The AOFAS scales were, at the time, an admirable attempt to standardise assessments of patients with foot and ankle disorders.

However, numerous studies have evaluated the validity and reliability of the AOFAS scales and have revealed important concerns. For example, one study found that the AOFAS scales correlated poorly with the extensively validated Medical Outcomes Study Short Form-36 (SF-36) (SooHoo et al 2006a). In this study of 91 participants, Pearson correlation coefficients ranged from 0.02 to 0.36 for the overall study sample. Correlations of this magnitude suggest poor construct validity of the scales. In addition, a small study of 25 participants showed that components of the SF-36, a generic outcome measure, had levels of responsiveness approaching that of the AOFAS and as such, the SF-36 could be used instead to monitor outcomes without loss of sensitivity (SooHoo et al 2006a). Further validity and reliability testing of the AOFAS Hallux Metatarsophalangeal-Interphalangeal Scale and Lesser Toe Metatarsophalangeal-Interphalangeal Scale was done in a small study of 11 people with rheumatoid arthritis (Baumhauer et al 2006). Although the scales were reliable, their validity was questionable with certain subscales correlating poorly with another foot-specific outcome measure, the well-validated Foot Function Index (FFI).

In addition, the agreement between prospective and retrospective AOFAS Hallux Scale assessments has been assessed. Poor agreement was found between prospective and retrospective evaluations of hallux surgery, indicating they could not be used interchangeably (i.e. a prospective assessment should not be compared with a retrospective assessment) (Schneider & Knahr 2005). Retrospectively acquired AOFAS data have also been shown to overestimate the benefit of surgery (Toolan et al 2001, Schneider & Knahr 2005). Accordingly, these studies highlight that prospective rather than retrospective study designs are preferable. Another study showed that population distributions of the AOFAS scales could be badly skewed; therefore the use of parametric statistical tests to analyse AOFAS scores should be viewed with great caution (Guyton 2001).

One recent study has reported validity of the AOFAS scales in a more positive light. This study compared the subjective component of the AOFAS scales with the Foot Function Index in an attempt to evaluate their criterion validity (Ibrahim et al 2007). The researchers found that AOFAS scales demonstrated moderate correlation (Pearson correlation coefficient = –0.68) suggesting acceptable criterion validity, although this component of the study had a small sample of 45. The study also attempted to evaluate test–retest reliability on 37 participants (8 of the original 45 participants dropped out). They reported no significant difference ($p = 0.27$) in the group mean AOFAS scores measured at baseline and then again after 2 weeks. However, this analysis did not use the more modern ICC approach, in which individual scores are correlated (i.e. true agreement), so these findings should be viewed with caution.

In summary, it seems that the AOFAS scales lack sound methodological construct, and as such, have questionable validity. This is supported by a recent publication by Suk and colleagues that extensively assessed and compared the AOFAS scales with other foot and ankle outcomes (Suk et al 2005). The AOFAS scales were rated highly for their ease of use (clinical utility), however, they were rated poorly for their methodological qualities. Clearly, although being widely used, the AOFAS scales (Clinical Rating Systems) require further development and validation. Accordingly, these instruments cannot currently be recommended for assessing outcomes relating to the foot and ankle.

American College of Foot and Ankle Surgeons scoring scale

The American College of Foot and Ankle Surgeons (ACFAS) developed a scale that is similar to the AOFAS scale discussed in the previous section. The ACFAS scale has four modules covering major areas of the foot and ankle, including: (i) the first metatarsophalangeal joint and first ray, (ii) the forefoot (excluding the first ray), (iii) the rearfoot (including flatfoot), and (iv) the ankle. Similar to the AOFAS scales, it attempts to combine some patient orientated measures, such as pain and appearance, with clinician-based assessments, such as radiographic and range-of-motion measures.

Although a 'user guide' was published in 2005 (Thomas et al 2005) and the first two of these modules were published in 2002 (Zlotoff et al 2002a, b), the ACFAS scale has been rightly criticised for not having been scientifically validated (Lavery & Armstrong 2006). Although the user guide states that the instrument was undergoing 'several tests to validate the design of this tool' (Thomas et al 2005, p. 316) no data have yet been presented to confirm its validity or reliability. Until adequate validity and reliability tests are done and appropriately reported, the use of this instrument is not recommended.

Patient-reported outcome measures: foot specific

Over the past decade, there has been a relative explosion of foot-specific outcome measures. The first properly validated questionnaire, the Foot Function Index, appeared in 1991 (Budiman-Mak et al 1991). Since then, many more have been reported and are used by clinicians and researchers. However, many have not been appropriately validated or used extensively. A discussion of all of these outcome measures would be exhaustive; therefore this section presents a detailed discussion of four foot-specific measures:

- American Academy of Orthopaedic Surgeons (AAOS) Foot and Ankle Questionnaire
- Foot Function Index (FFI)
- Foot Health Status Questionnaire (FHSQ)
- Manchester Foot Pain and Disability Index (MFPDI).

These questionnaires satisfy the following criteria:

- Easily accessible and well supported
- Well validated
- Have been used in clinical research.

Therefore the questionnaires discussed below are currently the best validated and most widely used measures of foot-specific health outcome assessment. Following the detailed discussion of these questionnaires is a list of further resources for those interested in more details. In addition, a list of other outcome measures is presented, including condition-specific outcome measures.

American Academy of Orthopaedic Surgeons Foot and Ankle Questionnaire

The AAOS has developed a series of musculoskeletal outcome measures that relate to different parts of the lower limb (American Academy of Orthopaedic Surgeons 2007). One of these instruments is the AAOS Foot and Ankle Questionnaire (American Academy of Orthopaedic Surgeons 2005), which has undergone relatively extensive validation. It has been tested for reliability, validity and sensitivity to change (Johanson et al 2004), and normative values from the general population have also been calculated (Hunsaker et al 2002). Validity testing was conducted on 290 patients with a broad range of foot problems. The AAOS Foot and Ankle Questionnaire demonstrates good internal consistency for most subscales (Cronbach's α ranging from 0.83 to 0.91), except for one subscale relating to stiffness and swelling (Cronbach's α 0.61). Test–retest reliability has been reported as good to excellent for all subscales (Pearson $r = 0.70–0.99$) (Johanson et al 2004). In an extensive comparison with other foot and ankle outcomes by Suk and colleagues (2005) the AAOS Foot and Ankle Questionnaire was given a high rating for its methodological qualities but only a moderate rating for its ease of use (clinical utility).

The AAOS Foot and Ankle Questionnaire has 20 items or questions that combined form the Foot and Ankle Core Scale and another five questions that form the Shoe Comfort Scale. The Core Scale can be further subdivided into four subscales: Pain (9 items), Function (6 items), Stiffness and Swelling (2 items) and Giving Way (3 items). A computerised spreadsheet for scoring is freely available on the AAOS website (American Academy of Orthopaedic Surgeons 2007). Patient scores are entered into this spreadsheet and the overall scores for each scale are automatically computed. **Figure 4.2** shows an example of the type of question presented in the AAOS Foot and Ankle Questionnaire.

There are few published reports of the AAOS Foot and Ankle Questionnaire being used in outcomes research. Thordarson et al (2005) investigated women undergoing hallux valgus surgery to ascertain age-adjusted baseline (i.e. pre-operative) data and compared these values with the normative data previously calculated by the AAOS (Hunsaker et al 2002). Another study used the questionnaire to evaluate health-related quality of life in patients with diabetes and foot ulcers (Evans & Pinzur 2005).

During the **past week**, please tell us about how painful your foot/ankle was during the following activities.
(Circle ONE response on each line, that best describes your average ability).

	Not painful	Mildly painful	Moderately painful	Very painful	Extremely painful	Could not do because of foot/ankle pain	Could not do for other reasons
Walking on uneven surfaces?	1	2	3	4	5	6	7

Figure 4.2 An example of a question used in the AAOS Foot and Ankle Questionnaire (taken from the Foot and Ankle Core Scale).

Despite the AAOS Foot and Ankle Questionnaire having undergone extensive validation testing, there are still some methodological concerns. For example, the original test–retest reliability was only done using Pearson's correlation coefficient, which unfortunately does not take into account systematic differences between the test and retest measurements (Terwee et al 2007). To address this concern, ICCs should be used to evaluate test–retest reliability. Newer validation techniques, such as the Rasch analysis (validation process using item response theory), would also be useful to ensure the questionnaire is robust from a construct point of view. Finally, there are currently no data on the amount of change required for the AAOS Foot and Ankle Questionnaire that is considered important (i.e. the Minimal Important Difference) to patients.

In summary, the AAOS Foot and Ankle Questionnaire appears to be a well-constructed outcome measure and has received reasonably extensive validity testing. It is readily available and the addition of an easily accessible scoring spreadsheet should make this instrument relatively easy to use. However, compared with other foot-specific questionnaires (e.g. FHSQ, FFI and MFPDI) it has had limited use in outcome studies and clinical trials. Therefore the AAOS Foot and Ankle Questionnaire is still somewhat untested. The questionnaire should also be further assessed using newer validation techniques (e.g. Rasch analysis) and should undergo further evaluation of test–retest reliability using ICCs.

Note: Further information about the AAOS Foot and Ankle Questionnaire can be obtained from the AAOS Lower Limb Outcome Instrument website (www.aaos.org/research/outcomes/outcomes_lower.asp) (American Academy of Orthopaedic Surgeons 2007).

Foot Function Index

The FFI was originally designed to measure the impact of foot pathology on function in terms of pain, disability and activity restriction in people with rheumatoid arthritis (Budiman-Mak et al 1991). During its initial validation it was examined for test–retest reliability, internal consistency, and construct and criterion validity. It demonstrated good test–retest reliability (ICCs ranging from 0.69 to 0.87) and a high degree of internal consistency (Cronbach's α ranging from 0.73 to 0.95). It has also been established that the original FFI has moderate to high levels of correlation with the SF-36, a commonly used generic health status measure (SooHoo et al 2006b). The pain subscale has also been shown to be a reliable side-to-side measure in orthopaedic intervention trials, where the foot that is not operated on serves as an internal control (Saag et al 1996). In the comparison with other foot and ankle outcomes by Suk and colleagues (2005) (mentioned above in the AAOS Foot and Ankle Questionnaire section) the original FFI was given a high rating for its methodological qualities but only a moderate rating for its ease of use (clinical utility).

The FFI was initially developed to assess the effect of foot orthoses on foot pathology in people with rheumatoid arthritis. However, its developers suggest its use need not be restricted to this group (Budiman-Mak et al 1995, Conrad et al 1996). The original FFI had three domains or subscales: Activity Limitation, Pain and Disability. Each domain contained a number of items or questions (five for Activity Limitation, nine for Pain, and nine for Disability) beside which respondents placed a mark representing their responses on a VAS. **Figure 4.3** provides an example from the *Pain* domain of the original FFI. The VAS ranged from the lowest end of the spectrum (e.g. 'No pain') to the highest end of the spectrum (e.g. 'Worst pain imaginable') and had corresponding verbal anchors at these extremes. If the respondent did not perform the activity in question, they ticked 'not applicable' (NA), which removed that question from the scoring.

HOW SEVERE WAS YOUR <u>FOOT</u> PAIN: NA

At its worst? ---- No pain —————— Worst pain imaginable —

Figure 4.3 An example of a question used in the original FFI (taken from the Pain domain).

After completion, each question was scored by measuring the mark placed by the respondent on the VAS, which was then assigned a score between 0 and 9 (i.e. 10 equal segments on the VAS). Once each question was scored, the scores were added and then divided by the number of applicable questions in that domain ('NA' questions were not scored and therefore did not enter into the equation). This was repeated for each domain and then an *overall* FFI could be computed by adding all of the domain scores and dividing by three (i.e. three domains). The scores for each domain ranged from 0 to 100, with 0 representing the best and 100 representing the worst possible scenarios. Similarly, the *overall* FFI score ranged from 0 to 100.

In its original form, the FFI was a relatively time-consuming and complex instrument. There were also some criticisms levelled at this version, particularly with the Activity Limitation domain and its use in individuals without significant activity limitation (Agel et al 2005, Landorf & Keenan 2002). In response to this, it was converted to a simpler five-point verbal rating scale version (the FFI-5pt) (Kuyvenhoven et al 2002). This version only consists of the Pain and Disability domains because the developers thought that the Activity Limitation domain was, on the whole, not applicable to their respondents (206 patients, 45 years of age or older with non-traumatic foot complaints). Basically, the VAS provided for each item in the original version was changed to a five-point verbal rating scale. In this form, it is easier to administer and code, thus making it less time-consuming to use. The FFI-5pt has been found to have the following characteristics: clinimetric properties similar to the original FFI; high internal consistency (Cronbach's α ranging from 0.88 to 0.94); good agreement with the original version (ICCs 0.64–0.79); and acceptable test–retest reliability (ICCs 0.70–0.83) (Kuyvenhoven et al 2002).

The FFI has subsequently been further revised – the FFI-R (Budiman-Mak et al 2006). The FFI-R has four subscales: Pain and Stiffness, Psychosocial, Disability, and Activity Limitation. Similar to the FFI-5pt, the FFI-R uses a Likert-type rating scale rather than the VAS system used in the original FFI. An example from the pain domain of the FFI-R is shown in **Figure 4.4**.

Now both short (34 items) and long (68 items) versions are available. A Rasch analysis (a more modern validation process using item response theory) of the FFI-R has also recently been conducted (Budiman-Mak et al 2006). This analysis found the FFI-R to have adequate construct validity with significant (but low) correlation ($r = 0.306$, $p = 0.018$) with 50-foot walk time. Further, it was found to be reliable (person reliability $r = 0.96$ and item reliability $r = 0.93$). The developers concluded that the FFI-R is a highly reliable instrument for assessing patients with foot problems ranging from low to high severity (Budiman-Mak et al 2006). However, further validity testing has been recommended by the developers on larger, more diverse samples. Finally, there are currently no data on the amount of change required for the FFI (both the original and revised versions) that is considered important (i.e. the Minimal Important Difference) to patients.

In summary, the FFI appears to be a highly useful instrument that has been well developed and validated. Although the revised version of the FFI (the FFI-R) has not yet been extensively used in clinical studies, the original FFI has been used across a range of pathologies, including investigations of Paget's disease (Williams et al 2006) and rheumatoid arthritis (Bal et al 2006, Conrad et al 1996, Kadambande et al 2007, van der Leeden et al 2006, Williams et al 2007, Woodburn et al 2002). The FFI has also been used in a relatively large number of outcome studies evaluating the effectiveness of interventions for foot problems, including tibial sesamoidectomy (Lee et al 2005), footwear (Williams et al 2007) and foot orthoses (Caselli et al 1997a,b, Conrad et al 1996, Gross et al 2002, Pfeffer et al 1999, Slattery & Tinley 2001, Woodburn et al 2002). The developers have made significant efforts to revise and validate the FFI, and further validation of the newer FFI-R will only strengthen this instrument as an appropriate outcome measure relating to foot problems.

Foot Health Status Questionnaire

The Foot Health Status Questionaire (FHSQ) was primarily developed to assess patients undergoing surgical treatment for common foot conditions; however, it was validated (content, criterion and construct validity) across a wide spectrum of pathologies including skin, nail and musculoskeletal disorders (Bennett et al 1998). It has a high test–retest reliability (ICCs ranging from 0.74 to 0.92) and high degree of internal consistency (Cronbach's α ranging from 0.85 to 0.88). Although it was originally designed with surgical outcomes in mind, it can be used to assess general foot conditions, such as skin conditions and musculoskeletal pain (Bennett et al 1998, Bennett & Patterson 1998). In the comparison with other foot and ankle outcomes by Suk and colleagues (2005) (mentioned previously in the AAOS Foot and Ankle Questionnaire section) the FHSQ was rated the highest in quality (methodological quality and clinical utility) of 25 foot and ankle outcome measures.

DURING THE PAST WEEK, HOW SEVERE WAS YOUR FOOT PAIN:

	No pain	Mild pain	Moderate pain	Severe pain	Very severe pain	Worst pain imaginable
At its worst?	1	2	3	4	5	6

Figure 4.4 An example of the style of question used in the FFI-R (taken from the Pain domain).

The FHSQ has four domains: Pain, Function, Footwear and General Foot Health. Each domain has a series of questions (four for Pain, four for Function, three for Footwear, and two for General Foot Health), and each question has a series of Likert scale-type responses (e.g. None, Very mild, Mild, Moderate, Severe). The respondent circles the most appropriate response (see **Figure 4.5** for an example from the Pain domain).

What level of foot pain have you had <u>during the past week?</u>

	(Circle number)
None	1
Very mild	2
Mild	3
Moderate	4
Severe	5

Figure 4.5 An example of a question used in the Foot Health Status Questionnaire (taken from the Pain domain).

The score for each question is then entered into a computer program (FHSQ, version 1.03), which then transforms the raw results and sums them into each domain. Like the FFI, the scores range from 0 to 100; however, 100 represents the best and 0 represents the worst scenario, the opposite to a VAS or the FFI.

There have been some criticisms of the FHSQ. Budiman-Mak and colleagues (2006) point out that it was validated on a relatively small sample (111 participants) and it is lacking in some areas of its theoretical development and validation. In addition, Landorf & Keenan (2002) reported that the General Foot Health domain may not be very discriminating between patients due to the limited number of questions (there are only two questions in this domain). There are currently no data on the amount of change required for the FHSQ that is considered important (i.e. the Minimal Important Difference) to patients.

Notwithstanding these concerns, the FHSQ seems to be a robust instrument to measure foot health status, and has now been used as an outcome measure in a number of published studies relating to a wide array of clinical problems. These studies include evaluations of: surgical interventions (Bennett et al 2001); foot orthoses for haemophilia (Slattery & Tinley 2001), painful pes cavus (Burns et al 2006) and plantar heel pain (Rome et al 2004, Landorf et al 2006); other conservative interventions for plantar heel pain (Radford et al 2006, 2007); and footwear for people with rheumatoid arthritis (Williams et al 2007).

In summary, the FHSQ has been widely used as a health status measure in outcome studies relating to foot problems. It has been well validated and is easy to use. The FHSQ has been used by clinicians in everyday practice and as an outcome measure in research, including assessments in which it was sent to participants via post to be completed at home (Landorf et al 2006). Accordingly, it is regarded as a useful health status measuring instrument for foot problems, and can be used with confidence. However, with the aforementioned criticisms in mind and with the knowledge that newer validation techniques exist (e.g. Rasch analysis), it requires ongoing validation.

Note: Further information about the FHSQ can be obtained from the Foot Health Status Questionnaire website (www.fhsq.homestead.com) (Bennett 2007).

Manchester Foot Pain and Disability Index (MFPDI)

The MFPDI is a self-administered questionnaire developed by Garrow and colleagues (2000) to assess foot pain and disability. It demonstrates good criterion validity when compared with similar items of the ambulation subscale of the Functional Limitation Profile Questionnaire and has excellent internal consistency (Cronbach's α 0.99). The initial validation was performed on 45 rheumatology patients, 33 patients attending their general practitioner for foot-related problems and 1000 responders to a population survey of foot disorders (Garrow et al 2000). Because the initial validation did not specifically target older people, further validation was carried out by Menz and co-workers (Menz et al 2006). In a sample of 108 community-dwelling older people with disabling foot pain, they found that the MFPDI had high internal consistency (Cronbach's α 0.89) and that its subscales were significantly associated with the SF-36 mental health subscale (r = 0.20, p = 0.039) and general health subscale (r = 0.21, p = 0.029). At this stage, however, the MFPDI seems to have not been assessed for test–retest reliability.

The MFPDI has four subscales associated with foot pain: ambulation, pain, personal appearance and difficulties experienced in performing work or leisure-related activities. There are a total of 19 questions or items in these four subscales. Each question is prefaced by the statement 'because of pain in my feet' and questions are answered relative to 'during the past month'. Respondents are asked to grade the severity of their foot problem by marking whether the disability associated with the problem is present 'none of the time' (scored 0), 'on some days' (scored 1) or 'on most or every day' (scored 2). The scores are then added up to generate total scores for each subscale and then these scores are expressed as a percentage. An example of the type of question presented in the MFPDI is shown in **Figure 4.6**.

random community sample, and Menz & Morris (2005) used it to investigate the association between foot problems and co-morbidities to the presence of disabling foot pain in retirement village residents.

In summary, the MFPDI has been used in an increasing number of studies. It has quickly gained a reputation for being a useful health status measuring instrument for foot problems. The MFPDI has the added advantage of being able to generate a simple case definition of disabling foot pain if individuals with this level of pain need to be targeted (e.g. in research). Because of the relative simplicity of the MFPDI, it seems to be particularly useful for larger projects and for postal surveys. It has undergone significant validation, although it appears that test–retest reliability still needs to be assessed. Further validation using newer validation techniques (e.g. Rasch analysis) would also be useful. Finally, there are currently no data on the amount of change required for the MFPDI that is considered important (i.e. the Minimal Important Difference) to patients.

	During the past month this has applied to me		
Because of pain in my feet:	None of the time	On some days	On most/ everyday(s)
I avoid walking outside at all			

Figure 4.6 An example of a question used in the MFPDI (taken from the Pain subscale).

The MFPDI is being or has been used in a number of studies, including: an evaluation of foot pain in individuals with Ehlers–Danlos syndrome (Berglund et al 2005); an investigation of pes planovalgus in rheumatoid arthritis (Turner et al 2003); a randomised trial evaluating the effectiveness of a patient self-management programme for basic footcare in older people (Waxman et al 2003); a large cross-sectional survey on a community sample in Cheshire, England (Garrow et al 2004); a study evaluating the epidemiology and management of osteoarthritis in older adults (Thomas et al 2004); and an investigation to determine the cause of foot pain in retirement village residents (Menz & Morris 2005). Its use as an outcome measure in clinical trials evaluating the effectiveness of interventions for foot problems is limited to date. Because of its simplicity and ease of use, however, it has mostly been used in larger investigations, such as mail-out surveys, and cross-sectional and predictive studies in older people.

An advantage of the MFPDI is that it can be used to define *disabling* foot pain in individuals participating in a study. Garrow and colleagues (2004) developed this classification for a large postal survey of 3417 individuals in England. The definition used in this study (i.e. the case definition of disabling foot pain) was that individuals were required to have had: foot pain in the past month and currently had pain, and that they marked at least one disability item on the MFPDI indicating that the disability was present at least 'some of the time'. This definition can, therefore, be used in studies where a classification needs to be made for those people with disabling foot pain. For example, Garrow and colleagues (2004) used this definition to assess the association of certain health problems to disabling foot pain in a large

A summary of the four foot-specific health status measures discussed above is presented in Table 4.3. Box 4.1 contains a list of useful resources for foot-specific health outcome measures. These resources cover both specific instruments and important issues relating to quality (e.g. methodological issues). The list is provided to assist readers that are either new to the health outcome area or simply want further information. In addition, less commonly used outcome measures will be discussed in some of these resources.

Patient-reported outcome measures relating to the feet: condition-specific

This section briefly discusses outcome measures that relate to either specific conditions where there is a high prevalence of feet being involved in the disease process (e.g. rheumatoid arthritis) or the condition directly affects the feet (e.g. hallux valgus). Many health status and quality-of-life instruments relate to specific populations or medical conditions. For

Table 4.3 Commonly used foot-specific health status measures

Outcome measure	*Applicability*	*Domains/subscales*	*Validity testing*	*Reliability testing*	*Concerns*
American Academy of Orthopaedic Surgeons (AAOS) Foot and Ankle Questionnaire	Applicable for musculoskeletal conditions of the foot and ankle	1. Global Foot and Ankle Scale (includes (i) Pain, (ii) Function, (iii) Stiffness and Swelling, and (iv) Giving Way) 2. Shoe Comfort Scale	Yes	Yes	At this stage, few published studies have used it and there has been little critical analysis. Should also undergo further validation (e.g. Rasch analysis and reliability testing (ICCs))
Foot Function Index (FFI)	Applicable for a broad spectrum of foot health issues. However, the original version was developed and validated on people with rheumatoid arthritis and the revised version (FFI-R) was validated on a sample of US war veterans. Has been used in clinical intervention trials	*Original FFI* 1. Activity Limitation 2. Pain 3. Disability (An overall FFI could also be computed by combining the above three domains) *Revised FFI (FFI-R)* 1. Pain and Stiffness 2. Psychological Stress 3. Disability 4. Activity Limitations	Yes	Yes	Initial version criticised because it had some scoring issues when used for people with less severe foot health issues. Should also undergo further validation on a broader sample
Foot Health Status Questionnaire (FHSQ)	Applicable for a broad spectrum of foot health issues. Has been used in clinical intervention trials	1. Pain 2. Function 3. Footwear 4. General Foot Health	Yes	Yes	General Foot Health domain may not adequately discriminate between individuals. Should also undergo further validation (e.g. Rasch analysis)
Manchester Foot Pain and Disability Index (MFPDI)	Applicable for a broad spectrum of foot health issues. Has been used successfully in large cross-sectional surveys and as an instrument to define disabling foot pain	1. Ambulation 2. Pain 3. Personal appearance 4. Difficulties experienced in performing work or leisure-related activities	Yes	No	Has not been used extensively in trials evaluating effectiveness of interventions. Should also undergo reliability testing and further validation (e.g. Rasch analysis)

example, health-related quality-of-life measures have been developed for rheumatoid arthritis (de Jong et al 1995) and ankylosing spondylitis (Doward et al 2003), both of which have a predilection for affecting the feet. Although these instruments do not relate explicitly to the foot, they can often be used to provide a broader picture of an individual's health status, similar to generic outcome measures.

Further, a growing number of condition-specific outcome measures that relate to foot problems are

Box 4.1 Useful resources relating to foot-specific health outcome measures

1. Martin R L, Irrgang J J 2007 A Survey of Self-reported Outcome Instruments for the Foot and Ankle. Journal of Orthopaedic and Sports Physical Therapy 37(2):72–84*†
2. Suk M, Hanson BP, Norvell D C et al 2005 AO Handbook – musculoskeletal outcome measures and instruments. Basel, Thieme*
3. Button G, Pinney S 2004 A meta-analysis of outcome rating scales in foot and ankle surgery: is there a valid, reliable, and responsive system? Foot & Ankle International 25(8):521–525†
4. Martin R L, Irrgang J J, Lalonde K A et al 2006 Current Concepts Review: Foot and Ankle Instruments. Foot & Ankle International 27(5):383–390†
5. Parker J, Nester C J, Long A F et al 2003 The problem with measuring patient perceptions of outcome with existing outcome measures in foot and ankle surgery. Foot & Ankle International 24(1):56–60‡
6. McDowell I 2006 Measuring health: a guide to rating scales and questionnaires, 3rd edn. Oxford, Oxford University Press‡
7. Terwee C B, Bot S D, de Boer M R et al 2007 Quality criteria were proposed for measurement properties of health status questionnaires. Journal of Clinical Epidemiology 60(1):34–42‡
8. Scientific Advisory Committee of the Medical Outcomes Trust 2002 Assessing health status and quality-of-life instruments: Attributes and review criteria. Quality of Life Research 11(3):193–205‡

*Key resource for choosing a foot-specific instrument.
†Resource that discusses many other foot-specific outcome measures not covered in this chapter.
‡Key resource for understanding methodological issues relating to health outcome measures.

becoming available. Helliwell and co-workers developed the Foot Impact Scale for Rheumatoid Arthritis, which has been well validated, including using Rasch analysis (Helliwell et al 2005). This instrument is highly specific to both a condition, rheumatoid arthritis, and a region, the foot. As such, it is likely to be very responsive to clinically meaningful changes in patients with involvement of the feet due to rheumatoid arthritis, although this component of the validation process still requires investigation. Two instruments have also been developed and validated to assess health-related quality of life in people with onychomycosis (Lubeck et al 1999, Potter et al 2006). Finally, Dawson and colleagues (2006) recently developed the Manchester-Oxford Foot Questionnaire (MOXFQ) to assess the outcomes of foot surgery, which they validated on patients undergoing hallux valgus surgery. This instrument has been found to be responsive to change and estimates of minimal clinically important differences have been calculated (Dawson et al 2007).

In summary, condition-specific outcome measures that relate to the feet are becoming increasingly available. The main reason for their development is that they are often more responsive to change (i.e. patient's foot health status changing over time) compared with generic outcome measures, or indeed instruments that concentrate on the foot more generally. Condition-specific instruments will most likely continue to be developed; however, caution is required to avoid multiple instruments being released that measure essentially the same constructs. A smaller number of well-validated instruments that have unique properties will be more beneficial than a large number with few differences. In future, researchers must carefully consider this point before embarking on developing yet another outcome measure.

Patient-reported outcome measures: generic

This section introduces readers to generic outcome measures. Because there are a number of well validated and widely used measures, only brief mention will be made of some of the more important generic health status instruments. With the earlier discussion relating to outcome measures in mind, it should be clear that foot problems, like other disorders of the human body, need to be evaluated in the broader context of health status. Accordingly, health status should be measured not only with specific health status instruments, but with generic measures as well. In the clinical setting, generic measures may be less important compared with foot-specific instruments; however, in research, it is widely accepted that it is essential to evaluate health status both with specific and generic measures. One of the main benefits of generic measures is that they allow comparison across conditions; something that, by definition, region- or condition-specific instruments cannot.

There are many generic instruments that measure health status, including the Sickness Impact Profile (Bergner et al 1976, Bergner et al 1981) and the Nottingham Health Profile (Hunt et al 1985), which were developed relatively early on in the history of the health-outcomes movement. More recently, health-related quality-of-life instruments have been developed using broader notions of health and its impact on an individual's quality of life. For example, one instrument that has received wide attention is the European Quality of Life Group's (EuroQoL's) EQ-5D (European Quality of Life Group 2007). The EQ-5D has been well validated and used for a vast array of conditions and interventions. Further, it has the added advantage of being able to generate a single index, which can be useful in cost-effectiveness studies. In addition to the EQ-5D, the World Health Organization Quality of Life (WHOQOL) instrument was developed to assess quality of life across different cultures (World Health Organization Australian Field Centre 2007, World Health Organization 2007). It is a well-developed instrument that has been extensively validated in many countries. It is culturally sensitive and can be used to compare quality-of-life issues between different countries.

However, by far the most commonly used instrument is the SF-36, developed during the Medical Outcomes Study (www.sf-36.org 2007). It has been extensively validated in many countries (including Australia, the UK and the USA) and against a variety of medical conditions, and is one of the most widely used instruments to measure health status (McHorney et al 1994, McHorney et al 1993, Tarlov et al 1989, Ware & Sherbourne 1992). The SF-36 has been used in research related to common musculoskeletal disorders, such as neck (Irnich et al 2001) and knee pain (Hinman et al 2003). It has also been specifically used in studies evaluating interventions for foot problems (Buchbinder et al 2002, Burns et al 2006, Davies et al 2000, Dawson et al 2006).

Summary

Health outcome assessment is an important component of clinical practice and health research. Surrogate and clinician-based outcome measures have traditionally been used to measure health problems. However, more recently, health-status assessment using patient-reported questionnaires has gained acceptance as a better method to assess the effect of a patient's health on their quality of life. Such assessment, using valid and reliable questionnaires, emphasises the manifestations of an illness from the consumer's perspective. Health status instruments fall into one of two categories, either generic or specific. It is generally recommended that both generic and specific instruments are used when measuring health outcomes, particularly in research. There are many generic instruments available; however, the SF-36 is one of the most commonly used in clinical trials. With respect to foot-specific health status measures, four instruments have acceptable validity, are readily available and are in use: AAOS Foot and Ankle Questionnaire, FFI, FHSQ and MFPDI. Due to relatively extensive validity testing on these instruments, they can be recommended as appropriate measures of foot-specific health status in clinical practice or research studies. In addition to these measures, the simple VAS can also be used, either in isolation to measure specific constructs, such as pain, or, more appropriately, as a complement to broader health status measurement. Finally, use of clinician-based outcome measures such as the AOFAS Clinical Rating Scales should be discouraged because of current validity concerns.

References

Agel J, Beskin J L, Brage M et al 2005 Reliability of the foot function index: a report of the AOFAS outcomes committee. Foot & Ankle International 26(11):962–967

American Academy of Orthopaedic Surgeons 2005 AAOS Foot and Ankle Questionnaire (version 2.0). Available at: www.aaos.org/research/outcomes/Foot_Ankle.pdf (accessed 23 April 2007)

American Academy of Orthopaedic Surgeons 2007 AAOS Lower Limb Questionnaires. Available at: www.aaos.org/research/outcomes/outcomes_lower.asp (accessed 23 April 2007)

Bal A, Aydog E, Aydog S T et al 2006 Foot deformities in rheumatoid arthritis and relevance of Foot Function Index. Clinical Rheumatology 25(5):671–675

Baumhauer J, Nawoczenski D A, DiGiovanni B F et al 2006 Reliability and validity of the American Orthopaedic Foot and Ankle Society Clinical Rating Scale: a pilot study for the hallux and lesser toes. Foot & Ankle International 27(12):1014–1019

Bennett P J 2007 The Foot Health Status Questionnaire. Available at: www.fhsq.homestead.com/ (accessed 9 April 2007)

Bennett P J, Patterson C 1998 The Foot Health Status Questionnaire (FHSQ): a new instrument for measuring outcomes of footcare. Australasian Journal of Podiatric Medicine 32(3):87–92

Bennett P J, Patterson C, Dunne M P 2001 Health-related quality of life following podiatric surgery. Journal of the American Podiatric Medical Association 91(4):164–173

Bennett P J, Patterson C, Wearing S et al 1998 Development and validation of a questionnaire designed to measure foot-health status. Journal of the American Podiatric Medical Association 88(9):419–428

Berglund B, Nordström G, Hagberg C et al 2005 Foot pain and disability in individuals with Ehlers–Danlos syndrome (EDS): Impact on daily life activities. Disability and Rehabilitation 27(4):164–169

Bergner M, Bobbitt R A, Carter W B et al 1981 The Sickness Impact Profile: development and final revision of a health status measure. Medical Care 19(8):787–805

Bergner M, Bobbitt R A, Pollard W E et al 1976 The Sickness Impact Profile: validation of a health status measure. Medical Care 14(1):57–67

Bombardier C, Melfi C A, Paul J et al 1995 Comparison of a generic and a disease-specific measure of pain and physical function after knee replacement surgery. Medical Care 33(4):AS131–144

Bowling A 2005 Measuring health: a review of quality of life measurement scales. Open University Press, Maidenhead

Bowling A, Ebrahim S 2005 Handbook of health research methods: investigation, measurement and analysis. Open University Press, Maidenhead

Boynton P M, Greenhalgh T 2004 Selecting, designing, and developing your questionnaire. British Medical Journal 328(7451):1312–1315

Buchbinder R, Ptasznik R, Gordon J et al 2002 Ultrasound-guided extracorporeal shock wave therapy for plantar fasciitis: a randomized controlled trial. Journal of the American Medical Association 288(11):1364–1372

Budiman-Mak E, Conrad K J, Roach K E 1991 The Foot Function Index: a measure of foot pain and disability. Journal of Clinical Epidemiology 44(6):561–570

Budiman-Mak E, Conrad K J, Roach K E et al 1995 Can foot orthoses prevent hallux valgus deformity in rheumatoid arthritis?: a randomised clinical trial. Journal of Clinical Rheumatology 1(6):313–321

Budiman-Mak E, Conrad K, Stuck R et al 2006 Theoretical model and Rasch analysis to develop a revised Foot Function Index. Foot & Ankle International 27(7):519–527

Burns J, Crosbie J, Ouvrier R et al 2006 Effective orthotic therapy for the painful cavus foot: a randomized controlled trial. Journal of the American Podiatric Medical Association 96(3):205–211

Caselli M A, Clark N, Lazarus S et al 1997a Evaluation of magnetic foil and PPT Insoles in the treatment of heel pain. Journal of the American Podiatric Medical Association 87(1):11–16

Caselli M A, Levitz S J, Clark N et al 1997b Comparison of viscoped and PORON for painful submetatarsal hyperkeratotic lesions. Journal of the American Podiatric Medical Association 87(1):6–10

Collins S L, Moore A, McQuay H J 1997 The Visual Analogue Pain Intensity Scale: what is moderate pain in millimetres? Pain 72:95–97

Conrad K J, Budiman-Mak E, Roach K E et al 1996 Impacts of foot orthoses on pain and disability in rheumatoid arthritics. Journal of Clinical Epidemiology 49(1):1–7

Davies S, Gibby O, Phillips C et al 2000 The health status of diabetic patients receiving orthotic therapy. Quality of Life Research 9:233–240

Dawson J, Coffey J, Doll H et al 2006 A patient-based questionnaire to assess outcomes of foot surgery: validation in the context of surgery for hallux valgus. Quality of Life Research 15(7):1211–1222

Dawson J, Doll H, Coffey J et al 2007 Responsiveness and minimally important change for the Manchester-Oxford Foot Questionnaire (MOXFQ) compared with AOFAS and SF-36 assessments following surgery for hallux valgus. Osteoarthritis and Cartilage 15(8):918–931

de Jong Z, van der Heijde D, McKenna S et al 1995 Development and validation of an R-A specific quality of life measure (RAQoL). Arthritis and Rheumatism 38(Suppl):S175

Doward L C, Spoorenberg A, Cook S A et al 2003 Development of ASQoL: a quality of life instrument specific to ankylosing spondylitis. Annals of Rheumatic Diseases 62(1):20–26

Duncan G H, Bushnall M C, Lavigne G J 1989 Comparison of verbal and Visual Analogue Scales for measuring the intensity and unpleasantness of experimental pain. Pain 37:295–303

European Quality of Life Group 2007 EQ-5D. Available at: at http://www.euroqol.org/ (accessed on 25 April 2007)

Evans A R, Pinzur M S 2005 Health-related quality of life of patients with diabetes and foot ulcers. Foot & Ankle International 26(1):32–37

Fayers P M, Hays R D 2005 Assessing quality of life in clinical trials. Oxford University Press, Oxford

Ferraz M B, Quaresma M R, Aquino L R et al 1990 Reliability of pain scales in the assessment of literate and illiterate patients with rheumatoid arthritis. Journal of Rheumatology 17(8):1022–1024

Friedman L M, Furberg C D, DeMets D L 1998 Fundamentals of clinical trials. Springer, New York

Garrow A P, Papageorgiou A C, Silman A J et al 2000 Development and validation of a questionnaire to assess disabling foot pain. Pain 85(1–2):107–113

Garrow A P, Silman A J, Macfarlane G J 2004 The Cheshire Foot Pain and Disability Survey: a population survey assessing prevalence and associations. Pain 110(1–2):378–384

Gebski V J, Marschner I, Keech A C 2002 Specifying objectives and outcomes in clinical trials. Medical Journal of Australia 176:491–492

Gross M T, Byers J M, Krafft J L et al 2002 The impact of custom semirigid foot orthotics on pain and disability for individuals with plantar fasciitis. Journal of Orthopaedic & Sports Physical Therapy 32(4):149–157

Guyatt G, Rennie D 2002 User's guide to the medical literature: essentials of evidenced-based medicine. American Medical Association, Chicago

Guyton G P 2001 Theoretical limitations of the AOFAS scoring systems: an analysis using Monte Carlo Modeling. Foot & Ankle International 22(10):779–787

Hawker G, Melfi C, Paul J et al 1995 Comparison of a generic (SF-36) and a disease specific (WOMAC) (Western Ontario and McMaster Universities Osteoarthritis Index) instrument in the measurement of outcomes after knee replacement surgery. Journal of Rheumatology 22(6):1193–1196

Helliwell P, Reay N, Gilworth G et al 2005 Development of a foot impact scale for rheumatoid arthritis. Arthritis & Rheumatism. 53(3):418–422

Herbert R, Jamtvedt G, Mead J et al 2005 Practical evidence-based physiotherapy. Elsevier, Edinburgh

Hinman R S et al 2003 Efficacy of knee tape in the management of osteoarthritis of the knee: blinded randomised controlled trial. British Medical Journal 327(7407):135–130

Hunsaker F G, Crossley K M, McConnell J et al 2002 The American Academy of Orthopaedic Surgeons Outcomes Instruments: normative values from the general population. Journal of Bone and Joint Surgery (Am) 84(2):208–215

Hunt S M, McEwen J, McKenna S P 1985 Measuring health status: a new tool for clinicians and epidemiologists. Journal of the Royal College of General Practitioners 35:185–188

Huskisson E C 1974 Measurement of pain. The Lancet 2:1127–1131

Ibrahim T, Beiri A, Azzabi M et al 2007 Reliability and validity of the subjective component of the American Orthopaedic Foot and Ankle Society Clinical Rating Scales. Journal of Foot and Ankle Surgery 46(2):65–74

Irnich D, Behrens N, Molzen H et al 2001 Randomised trial of acupuncture compared with conventional massage and 'sham' laser acupuncture for treatment of chronic neck pain. British Medical Journal 322(7302):1574–1579

Jenkinson C, McGee H 1998 Health status measurement – a brief but critical introduction. Radcliffe Medical Press, Oxford

Jensen M P, Chen C, Brugger A M 2003 Interpretation of Visual Analog Scale ratings and change scores: a reanalysis of two clinical trails of postoperative pain. Journal of Pain 4(7):407–414

Jensen M P, Martin S A, Cheung R 2005 The meaning of pain relief in a clinical trail. Journal of Pain 6(6):400–406

Jensen M P, Turner J A, Romano J M et al 1999 Comparative reliability and validity of chronic pain measures. Pain 83:157–162

Johanson N A, Liang M H, Daltroy L et al 2004 American academy of orthopaedic surgeons lower limb outcomes assessment instruments. Reliability, validity, and sensitivity to change. Journal of Bone and Joint Surgery (Am) 86(5):902–909

Kadambande S, Debnath U, Khurana A et al 2007 Rheumatoid forefoot reconstruction: 1st metatarsophalangeal fusion and excision arthroplasty of lesser metatarsal heads. Acta Orthopaedica Belgica 73(1):88–95

Kahl C, Cleland J A 2005 Visual Analogue Scale, Numeric Pain Rating Scale and the McGill Pain Questionnaire: an overview of psychometric properties. Physical Therapy Reviews 10:123–128

Kane R L 1997 Understanding health care outcomes research. Jones and Bartlett Publishers, Boston

Kantz M E, Harris W J, Levitsky K et al 1992 Methods for assessing condition-specific and generic functional status outcomes after total knee replacement. Medical Care 30(5 Suppl):MS240–252

Keller R B, Rudicel S A, Liang M H 1993 Outcomes research in orthopaedics. Journal of Bone and Joint Surgery 75-A(10):1562–1574

Kelly A-M 1998 Does the clinically significant difference in Visual Analogue Scale Pain scores vary with gender, age, or cause of pain? Academic Emergency Medicine 5(11):1086–1090

Kelly A-M 2001 The minimum clinically significant difference in Visual Analogue Scale Pain score does not differ with severity of pain. Emergency Medicine Journal 18(3):205–207

Kitaoka H B, Alexander I J, Adelaar R S et al 1994 Clinical rating systems for the ankle-hindfoot, midfoot, hallux, and lesser toes. Foot & Ankle International 15(7):349–353

Knott C, Beyer J, Villarruel A et al 1994 Using the OUCHER: developmental approach to pain assessment in children. MCN. American Journal of Maternal Child Nursing 19:314–320

Kuyvenhoven M M et al 2002 The Foot Function Index with verbal rating scales (FFI-5pt): a clinimetric evaluation and comparison with original FFI. Journal of Rheumatology 29(5):1023–1028

Landorf K B, Keenan A-M 2002 An evaluation of two foot-specific, health-related quality-of-life measuring instruments. Foot & Ankle International 23(6):538–546

Landorf K B, Keenan A-M, Herbert R D 2006 Effectiveness of foot orthoses to treat plantar fasciitis: a randomized trial. Archives of Internal Medicine 166(12):1305–1310

Lavery L, Armstrong 2006 ACFAS scoring scale: ready, fire, aim? Journal of Foot and Ankle Surgery 45(4):284–285

Lee S, Gorter K J, Zuithoff P et al 2005 Evaluation of hallux alignment and functional outcome after isolated tibial sesamoidectomy. Foot & Ankle International 26(10):803–809

Lubeck D P, Gause D, Schein J R et al 1999 A health-related quality of life measure for use in patients with onychomycosis: a validation study. Quality of Life Research 8(1–2):121–129

McDowell I 2006 Measuring health: a guide to rating scales and questionnaires. Oxford University Press, Oxford

McHorney C A, Ware J E Jr, Lu J F et al 1994 The MOS 36-item short-form health survey (SF-36): III. Tests of data quality, scaling assumptions, and reliability across diverse patient groups. Medical Care 32(1):40–66

McHorney C A, Ware J E, Jr. Raczek A E 1993 The MOS 36-item short-form health survey (SF-36): II. Psychometric and clinical tests of validity in measuring physical and mental health constructs. Medical Care 31(3):247–263

Melzack R 1975 The McGill Pain Questionnaire: major properties and scoring methods. Pain 1:277–299

Menz H B Morris M E 2005 Determinants of disabling foot pain in retirement village residents. Journal of the American Podiatric Medical Association 95(6):573–579

Menz H B, Tiedemann A, Kwan M M S et al 2006 Foot pain in community-dwelling older people: an evaluation of the Manchester foot pain and disability index. Rheumatology 45(7):863–867

Muldoon M F, Tiedemann A, Kwan M M et al 1998 What are quality of life measurements measuring? British Medical Journal 316:542–545

Murphy D F, McDonald A, Power C et al 1988 Measurement of pain: a comparison of the Visual Analogue with a Nonvisual Analogue Scale. Clinical Journal of Pain 3(4):197–199

Patrick D L, Deyo R A 1989 Generic and disease-specific measures in assessing health status and quality of life. Medical Care 27(3):S217-S232

Peat J K 2001 Health science research: a handbook of quantitative methods. Allen & Unwin, Crows Nest, NSW

Pfeffer G et al 1999 Comparison of custom and prefabricated orthoses in the initial treatment of proximal plantar fasciitis. Foot & Ankle International 20(4):214–221

Portney L G, Watkins M P 2008 Foundations of clinical research: applications to practice. Peason Prentice Hall, Upper Saddle River, NJ

Potter L, Bacchetti P, Deland J et al 2006 The OnyCOE-t questionnaire: responsiveness and clinical meaningfulness of a patient-reported outcomes questionnaire for toenail onychomycosis. Health and Quality of Life Outcomes 4(1):50

Price D D, Harkins S W 1987 Combined use of experimental pain and Visual Analogue Scales in providing standardized measurement of clinical pain. Clinical Journal of Pain 3(1):1–8

Price D D, McGrath P A, Rafii A et al 1983 The validation of Visual Analogue Scales as ratio scale measures for chronic and experimental pain. Pain 17:45–56

Radford J A, Landorf K B, Buchbinder R et al 2006 Effectiveness of low-Dye taping for the short-term treatment of plantar heel pain: a randomised trial. BMC Musculoskeletal Disorders 7:64

Radford J A, Landorf K B, Buchbinder R et al 2007 Effectiveness of calf muscle stretching for the short-term treatment of plantar heel pain: a randomised trial. BMC Musculoskeletal Disorders 8:36

Revill S I, Robinson J O, Rosen M et al 1976 The reliability of a linear analogue for evaluating pain. Anaesthesia 31:1191–1198

Rome K, Gray J, Stewart F et al 2004 Evaluating the clinical effectiveness and cost-effectiveness of foot orthoses in the treatment of plantar heel pain: a feasibility study. Journal of the American Podiatric Medical Association 94(3):229–238

Saag K G, Saltzman C L, Brown C K et al 1996 The Foot function index for measuring rheumatoid arthritis pain: evaluating side-to-side reliability. Foot & Ankle International 17(8):506–510

Schneider W, Knahr K 2005 Poor agreement between prospective and retrospective assessment of hallux surgery using the AOFAS hallux scale. Foot & Ankle International 26(12):1062–1066

Schunemann H J, Guyatt G H 2005 Commentary – goodbye M(C)ID! HELLO MID, where do you come from? Health Services Research 40(2):593–597

Scientific Advisory Committee of the Medical Outcomes Trust 2002 Assessing health status and quality-of-life instruments: attributes and review criteria. Quality of Life Research 11(3):193–205

Scott J, Huskisson E C 1976 Graphic representation of pain. Pain 2:175–184

Scott J, Huskisson E C 1979a Accuracy of subjective measurement made with or without previous scores: an important course of error in serial measurement of subjective states. Annals of Rheumatic Diseases 38:558–559

Scott J, Huskisson E C 1979b Vertical or horizontal visual analogue scales. Annals of Rheumatic Diseases 38:560

SF-36.org 2007 SF-36. Available at: www.sf-36.org/ (accessed 28 April 2007)

Slattery M, Tinley P 2001 The efficacy of functional foot orthoses in the control of pain in ankle joint disintegration in hemophilia. Journal of the American Podiatric Medical Association 91(5):240–244

SooHoo N, Vyas R, Samimi D 2006a Responsiveness of the foot function index, AOFAS clinical rating systems, and SF-36 after foot and ankle surgery. Foot & Ankle International 27(11):930–934

SooHoo N F, Samimi D B, Vyas R M et al 2006b Evaluation of the validity of the foot function index in measuring outcomes in patients with foot and ankle disorders. Foot & Ankle International 27(1):38–42

Spilker B 1991 Guide to clinical trials. Raven Press, New York

Staquet M J, Hays R D, Fayers P M 1999 Quality of life assessment in clinical trials. Oxford University Press, Oxford

Streiner D L, Norman G R 1995 Health measurement scales: a practical guide to their development and use. Oxford University Press, Oxford

Suk M, Hanson B P, Norvell D C et al 2005 AO Handbook – musculoskeletal outcome measures and instruments. Thieme, Basel

Tarlov A R, Ware J E Jr, Greenfield S et al 1989 The medical outcomes study: an application of methods for monitoring the results of medical care. Journal of American Medical Association 262(7):925–930

Terwee C B, Bot S D, de Boer M R et al 2007 Quality criteria were proposed for measurement properties of health status questionnaires. Journal of Clinical Epidemiology 60(1):34–42

Testa M A, Simonson D C 1996 Assessment of quality-of-life outcomes. New England Journal of Medicine 334(13):835–840

Thomas E, Wilkie R, Peat G et al 2004 The North Staffordshire Osteoarthritis Project – NorStOP: prospective, 3-year study of the epidemiology and management of clinical osteoarthritis in a general population of older adults. BMC Musculoskeletal Disorders 5(1):2

Thomas J L, Christensen J C, Mendicino R W; American College of Foot and Ankle Surgeons (ACFAS) et al 2005 ACFAS scoring scale user guide. Journal of Foot and Ankle Surgery 44(5):316–335

Thordarson D B, Ebramzadeh E, Rudicel S A et al 2005 Age-adjusted baseline data for women with hallux valgus undergoing corrective surgery. Journal of Bone and Joint Surgery (Am) 87(1):66–75

Toolan B C, Wright Quinones V J, Cunningham B J et al 2001 An evaluation of the use of retrospectively acquired preoperative AOFAS clinical rating scores to assess surgical outcome after elective foot and ankle surgery. Foot & Ankle International 22(10):775–778

Turner D E, Woodburn J, Helliwell P S et al 2003 Pes planovalgus in RA: a descriptive and analytical study of foot function determined by gait analysis. Musculoskeletal Care 1(1):21–33

van der Leeden M, Steultjens M, Dekker J H et al 2006 Forefoot joint damage, pain and disability in rheumatoid arthritis patients with foot complaints: the role of plantar pressure and gait characteristics. Rheumatology 45(4):465–469

Ware J E, Sherbourne C D 1992 The MOS 36-item short-form health survey (SF-36). I. Conceptual framework and item selection. Medical Care 30(6):473–483

Waxman R, Woodburn H, Powell M et al 2003 FOOTSTEP: a randomized controlled trial investigating the clinical and cost effectiveness of a patient self-management program for basic foot care in the elderly. Journal of Clinical Epidemiology 56(11):1092–1099

Williams A E, O'Neill T W, Mercer S et al 2006 Foot pathology in patients with Paget's disease of bone. Journal of the American Podiatric Medical Association 96(3):226–231

Williams A E, Rome K, Nester C J 2007 A clinical trial of specialist footwear for patients with rheumatoid arthritis. Rheumatology 46(2):302–307

Woodburn J, Barker S, Helliwell P S 2002 A randomized controlled trial of foot orthoses in rheumatoid arthritis. Journal of Rheumatology 29(7):1377–1383

World Health Organization Australian Field Centre 2007 WHOQOL. Available at: www.psychiatry.unimelb.edu.au/qol/whoqol/index.html (accessed 25 April 2007)

World Health Organization 1958 The first ten years of the World Health Organization. WHO, Geneva

World Health Organization 2007 WHOQOL. Available at: www.who.int/substance_abuse/research_tools/whoqolbref/en/ (accessed 25 April 2007)

Zlotoff H J, Christensen J C, Mendicino R W et al 2002a ACFAS universal foot and ankle scoring system: forefoot (module 2). Journal of Foot and Ankle Surgery 41(2):109–111

Zlotoff H J, Christensen J C, Mendicino R W et al 2002b ACFAS universal foot and ankle scoring system: first metatarsophalangeal joint and first ray (module 1). Journal of Foot and Ankle Surgery 41(1):2–5

Part 2

Systems examination

CHAPTER

5

The medical and social history

I Reilly

Chapter contents

Introduction

Conditions affecting the lower limb may be caused by, or have ramifications for, the patient's general health and well-being. The clinician must therefore be aware of the patient's medical and social history as they may have implications for the diagnosis and management of lower limb problems. Taking a history is a highly skilled exercise and one that requires practice to achieve and maintain competency. Information gleaned from a skilled enquiry is the first step towards making the correct diagnosis, directing further investigations and facilitating the formulation of an appropriate treatment plan. A properly taken medical and social history is concerned with the patient as a whole and not just the lower limb complaint with which the patient has presented. The approach outlined in this chapter forms the basis of a holistic approach to patient care.

Purpose of the medical and social history

History taking is as important as any diagnostic test or physical examination. It is the least expensive of all investigations and time spent on obtaining a thorough history is rarely wasted. Diseases or abnormalities of the lower limb often present with a history of signs and symptoms which will allow the practitioner to make a provisional diagnosis. Once a history has been taken, physical examination and diagnostic tests can then be used to confirm the diagnosis and stage the severity of the condition. A comprehensive history taking therefore initiates the diagnostic process and helps the practitioner to formulate and implement an effective management plan.

An inadequate history of the patient's health status may have the following consequences:

1. The patient is placed at risk.
   With an inadequate knowledge of the patient's medical history, inappropriate or unsafe treatment may be provided. The actual risk of causing a bacteraemia in a patient with a prosthetic joint (which could infect and then loosen the joint) by performing nail surgery remains unquantified but a theoretical risk certainly exists. Bacteraemia in patients with a history of endocarditis or rheumatic valvular disease may lead to bacterial growth on the previously damaged heart valves or endocardium. Inadequate knowledge of the

patient's existing medication could lead to adverse inter-drug reactions with newly prescribed treatment. If drugs are prescribed (or omitted) in the absence of a detailed medical history, an existing condition may be exacerbated. For example, aspirin and non-steroidal anti-inflammatory drugs (NSAIDs) may precipitate asthma attacks.

2. The practitioner is placed at risk.
Inadequate history taking may place the practitioner at risk when handling tissue fluids or products. A history of jaundice should alert the practitioner to the possibility of hepatitis, whereas a history of haemophilia, blood transfusion, foreign travel or intravenous drug use may place the patient – and thus the practitioner – at risk from a blood-borne infection.

3. Poor treatment outcomes.
Treatment may fail or cause the patient's presenting condition to worsen because inadequate history taking has prevented accurate diagnosis of the presenting foot complaint. For example, pain and swelling in the calf of a 39-year-old woman, which develops after sport, may be nothing more than local oedema or muscle strain. But if the practitioner finds there is also a history of cigarette smoking, use of the contraceptive pill and recent immobilisation, the differential diagnosis would include deep vein thrombosis, a potentially life-threatening condition that requires quite different management to a pulled muscle.

4. An increased risk of clinical emergencies.
Individuals may be placed at risk by certain treatments, drugs or procedures that are usually considered routine. Adequate history taking will identify those patients who have previously developed adverse reactions. Poor history taking may result in a request for an inappropriate antibiotic prescription from a general practitioner for a patient who is sensitive to penicillin. Hypersensitivity reactions to medicaments (e.g. iodine allergy) or dressings (e.g. zinc oxide strapping) may be known to the patient and should be noted because of the risk of anaphylaxis.

All these factors have implications for cost and litigation.

Format of the medical and social history enquiry

A systematic approach to history taking will ensure that the practitioner covers all relevant areas in the enquiry process. The medical history and systems enquiry presented is based on the hospital assessment or clinical clerking system. Findings recorded with this system (Box 5.1) will determine the need for further clinical or laboratory investigation and indicate the patient's suitability for a range of treatments.

Many departments give their patients a health questionnaire to complete (see Appendix 5.1). This can be sent to the patient before the initial visit or, more commonly, before they see the practitioner again. The use of questionnaires gives patients time to consider their answers and reduces the time spent in taking a medical history during the consultation.

Box 5.1 The medical history and systems enquiry

Part 1. Medical history

- Current health status
- Past and current medication
- Past medical history

Part 2. Family history

Part 3. Personal social history

- Home circumstances
- Occupation
- Sports and hobbies
- Foreign travel

Part 4. The systems enquiry (CRAGCEL)

- Cardiovascular system
- Respiratory system
- Alimentary system
- Genitourinary system
- Central nervous system
- Endocrine system
- Locomotor system

Medical history

Current health status

Before history taking begins, the practitioner will gain some impressions about the patient's current health status from simple observation. Patients should be observed from the moment they enter the consulting room. Diseases of nerves, muscle, bone and joints may be manifested by a patient's gait or posture. For example, upper and lower motor neurone lesions may cause an ataxic gait, in which coordination and balance are impaired. Patients with acute foot or leg pain will walk with a limp as they try to 'guard' the injured part. Patients with chronic foot disorders may shuffle rather than stride because a propulsive gait could cause more pain. Gait disorders in children are best visualised as the child walks into the room to meet the practitioner; children often become self-conscious when asked to walk on demand.

The consultation should begin with a handshake as considerable information can be gleaned from this simple contact. Wasting of the thenar eminence and intrinsic musculature of the hand occurs with rheumatoid arthritis and with some genetic disorders such as Friedreich's ataxia and Charcot–Marie–Tooth disease. Disorders of skin and nails may manifest themselves in the hand: for example, psoriasis and eczema may cause hypertrophy and anhydrosis of the skin; pulmonary or cyanotic heart disease may cause clubbed or hippocratic nails.

The patient's facial appearance and expression is also of interest to the practitioner. The tense tired face of those in chronic pain will appear similar to those suffering from depression. Parkinson's disease or long-term use of psychotropic drugs reduce facial expressions, whereas the thyrotoxic patient, with characteristic protruding eyes, will be striking for their 'angry' appearance. Patients on long-term steroid therapy can develop a 'moon' face. Hypothyroidism will lead to a loss of hair from the outer third of the eyebrows, baldness, and coarse, thickened facial skin. Acromegaly, in which there is an excess of growth hormone production due to a disorder of the pituitary gland, will give rise to a heavy 'lantern' jaw. Cyanotic blue lips are a sign of poor cardiac function. Small plaques of brown lipid under the eyes, seen in hyperlipidaemia, are associated with atherosclerosis.

Weight abnormalities affect the lower limb and should be noted on the first meeting with the patient. Obesity is associated with recalcitrant heel pain and other postural symptoms. Seriously underweight patients may have a range of systemic conditions or they could be poorly nourished due to alcoholism, drug misuse or anorexia nervosa. Fatigue and weight changes are symptoms of many systemic illnesses and are always worthy of note, especially if weight change seems to be rapid.

The following questions will reveal important information about the patient's general health:

- Are you feeling well?
- Are you under the doctor or consultant for any treatment currently?
- Do you sleep well at night?
- Do you feel tired during the day?
- Is your weight stable?

For women:

- Could you be pregnant?

In general, patients who are unwell are not good candidates for invasive procedures or treatments that are likely to demand close compliance on their behalf.

Past and current medication

Information about the patient's previous and current drug therapy can provide useful information about the patient's health. Patients should be asked if they are currently taking, or have taken in the past, any tablets or other medicines, or if they are using or have used any ointments or creams prescribed by their doctor. It is not uncommon for patients to have taken prescribed drugs for many years with no clear understanding about why they are/were taking them. Refer to the *British National Formulary* (BNF) or another pharmacological text if you are unfamiliar with any drugs that the patient is taking.

Large doses or prolonged use of certain medications can be associated with significant adverse drug reactions with relevance to the lower limb. Most drugs produce several effects, but the prescriber usually wants a patient to experience only one (or a few) of them; the other effects may be regarded as undesired. Although most people use the term 'side effect', the term 'adverse drug reaction' is more appropriate for effects that are undesired, unpleasant, noxious or potentially harmful. For example, prednisolone, commonly used in the treatment of rheumatoid arthritis, can reduce skin thickness and impair wound healing. Bendroflumethiazide, a useful diuretic for the treatment of cardiac failure or hypertension, can cause hyperuricaemia, which may result in gout-like symptoms. Warfarin, an oral anticoagulant used for the treatment and prophylaxis of venous thrombosis and pulmonary embolism, increases clotting time and has obvious implications if surgical treatment is planned. Other examples of adverse drug reactions are listed in Table 5.1.

Patients should also be asked if they are currently taking or have taken in the past any tablets or medicine or used any ointments or creams which they have purchased from a chemist. Self-prescribed medication is of interest to the practitioner not least because the quantities used may be quite variable, with the possibility of chronic overdosing. For example, repeatedly exceeding the recommended daily dosage of vitamins A and D supplements may

Table 5.1 Adverse effects of drugs affecting the lower limb

Drug	*Therapeutic use*	*Side effects*
Beta-blockers	Hypertension	Coldness of extremities
Calcium channel blockers	Hypertension	Ankle oedema
Angiotensin-converting enzyme (ACE) inhibitors	Hypertension	Muscle cramps
Propanolol	Hypertension	Paraesthesia
Furosemide	Hypertension	Bullous eruptions
Salbutamol	Asthma	Peripheral vasodilatation
The contraceptive pill	Contraception	Increased risk of deep vein thrombosis
Colchicine	Gout	Sensorimotor neuropathy
Indometacin	Arthritis	Sensorimotor neuropathy
Corticosteroids	Inflammation	Osteoporosis, skin atrophy
Aspirin	Pain management	Purpura
Metronidazole	Anaerobic infections	Sensorimotor neuropathy
4-quinolones	Infection	Damage to epiphyseal cartilage
Chloramphenicol	Infection	Peripheral neuritis
Nalidixic acid	Infection	Bullous eruptions

lead to ectopic calcification in tendon, muscle and periarticular tissue.

The practitioner should be alert to the possibility of a patient developing an allergy or adverse reaction to medications used during treatment. In particular, details of any adverse reactions, either by the patient or any member of the patient's family, to previous local anaesthetic injections and other drugs (e.g. penicillin) should be sought and explored. A type I hypersensitivity reaction, which may lead to anaphylactic shock, is of most concern. It is not known why some individuals are predisposed to anaphylaxis, though genetic mechanisms are certainly involved since there is a strong familial disposition. In some individuals, contact with certain allergens will stimulate the production of an antibody of the immunoglobulin E (IgE) class, which has the ability to adhere to mast cells in tissues and basophils in the circulation. When an individual sensitised in this way is exposed on a second occasion to the allergen, the allergen combines with the IgE antibodies on the surface of the mast cells. This causes immediate destruction of the mast cell, which releases its contents, specifically histamine, serotonin, platelet-activating factor and slow-reacting substance. If the exposure to the allergen is systemic, hypotension, bronchiole constriction, laryngeal oedema, swelling of the tongue, urticaria, vomiting and diarrhoea may follow. Thankfully, fatal anaphylaxis is rare. When it does occur it usually follows entry of an antigenic drug into the circulation of a sensitised individual. Insect stings are also an important cause of anaphylactic fatality. A local type I hypersensitivity reaction may be caused by local anaesthetic agents but this is rare. In such cases the skin around the area of the injection shows an immediate, localised inflammatory reaction.

Of particular concern to the podiatric practitioner is the potential for overdosage of local anaesthetics, which can lead to convulsions as a result of central nervous system depression. This may be followed by a profound drop in blood pressure and life-threatening cardiovascular depression. In such circumstances oxygen must be administered to support the patient. The risk of such a clinical emergency can be minimised by adhering to the maximum safe dose for the various local anaesthetic agents and always having oxygen available.

Use of recreational drugs should be recorded. Amphetamines, like many mood stimulants, have a vasoconstrictive effect. The use of injectable drugs places the patient at risk of hepatitis and human immunodeficiency virus (HIV) infection. Long-term or heavy use of tobacco can affect wound healing due to the immediate vasoconstrictive effect of nicotine as well as the long-term effects on increased platelet adhesiveness and atherosclerosis. Tobacco smokers are also at greater risk of bronchitis, asthma and lung cancer. Questions to ask are:

- Do you smoke?
- What do you smoke – cigarettes, cigars, a pipe?
- How many do you smoke a day?
- How long have you smoked?
- Have you tried to stop?
- Are you exposed to passive smoking at home?

Heavy alcohol consumption can affect the peripheral sensation, immune response, postoperative wound healing and the metabolism of local anaesthetics, as well as having implications for treatment compliance. Alcohol consumption is generally measured in units. One unit of alcohol is equivalent to one glass of wine, a single measure of spirits or half a pint of beer. More than four units of alcohol per day is noteworthy. Unfortunately, it is likely that those patients misusing alcohol are least likely to be forthcoming about their alcoholism. Where alcohol misuse is suspected, questions should be asked in a permissive manner. The CAGE system is useful here – two or more positive replies identifies problem drinkers; one is an indication for further enquiry about a person's drinking. Ask if they:

- have **C**ut down on drinking – have tried repeatedly without success
- are **A**nnoyed by criticism about drinking habits
- have **G**uilty feelings about drinking
- need an **E**ye opener drink needed in the morning.

The patient should also be asked about dry retching in the morning, as this is a symptom of alcohol withdrawal. Drinking before 10 a.m. is an important finding as it is associated with chronic alcoholism.

Past medical history

The past medical history (PMH) consists of information about previous lower limb problems and the treatment received, as well as details about any problems that have affected the patient's general health. The nature of previous podiatric treatment, the name of the practitioner, details of relevant investigations such as X-rays, and the patient's view of the treatment's success should be recorded. This information may prevent the repetition of tests or treatments which have previously been ineffective. The patient should then be asked:

- Have you been off work due to illness for more than 1 week in the past 6 months?
- Have you ever been admitted to hospital?
- Have you ever had an operation?
- Have you ever been under the care of a consultant or a hospital specialist?
- Did you have any major childhood illnesses?

These questions will hopefully prompt the patient into recollecting any previous incidents of illness or surgery. Hospital records can provide this information but they are not always available. Questioning should follow a sequence that moves from the patient's childhood to the present.

Hospitalisations for operations or injuries should be recorded and any complications noted (Case history 5.1). In females, a particularly common procedure is hysterectomy, which has implications for the lower limb in that the effect on hormone balance can lead to premature osteoporosis. This may manifest clinically as vertebral collapse, leading to spinal

Case history 5.1

A 23-year-old secretary presented with pain in the first metatarsophalangeal joint. The pain was aching in nature, severe and worse on exercise. The range of motion of the joint was reduced, with painful crepitus evident on dorsiflexion. Further enquiry elicited a history of trauma from a fall in a horse-riding accident 2 years ago.

Diagnosis: Traumatic arthritis. An X-ray revealed a compression fracture to the head of the first metatarsal, which has predisposed degeneration of the joint.

deformity and possible neural compression. Injuries may often appear to be unrelated to the patient's presenting complaint but it must be remembered that the lower limb functions as one unit and if one component of the unit is damaged, it can lead to compensations elsewhere in the lower limb. If a patient is still under the care of a hospital consultant it is prudent to inform the consultant before any treatment is given that may affect other body systems.

Family history

A pedigree chart may be used to record details of major illnesses and lower limb problems of the immediate family (Fig. 5.1). Conventions exist regarding the symbols used in the charts. The author's favourite quote from a patient was that 'they don't make old bones in my family!'

Many cardiovascular, alimentary, neurological and endocrine disorders can be inherited and therefore the use of pedigree charts is particularly useful in paediatrics. Enquiry about the medical history of the immediate family may reveal a predisposition to a range of systemic diseases, a good example of which is non-insulin-dependent diabetes. It can also be of value to record the cause of death of immediate family. Certain lower limb pathologies can be inherited or seem to have a familial predisposition, especially diseases that are neurological in nature such as Friedreich's ataxia and Charcot–Marie–Tooth disease. The diagnosis in a patient presenting with difficulty walking will be influenced by a positive family history of a condition such as these. All forms of spina bifida should be noted even if the problem has been labelled as spina bifida occulta (impaired gait, pes cavus and plantar ulceration have been found to appear late in cases of spina bifida occulta). The patient should be asked if anyone else in the family has suffered from leg or foot problems. This information will help to determine the inherited nature of any foot condition and, in the case of pes cavus, hallux valgus and lesser digit deformity, could indicate the degree of severity that the patient's presenting condition may eventually achieve.

The ethnic origin of the patient should also be noted. Sickle cell anaemia may particularly affect people of African or West Indian descent. Thalassaemia, another haemolytic anaemia, can affect patients from the Mediterranean and Southeast Asia.

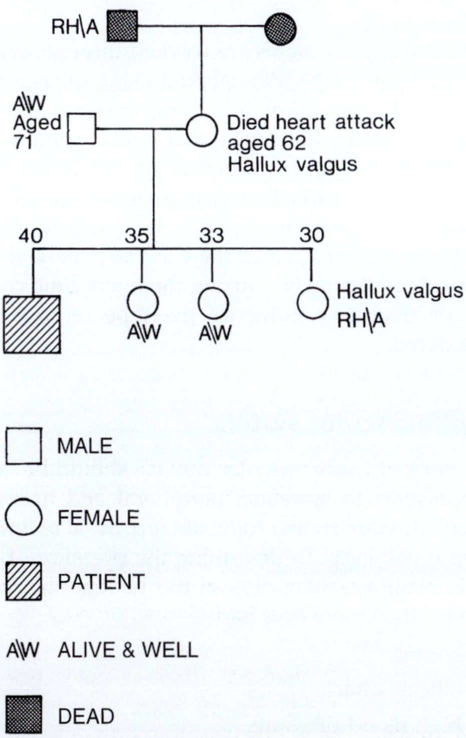

Figure 5.1 A pedigree chart.

Personal social history

Home circumstances

It is important to consider the patient's home situation. With some types of treatment patients are required to reduce their activity level to a minimum, change dressings or administer treatments at home. In the case of surgical treatment the practitioner must establish who is going to transport the patient to and from surgery and who is going to assist them through the immediate postoperative recovery period. Lack of home support may rule out certain forms of treatment.

Occupation

A patient's occupation may be a contributory cause of the lower limb problem and may influence the treatment that can be given (Case history 5.2). Some patients may experience particular difficulties in taking time from work to attend for treatment. The nature of the work should be determined (what they *actually* do) and special footwear requirements should be noted. The types of surface that the patient stands and walks on during the day can be exciting factors. Bare concrete floors will exacerbate chilblains, whereas patients whose occupation involves standing on ladders will often suffer from chronic medial longitudinal arch pain.

Case history 5.2

A 27-year-old female sales executive attended the clinic with heel pain. The pain was on the anteromedial aspect of the plantar heel pad and had been present for some time. Point tenderness at the origin of the medial band of the plantar fascia was elicited. Examination revealed a hyperpronatory foot type.

Diagnosis: Plantar fasciitis. However, the patient was required to wear fashionable court shoes for her employment. She was unwilling to compromise on the style of footwear she wore and provision of a suitable orthotic was impossible. The patient was subsequently prescribed stretching exercises and cortisone injections.

Case history 5.3

A 23-year-old man attended clinic after 6 months of working as a volunteer in India. For some of the time in India he walked around barefoot and recalls occasionally having to remove splinters and small stones from his sole. He presented with a pruritic, inflamed lesion with a central black dot, under the free edge of the hallucal toe nail of his left foot.

Diagnosis: A tropical parasitic infection with the jigger or sand flea, *Tunga penetrans*. Originally a native of the New World, it is now widely disseminated in Africa and Asia. A fertilised female, gaining access to human skin, burrows beneath the surface where it becomes engorged with blood. The site of penetration is usually found under the toe nail of the barefooted patient, but can occur on the plantar aspect of the foot. The central black dot is the flea's abdominal segments. Treatment is by incision and prophylactic antisepsis.

Sports and hobbies

Active sportsmen and women may make the association between their sport and a lower limb problem, but those who participate in occasional sporting activities and hobbies may not. Patients who participate in infrequent sporting activities may not think of informing the practitioner of these activities. However, these patients are often more prone to injury because they are often not as fit and do not follow appropriate warm-up and warm-down regimens. These patients are more likely to develop hamstring or calf muscle injury due to poor flexibility – the so-called weekend warrior. Details of any sporting hobby should therefore be sought from the patient. The assessment of the patient with a sports injury is considered in detail in Chapter 15.

Foreign travel

Details of foreign travel should be recorded in case the patient has acquired an infection while abroad. In particular, recent travel to tropical countries and details of any foot injuries sustained while walking barefoot should be recorded (Case history 5.3). Ask if the visit was urban or rural and whether they had any specific vaccinations.

The systems enquiry

The systems enquiry is the key part of the medical history. It seeks to discover if the patient has any systemic conditions, particularly those that may affect the patient's lower limb problem, and to unearth any signs and symptoms which the patient has not complained of spontaneously. The systems enquiry may reveal significant symptomatology which the practitioner is either inexperienced in or unqualified to diagnose. In such circumstances the patient should be informed that a second opinion is recommended. The subsequent referral for a second opinion should be seen as part of the patient's overall treatment plan.

All the body systems are worked through in a set order, which can be remembered using the acronym 'CRAGCEL' (see Box 5.1). The systems enquiry involves asking questions that will seem, to the patient, to be quite unrelated to the lower limb problem. It is important that patients are advised before the enquiry begins that the purpose of the questions is to ensure that there are no general health problems that may be causing the lower limb condition or that may influence the type of treatment considered.

Cardiovascular system

A history of cardiovascular disease should be taken with respect to systemic, peripheral and haematological disease states, followed up by a review of symptomatology. To determine the presence of systemic cardiovascular disease the patient should be asked if they have ever had:

- angina
- a heart attack
- high blood pressure
- heart failure

- irregular heart rhythms
- rheumatic fever.

Ischaemic heart disease describes two clinical syndromes: angina pectoris and myocardial infarction (MI). Angina occurs as a result of atherosclerosis of the arteries to the myocardium and often coexists with atherosclerosis of the arteries to the lower limb. MI is a gross necrosis of the myocardium due to interruption of the blood supply to the area.

Hypertension is a risk factor for many life-threatening conditions such as MI, renal failure and cerebral vascular accidents (strokes). An increase in blood pressure is often asymptomatic and many hypertensive people do not realise they have the condition until they develop symptoms (e.g. transient ischaemic attacks) or routine screening reveals a diastolic blood pressure above 90 mmHg. Practitioners should routinely take their patients' blood pressure, not least because the stress caused by treatment or examination may provoke a clinical emergency in a patient with uncontrolled hypertension.

Congestive heart failure (CHF) results from the inability of the heart to sufficiently supply oxygenated blood to the tissues. Causes include valvular heart disease, myocardial disease and hypertension (Case history 5.4). Arrhythmias may present as bradycardia (slow heartbeat) or tachycardia (fast heartbeat) with varying degrees of irregularity. Certain rhythms such as ventricular tachycardia predispose to cardiac arrest.

Rheumatic fever is a febrile disease occurring as a sequel to group A haemolytic streptococcal infections. It is characterised by inflammatory lesions of connective tissue structures, especially of the heart and blood vessels, and predisposes to bacterial endocarditis.

Having recorded disease states of which the patient is aware, enquire further about any systemic cardiovascular symptoms. Ask the patient if they:

- suffer from chest pains
- are ever short of breath
- experience palpitations
- find that their ankles swell
- are prone to fainting.

The most important cardiovascular symptom to elicit is chest pain (Table 5.2) because of the range of pathologies responsible for its occurrence. The differential diagnosis includes MI, angina pectoris, pneumonia, pericarditis and oesophageal reflux. The pain of angina is tight and pressure-like, precipitated by exercise and relieved by rest, and usually lasts for only a few minutes. The pain in an MI is similar in nature but is much more intense, lasting from 30 minutes to 3 hours.

Dyspnoea (shortness of breath) may occur as a result of pulmonary oedema. In CHF there is an inadequacy in the supply of oxygenated blood. To compensate for this, first the heart rate and then the volume of blood filling the left ventricle increases. Because it takes longer to fill the left ventricle, the pressure in the whole cardiac pulmonary system 'backs up', causing pulmonary congestion, reduced blood gas exchange and eventually pulmonary oedema. Pulmonary oedema and shortness of breath are, therefore, signs and symptoms of left-sided heart failure.

Right-sided heart failure is almost always associated with left-sided heart failure and gives rise to peripheral oedema. The right side of the heart can no longer deal with the volume of venous blood returning to the heart for transportation to the lungs and a 'back up' of pressure occurs in the systemic circulation, resulting in transudation of fluid into the peripheral connective tissue. Gravity will force most of the transudate to collect bilaterally in the feet and ankles. Initially, the patient will notice that the swelling reduces at night when the legs are recumbent. In chronic right-sided heart failure, the peripheral oedema will eventually be infiltrated by fibrous tissue that cannot be reduced by elevation (non-pitting oedema).

Syncope (fainting) is a transient loss of consciousness. Cardiac disease such as arrhythmias and aortic stenosis can cause syncope by decreasing the cerebral blood supply. Other less-specific systemic cardiac

Case history 5.4

A 65-year-old woman attended the podiatry clinic complaining of weak muscles in her legs. She had noticed the weakness for some time, stating that if her symptoms continued to deteriorate she would have to give up her job as a school playground supervisor. Further questioning revealed that her weakness could more accurately be described as fatigue and heaviness of her legs walking to and from work. The patient had also noticed that climbing stairs causes a tight squeezing pain in her chest. Sitting down relieved the pain but prolonged sitting tended to make her ankles swell.

Diagnosis: Congestive heart failure. This condition can have a direct effect on the ability of the muscles to function under strain.

Table 5.2 Common causes of chest pain

Cause	*Common symptoms*	*Common signs*
MI	Central, crushing pain that radiates into the arms and jaw. Nausea, vomiting, anxiety and sweating	Pain, sweating, tachycardia
Angina	Heavy central chest pain precipitated by activity and stress and relieved by rest	May be absent
Pulmonary embolus	Central or pleuritic chest pain. Sudden onset shortness of breath	Tachycardia, tachypnoea, hypotension
Pleurisy	Sharp, localised stabbing pain exacerbated by breathing, coughing and movement	Fever
Dyspepsia	Central epigastric sharp or burning pain which can radiate to the back	Epigastric tenderness
Musculoskeletal	Localised pain exacerbated by breathing, coughing and movement	Localised tenderness

symptoms include fatigue and decreased exertional tolerance.

To determine the presence of peripheral vascular disease the patient should be asked if they have ever had:

- a thrombosis or blood clot (deep vein thrombosis [DVT])
- night cramps
- an ulcer on their leg or foot
- varicose veins and/or surgery.

Whereas cardiac problems may affect lower limb perfusion, peripheral vascular disease can occur in the absence of cardiac symptoms. The general enquiry may have already revealed sleeping problems, but the cardiovascular system investigation should determine whether sleep disturbance is due to cramping pain in the legs. Nocturnal cramps are a consequence of increased permeability of the microcirculation that accompanies the warming of the legs under bedding. In the presence of any impairment of the venous system, toxic metabolites will accumulate, increasing carbon dioxide tension while lowering oxygen levels. Muscle ischaemia follows, manifesting as a painful tautness of muscle fibre.

Also enquire further about any peripheral vascular symptoms. Ask the patient if they:

- get cramp at night
- get muscle cramps while walking
- suffer from chilblains
- notice their feet change colour if it is particularly cold.

All the above factors are signs and symptoms of peripheral vascular disease. Assessment of the vascular status of the lower limb is covered in detail in Chapter 6.

Haematological disorders should be considered. To determine the presence of haematological disease patients should be asked if they have:

- anaemia
- haemophilia
- any other blood disorder.

Anaemia occurs when red blood cells or haemoglobin content decreases because of blood loss, impaired production or excessive destruction of red blood cells. Tissue hypoxia results from anaemia and this in turn leads to cardiovascular and pulmonary compensations. Clinical symptoms depend on the severity and duration of the anaemia. Severe anaemia is associated with weakness, vertigo, headaches, tiredness, gastrointestinal complaints and CHF.

Sickle cell disease is an inherited condition that can affect persons of African or West Indian descent. Those who inherit the gene from both patients have more than a 75% chance of developing the condition. Individuals with sickle cell disease are prone to ulceration around the malleoli, a complaint more characteristic of older people with venous insufficiency. In most cases, patients will know whether they have sickle cell anaemia, as from early childhood the digits of the hands and feet tend to swell and are very painful. The use of tourniquets carries an increased risk of complication. A tourniquet causes relative anoxia and this in turn causes occlusion in small vessels due to changes in the haemodynamic qualities of red blood cells, which may lead to small vessel infarction and possibly gangrene.

Respiratory system

To determine the presence of known systemic respiratory disease (Table 5.3) the patient should be asked if they have ever had:

- asthma
- chronic bronchitis
- emphysema
- pulmonary embolism.

Asthma presents as a dry, wheezing cough accompanied by dyspnoea. Exercise, infection or stress may provoke attacks. Patients may be treated with long-term corticosteroid therapy. Chronic bronchitis is associated with a history of cigarette smoking and peripheral atherosclerosis. Emphysema causes dyspnoea with varying degrees of exertion. In time the patient will develop right-sided heart failure and peripheral oedema. Pulmonary emboli may cause pleuritic chest pain and haemoptysis. It is a life-threatening condition that may follow prolonged postoperative bed rest.

Having recorded disease states of which the patient is aware, enquire further about any respiratory symptoms. Ask the patient if they:

- have shortness of breath
- have chest pain related to breathing or exercise
- have a cough (dry or productive)
- are coughing up blood.

Shortness of breath (dyspnoea) is one of the most common symptoms of respiratory disease. Pulmonary embolism (PE) secondary to a DVT may cause difficulty in breathing. Dyspnoea on exertion (DOE or exertional dyspnoea) indicates dyspnoea that occurs (or worsens) during activity. Respiratory illness associated with pulmonary inflammation and pressure on the pleural surfaces will lead to chest pain. The pleura (the serous membrane covering of the lungs and thoracic cavity) is richly endowed with sensory nerve endings. Stimulation of these nerves will cause a knife-like pain, which is intensified by deep breathing. Pulmonary hypertension and infection are commonly associated with chest pain. Coughing is a protective mechanism used to clear

Table 5.3 Clinical features and implications of respiratory diseases

Disease	*Clinical features*	*Clinical implications*
Asthma	Dyspnoea, wheezing, cough	Attacks may be provoked by exercise, infection or stress. May be treated with long-term corticosteroid therapy
Chronic bronchitis	Cough with expectoration of sputum for at least 3 months in 2 successive years	Commonly a history of cigarette smoking carries an accompanying risk of peripheral atherosclerosis
Emphysema	Dyspnoea with varying degrees of exertion	Patient will have limited exercise potential; in time this leads to right-sided heart failure and peripheral oedema
Pulmonary embolism	Pleuritic chest pain and haemoptysis	A life-threatening condition which may follow prolonged postoperative bed rest

Case history 5.5

A 19-year-old man presented with poor hygiene and digital ulcers on his left foot. The ulcers arose from neglected chilblains. A social history reveals that he had been homeless since leaving school some years ago. A cough of 2 months' duration is noted with the sputum yellow in colour and tinged with blood, indicating haemoptysis.

Diagnosis: Tuberculosis. A chest X-ray revealed a number of calcified granulomas and a small cavity consistent with a tuberculosis infection.

Case history 5.6

A 32-year-old man presented with low back pain that was worse at night or after inactivity. He also had heel pain and neck pain, loss of appetite, mouth ulcers and moderate weight loss. Examination revealed joint pain and swelling in the shoulders, knees and ankles.

Diagnosis: Ankylosing spondylitis. This condition was confirmed by X-rays and blood tests. It is a progressive inflammatory disease that usually affects young men. Common symptoms are recurring mouth ulcers (aphthae) and fatigue. There is often a positive family history with 95% of patients carrying the HLA-B27 antigen.

foreign material or mucus. The causes of coughing can be:

- mechanical, e.g. inhalation of dust
- inflammatory, e.g. mucous membrane oedema
- non-pulmonary, e.g. pulmonary embolism
- malignancy, e.g. dry cough
- drug-induced, e.g. ACE inhibitors.

The coughing up of bloody sputum is always considered an abnormal finding. Massive haemoptysis is a life-threatening condition that follows pulmonary neoplasm, mitral stenosis, pulmonary hypertension and tuberculosis (Case history 5.5).

A social and environmental history may also be relevant. The patient should be asked if they:

- have ever had asthma or an allergy to any airborne substances such as house dust or pollen
- use any chemicals at work
- are exposed to chemical vapours
- live or work with people who smoke cigarettes.

Alimentary system

Gastrointestinal disorders are extremely common and have many implications for the lower limb and its treatment (Case history 5.6). To determine the presence of gastrointestinal disease the patient should be asked if they have ever had:

- toothache or gum swelling
- any diet or bowel problems
- indigestion or stomach ache
- stomach problems, for example upset stomach after taking aspirin.

The enquiry should start with questions about the mouth and then progress to the stomach, intestines and bowel (Case history 5.6). Patients should be asked if they are currently suffering from toothache or gum disease. This question will establish the presence of any potential nidus of infection in the oral cavity – dental disease presents a risk of bacteraemia. Information about previous dental care may reveal that the patient has to take antibiotics before undergoing dental treatment. A known side effect of NSAIDs is gastrointestinal irritation. This is significant when these drugs are used for prolonged periods. Whereas the majority of people will suffer occasional indigestion, a history of dyspepsia provoked by small doses of alcohol or analgesics may indicate gastrointestinal sensitivity.

The character of any abdominal pain, its location, precipitating factors and radiation of the pain should be considered. The pain in gastritis is burning or gnawing in character and is localised to the epigastrium but may radiate to the back. Gastritis pain is precipitated by ingestion of alcohol, aspirin or fasting for long periods. Food consumption will rapidly relieve the pain. Chronic gastritis will eventually progress to peptic ulcerative disease. Pain arising from the biliary tract leads to a full or cramping sensation in the upper quadrant just behind the right rib cage. It will occasionally radiate to the right shoulder, will not be relieved by ingestion of food, and may be exacerbated by the ingestion of fatty food.

The commoner forms of liver disease are rarely accompanied by specific abdominal pain, although in most hepatic conditions the liver may be tender and enlarged on examination. A history of jaundice is common with most liver diseases. Jaundice is a syndrome characterised by deposition of yellow bile pigment in the skin, conjunctivae, mucous membranes and urine. If the liver is damaged and its function impaired by cirrhosis, first-pass metabolism will not operate effectively. First-pass metabolism refers to the removal of drugs from the hepatic portal circulation and their subsequent metabolism in the liver. Certain drugs, for example the opioid antagonist naloxone, are almost completely eliminated by first-pass metabolism. If first-pass metabolism is impeded, an increase in circulating concentrations of the drug will follow. The maximum safe dose that can be administered will have to be reduced in these cases. Liver disease is also significant when the use of amide local anaesthetics (e.g. prilocaine, mepivacaine, bupivacaine) is being considered as they are metabolised by the liver.

Chronic alcohol misuse can increase the activity of the liver's phase I oxidase enzymes, which are responsible for the metabolism of drugs such as paracetamol, warfarin, barbiturates and benzodiazepines. This increase in enzyme activity and drug metabolism will significantly reduce the therapeutic effect of these drugs. Combined alcohol and drug ingestion, however, will have the immediate effect of enhancing the therapeutic effect of oral hypoglycaemics, benzodiazepines and tricyclic antidepressants, which could produce potentially life-threatening effects.

A history of regular nausea, vomiting or dysphagia (difficulty in swallowing) will always demand an explanation. These clinical features may be due to central nervous system problems (e.g. intracranial tumours, meningitis), endocrine disorders (e.g. myxoedema, diabetic ketoacidosis) or systemic or gastrointestinal tract infections. Constipation and diarrhoea are common complaints that are usually benign and self-limiting. Where there is an underlying disease the problem is usually accompanied by fever, severe pain and blood loss. Although not specifically relevant to the lower limb, a history of altered bowel habit is important when making an assessment of the patient's general health and can influence the types of drug that may be used.

Genitourinary system

The kidneys regulate the body's electrolyte and fluid balance. This has implications for lower limb circulation and oedema, both important for wound healing. Polyuria (excessive urination) is associated with diabetes, cardiac failure or cortisol deficiency, all of which will affect healing.

To determine the presence of genitourinary disease the patient should be asked if they:

- have any 'waterworks' problems (such as pain)
- have their sleep disturbed by the need to go to the toilet
- have had any sexually transmitted infections.

Renal pain is a symptom of gross structural disease of the kidney, such as kidney stones or a blood clot passing down the ureter. Infection or malignancy may also cause pain in the area of the renal angle (Fig. 5.2) as well as more anteriorly in the abdomen. Leg and ankle swelling is an important finding, which may be related to kidney disease and indeed could be the first clinical sign of a renal problem. Renal dysfunction that leads to a massive loss of protein into the urine will disrupt normal capillary haemodynamics, causing reduced transudation of fluid. Fluid will pool in the tissues rather than returning back into the capillary circulation. Oedema of the dependent limb will result, particularly around the ankles. However, it should be remembered that renal dysfunction is not the only cause of ankle oedema. Breathlessness on exertion, weight loss, nausea and vomiting also occur in renal failure and may further confuse the clinical picture. A symptom that is renal-specific is disturbed micturition (Table 5.4). Frequency of urination is dependent upon fluid intake and specific drugs within food and drink. Most people urinate four to six times every 24 hours, mostly in the daytime.

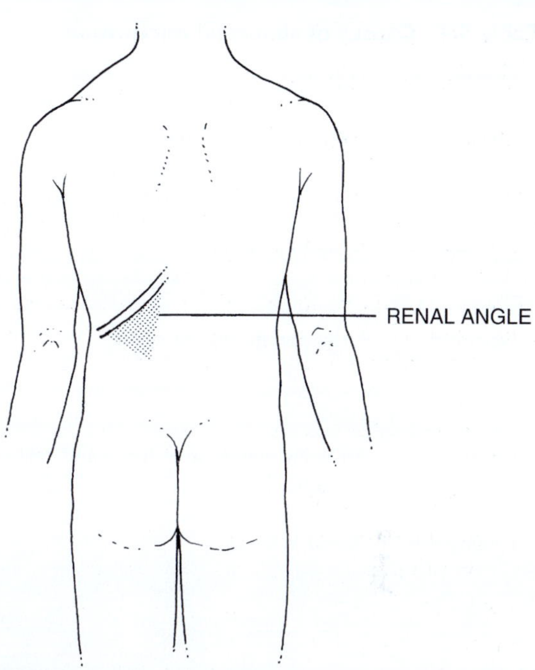

Figure 5.2 The renal angle.

Patients should be asked if they experience any pain or problems passing urine and whether their sleep is disturbed by the need to pass urine. A positive response to these questions requires further investigation, as the kidneys may affect bone metabolism as well as blood pressure and water regulation.

Table 5.4 Causes of abnormal micturition

Abnormality	*Definition*	*Causes*
Polyuria	Frequent micturition	Diabetes mellitus, diminution in bladder's effective filling capacity due to infection, foreign bodies, stones or tumour
Dysuria	Painful urination	Irritation and inflammation of bladder or urethra usually due to bacterial infection
Nocturia	Urination during the night	May reflect early renal disease. Decrease in concentrating capacity may be associated with cardiac or hepatic failure
Oliguria	Straining, decrease in force and calibre of urinary stream	Obstruction distal to the bladder. In men it is most commonly due to prostatic obstruction
Haematuria	Blood in urine	Haematuria without pain: renal or prostatic disease, bladder or kidney tumour. With pain: ureteral stone or bladder infection

Case history 5.7

A 42-year-old man attended clinic with jaundice. He complained of a fever and malaise, nausea and vomiting. His urine was tested which was found to be dark in colour. He had a 'home' tattoo made by his previous girlfriend who had been an intravenous drug user.

Diagnosis: Hepatitis C. This is an inflammation of the liver caused by the hepatitis C virus.

Sexually transmitted infections

The practitioner should use the systems enquiry and medical and social history to determine whether the patient is in a high-risk group for blood-borne infections such as hepatitis B or HIV. Reiter's disease, gonorrhoea, HIV and syphilis are all sexually transmitted infections (Case history 5.7). Practitioners investigating a lower limb complaint may find it difficult to enquire about sexually related problems (Table 5.5). However, as these conditions can lead to an array of lower limb symptoms, questions about them must be included in the systems enquiry. After enquiring about the urinary system, the patient should be asked if they have ever had any sexually transmitted infections, skin problems or discharge.

Table 5.5 Lower limb signs and symptoms associated with sexually transmitted diseases

Disease	*Lower limb signs and symptoms*
Reiter's syndrome	Asymmetrical arthralgia of hip, knee, ankle and metatarsophalangeal joint; 'sausage toe'; keratoderma blenorrhagica
HIV infection	Kaposi's sarcoma – a widespread skin or mucous membrane lesion appearing as a pink or red macule or violaceous plaques and nodules on the face, trunk and limbs. May appear wart-like
Gonococcal arthritis	Acute joint pain, swelling and stiffness. Usually accompanied by urethritis, dysuria and haemorrhagic vesicular skin lesions. Serious joint damage may result if the condition is not properly treated

Central nervous system

Diseases of the nervous system may cause pain in the lower limb, deformity or gait abnormalities. Comprehensive history taking is essential (Case history 5.8). To determine the presence of central nervous system disease the patient should be asked if they:

- have any known neuromuscular disorder
- have had a head injury
- have had a stroke
- have epilepsy.

Record details of a family history of epilepsy or neuromuscular disease. General neurological symptoms may be significant. Patients should be asked if they get frequent headaches. While stress-related headaches, migraine and extracranial causes such as cervical spondylosis account for the majority of headaches, cranial arteritis is an important cause in elderly people. Brain tumours (slow onset) and subarachnoid bleeding (sudden onset) must be considered in severe headaches.

Fainting, dizziness and visual disturbance may occur in association with headaches. The basis for most fainting episodes is inadequate blood supply to the brain and is commonly cardiac or cerebrovascular in origin. Anaemia, hypoglycaemia and emotional stress can also explain a temporary loss of consciousness.

Having recorded disease states of which the patient is aware, enquire further about any peripheral neurological symptoms. Ask the patient if they:

- ever get shooting pains in their arms or legs
- find their hands or feet go numb
- have a tremor
- have ever noticed any weakness or sluggishness of the arms or legs.

Case history 5.8

A 40-year-old factory worker presented with bilateral weakness in his legs. The history revealed that the weakness occurred intermittently but was not related to exercise or activity. Four years earlier he had suffered from blurred vision in his right eye and transient bouts of tingling in his right arm. He had not sought a medical opinion for these symptoms for fear of losing his driving licence. The podiatrist suspects a progressive central nervous system disorder.

Diagnosis: Multiple sclerosis. The patient was subsequently referred for a neurological assessment.

The major diseases associated with abnormal function of the somatic nervous system are myasthenia gravis and muscle spasticity. Myasthenia gravis is an autoimmune disease that affects the neuromuscular junctions and is characterised by weakness and fatigue after brief activity. Muscle spasticity is characterised by increased muscle tone in the skeletal muscles and is often treated with muscle relaxants.

Peripheral neuropathy may be either acquired or inherited. Acquired peripheral neuropathies are grouped into three broad categories:

- Those caused by systemic disease
- Those caused by trauma from external agents
- Those caused by infections or autoimmune disorders affecting nerve tissue.

Causes of peripheral neuropathy are summarised in Box 5.2. Numbness and paraesthesia, loss of muscle bulk or weakness are significant findings. If the patient's response is positive, peripheral neuropathy, which can result from a range of causes, should be considered. It is essential to establish the course of

Box 5.2 Causes of peripheral neuropathy

- Hereditary neurological disease – Charcot–Marie–Tooth disease, Friedreich's ataxia
- Systemic disorders:
  - Inflammatory disorders – rheumatoid arthritis, systemic lupus erythematosus, vasculitis, sarcoidosis, amyloidosis
  - Endocrine – diabetes mellitus, hypothyroidism, hypocalcaemia
  - Renal failure
- Compression
  - Nerve root compression of the sciatic or femoral nerve
  - Distal nerve compression of the popliteal, common peroneal and anterior tibial nerves
- Nutritional disorders
  - Pernicious anaemia, or thiamine or vitamin B_6 deficiency
  - Chronic alcohol misuse
- Infections – tuberculosis, acquired immune deficiency syndrome (AIDS), leprosy, syphilis
- Tumour – bronchogenic carcinoma, myeloma, lymphoma
- Toxic agents – carbon monoxide, solvents, industrial poisons, lead
- Medication – isoniazid, metronidazole, nitrofurantoin

the symptoms and consider them in the light of the patient's age. Slow progressive weakness of the limbs over a period of many years in a young person may point to muscular dystrophy, whereas a more acute onset may indicate a demyelinating disorder or spinal cord compression.

The significance of some symptoms in the neurological enquiry are difficult to interpret because the enquiry relies on the patient's subjective account (Case history 5.8). However, inadequate assessment of the neurological basis of foot pathology can lead to inappropriate treatment through missed diagnosis. Neurological assessment of the lower limb is covered in detail in Chapter 7.

Endocrine system

Disorders of the endocrine system may be divided into those conditions which present relatively frequently (and are of regular concern) and those which are rare (Case history 5.9). To determine the presence of endocrine disease the patient should be asked if they have had:

- sugar diabetes
- thyroid problems.

In the assessment of the lower limb, diabetes mellitus, thyroid disease, growth disorders, obesity and problems associated with the menopause are particularly relevant. Routine questioning about endocrine symptomatology should begin with asking the patient if they:

- ever suffer from a thirst that they find hard to quench no matter how much they drink
- have a stable weight.

Case history 5.9

A 40-year-old male steelworker sought the opinion of a podiatrist when he began to develop corns on the dorsal aspect of both fifth proximal interphalangeal joints. The patient reported that his industrial boots no longer fitted properly and joked that he must still be growing as his protective headwear and gloves did not feel quite right. Further questioning revealed a tendency to sweat profusely even when sitting quietly, regular headaches and joint pains. His wife had remarked that his features had become more rugged.

Diagnosis: Acromegaly. A urine sample demonstrated glycosuria and his blood pressure was elevated to 190/110 mmHg.

Diabetes is a disease of either insulin deficiency or peripheral resistance to insulin action. Insulin produced by the beta cells of the pancreas decreases blood glucose by inhibiting glycogen breakdown and facilitating the entry of glucose into tissue cells. When peripheral tissues fail to utilise glucose, blood glucose levels rise and glucose is excreted in the urine. Because the body will continue to need a source of energy, homeostasis provokes breakdown of body fat and muscle tissue. This process of 'accelerated starvation' can be quite abrupt in children, causing anorexia, nausea, coma and, if untreated, death. In older patients it is more gradual and, indeed, the first presenting symptom may be one of the complications of the disease.

Thirst, polyuria and weight loss are the three most common symptoms of diabetes. These three features may also occur with other conditions such as diabetes insipidus, hypercalcaemia and renal failure (Table 5.6). The thirst associated with diabetes is a result of the osmotic diuretic effect of glucose, although it is difficult to be precise as to what is excessive thirst. An increased volume and frequency of urination will lead to a corresponding increase in fluid intake. The

Table 5.6 Causes of thirst and polyuria

Cause	*Physiological reason*
Diabetes mellitus	Osmotic diuretic effect of glucose
Diabetes insipidus	Kidney disease prevents normal concentrating of urine or pituitary gland disorders cause a deficiency of antidiuretic hormone
Hypercalcaemia	Result of hyperparathyroidism where hypercalcaemia causes reversible impairment of renal concentrating mechanism
Hypocalcaemia	Often a side effect of diuretic therapy, it leads to impaired concentrating ability in the kidney
Excess salt intake	Osmotic diuretic effect of increased sodium level
Renal failure	Normal concentrating function of kidney lost

patient is often aware that sleep is regularly disturbed by the need to urinate and a history of polyuria should always be followed up by glucose testing of the urine. Although people with diabetes often believe that their decreasing weight is due to polyuria, it is in fact a result of accelerated fat and protein catabolism.

The thyroid hormones triiodothyronine and tetraiodothyronine (T_3 and T_4) are essential for normal growth and development and have many effects on body metabolism, the most obvious being to stimulate the basal metabolic rate. In thyroid disease there is either inadequate or excessive production of thyroid hormones. The clinical features of hyperthyroidism are listed in Box 5.3.

The clinical features of hyperthyroidism such as muscle weakness, tachycardia, weight loss and sleep disturbance may have already been picked up from the systems enquiry. Other features associated with the condition may not have been highlighted, for example heat intolerance, hand tremor and irritability. If hyperthyroidism is suspected, the patient should be asked:

- Do you find that you cannot tolerate hot rooms or buildings?
- Have you noticed a change in your handwriting?
- Do your hands shake?
- Do your hands and feet get excessively sweaty?

Hyperthyroidism is an important systemic cause of hyperhydrosis of the feet and hands. Other lower limb signs and symptoms include infiltration of non-pitting mucinous ground substance on the anterior surface of the tibia, which causes intense itching and erythema. This so-called pretibial myxoedema (a confusing term since myxoedema suggests hypothyroidism) is more accurately described as an infiltrative dermopathy. Hyperthyroidism can cause tarsal tunnel syndrome and must be considered as a differential diagnosis for this condition, especially as the dermopathy will remain even after thyroid function is stabilised.

Box 5.3 Clinical features of hyperthyroidism

- Weight loss (with a normal appetite)
- Heat intolerance
- Fatigue
- Cardiac palpitations
- Irritability
- Hand tremors
- Sleep disturbance
- Bulging eyes
- Goitre
- Diarrhoea
- Generalised muscle weakness

Inadequate levels of circulating thyroid hormone will lead to hypothyroidism. This condition may be discovered by asking the patient:

- Have you noticed any hair loss from your head or eyebrows?
- Are you troubled by dry scaly skin on your head or face?
- Have you noticed your hands or face getting puffy?
- Do you feel you have generally slowed down?
- Are you getting forgetful?
- Do you notice the cold?
- Has your weight increased?

In hypothyroidism the facial expression is dull and the features puffy with swelling around the eye sockets due to infiltration of mucopolysaccharides. The eyelids will droop due to decreased adrenergic drive and the skin and hair will be coarse and dry. The tongue may be enlarged, the voice hoarse and speech slow. Tarsal and carpal tunnel syndrome, caused by the infiltration of mucopolysaccharides, are common clinical features. Either form of thyroid disease renders the patient a poor candidate for foot surgery because it reduces the ability to deal with stress. Cardiac arrhythmias or metabolic imbalance may occur in stressful situations. Screening for thyroid disease is therefore essential and the above enquiry should be included in any presurgery assessment.

Disorders of the adrenal gland should also be considered. The adrenal gland has two functionally distinct parts, the cortex and the medulla. The more important of the two, the adrenal cortex, is essential for life as it produces glucocorticoids and mineralocorticoids, which maintain blood volume during stress. The patient should be asked:

- Do you ever feel faint or dizzy when standing up after sitting for some time?
- Have you noticed any coloured patches or streaks developing on your skin?
- Have you had any problems with increased facial hair?
- Do you bruise easily?

The adrenal cortex is susceptible to either hypo- or hyperfunction. Hypofunction or Addison's disease is an autoimmune condition, and the majority of clinical features are due to deficiency in glucocorticoids and mineralocorticoids (Table 5.7). The most relevant aspect of Addison's disease is the reduction in the level of cortisol. This hormone is normally produced in response to stress. Cortisol deficiency will reduce resistance to infection and trauma. Cushing's disease presents as an overproduction of glucocorticoids or by excessive use of cortisol or other steroid hormones. High levels of cortisol increases carbohydrate production and leads to truncal obesity and development of a moon face. Purple striae or stretch marks will develop on the abdomen. Thinning of the skin and increased risk of infection are important lower limb features of Cushing's disease. Osteoporosis may occur as a sequel to disruption of normal kidney function. An increased production of androgens may cause hirsutism. Secondary diabetes mellitus may also occur as a sequel to Cushing's disease.

Overactivity of the anterior pituitary gland will increase circulating levels of growth hormone, which results in excessive growth of feet, hands, jaw and soft tissue acromegaly. Excess growth hormone leads to glycogenesis: approximately 30% of people with acromegaly develop diabetes mellitus. Hypertension, due to inadequate renal clearance of phosphates, also affects 30% of people with acromegaly. The majority of people with acromegaly (see Case history 5.9) have constant headaches and joint pains. The condition, although rare, has significant foot health implications with a catalogue of signs and symptoms that will become apparent during virtually every stage of the functional enquiry.

Table 5.7 Clinical features associated with disorders of the adrenal glands

Disorder	*Clinical features*
Adrenal undersecretion (e.g. Addison's disease)	*Common features*: tiredness generalised weakness lethargy anorexia weight loss dizziness and postural hypotension pigmentation *Less common features*: hypoglycaemia loss of body hair depression
Adrenal oversecretion (Cushing's disease)	Truncal obesity (moon face, buffalo hump, protuberant abdomen) Thinning of skin Purple striae Excessive bruising Hirsutism Hypertension Glucose intolerance Muscle weakness and wasting, especially of proximal muscles Back pain (osteoporosis and vertebral collapse) Psychiatric disturbances

Locomotor system

Many authors argue that there is no other medical speciality that interfaces with podiatry as closely as rheumatology. Approximately 20% of patients with rheumatoid arthritis present initially with foot and ankle symptoms, and most patients will eventually develop foot and ankle symptoms. Gout has a predilection for the first metatarsophalangeal joint and osteoarthritis is so common in the same joint that it has its own name – hallux limits. The main rheumatological conditions affecting the lower limb are listed at Table 5.8. However, remember that rheumatology

Table 5.8 Rheumatological conditions affecting the lower limb

Diffuse connective tissue disease	Rheumatoid arthritis Systemic lupus erythematosus Seronegative spondyloarthropathies
Degenerative joint disease	Osteoarthritis
Crystal induced arthropathies	Gout Pseudogout (calcium pyrophosphate dihydrate deposition (CPDD))
Non-articular rheumatism	Fibrositis Tendonitis Pain syndromes

Case history 5.10

A 45-year-old female teacher presented with pain under the balls of both feet. She complained of general malaise and going to bed much earlier in the evening than she used to. She described stiffness in her hands and knees, which was worse in the morning, but improved after a hot bath and an aspirin. On examination the small joints of her hands and feet were swollen, leading the practitioner to suspect a systemic rather than local mechanical cause.

Diagnosis: Rheumatoid arthritis. This was confirmed by a blood test, which showed a raised ESR (erythrocyte sedimentation rate) and rheumatoid factor.

is concerned with diseases of connective tissue and you will see that such pathology is likely to present at multiple sites.

To determine the presence of musculoskeletal disease the patient should be asked if they have had:

- any form of arthritis
- any joint swelling or stiffness
- back, hip, knee, ankle or foot pain
- limb pain during any specific activity
- fractures of any bones in the legs or feet
- strained or injured muscles in the legs.

The aim of the locomotor enquiry is to broaden the practitioner's outlook beyond the specific presenting complaint to a broader view of the locomotor system. The patient's account of spine pain and pain involving areas other than that of the presenting complaint should be obtained. Information from the locomotor enquiry will help the practitioner consider pathology which may have a systemic origin (Case history 5.10). Assessment of the locomotor system is detailed in Chapter 10.

Summary

Accurate diagnosis, which includes taking the patient's medical and social history, forms the basis for formulation of an effective treatment plan. A format for history taking has been presented which covers all aspects of the patient's current and past medical status. It has been emphasised that the personal social history is as important as the medical history, since it enables an assessment to be made about aspects of the patient's lifestyle which could influence any proposed treatment. The approach outlined in this chapter will ensure that a broad range of factors are taken into consideration when making a diagnosis and drawing up a treatment plan.

Further reading

British National Formulary (BNF), updated twice yearly. British Medical Association (BMA) and Royal Pharmaceutical Society of Great Britain (RPSGB), London

Davey P 2006 Medicine at a glance, 2nd edn. Blackwell Publishing, Oxford

Fishman J, Fishman L, Grossman A 2005 History taking in medicine and surgery. PasTest, Knutsford

Gleadle J 2003 History and examination at a glance. Blackwell Science Ltd, Oxford

Greenberger N, Hinthorn D 1993 History taking and physical examination: essentials and clinical correlates. Mosby Year Book, St Louis

Levy L A, Hetherington V J 2006 Principles and practice of podiatric medicine. Data Trace Publishing Company, Maryland

Munro J F, Campbell I W 2000 McLeod's clinical examination, 10th edn. Churchill Livingstone, Edinburgh

Seidel H M, Ball J W, Benedict G W et al 2006 Mosby's guide to physical examination, 6rd edn. Mosby, St Louis

Seymour P, Siklos C 2004 Clinical clerking: a short introduction to clinical skills, 3rd edn. Cambridge University Press

Tally N, O'Connor S 1989 Clinical examination. Blackwell Scientific, Oxford

Turner R, Blackwood R 1991 Lecture notes on history taking and examination, 2nd edn. Blackwell Science, Oxford

Zier B 1990 Essential of internal medicine in clinical podiatry. W B Saunders, Philadelphia

Appendix 5.1: Medical Health Questionnaire

Please complete the health questionnaire in your own time. Take as long as you feel you need. If there are any areas of the form that you are not clear about, please ask the practitioner for help. It is important that we know about all aspects of your health as this may affect your legs and feet and may be important when deciding the best form of treatment for you.

Your foot/leg problem

Have you had any previous treatment for your feet? Yes ❑ No ❑

Who provided the treatment? ______

Were any X-rays taken? Yes ❑ No ❑

Were any blood samples taken? Yes ❑ No ❑

Your general health

Are you generally well? Yes ❑ No ❑

Are you seeing a doctor or consultant currently? Yes ❑ No ❑

Are you sleeping well? Yes ❑ No ❑

What is your weight? ____________

For women, could you be pregnant? Yes ❑ No ❑

Past medical history

Has your weight recently changed? Yes ❑ No ❑

If Yes, how has your weight changed? ______________________

Are you taking any medication or tablets? Yes ❑ No ❑

If Yes, please list:

____
____
____
____

Are you allergic to anything? Yes ❑ No ❑

If Yes, please list:

____
____
____
____

Do you smoke? Yes ❑ No ❑

If Yes, how many do you smoke per day? ______________________

Have you ever:

Been off sick from work for more than a week? Yes ❑ No ❑

Been admitted to hospital? Yes ❑ No ❑

Undergone an operation? Yes ❑ No ❑

Been under the care of a hospital consultant? Yes ❑ No ❑

If Yes, please give details: _________

Do you take any recreational drugs? Yes ❑ No ❑

Have you ever been injured at work? Yes ❑ No ❑

Did you have any major childhood illnesses? Yes ❑ No ❑

If Yes, please state which ones:

____
____
____
____

Family history

Does anyone in your family suffer from foot or leg problems Yes ❑ No ❑

Please place a circle (and state whom) if a **member of your family** suffered from any of these illnesses:

Haemophilia Yes/No

Family member affected ______________________

Sickle cell disease Yes/No

Family member affected ______________________

Diabetes Yes/No

Family member affected ______________________

Rheumatoid arthritis Yes/No

Family member affected ______________________

Epilepsy Yes/No

Family member affected ______________________

Social history

What is your occupation? ________

Do you participate in sporting activities? Yes ❑ No ❑

If Yes, please state which sports and how regularly you participate:

____

____

____

____

Heart and circulatory problems

Have you ever had:

A heart attack Yes ❑ No ❑

Angina Yes ❑ No ❑

High blood pressure Yes ❑ No ❑

Heart failure Yes ❑ No ❑

Irregular heart rhythms Yes ❑ No ❑

Rheumatic fever Yes ❑ No ❑

A thrombosis or blood clot Yes ❑ No ❑

Night cramps Yes ❑ No ❑

Muscle cramps when walking short distances Yes ❑ No ❑

An ulcer on your leg or foot Yes ❑ No ❑

Chilblains Yes ❑ No ❑

Varicose veins and/or surgery for veins Yes ❑ No ❑

Anaemia Yes ❑ No ❑

Hepatitis or jaundice Yes ❑ No ❑

Haemophilia Yes ❑ No ❑

Any other blood disorder Yes ❑ No ❑

Do you suffer from:

Chest pains Yes ❑ No ❑

Shortness of breath Yes ❑ No ❑

Palpitations Yes ❑ No ❑

Swollen ankles Yes ❑ No ❑

Regular fainting Yes ❑ No ❑

Respiratory problems

Have you ever had:

Asthma Yes ❑ No ❑

Chronic bronchitis Yes ❑ No ❑

Emphysema Yes ❑ No ❑

A blood clot on the lung Yes ❑ No ❑

Have you ever had a cough for several months? Yes ❑ No ❑

Do you ever bring up blood when you cough? Yes ❑ No ❑

Diet and digestive problems

Are you troubled by toothache or gum swelling? Yes ❑ No ❑

Do you have any diet or bowel problems? Yes ❑ No ❑

Do you suffer from indigestion or stomach ache? Yes ❑ No ❑

Do painkillers such as aspirin upset your stomach? Yes ❑ No ❑

Genitourinary problems

Have you ever had any 'waterworks' problems? Yes ❑ No ❑

Have you ever had jaundice or hepatitis? Yes ❑ No ❑

Is your sleep disturbed by the need to go to the toilet? Yes ❑ No ❑

Have you ever had any sexually transmitted infections? Yes ❑ No ❑

Are you in a high risk group for blood-borne infections, such as hepatitis B or HIV? Yes ❑ No ❑

If you are a woman:
Are you or could you be pregnant? Yes ❑ No ❑

Are you taking hormone replacement therapy or the contraceptive pill? Yes ❑ No ❑

Have you had your menopause? Yes ❑ No ❑

Have you had a hysterectomy? Yes ❑ No ❑

Head and nerve problems

Have you ever injured your head or spine? Yes ❑ No ❑

Do you suffer from migraines or regular headaches? Yes ❑ No ❑

If Yes, how frequently? ___________

Do you ever get numbness, weakness, tingling, heaviness or shooting pains in your legs and feet? Yes ❑ No ❑

Do you ever get blackouts or feel faint? Yes ❑ No ❑

Glandular problems

Do you have sugar diabetes? Yes ❑ No ❑

Do you have thyroid problems? Yes ❑ No ❑

Are you always thirsty? Yes ❑ No ❑

Do your hands and feet get particularly sweaty? Yes ❑ No ❑

Are you particularly sensitive to cold? Yes ❑ No ❑

Do you bruise easily? Yes ❑ No ❑

Bone and joint problems

Do you have any arthritis? Yes ❑ No ❑

Do you ever get any aches and pains in your joints? Yes ❑ No ❑

Do you have any arthritis or long-standing muscle injuries? Yes ❑ No ❑

Thank you for completing this questionnaire. Please add any further information that you think may be of use.

____

____

CHAPTER 6

Vascular assessment

S Rees

Indicates figures on DVD, including colour

Indicates video of assessment on DVD

Chapter contents

Introduction

Assessment of vascular status is an essential part of the examination of the lower limb. This chapter begins by explaining the purpose of a vascular assessment and then proceeds to an overview of the anatomy and physiology of the cardiovascular system (CVS). An evidence-based approach has been used to describe evaluation of the CVS, with particular emphasis on the vascular status of the lower extremity. The diagnostic prediction of clinical tests, as well as ranges of expected and abnormal values are included. Simple non-invasive tests are described, which can be carried out by the practitioner using the minimum of equipment. The indications and limitations of hospital and laboratory tests are also outlined.

Purpose of a vascular assessment

The vascular status of the lower limb bears a direct relationship to tissue viability. Furthermore, peripheral arterial disease has been shown to be associated with an increase in morbidity and mortality (Criqui et al 1992, Lange et al 2005, Leibson et al 2004). Accordingly, the assessment of the peripheral circulation may perform a useful screening function by detecting previously unidentified vascular abnormalities.

Information gained from a vascular assessment can be used to identify:

- whether the blood supply to and from a limb is adequate for normal function and tissue viability.

- vascular problems and the functional site, that is, is it an arterial venous, insufficiency or a combination lymphatic.
- whether there are any vascular abnormalities which could affect healing or the choice of treatment for another condition.
- those patients in whom vascular conditions require further investigation, treatment or referral to a specialist.

Overview of the cardiovascular system

Anatomy of the cardiovascular system

The cardiovascular (CVS) consists of a closed system of vessels through which blood and lymph are pumped around the body by means of the heart.

The heart

The heart is constructed as a double pump in series: the right side pumps blood through the lungs for oxygenation (pulmonary circulation) and the left side pump supplies the systemic circulation. The heart is lined by endocardium and surrounded by a tough, non-extensible pericardium. The endocardium forms the cusps of one-way valves, called the tricuspid and bicuspid (mitral) valves, which control the flow of blood through the heart. It also forms semilunar valves, which control the entry of blood into the vessels leaving the heart. Closure of these valves is responsible for the two heart sounds, 'lub' 'dup', which can be heard through a stethoscope applied to the chest wall. Illustrates the major structures of the heart.

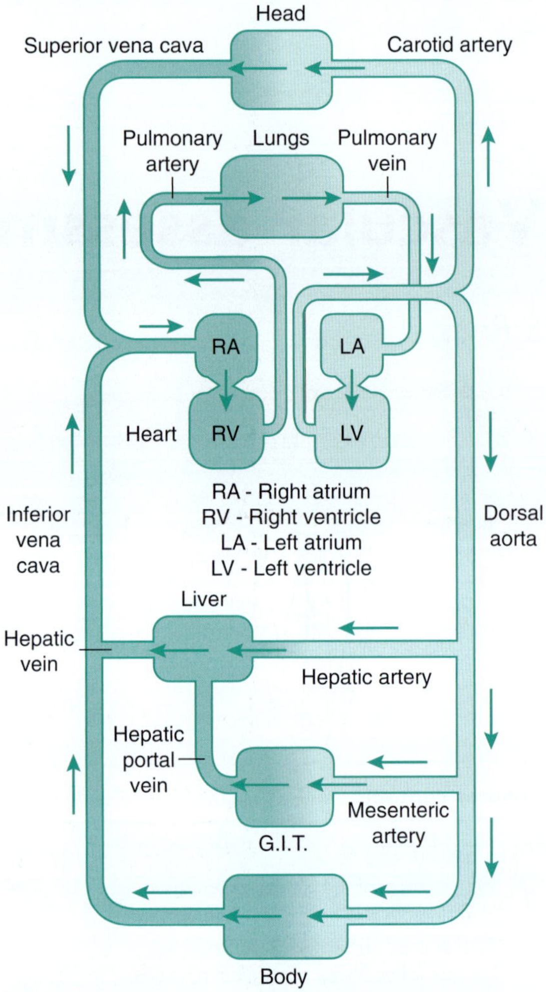

Figure 6.1 The major vessels of the cardiovascular system. In the body proper, the dorsal aorta and the vena cavae run in the central axis, but for purposes of clarity they are shown to the right and left of the body, respectively. RA = right atrium, RV = right ventricle, LA = left atrium, LV = left ventricle, GIT = gastrointestinal tract.

Peripheral circulation

The blood flows via a system of vessels of varying diameters (Table 6.1). The major arterial and venous vessels in the lower limb are shown in Figure 6.2.

Arterial tree

Blood is transported to the tissues is via arteries. These branch into consecutively smaller vessels called arterioles which eventually supply the capillary beds. The walls of arteries consist of three layers, from inner to outer, the tunica intima, tunica media and tunica adventitia (Fig. 6.3A). The interface of the vessel with the streaming blood is lined with endothelial cells to form a smooth surface to prevent adhesion of blood components. These cells secrete a variety of substances essential for maintenance of the vessel wall and circulatory function. All the vessels have some smooth muscle in the tunica media to enable them to change diameter, but arterioles have the greater proportion (primarily under sympathetic control).

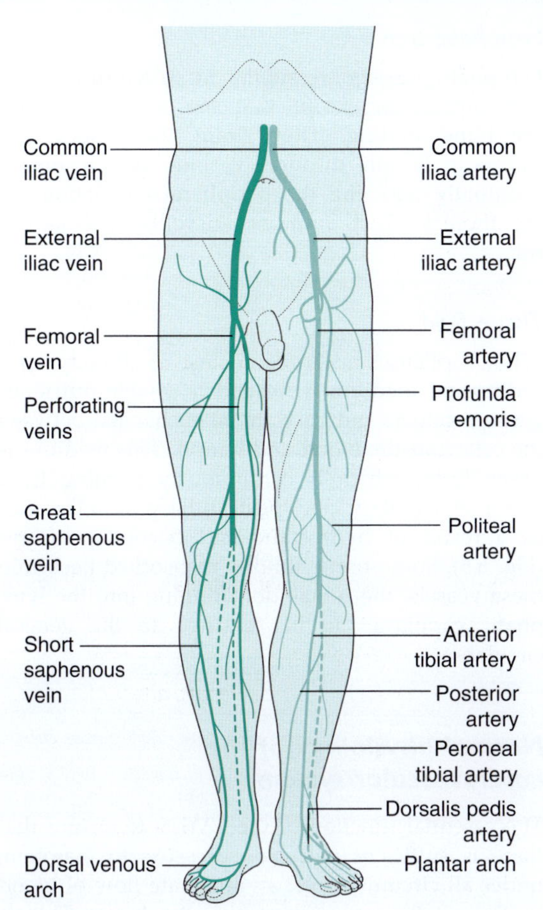

Figure 6.2 Anatomy of the major arterial and venous circulations in the lower limb.

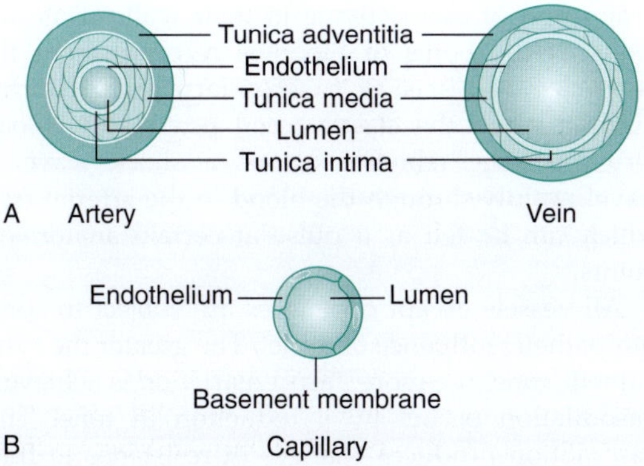

Figure 6.3 **A** Cross-section through an artery and vein showing tunica intima, media and adventitia **B** Cross-section through a capillary. Note the relative proportions of wall thickness in the artery and vein and the single cell thick capillary.

Table 6.1 Anatomy of peripheral vessels

Vessel	*Diameter*	*Wall thickness*
Aorta	25 mm	2 mm
Artery	4 mm	1 mm
Arteriole	30 μm	20 μm
Capillary	6 μm	1 μm
Venule	20 μm	2 μm
Vein	5 mm	500 μm
Vena cava	30 mm	1.5 mm

Venous tree

Blood is drained from the tissue beds by venules, which join to form the veins, a system with larger capacitance than the arteries. The three layers seen in the arterial wall are also present in veins but the proportions differ, as can be seen in Figure 6.3A. Veins are found either in the superficial fascia or deep to the muscle. Communicating veins allow drainage from the superficial to deep veins. The vascular endothelium is specialised to form semilunar valves. These prevent backflow of blood and are especially important in the perforating veins. The systemic veins of the lower limb drain into the inferior vena cava and return the deoxygenated blood back to the heart.

Capillary bed

Networks of capillaries link the arterioles and venules. They are the smallest and most numerous vessel, having only a thin-walled endothelium (Fig. 6.3B). Capillaries facilitate delivery of oxygen and nutrients to local tissues and no cell is far from a capillary bed. Precapillary sphincters in short vessels called metarterioles control capillary bed perfusion. Capillaries can be bypassed by arterio-venous (AV) anastomoses or 'shunts' which are vessels forming a direct link between an arteriole and a venule (Fig. 6.4A). At cutaneous sites exposed to extremes of temperature, such as fingertips, apices of toes, nose and earlobes, the AV anastomoses are numerous and form specialised structures under the nail beds called glomus bodies or Sucquet–Hoyer canals (Fig. 6.4B). Shunting of blood from the superficial to deep, thus bypassing cutaneous regions, helps to preserve core body temperature.

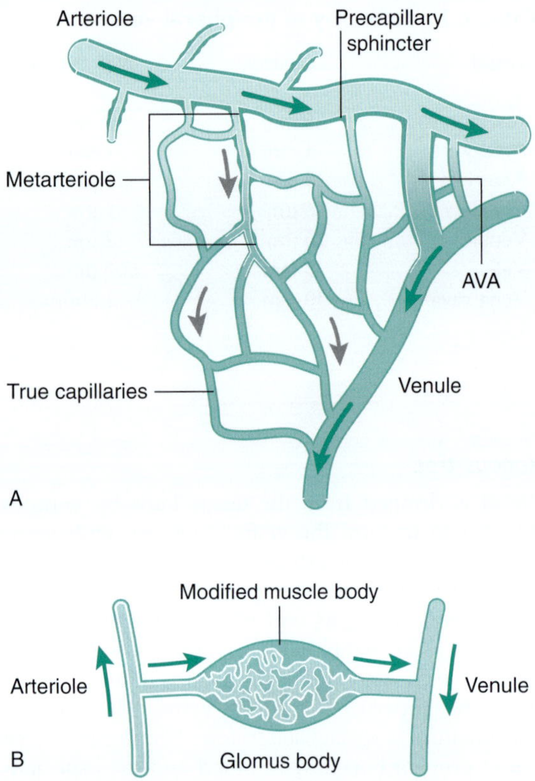

Figure 6.4 **A** Diagram of the microcirculation showing an arteriole and a venule connected by an arteriovenous anastomosis (AVA) and a capillary network. The AVA is a shorter, tortuous, muscular vessel of a larger calibre. The capillary network comprises metarterioles, which have a muscular coat, and the distal portion of the capillary network, which consists solely of endothelial cells **B** The specialised AVA under the nail bed (glomus body).

Microcirculation

The smaller diameter vessels collectively form the microcirculation.

Collaterals

Most microcirculations are served by more than one branch of the arterial tree. These parallel branches are called collaterals and may anastomose freely or hardly at all, the degree of communication varying from tissue to tissue. The lack of anastomoses in the coronary circulation is responsible for the catastrophic effects of an occlusion in the left coronary artery.

Lymphatic tree

Lymphatic vessels are similar in structure to veins and capillaries, except that the smallest vessels are blind ending. They drain the tissues and transport lymph through various lymph nodes, eventually rejoining the peripheral circulation via the thoracic duct. Immune surveillance is a key role.

Tissue fluid

While capillaries bring blood close to all body cells, a diffusion medium is needed to enable nutrients, waste products and gases to be exchanged between the cells and the blood and lymph. This medium is tissue fluid, which is continuously forming from blood at capillary and postcapillary venular sites as a result of hydrostatic and oncotic pressures (Fig. 6.5). Some tissue fluid is reabsorbed back into these vessels, the remainder draining into the lymphatic capillaries to be returned to the general circulation.

Normal physiology of the cardiovascular system

The essential function of the CVS is to ensure that there is sufficient perfusion pressure to maintain, under all circumstances, an adequate flow of blood to the vital organs, especially the brain. This is achieved by alteration of the rate and force of contraction of the myocardium and by varying the diameter throughout the peripheral circulation.

The aorta and pulmonary arteries have a large proportion of elastic tissue in their walls. This distends as the bolus of blood is received from the ventricles and acts as a secondary pump during diastole when the elastic recoil propels the blood forwards. The rebound causes a shock wave to travel rapidly through the blood in the arterial tree, which can be felt as a pulse at certain anatomical points.

All vessels except capillaries are subject to some sympathetic influence or 'tone'. The greater the sympathetic tone, the more vasoconstriction is achieved. Vasodilation occurs by a reduction in tone. This vasomotion produces changes in resistance to flow (peripheral resistance) and thus modifications in the work the heart has to do (afterload). The greatest effect is produced in the arterioles, which allow the CVS to control distribution of blood and, together with the heart, form the effector organs for blood pressure homeostasis.

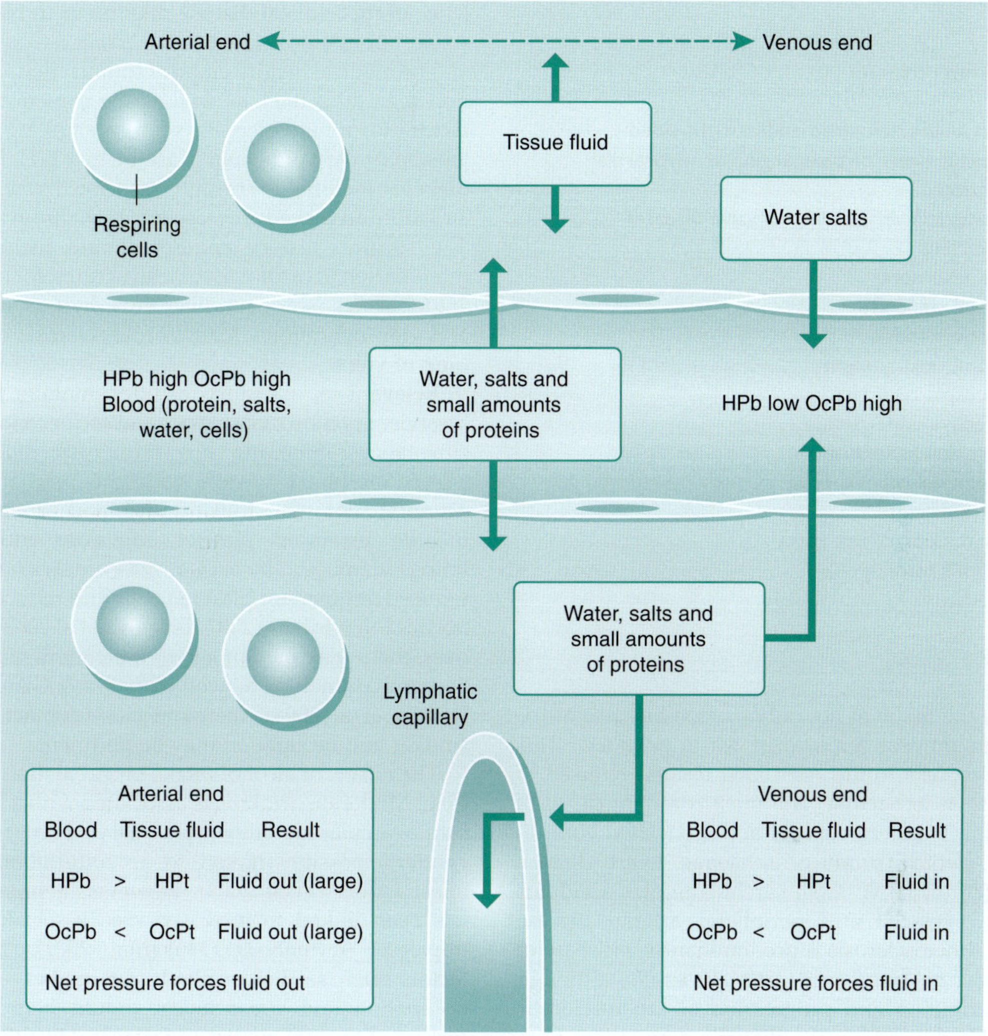

Figure 6.5 The process of formation and reabsorption of tissue fluid in an ideal capillary. Movement of fluid in and out of the capillary will vary according to the precise balance of pressures along the capillary at any one time.

The vascular assessment

VIDEO

The assessment of each part of the vascular tree includes the following:

- History, current medication and lifestyle factors
- Symptoms
- Signs
- Clinical tests
- Hospital/laboratory tests.

General overview of the cardiovascular system

Central problems such as congestive heart failure, ischaemic heart disease (angina and/or myocardial infarction), as well as systemic problems such as the anaemias may all influence the circulation to and from the lower limb (Box 6.1).

History and medication

History taking is discussed in detail in Chapter 5. Any factors which compromise tissue perfusion will

Box 6.1 Cardiac conditions which may affect lower limb perfusion

- Heart failure: left-sided and/or right-sided
- Ischaemic heart disease: angina or myocardial infarction
- Rheumatic fever (leading to valve disease)
- Myocarditis
- Valve disorders:
  - mitral stenosis
  - aortic stenosis
  - mitral regurgitation
  - tricuspid regurgitation
  - infective endocarditis
- Congenital heart disease:
  - septal defects
  - valve defects
  - coarctation of the aorta
  - Fallot's tetralogy

deprive the tissue of not only oxygen but also nutrients and prevent removal of waste products. This causes hypoxia to the associated tissues, referred to clinically as ischaemia. The most common cause of ischaemia is atherosclerosis and associated complications, which produce ischaemic heart disease (IHD) (coronary vessels), cerebrovascular accidents (cerebral vessels) and peripheral arterial disease (PAD). Atherosclerosis is predominantly a disease of large and medium-sized arterial vessels, although the distribution and progression of atherosclerotic disease is different in the diabetic population, with some small arteries affected (Aboyans et al 2006). Prognosis is thought to rely more on the predisposition of plaque erosion and/or rupture, than on the extent of atheromatous disease (Falk et al 1995, Libby 2001).

The presence of atheromatous disease anywhere in the body should alert the clinician to consider atherosclerosis in other areas, that is, the presence of angina may predict atherosclerosis in the vessels supplying the lower limb (Fisicaro 2003). The segments between the descending aorta and the popliteal artery are most likely to develop such disease. Below the level of the knee, the vessels are small arteries, which are generally not affected by clinically relevant atherosclerosis in the non-diabetic population. However, the majority of studies performed have been in the Caucasian population, and an extensive review of PAD and ethnicity indicated that prevalence of more distal disease may occur in black and Asian populations (Hobbs et al 2003).

The medical history enquiry should elicit information regarding IHD, as well as the presence of risk factors for atherosclerosis, such as smoking, hypertension or dyslipidaemia (Case history 6.1). Primary diabetes mellitus is strongly associated with earlier and more advanced atherosclerosis (Kallio et al 2003). The surgical history enquiry should include any intervention to cardiovascular structures, for example angioplasties (coronary, iliac, etc.), bypass surgeries and vein operations, for example sclerosis or stripping of veins.

Relevant social history includes smoking, alcohol, lifestyle, psychosocial stresses and socioeconomic circumstances. Smoking has numerous deleterious effects on blood vessels with the mechanism of action(s) not yet fully understood. Pathologies include increased platelet adhesion, endothelial lining damage, increased vasoconstriction and reduced antioxidant plasma levels and reduced fibrinolysis (Newby et al 2001, Tsuchiya et al 2002). Moreover, there may be damage to the endothelial lining by passive smoking as well (Barnoya & Glantz 2005, Otsuka et al 2001), therefore close contact with a smoker and occupation may be pertinent.

The effects of alcohol intake on circulation are less clear. Moderate drinking is associated with a lowered cardiovascular mortality (Mukamal et al 2005) for both genders, possibly linked to an anti-inflammatory effect (Albert et al 2003). However, a high intake has been linked to increased risk, associated with impaired fibrinolysis (Mukamal 2001). Lifestyle factors such as diet (e.g. salt, fat intake), exercise, occupation and stress levels should help form a picture of general mental and physical health, mobility and risk levels. Socioeconomic risk factors for cardiovascular disease include low socioeconomic status (Steptoe et al 2002) and low education levels (Grazuleviciene et al 2002).

Drugs may indicate cardiovascular disease is present (e.g. diuretic therapy), or influence circulation as a side effect. Many of the antihypertensive drug regimens such as diuretics, beta-blockers and calcium antagonists can affect the peripheral circulation. Diuretics act on various parts of the nephron in the kidney to reduce water and salt reabsorption, initially reducing preload and cardiac output and later affecting peripheral resistance, with both mechanisms reducing blood pressure. Beta-blockers prevent the stimulatory action of endogenous catecholamines on the heart, again reducing cardiac output and blood pressure. Even selective agents, such as atenolol, may cause some peripheral vasoconstriction. Calcium antagonists act by interfering with the process of vascular smooth muscle contraction, reducing peripheral resistance and so reducing blood pressure. Some act more peripherally than centrally, for example amlodipine and have some vasodilatory influence (currently not licensed for PAD).

Lipid-lowering drugs indicate risk factors for thrombotic disease, given the relationship between dyslipidaemia (high low-density lipoprotein (LDL), low high-density lipoprotein (HDL), high triglycerides, low apolipoproteins) formation of atheroma and cardiovascular disease (Hobbs 2003). The most common are the statin and fibrate drug groups. Anti-platelet drugs are most commonly taken for IHD (to prevent and/or to manage), and are also used for management of transient ischaemic attacks, stroke, PAD, and after some vascular surgeries e.g. angioplasty stunt. Taking an anti-platelet indicates risk of, or the presence of thrombotic disease and should alert the clinician to enquire about the nature of the problem. The most common drug is aspirin, but clopidogrel and dipyridamole are also used. Anticoagulation therapy, usually warfarin (non-acute), indicates cardiovascular disease such as atrial fibrillation, valve disease/replacement, history of deep vein thrombosis or pulmonary embolism, and it is sometimes used for the management of stroke.

Case history 6.1

A West Indian man aged 74 years presented with hard skin on the balls of his feet and a burning sensation. His medical and social history revealed that he had an aortic aneurysm resected at age 72, and he was a smoker. His brother has type 2 diabetes and he thinks he was last checked for diabetes about a year ago. He was taking bendroflumethiazide (bendrofluazide) 25 mg od to control hypertension, aspirin 75 mg od, atorvastatin 10 mg od and co-codamol 15/500 (osteoarthritis and back pain) as required.

Symptomatic history revealed the burning occurred mainly at rest and in bed and was similar in severity in both feet, but worse in the toes. There was no history of injury or previous ulceration. Mobility was poor due to osteoarthritis in both knees making a diagnosis of claudication difficult. A vascular assessment found telangiectases and haemosiderosis with normal skin texture and condition in both lower limbs, apart from dry skin. Varicose veins were present in the right leg, and hair was absent from legs and the feet, both of which felt cold. The fatty pad under the metatarsal heads was reduced and diffuse callus present with general plantar forefoot inflammation. All lower extremity pulses were palpable, regularly irregular with reduced PT pulses. His blood pressure (BP) was 145/96 mmHg. The ankle–brachial pressure index (ABPI) in the right leg was 0.9 and in the left leg was 0.75. Buerger's test was positive for the left leg, with a flush occurring after 30 seconds.

Differential diagnoses for the pain are rest pain (although not present all the time and not 'severe'), popliteal aneurysm (can occur bilaterally), pain from inflammation associated with the callosities or unprotected metatarsal heads (you would expect this to feel worse on walking), neuropathic pain from an undiagnosed cause, for example family history of diabetes, so he could have latent diabetes, or neuropathic symptoms as a side effect from the atorvastatin. Spinal stenoses can also cause burning feet as part of 'root pain'. Combinations could include rest pain which is not felt as severe because of co-morbid sensory neuropathy. Venous disease can cause 'restless legs', which can be reported as 'burning feet/legs'.

The findings imply there is an arterial deficit, with venous signs being relatively mild. The reduced PT pulses, left ABPI result and positive Buerger's test all imply femoropopliteal (or distal) stenoses. No popliteal mass was found. His risk factors for atherosclerotic disease are hypertension, history of aortic aneurysm, smoking and raised lipids (as per the atorvastatin). An aortic aneurysm does increase the risk for popliteal aneurysm, hence its inclusion in the differential diagnosis. A West Indian background may predispose to more distal atherosclerosis, that is infragenicular.

The case warrants a referral to the general practitioner (GP) for modification of risk factors, namely blood pressure control (still higher than ideal despite the drug therapy, but only a one off reading) and help to stop smoking. A check-up for latent diabetes, a second opinion regarding suspicion of peripheral vascular disease and assistance with pain management are also required. In this scenario in the UK, it is not mandatory for a GP to refer on for a vascular opinion. Improved lifestyle and pain control should help mobility and encourage the development of a collateral circulation. If tissue viability becomes seriously threatened, angioplasty or bypass interventions may be considered.

Central symptoms

Angina and myocardial infarction (MI)

Pain in the chest on exercise or other stress indicates inadequate blood supply to the myocardium. The pain of angina can vary from a mild discomfort to an intense crushing sensation. It may radiate into the left arm or to the lower jaw. Unstable angina may be prodromal to an acute heart attack.

The chief distinguishing feature of an acute MI, as opposed to an angina pectoris attack is that the latter lasts only minutes and is usually relieved within 5 minutes of rest or by sublingual glyceryl trinitrate. There are many other causes of chest pain and while few closely mimic angina, indigestion and other gastrointestinal disorders may be confused with angina (Ch. 5). It is noteworthy that diabetic autonomic neuropathy, as well as age can mask symptoms of IHD, and silent heart attacks do occur (Fornengo et al 2006).

Breathlessness (dyspnoea)

Shortness of breath (SOB) is an important cardiac symptom/sign (it may be evident while in your surgery), as well as reflecting respiratory disease. It is a typical feature of angina and heart failure (left-sided or congestive).

Palpitations

The awareness (usually unpleasant) of one's own heart beat can point to a cardiac arrhythmia. However, this is a common symptom, which often has no cause, or is associated with emotional stress or stimulatory substances, such as caffeine.

Fatigue

Significant cardiovascular disease, for example heart failure, or severe anaemia will cause fatigue, since muscle and brain tissue will be hypoxic.

Signs

Oedema

Any factor which interferes with the normal process of tissue fluid formation and reabsorption may cause fluid to accumulate in the tissues. This is referred to as oedema, which will be observable in the peripheral tissues as swelling. It can be due to local factors, such as trauma or occluded drainage vessels, or to central factors such as right sided or congestive heart failure or renal disease. An important exacerbating factor is the renin–angiotensin–aldosterone system, which is triggered by a low cardiac output. This will cause renal retention of salt and water, thus imposing an even greater load on the failing heart.

Cyanosis

Central cyanosis is the bluish discoloration of lips, tongue and mucous membranes and indicates that arterial blood is inadequately oxygenated. It may be due either to defects in the pump such as a congenital hole in the heart, cardiac failure, or to deficiencies of ventilation such as chronic obstructive airways disease. Severe cardiac and respiratory failure will also cause peripheral cyanosis.

Pallor

A pale appearance, noticeable in the face, palmar or plantar areas, the conjunctiva or nail bed may indicate anaemia, but this is not a sensitive observation (Nardone et al 1990).

The tongue

Abnormalities associated with the anaemias include inflammation of the tongue (glossitis), which may appear smooth and either pale (pernicious anaemia) or bright red (vitamin B group deficiency).

The nails

Iron-deficiency anaemia may cause koilonychia (spoon-shaped nails), a sign also associated with connective tissue disease (Fawcett et al 2004). Clubbing of the finger nails may be due to subacute infective endocarditis or congenital cyanotic heart disease. It is also associated with a variety of other, primarily respiratory causes (Fawcett et al 2004). Splinter haemorrhages appear as subungual small brown/black splinters and can be associated with vasculitis (inflammation of a blood vessel(s)), although trauma is a common cause. If pathological, a local cause such as a digital septic thrombosis should be considered, as should widespread involvement of arteries of all organs, including coronary, splanchnic and cerebral, which can occur, for example in aggressive rheumatoid arthritis. Splinter haemorrhages may also indicate subacute bacterial endocarditis (Fawcett et al 2004).

Clinical tests

Heart rate and rhythm

Heart rate and rhythm are normally assessed by taking the pulse at the wrist (radial artery), with a normal adult resting rate at between 60 and 80 beats per minute. Arrhythmias are abnormal heart rates/rhythms and can be physiological or pathological, depending on the cause. A change in pace, but where sinus rhythm is sustained, may reflect a physiological response by the pacemaker for the heart, the sinoatrial node. Heart rates of less than 60 beats per minute are classified as bradycardia and those over 100 beats per minute as tachycardia. Athletes are an example of physiological bradycardia, whereas the bradycardia due to a complete heart block in the atrioventricular septum is pathological. Thyroid hormones, if present in excess, increase the affinity of beta$_1$-receptors to catecholamines and so induce tachycardia, as seen in hyperthyroidism. Rhythm is denoted as regularly regular (sinus rhythm), regularly irregular (a repeating irregularity, for example ectopic beats) or irregularly irregular, for example atrial fibrillation.

Pulse amplitude may be assessed centrally via the carotid artery. Small volume may reflect vessel stenosis, tachycardia and cardiac failure. A large amplitude or 'bounding' pulse is a pathological finding, with causes including a high output state, for example thyrotoxicosis or aortic valve regurgitation.

Blood pressure

Systemic hypertension has no known cause in 95% of cases (essential hypertension) and is usually asymptomatic unless very severe. Hypertension may be defined as persistent raised blood pressure above 140/90 mmHg (National Institute for Health and Clinical Excellence (NICE) 2006). High blood pressure can damage vital organs, such as the eye and kidney and, owing to blood vessel damage, MI, stroke and peripheral vascular disease may ensue.

Manual (see Box 6.2) or automated equipment may be used to obtain readings, with equally good repeatability, but with the precaution that differences in readings between devices may seem clinically relevant (Sims et al 2005). The British Hypertension Society recommend several readings are taken before 'persistent' high blood pressure is diagnosed. It is now commonplace for people to monitor their own blood pressure at home or have ambulatory blood pressure monitoring via a 24 hour tape, thus obtaining a more accurate mean value taken over 24 hours. The upper normal limit is lower in children and higher in elderly people. Assessment also includes determination of risk factors e.g. bodyweight, salt intake etc.

Box 6.2 Taking blood pressure – manual technique

The patient should be rested and seated comfortably with one arm flexed at the elbow and resting at heart level on a flat surface. It is conventional to use the right arm as the best representation of central blood pressure:

- The brachial pulse should be palpated.
- A sphygmomanometer cuff is wrapped around the arm, 2–3 cm above the elbow crease.
- The pressure cuff should be inflated until the brachial pulse can no longer be palpated. The value of this pressure should be noted and the pressure released rapidly.*
- The diaphragm of the stethoscope is placed on the brachial artery in the antecubital fossa and the pressure cuff re-inflated to the same value as previously obtained. Nothing will be heard at this stage. All vessels will be occluded so that no blood can flow through the artery.
- The pressure should be released slowly and steadily (2 mm/s), watching the needle on the manometer face. As the pressure falls to the level of the patient's systolic blood pressure a knocking sound will be heard in the stethoscope. At this stage the pressure in the cuff is sufficient to prevent flow of blood during diastole, but not during systole, so that systolic flow can be heard. The value when the first sound returns is recorded as the systolic blood pressure.
- The pressure should continue to be released. The sounds will first increase then decrease in intensity and finally disappear. At this stage the pressure in the cuff is insufficient to occlude the artery at any stage in the cardiac cycle and this point is taken as the value for the diastolic blood pressure.
- The practitioner should ensure that the cuff is deflated completely.
- The mean of three recordings should be taken.

Pitfalls

- The rubber tubing may wear out.
- The valve may be faulty.
- The cuff may be the wrong size for the diameter of the limb.
- The arm may not be at heart level.

*With experience many clinicians will guess the point of cut-off for inflation and if when the cuff is released, no sound is still heard, the cuff is inflated further.

Clinical examination of the heart

Useful information is gleaned from examining the precordium. Techniques of palpation and listening with a stethoscope are used to detect abnormalities such as flow disturbances, for example valve regurgitation and murmurs.

Blood tests

Assessment of cardiovascular problems may be assisted by lipid profiles and a full blood count (indicating anaemias, platelet disorders, infection). Following an MI, necrotic myocardial cells produce markers of cardiac damage such as troponin and creative kinase (peaks 24 hr post infection).

Hospital tests

These are performed to confirm diagnosis, establish extent of disease and to identify the exact site(s) of a problem as a prerequisite to medical and/or surgical management.

Non-invasive imaging

- Chest X-ray
  A plain radiograph of the chest may show enlargement of the heart, pericardial effusion and calcification of heart structures and vessels.
- Electrocardiogram (ECG)
  The electrical activity of the heart is recorded using limb and chest leads attached to the skin. Many pathologies of the heart, such as MI or ventricular enlargement in a failing heart, will alter the normal PQRS waveform. Exercise may be used to highlight problems not apparent at rest.
- Echocardiography
  This uses reflected ultrasound waves to construct an image of the heart, which can inform about some structural, for example valve disease, and functional abnormalities, for example cardiomyopathies. Anatomical barriers restrict full access to the heart. Haemodynamics can be observed by Doppler imaging, which may be enhanced by 'stress' via exercise or cardiac stimulants, or by introducing contrast agents.
- Cardiac magnetic resonance imaging (MRI)
  Magnetic fields and radiowaves (non-ionising radiation) in conjunction with an ECG are used to obtain cardiac images (chambers and flow dynamics) which can help diagnose congenital heart disease, valve pathologies, abnormal masses and pericardial disease. This may be performed with or without contrast material. Intravenous gadolinium can be used to highlight blood vessels. MRI cannot visualise vessel calcification.
- Cardiovascular computed tomography (CT)
  Ultrafast slices are taken to overcome the movement of the beating heart. It is helpful to assess coronary calcification and thus the risk level for coronary artery disease.

Invasive imaging techniques

- Coronary angiography
  A radiopaque catheter is introduced into a vein in the groin or arm and threaded through to the heart under real time X-ray images. Contrast material can then be injected, allowing visualisation of the coronary vessels by X-ray fluoroscopy, illustrating regions of stenosis. Chamber pressures may be measured and blood samples taken for information on oxygen saturation and metabolite levels, for example lactate. People can react to the contrast material and there is a small risk of other serious complications, for example MI or cerebrovascular accident (CVA). Image enhancement by 'subtracting' a series of images taken before contrast injection, removes the non-iodinated background structures and improves image quality (digital subtraction angiography).
- Intravascular ultrasound
  Specially designed long, thin catheters attached to ultrasound equipment allows visualisation of the lumen and subluminal surfaces. This can help assess the stage and vulnerability of plaques, as well as check on stents after surgery.
- Nuclear scans
  The volume of blood available for the myocardium and myocardial function may be assessed by nuclear imaging. Injected radiopharmaceutical agents, such as thallium-201 or technetium-99m, are taken up by the myocardial tissue, and images are taken using gamma cameras or positron emission tomography techniques.

Peripheral vascular system

Peripheral vascular disease (PVD) in the singular is often taken to mean the manifestations of atherosclerosis distal to the aortic arch. PAD or peripheral arterial occlusive disease (PAOD) are more accurate terms. The plural term peripheral vascular diseases refers to all anatomically relevant vascular pathologies. It is important to distinguish between an impoverished arterial supply, reduced venous drainage and impaired lymphatic drainage, although more than one pathology may be present.

Many authors have emphasised the central role of the clinical examination, which when performed competently, can provide information both sensitive and specific for PAD diagnoses (Boyko et al 1997, Criqui et al 1992). Of the non-invasive tests, the ABPI remains the global gold standard (Collins et al 2006, Hiatt et al 1995, Hirsch et al 2001, McDermott et al 2000, Newman et al 1993). Invasive tests are usually reserved for presurgical evaluation. The non-invasive assessment yields information to help confirm the presence of PAD, determine the extent and distribution of stenoses, monitor changes following interventions and/or over time, and make clinical judgements regarding healing potential. Despite the poor prognostic outlook and the plethora of clinical methods applied to PAD assessment, it remains under-diagnosed (Hirsch et al 2001).

One of the most important indicators for undertaking an assessment of lower limb circulation is the condition of diabetes mellitus. While the approach is broadly the same, it has been demonstrated that the reliability of key tests such as the ABPI, the toe brachial index and pulse waveform analysis may be compromised, particularly in the presence of diabetic neuropathy (Williams et al 2005). This will influence the interpretation of the test results.

Table 6.2 Causes of arterial insufficiency in the foot

Acute	*Extrinsic*: tight clothing tourniquet plaster cast trauma frostbite immersion foot *Intrinsic*: thrombosis embolus ruptured aneurysm oedema
Transient (usually lead to acute problems but may progress to chronic)	Raynaud's phenomenon Chilblains Hereditary cold fingers
Chronic	Atherosclerosis Vasculitis Thromboangiitis obliterans (Buerger's disease) Arteriolosclerosis?

Arterial insufficiency

Medical history

Conditions which can affect the arterial supply to the lower limb can be viewed as acute, chronic or transient (Table 6.2). Most arterial problems affecting the lower limb are chronic and involve the progressive narrowing of peripheral arteries, most commonly the aortoiliac bifurcation and the iliac segments. While this can result in claudication pain and to varying degrees poor tissue viability, only a small percentage of people (1–6% in 5 years, rising to 18% in 10 years) require surgery (Andreozzi & Martini 2004). Up to 5% develop critical ischaemia requiring amputation (Dormandy et al 1989, McDaniel & Cronenwett 1989), although this figure may double over 10 years (Andreozzi & Martini 2004). Age-related and generalised vessel disease is referred to as arteriosclerosis, involving thickening and hardening of the vessel wall.

The most common cause of PAD is atherosclerosis. This is a pathological process involving formation of a fatty plaque (atheroma) in the subintimal space of large and medium-sized arteries (Murphie 2001a). The atheroma itself may protrude into the lumen and reduce or obstruct flow. However, the greatest risk arises from predisposition of the overlying fibrous cap to ulcerate, promoting thrombus formation. This may cause further narrowing (stenosis) or even complete blockage of the vessel. In addition, fragments of the thrombus can embolise and be swept away, causing obstruction further down the arterial tree. Global risk factors for systemic atherosclerosis are similar and recognised in descending order as hypertension, hypercholesterolaemia and diabetes, with obesity and tobacco usage being other key factors (Bhatt et al 2006). A clinical history that indicates atherosclerotic complications assists in the assessment of vascular health. Angina, MI and coronary or peripheral bypass surgery all indicate the extent and stage of atherosclerotic disease. Aneurysm must also be taken into consideration, as the most frequent underlying pathology is atherosclerosis (Fig. 6.6). Furthermore, an association exists between aortic and popliteal aneurysms, so this must always be checked.

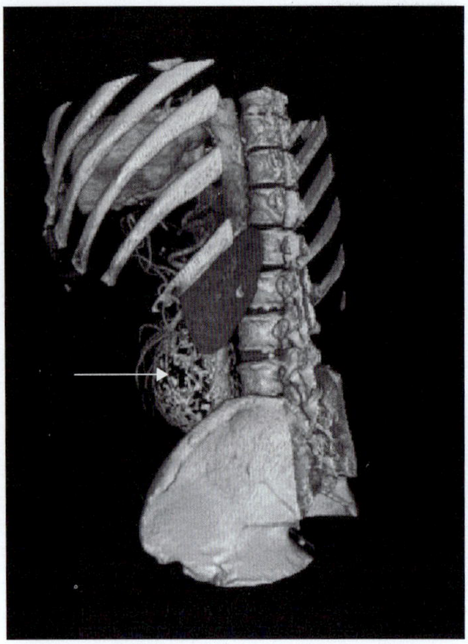

Figure 6.6 CT anteriogram showing a large abdominal aortic aneurysm.

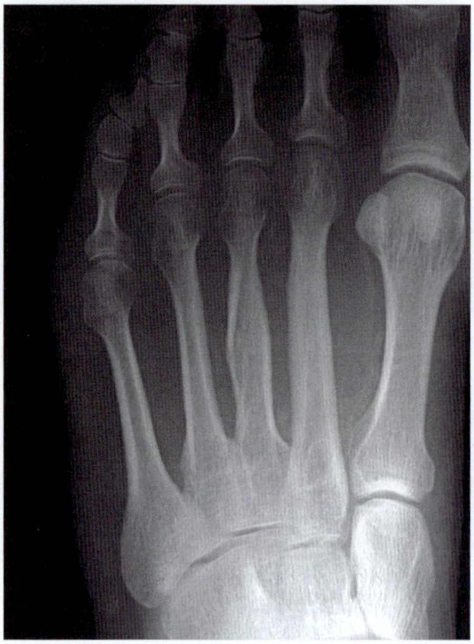

Figure 6.8 Vessel calcification (dorsalis pedis).

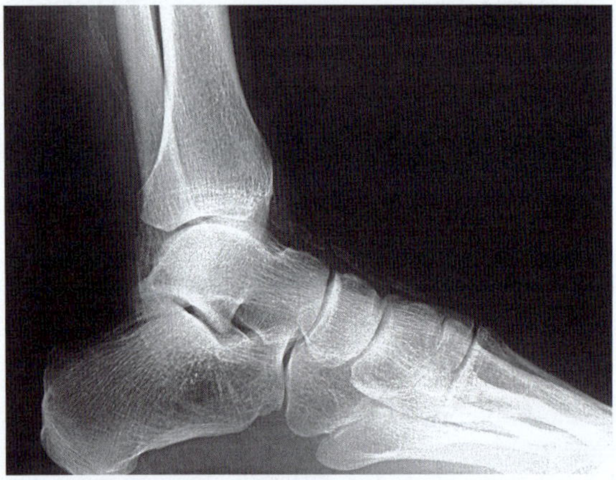

Figure 6.7 Vessel calcification (posterior tibial).

The clinician should be aware of pathological vascular calcification, as high levels in coronary vessels are linked to an increased risk of sudden death and MI (Greenland et al 2004, O'Rourke et al 2000). The clinical relevance in the lower limbs is poorly understood, but there are implications for test selection (see the sections on ABPI and toe pressures) and management of vasculopathies. Vessel wall calcification (Fig. 6.7) is most commonly seen in advanced atherosclerotic plaques, giving the 'sclerotic' or hardening component of the plaque in the subintimal space. The resulting rigidity will alter vascular resistance and elasticity. Normally mechanisms are in place to prevent abnormal calcium deposition in non-osseous tissues, for example via protective matrix proteins such as osteopontin. More research is needed to discover the pathogenesis of calcific damage.

A distinct process of dystrophic calcification can affect the smooth muscle layer of the vessel wall, often referred to as medial arterial calcification or Mönckeberg's sclerosis. The condition is associated with atrophy of the smooth muscle arising from autonomic neuropathy (Forst et al 1995, Gilbey et al 1989) and it follows that this is seen with age (Elliott & McGrath 1994) and diabetes (Chantelau et al 1997, Edmonds 2000, Watkins & Edmonds 1983). It generally affects arteries not associated with atherosclerosis, for example distal small arteries (Figs 6.7, 6.8) and breast and thyroid vessels, although it is found in the aorta. One study on a population of people with type 2 diabetes found medial sclerosis in 17% and intimal-type calcifications in 23% (Niskanen et al 1994). The calcium deposits are laid down upon the circumferential smooth muscle and it is this process which is attributed to non-compressible vessels in the diabetic population (Edmonds et al 1982). Atherosclerotic and medial wall calcification may coexist and both contribute to rigid and inelastic vessel walls.

Primary diabetes mellitus has deleterious effects on arteries, accelerating the atherosclerotic process and worsening the prognosis for cardiovascular morbidity and mortality (Kallio et al 2003). PAD is twice as likely to occur in the diabetic population (Wattanakit et al 2005). Amputation rates (Aksoy et al 2004, McAlpine et al 2005) and mortality associated with PAD are also increased (Leibson et al 2004). The pattern of diabetic atherosclerotic lesions varies from the non-diabetic population, in that extensive involvement of vessel segments is seen, as well as more distal occlusions, for example the posterior tibial artery (van der Feen et al 2002). Such multilevel disease not only has implications for tissue viability but also presents major problems for management (Faries et al 2001).

Renal disease has a number of effects on blood vessels and as a frequent complication of diabetes mellitus, kidney disease poses an additional threat to peripheral perfusion and tissue viability when these coexist. Medial arterial calcification is accelerated with significant renal disease (Leskinen et al 2002) and this is likely to be related to failure of calcium and phosphate regulation. Impaired vitamin D conversion and hyperparathyroidism will also contribute to disturbed mineral metabolism.

There appears to be little evidence for atherosclerosis in the microcirculation (Murphie 2001b). Although hyalinisation (arteriolosclerosis), thickening of basement membranes and functional abnormalities of small vessels have been observed, these changes occur mainly in renal and retinal vessels, and are not considered to have major effects on the vascular status of the foot. However, in the diabetic population, there has been considerable focus on abnormalities of the microcirculation, since this is suspected to contribute to the non-healing wound.

Less common causes of PAD include thromboangiitis obliterans, vasculitis, vasospastic disorders and embolic disease. Thromboangiitis obliterans is characterised by inflammatory changes in small and medium-sized arteries and veins. It mainly affects young men and there is a very strong association with smoking. All signs and symptoms of arterial ischaemia and superficial phlebitis of the hands and feet may be present. Eventually, distal necrosis occurs.

Vasculitis is inflammation of blood vessels seen in a large number of rheumatic and connective tissue diseases. Any vessel can be affected, with the most serious consequences being in the arterial tree, resulting in partial or total occlusion. Some of the conditions associated with vasculitis are:

- rheumatoid arthritis
- systemic lupus erythematosus (SLE)
- polymyositis
- dermatomyositis
- systemic sclerosis
- polyarteritis nodosa
- giant-cell arteritis
- erythema nodosum
- Henoch–Schönlein purpura.

Raynaud's disease and phenomenon (when linked to another disease) affects approximately 5% of the population and, in severe cases, may produce digital atrophy, necrosis and ulceration (Case history 6.2). Chilblains are also thought to rise from increased vasoreactivity to non-freezing cold. Arterial emboli can be composed of any obstructive body that lodges in the smaller vessels of the arterial tree, causing ischaemia distally. The most common embolus is formed by a thrombus fragment, for example from the heart during atrial fibrillation, from an aortic aneurysm or following an MI. Where smaller arteries branch or narrow, impaction occurs and in the lower limb, vulnerable sites include the common femoral bifurcation and the popliteal trifurcation.

Symptoms

An acute occlusion, for example femoral embolism, produces signs and symptoms known as the six Ps:

- Pain
- Pallor
- Pulselessness
- Paraesthesia
- Paralysis
- Perishing cold.

If the occlusion is prolonged (more than 6–8 hours), the tissues eventually suffer irreversible damage and this stage can be recognised by mottling, muscle tenderness, motor or sensory deficit and necrosis. Prompt embolectomy is required for limb salvage. Amputation may be required (Campbell et al 1998). Rarely, fat emboli may lodge in small/microvascular peripheral vessels causing vasculitis and necrosis, for example following vascular surgery. This can be seen in the foot.

Case history 6.2

A 35-year-old Caucasian woman presented in winter complaining of numbness and pain in her fingers and toes. Her general health is good, she gave up smoking 3 years ago (20/day for 12 years) and she drinks 30–40 units/week, believing this to assist her circulation. She denies taking recreational drugs. She takes the contraceptive pill and relates a long history of poor circulation from her teenage years. Her father has very poor circulation and a variety of health problems, but she does not know the cause. Occupation is in administration. She presently lives alone, having recently separated from her partner. Her footwear is inadequate for winter, and general hygiene is poor.

Symptomatic history revealed long-standing problems with fingers that turn white and numb in the cold and small wounds on the tips of fingers and toes which follow episodes of cold exposure. Recently one of the toes became infected, prompting her to seek help. She has joint pain in the hands and feet.

Generally she is thin and pale. Examination of the lower limbs revealed pale skin and cold toes. The lesser toes were held in flexion deformities. No hairs were present. The skin was tight, shiny and smooth. There were small, painful ulcers on the apices of the third and fourth toes bilaterally. One ulcer showed signs of infection. Pedal pulses were palpable but feeble. Popliteal pulses were within normal limits. ABPI at the dorsalis pedis artery for right and left foot was 1.0 and 0.97, respectively. Leg elevation tests were negative. No joint changes in the hands were evident. The nails were thin and broken, with pale nail beds and small erythematous patches on the finger tips, but no ulceration.

Differential diagnoses include autoimmune disorders such as rheumatoid arthritis, systemic lupus erythematosus or systemic sclerosis, all of which may cause joint pain and deformities of the hands and feet and are linked to Raynaud's phenomenon and vasculitis. The third decade is associated with the onset of such autoimmune conditions. The flexion position of the toes and skin changes can arise from systemic sclerosis (scleroderma). Raynaud's disease can occur in isolation as well. Rarely female carriers of Fabry's disease can present with arteriopathies and there are also rare cases of Buerger's disease among female smokers. The family history can be helpful with regard to such conditions, although the history provided here was insufficient.

Some features of an anaemia were present, which could be relevant to an autoimmune diagnosis, or in isolation could contribute to poor healing and immunity. Alcoholic disease must be deliberated, since typically the units confessed to are at least half of what the real intake is. This may link into an anaemia from malabsorption and also the apparent self-neglect. Thromboses in the microvasculature could cause peripheral ulceration and risk factors for thrombophilia should be taken into account, in this case the use of the contraceptive pill. If drugs were being injected into the dorsal venous arch (used when proximal veins have been destroyed by chronic drug misuse), local vasculitis can also result.

The findings of this vascular examination are helpful to exclude macrovascular disease and certainly this would be unusual in this age group. There are features consistent with microvascular disease, suggestive of Raynaud's disease/phenomenon and/or vasculitis. Blood tests, including full blood count, liver function tests, autoantibodies and rheumatoid factor, are required to establish a diagnosis, with consideration for other thrombophilia markers, for example homocysteine levels.

Chronic PAD may share some of these signs and symptoms and certainly pain on walking (see intermittent claudication), at rest (see rest pain) and in the extremities, can arise from chronic ischaemia. However, PAD is asymptomatic in 80–93% of cases (Fowkes et al 1991, Newman et al 1993), with smoking and diabetes mellitus associated with a higher probability of symptom absence (Eason et al 2005). Pain may develop suddenly following thrombosis overlying a plaque, but if atherosclerosis has been present long-term, symptoms may be less severe than for an acute embolism, since collateral vessels will have formed. The following types of ischaemic pain can occur (also see Fontaine's classification (Table 6.3)).

Intermittent claudication

Just as angina pectoris indicates insufficient blood supply to the myocardium, so intermittent claudication indicates inadequate blood supply to the periphery. The deficiency will be accentuated on exercise, occurring at a reproducible distance (the claudication distance) with a characteristic cramping or aching pain. Sometimes the complaint will be tightness,

Table 6.3 Fontaine's classification of peripheral vascular disease

Stage	*Symptoms*
I	Occlusive arterial disease but no symptoms (due to collaterals)
2	Intermittent claudication
3	Ischaemic rest pain (usually worse at night, relieved by dependency)
4	Severe rest pain with ulceration/necrosis (gangrene)

Box 6.3 PAD distribution according to claudication symptoms

- Buttock and hip – aortoiliac disease
- Thigh – common femoral, external iliac or aortoiliac artery
- Upper two-thirds of the calf – superficial femoral artery
- Lower one-third of the calf – popliteal artery
- Foot claudication – tibial or peroneal artery

fatigue or burning in the affected muscle group. The exercising muscles have to respire anaerobically and produce metabolites which are not cleared by the blood. These cause ischaemic pain, which forces the patient to stop the activity. Resting for a few minutes reduces the amount of metabolites produced and allows the patient to continue walking for a further period. It is typical of claudication pain to subside within 10 minutes of rest. The distance walked before onset of the pain is a good indication of the severity of the condition, which may affect mobility and quality of life (Dumville et al 2004). Accurate assessment and diagnosis of claudication may be achieved using the Edinburgh claudication questionnaire (Leng & Fowkes 1992), which has a high sensitivity and specificity of 91% and 99%, respectively.

The region of the ischaemic muscle pain can indicate the site of the occlusion (see Box 6.3), with symptoms typically one level below the constriction. Calf pain is common (Buckenham 2003), with thigh, hip, and buttocks affected when more extensive proximal lesions are involved. Non-arterial sources of pain should be considered, for example arthritis, degenerative spinal disease, not only as part of the differential diagnoses but also because such conditions may mask the presence of symptomatic PAD (Newman et al 2001). It should be borne in mind that patients with neuropathy may not complain of intermittent claudication.

Night cramps

If the blood supply is more severely compromised, the removal of gravity assisted flow in bed can initiate night cramps. These may be alleviated by dropping the legs over the side of the bed. The warmth of the bedclothes increases the metabolic rate of the tissues and so increases their demand for oxygen; however, this cannot be met and produces cramp. Using gravity to aid flow and cooling the limb helps to reduce metabolic activity. Many people experience cramps and/or 'restless legs' (nocturnal and during the day) not attributable to any vascular cause. Venous disease may cause leg pain and night cramps (Kroger et al 2002, Saarinen et al 2005).

Rest pain

This is the most severe symptom of critical limb ischaemia, characterised by unremitting debilitating pain, often in the heel, toes or soles. Here the blood supply is inadequate even at rest, mobility is impaired and the peripheral tissues require gravity for flow, with pain aggravated by elevation and concordantly worse at night (Halperin 2002). Dependency can alleviate the pain (Braunwald 2001, Woods 1991) and patients may report they have to sleep in a chair. Differential diagnoses should include painful neuropathies and musculoskeletal disorders.

Observation

While an experienced practitioner can glean considerable information from simple observation, it is important not to rely on these observations alone, but to view them as part of the whole picture. The patient should be seated on a couch in a comfortably warm room.

Colour

Table 6.4 lists the range of colour changes seen in the lower limb and their significance.

Tissue viability

- Skin condition

  If arterial supply is poor, the skin may appear thin and fragile and is sometimes described as 'parchment-like'.

Table 6.4 Interpretation of colour changes in the lower limb

Colour	*Causes*
Pink	Healthy circulation
White/pale	Cold, anaemia, chilblains, Raynaud's phenomenon, cardiac failure
White below demarcation line	Severe ischaemia
Blue (peripheral cyanosis)	Cold, chilblains, Raynaud's phenomenon, venous stasis
Blue seen with central cyanosis	Cardiac/respiratory failure
Hazy blue	Infection, necrosis, bruising
Red	Heat, exercise, extreme cold (cold-induced vasodilation), inflammation, infection (cellulitis), chilblains, Raynaud's phenomenon
Brown	Haemosiderosis, necrosis, melanoma
Black	Bruising, shoe dye, necrosis, melanoma

- Skin appendages
  These may shrink and even disappear, leaving the skin without natural moisture from sebum and anhidrotic from loss of sweat gland activity. Hairs may be absent, but this is also a common finding in people with normal circulation.
- Atrophy
  In chronic situations atrophy (wastage) of soft tissue, including muscle, will also be present. This may be observed in the pulp of the digits, which may appear 'pencilled' or on the plantar surface of the foot. In severe limb ischaemia, muscle tone will be lost and the limb will appear lifeless (Figs 6.9, 6.10).

Ischaemic ulcers

An impaired peripheral circulation makes ulcers more likely to develop as the tissues are unable to withstand the normal daily stresses on the lower limb. The characteristics of the wound can assist in diagnosis of the circulatory problem, since ulcers caused by ischaemia differ in many respects from those caused by other deficiencies such as poor drainage or neuropathy (see Chapter 18). Ischaemic ulcers are usually initiated by trauma, but this may be a minor injury. They are typically painful, unless there is neuropathy present, as for example in some diabetic patients. There is an impoverished inflammatory response of the surrounding tissues, which can appear tight, shiny and pale. The ulcer bed may have little or no granulation tissue, but slough is often present. Exudate is usually light, unless there is infection. The borders are well demarcated and they may

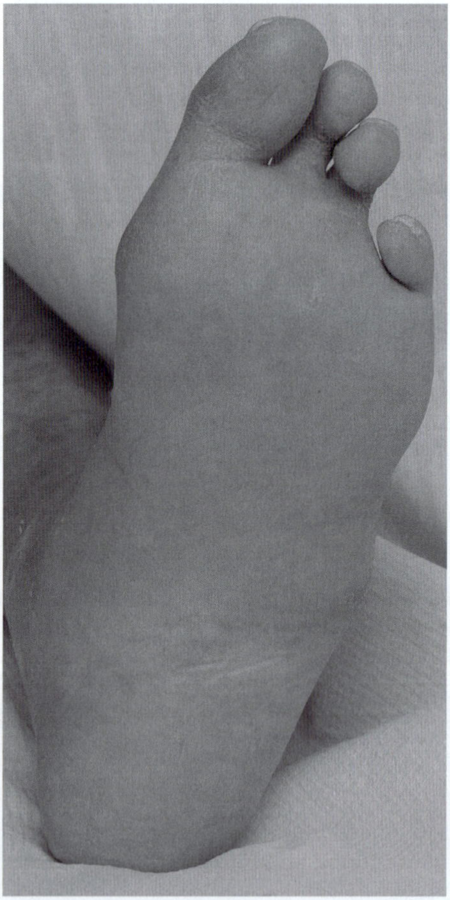

Figure 6.9 Severe ischaemia.

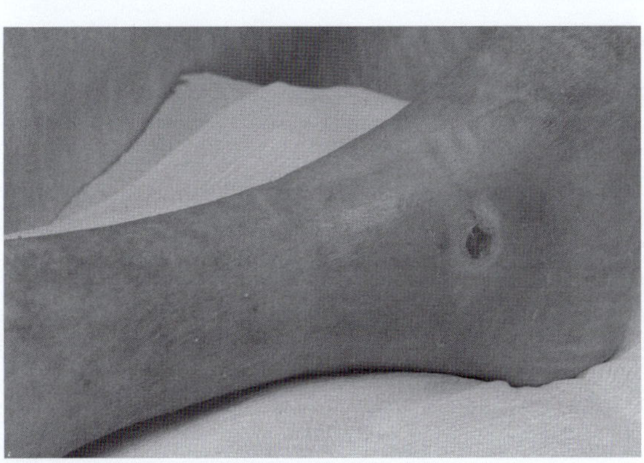

Figure 6.10 Ischaemic ulcer.

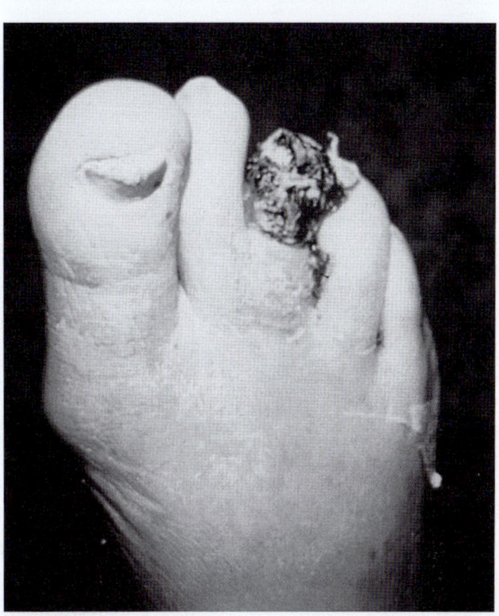

Figure 6.11 Gangrene.

have a 'punched out' appearance (Fig. 6.10). Such ulcers often occur first under the toe nails, on the apices of the toes or around the borders of the feet, a contributory factor usually being tight or ill-fitting footwear. Leg elevation may exacerbate the pain, whereas lowering the leg into dependency can improve the blood supply and improve the pain. Ischaemic ulcers are unlikely to heal unless there is an improvement in blood supply.

Nails

Poor blood supply will affect the nail texture, which may be crumbly, discoloured or thickened. If these signs are present the differential diagnosis should include dermatological conditions such as psoriasis (Ch. 8) and fungal infection.

Necrosis (gangrene)

Severe ischaemia, if unrelieved, will progress to necrosis or dry gangrene, with the most distal regions being affected first. The tissue will appear hard, black and mummified, with a clear demarcation line between dead and living tissue (Fig. 6.11). Ulceration and infection may cause a septic vasculitis, which again leads to ischaemia and necrosis, but here the tissue remains moist and usually has a distinctive smell. This is wet gangrene. Pus and infection of surrounding tissue is present. The presence of proximal arterial occlusion and poor collateral development may be contributing factors. Other causes of non-healing ulcers, such as venous disease, as well as vasospastic and immune disorders should be considered.

Oedema

Oedema is not usually associated with poor peripheral arterial supply. If present bilaterally, the cause is likely to be a central one such as congestive heart failure. Unilateral or localised oedema may be due to infection, trauma, allergy or impaired venous or lymphatic drainage (Table 6.5), such as during or after a deep vein thrombosis.

Clinical tests

The following tests should be repeated for both lower limbs. Some of these tests are of greater significance than others in aiding diagnosis and their utility is summarised in Table 6.6.

Temperature

The back of the practitioner's hands should be used to stroke the anterior surface of both limbs simultaneously from above the knee to the toes. The absolute temperature is not a helpful sign, given the variables of weather, clothing, exposure and natural variations in skin temperature (practitioner and patient). However, both limbs should feel similar at the respective levels of the limbs. Any difference between the two limbs of more than 2°C should be investigated further, since a unilateral cool/cold limb is moderately specific for arterial disease (see Table 6.6). It is

Table 6.5 Differential diagnosis of oedema of the lower limb

CAUSES			
Cardiac failure	*Venous stasis*	*Primary lymphoedema*	*Secondary lymphoedema*
Bilateral	Unilateral	Bilateral	Unilateral
Transudate	Transudate	Exudate	Exudate
Pitting	Pitting (unless very long-standing)	Non-pitting	Non-pitting (unless recent)
Acquired	Acquired	Congenital	Acquired
Post-MI	Post-immobilisation		Post-infection, radiotherapy, surgery, malignancy

important to establish that one leg is cooler, as opposed to one leg being warmer, perhaps because of venous problems or infection (this may not produce the expected rise in local tissue temperature if there is arterial insufficiency). A more quantitative measurement can be obtained by testing skin temperature with a handheld infrared thermometer.

Warm knees have been cited as a clinical indicator of arterial disease affecting the femoropopliteal segment (Zweiffler 1965, O'Brien et al 1990), although no large studies have been performed to clarify the diagnostic level of the test. It is believed that stenoses at mid-thigh level or distal to the adductor canal encourage a collateral circulation distributed around the knees, producing a local rise in temperature.

Capillary filling time

Capillary filling time (CFT) lacks sensitivity and has a poor to moderate specificity, which means it is not a very useful test. It is quick and easy to perform, which perhaps explains its enduring popularity. It is not the capillaries but the subpapillary venous plexus which is responsible for colour in the skin and is blanched by digital pressure. The time is noted in seconds for the blood to return after blanching. Normal colour should return within 2–3 seconds on a warm day and within 5 seconds on a cold day. Prolonged return of colour is taken as an insensitive and non-specific sign of a compromised circulation.

Leg elevation tests

Postural changes in circulation may be harnessed to help diagnose vascular conditions. Both tests described are quick and simple to perform. Buerger's test is reported as 100% sensitive for disease distal to the mid-thigh, that is if negative, occlusive disease can be ruled out in this segment. Venous filling time has a high specificity (McGee & Boyko 1998), meaning that if positive (abnormal), it is likely disease is present. It may not be practical to position some patients in a supine position and to raise the leg, for example in spine and hip disease.

Buerger's elevation/dependency test

- Stage 1
  The patient is supine and the leg is raised slowly to 45°. The leg is observed for rapid or severe pallor, implying inadequate supply without gravity assisting flow. In severe cases, draining of blood is observed as the limb is elevated. After 1–2 minutes, it is common to observe some loss of pink/red colour from the foot. However, in an ischaemic limb, the skin will appear white.
- Stage 2
  The limb is lowered into dependency and the time taken for the plantar surface/toes to return to the colour of the other limb is noted. If the blood supply is adequate, the plantar surface of the foot should regain its normal colour within 15–20 seconds. A delayed time of 20 seconds or more suggests that blood supply is inadequate, with severe ischaemia being likely if the delay is 40 seconds or more. If the colour on dependency is a dusky red, this is a serious sign, indicating that the tissues have been hypoxic during the test and a reactive vasodilation has provoked hyperaemia. The flush may start in the toes and spread proximally. Elevating both legs simultaneously can help to highlight discrepancies between limbs. Putting the couch into Trendelenburg's position can help reduce the manual labour involved in holding heavy limbs, with care to maintain patient safety in this position.
- Venous filling time
  In a healthy recumbent individual, venous filling in the legs depends on and is proportional to arterial inflow. A visible vein on the foot is identified (it can be marked if necessary) and the leg

Table 6.6 Diagnostic prediction of commonly used clinical tests for the investigation of lower extremity arterial disease

Examination result	*Study*	*No. of people*	*% Sensitivity* (+LR)*	*% Specificity* (–LR)*	*Interpretation*
History of IHD†	Stoffers et al 1996	2455	47.9 (2.3)	79.1 (0,7)	Moderate predictor of PAD, but if no history of vascular disease, PAD cannot be excluded
Abnormal PT pulse‡	Criqui et al 1985	613	71.2 (7.9)	91.3 (0.3)	Likely to be abnormal if disease present and a strong indicator of disease
Abnormal DP pulse‡	Criqui et al 1985	613	50 (1.9)	73.1 (0.7)	Mild predictor of disease when abnormal, but if normal cannot exclude disease
Abnormal PT and DP pulses‡	Christensen et al 1989 Stoffers et al 1996	132 2455	63–95 (3–44.6) 72.8 (if absent/ weak) (9)	73–99 (1–4) 91.9 (0.3)	Moderate to good predictor of disease and if normal moderately helpful in excluding disease
Abnormal femoral pulse	Johnston et al 1981 Stoffers et al 1996	78 2455 2455	38 6.9 (absent) 33.1(weak)	100 (∞) 98.9 66.9	Absent pulse confirms diagnosis of aortoiliac disease. A feeble pulse weakly suggests disease. Normality does not exclude disease.
Claudication pain	Stoffers et al 1996	2455	30.6	92.8	When present strongly indicates disease, but absence cannot exclude disease
Claudication pain and any abnormal pulse	Criqui et al 1985	613	4.8	99.6	Confirms diagnosis when present together.
Femoral arterial bruit	Criqui et al 1985 Stoffers et al 1996	613 2455	20 (5) 29.1 (5.7)	96 (1.2) 94.9 (0.1)	Strong indicator of disease. If no bruit, cannot exclude disease

Table 6.6 *Continued*

Examination result	*Study*	*No. of people*	*% Sensitivity* (+LR)*	*% Specificity* (–LR)*	*Interpretation*
ABPI < 0.9	Williams et al 2005 ABPI < 0.9 *and* TBI < 0.75	41 limbs (controls) 25 limbs (diabetes no neuropathy) 64 (diabetes neuropathy)	83 100 53	100 88 95	Result confirms vascular disease and if normal helps to exclude disease (see caveats in text) In diabetes without neuropathy, a result in the normal range excludes disease and if low, moderate prediction of disease A normal result cannot exclude disease in presence of neuropathy, but if low, good prediction of disease
Buerger's test	Insall et al 1989	55 limbs	100 (2.2)	54 (0)	Negative result (normal) rules out disease (distal to the adductor canal)
Venous filling time (>20 seconds)	Boyko et al 1997	631	22–25 (3.6–4.6)	94–95 (1.2–1.3)	Predicts disease when prolonged. Normal filling time does not exclude disease
Pole test Arteriogram + rest pain OR absolute ankle pressure ≤40 mmHg OR $TcPO_2$ ≤30 mmHg	Paraskevas et al 2006	57 limbs	95 (3.5)	73 (0.07)	Normal result helps to rule out disease. Abnormality moderate prediction of critical limb ischaemia
Toe Doppler absolute pressure <50 mmHg (optical method)	Kroger et al 2003	175	8 (2)	96 (1)	If abnormal, disease highly likely. If not, cannot exclude disease

Table 6.6 *Continued*

Examination result	*Study*	*No. of people*	*% Sensitivity* (+LR)*	*% Specificity* (–LR)*	*Interpretation*
Capillary refill time (>5 seconds)	Boyko et al 1997 (ABPI <0.05)	631	25–28 (1.6–1.9)	84–85 (0.5–0.6)	Moderate predictor of disease when prolonged. Normal filling time does not exclude disease
Unilateral cool skin	Boyko et al 1997 (ABPI <0.05) Stoffers et al 1997	631 2455	65–80 (1.2–1.5) 9.9 (5.8)	46–47 (0.4–0.7) 98.3 (1.1)	Wide range of sensitivity and specificity. Can predict disease when present, but do not use in isolation. If temperature equal, does not exclude presence of disease
Colour change (blue, pale, red)	Boyko et al 1997 (ABPI <0.05) Stoffers et al 1997	631 2455	24–32 (1.6–2) 35 (2.8)	84–85 (0.5–0.7) 87 (0.7)	Moderate predictor of disease when present. Absence does not exclude disease
Absent hair	Boyko et al 1997 (ABPI <0.05)	631	47–48 (1.6)	70–71 (0.8)	If hair present cannot exclude PAD. If absent, moderate predictor of disease
Atrophic skin	Boyko et al 1997 (ABPI <0.05)	631	43–50 (1.4–1.6)	70 (0.8–0.7)	If no atrophy, cannot exclude PAD. If skin is atrophic, moderate predictor of disease

Unless otherwise stated, ABPI <0.9 is the benchmark for PAD.
Positive and negative predictive values excluded dependence on disease prevalence.
Likelihood ratios (LRs) calculated from raw data as necessary.
*Sackett and Rennie 1992. LR = likelihood ratio (a high +LR (>10) rules in disease and a –LR <0.1 rules out disease).
†IHD = ischaemic heart disease.
‡'Abnormal' pulse is feeble or absent, PT = posterior tibial, DP = dorsalis pedis.

is elevated to 45° for at least 1 minute to establish venous drainage. The selected vein on the foot should collapse or 'gut' and even disappear. The foot is placed in the dependent position and if arterial inflow is normal, the vein will refill within 20 seconds (Boyko et al 1997) (Fig. 6.12). If the filling time is prolonged, the test indicates a failure of arterial supply. The test is highly specific for occlusive disease, but key limitations include finding a suitable vein. In patients with valve incompetence, leaking will hasten refilling, negating the test.

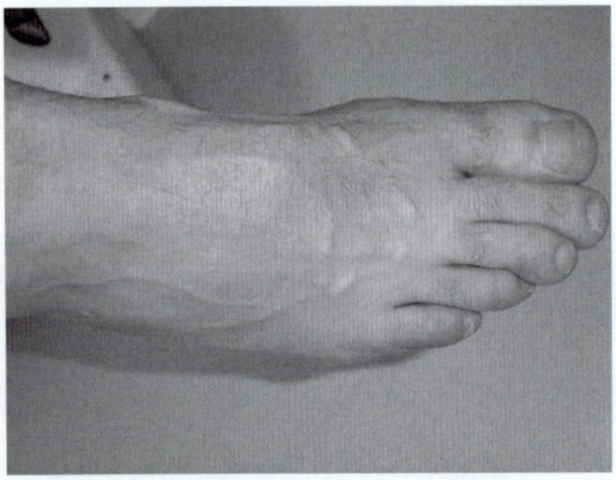

Figure 6.12 Checking venous filling time.

IMAGES

Allen's test

This is employed almost exclusively for the upper limb, but can be used to detect occlusion distal to the ankle. One leg is elevated and the dorsalis pedis artery is compressed with the practitioner's thumb. Maintaining pressure on the artery, the leg is lowered into dependency. If the posterior tibial artery is patent, the foot should return rapidly to its normal colour. The patency of the dorsalis pedis artery can be tested in a similar manner, by compressing the posterior tibial vessel.

Peripheral pulses

A pulse (wave) can be palpated wherever a large enough arterial vessel travels close to the skin surface, for example wrist, or can be compressed against an underlying structure, for example popliteal and femoral arteries. The main pulse points in the lower limb are indicated in **Figure 6.13**. The frequency of the pulse wave will be the same as the frequency of the heartbeat, or the ventricular systole. The practitioner should place the tips of the second, third and fourth digits over the pulse point to maximise the sensory feedback. Thumbs should not be used because the pulse from the thumb itself may confuse the result:

- Femoral pulse
  The external iliac artery becomes the femoral artery as it passes under the inguinal ligament and this is palpable by pushing against the ligament midway between the anterior superior iliac spine and the pubic symphysis.
- Popliteal pulse
  With the patient sitting or lying supine, bend the extended knee slightly and circle the knee using both hands, keeping the thumbs on the tibial tuberosity. Press the fingers into the lower popliteal fossa to compress the neurovascular bundle against the posterior tibia, which should allow you to detect the pulse. If the pulse is easily palpable, there must be a suspicion of aneurysm. Popliteal aneurysm is the most common aneurysm to affect the lower extremity, and, although rupture is rare, the bulge can encourage thrombotic occlusion, threatening circulation to the foot. This may produce a bounding pulse, or in more advanced cases a pulsating mass. The patient may be asymptomatic and signs of circulatory insufficiency are not always present, although popliteal aneurysms can produce acute ischaemia.
- Pedal pulses
  Two pulses are used to assess circulation in the foot. The dorsalis pedis (DP) artery pulse point lies on the dorsum of the midfoot, just lateral to the extensor hallucis longus tendon and palpation can be made easier by slight dorsiflexion of the foot (Woods 1991). The PT pulse is best felt under and just behind the medial malleolus. Of the pedal pulses, an abnormal PT is more useful to detect disease (Table 6.6). The more proximal locations of these vessels may be used, for example anterior tibial, or alternatives such as the peroneal artery. It is advised to take each pulse simultaneously on both limbs, since bilateral palpation enables the clinician to compare differences in strength and rhythm, while enhancing clinical efficiency. Beats per minute should be recorded, as well as rhythm (regular, regular, etc.). If the arteries are all patent and there is no vascular problem, then the findings should be identical at each site and between the limbs. If not, the pulses should be checked again. Inter-observer precision for peripheral pulse palpation is satisfactory to good, for present versus absent, but poor for present versus reduced (Lawson et al 1980, Myers et al 1987). It is rare for peripheral oedema to obscure the pulse, but the clinician may need to press more firmly and wait a few seconds for fluid dispersal before detection.

It is important to acknowledge that circulation may be healthy in the absence of one pulse (Beard 2000). Non-palpable pulses in healthy individuals may be from anatomical variation, under-development or congenital absence. The DP pulse is congenitally absent in 2% of the population and the PT pulse in 0.1% (Nuzzaci et al 1984, Robertson et al 1990). Inability to palpate a pedal pulse occurs most frequently for DP (8.1%), uncommonly for PT (2.9%), with clini-

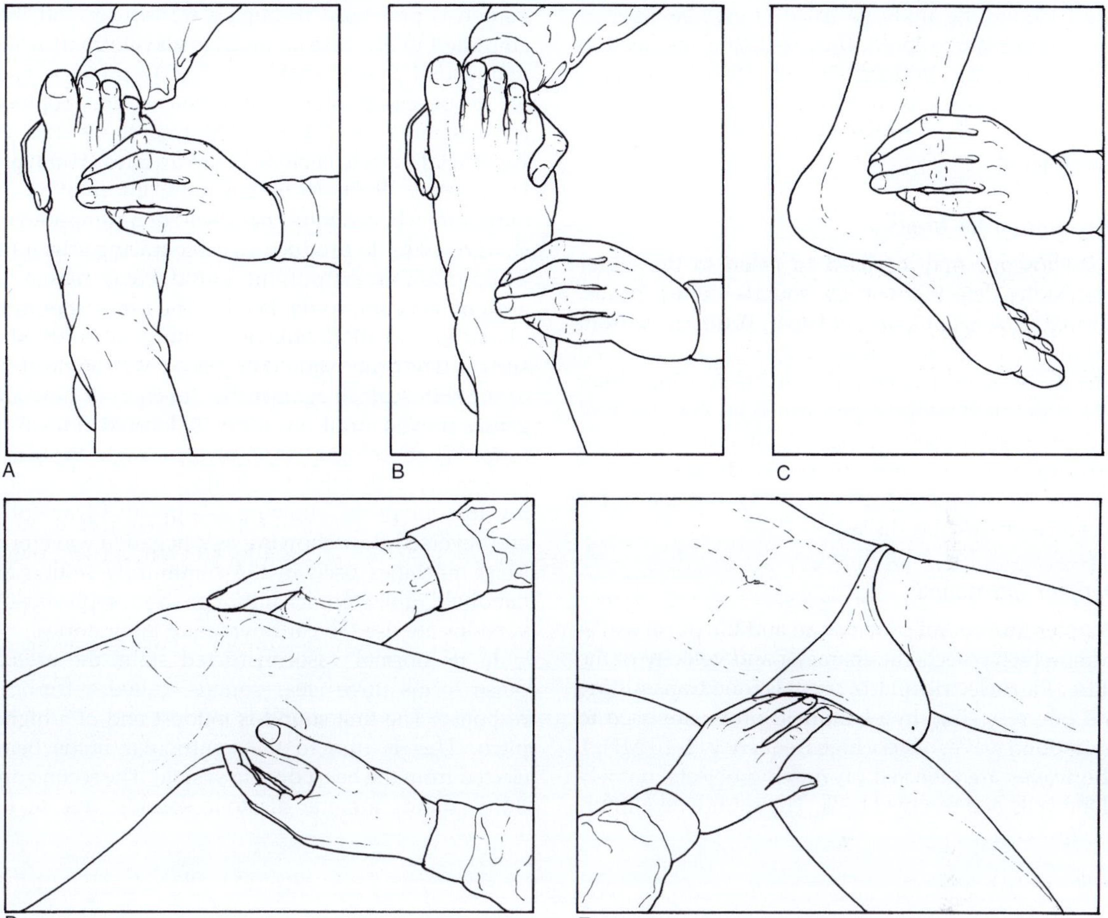

Figure 6.13 Location of pulses in the lower limb. **A** Dorsalis pedis. **B** Anterior tibial. **C** Posterior tibial. **D** Popliteal. **E** Femoral.

cal absence of both pedal pulses in healthy subjects being extremely rare, ranging from zero to 1.9% (Barnhorst & Barner 1968, Morrison 1933, Nuzzaci et al 1984). This helps to guide the clinician, since absence of both pulses can be taken seriously as a sign of vascular compromise.

Of course, peripheral pulse deficits may suggest that there is some occlusion in the arterial tree. The clinician should trace the pulse proximally to establish the region where the occlusion may be, for example move to the popliteal pulse if posterior tibial cannot be palpated. The PT artery is the major blood supply to the foot, so suspicion of compromise must be investigated. One paper heralded an abnormal/absent posterior tibial pulse as the single best discriminator of PAD (Criqui et al 1985). Pulses can be graded by using a score of 0–4, with 0 representing no pulse, 1 a feeble pulse, 2 a normal pulse, 3 a bounding pulse (abnormal) and 4 aneurysmal (rare below popliteal level). However, many grading systems are recognised.

In cases where a pedal pulse(s) is not palpable, Doppler auscultation can be employed. This is not a substitute for pulse palpation, which is an established technique for assessing lower extremity circulation. The value of listening to the Doppler waveform remains debatable. While the character of the pulse sounds will alter in the presence of disease, the number of variables affecting the quality/audibility of the sound reduce the benefit (Takahashi et al 2006). Khan and co-authors (2006) recommended a vascular patency scoring system, for which inclusion of the Doppler output increased the diagnostic accuracy. In practical terms, the clinician should consider placing a cuff around the ankle, so an ABPI may be taken at the same time (see later), thus reducing the need to relocate the pulse. In cases where disease is suspected but proximal examination fails to reveal abnormality, disease of the microvasculature should be investigated.

Auscultation for bruits

A stethoscope may be used to listen to the larger arteries to detect abnormal sounds called bruits. Normal flow is laminar and silent. Bruits arise from turbulence in arteries caused either by an increased velocity or an obstruction. Examination using either side of the stethoscope is performed on iliac, femoral and popliteal vessels, using a light touch to avoid inducing a bruit by direct pressure. The detection of a femoral bruit has a high specificity, indicating the presence of vascular disease.

Doppler ultrasound

Doppler ultrasound provides an audible pulse waveform, which reflects the character and velocity of the pulse. Piezoelectric quartz crystals (one transmitting and one receiving) in a handheld probe are used to emit sound waves of very high frequency (2–10 MHz). The waves are reflected off moving objects, namely blood cells and received back. The soundwave information is processed through a transducer and then amplified to produce an audible waveform. It is recommended that a 4 MHz or 5 MHz probe is used for deep vessels such as the femoral and popliteal arteries and an 8 MHz or 10 MHz probe is used for superficial vessels such as pedal arteries (Huntleigh Diagnostics 1999). To obtain more information the output may be fed into a handheld or a computerised chart recorder to produce a visible tracing (Fig. 6.14). To optimise the output, the sound waves require an airtight medium, so the head of the probe should be placed in a small globule of coupling gel on the skin surface. The probe should be placed at an angle of 45° to the skin surface against the direction of flow and gently moved until an artery is located (Figs 6.15, 6.16). When using a trace, always angle the probe proximally so that the systolic flow is detected as flow towards the probe, showing as a positive waveform, and reversed flow showing as a negative waveform. Most machines used in the community setting are handheld mini Doppler, although more sophisticated versions are used in cardiovascular laboratories.

In its normal vasoconstricted state, the arterial pulse forms three clear sounds, called a triphasic response. The first sound is loudest and of a higher pitch. This is due to the ventricular bolus being ejected from the heart during systole. The second and third sounds are the diastolic sounds, due to the

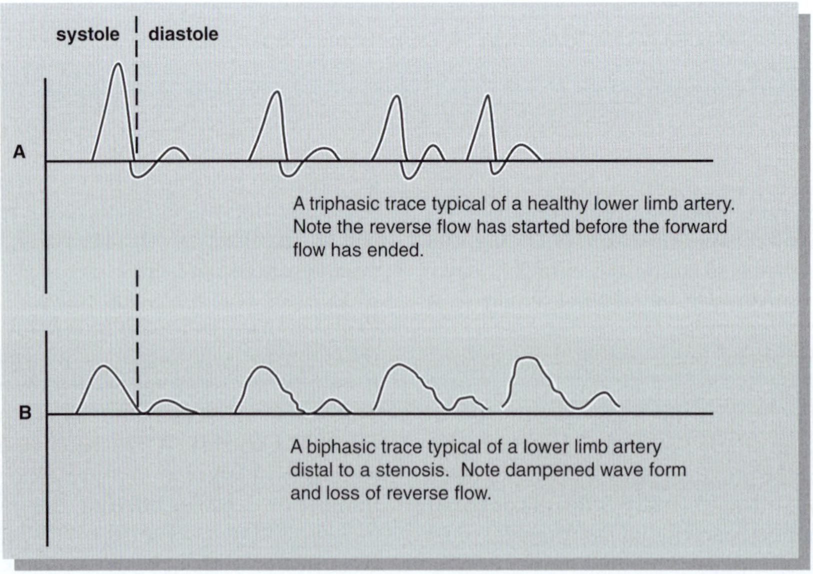

Figure 6.14 Doppler traces **A** Triphasic trace typical of a healthy lower limb artery. Note the reverse flow has started before the forward flow in the systolic phase has ended **B** A biphasic trace typical of a lower limb artery distal to a stenosis. Note dampened waveform and loss of reverse flow.

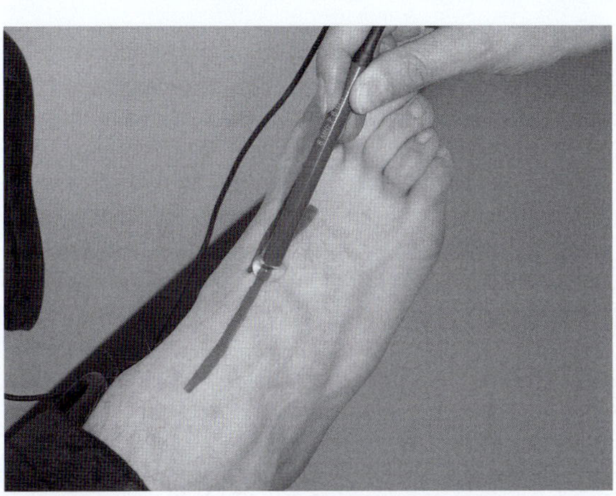

Figure 6.15 Doppler of dorsalis pedis artery.

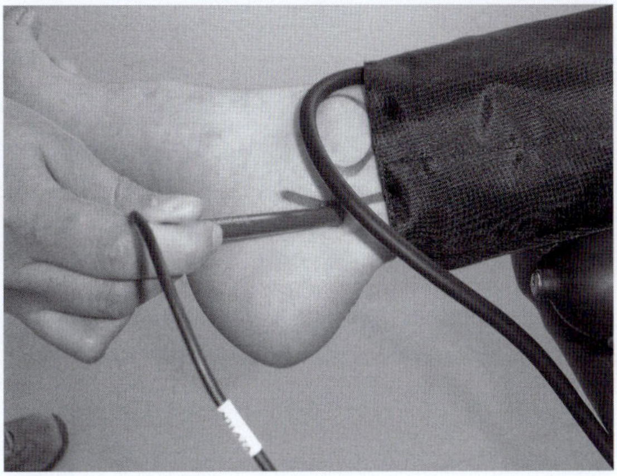

Figure 6.16 Doppler of posterior tibial artery.

reversal of flow caused by the elastic distension in the arteries and a final forward flow as the arteries rebound. The diastolic sounds correspond to the 'dicrotic notch' seen on Doppler traces, which will show two forward components and one reverse component (Fig. 6.14A). Loss of the reverse flow component or dampening of the waveform indicates disease (Fig.6.14B), although a diphasic response can be seen with ageing as the vessels lose compliance. Forward and reverse flow simultaneously suggests turbulence, as would occur just distal to a site of stenosis. A monophasic response indicates disease, but care must be taken first to ensure that the technique is not at fault. No signal will be heard in a state of acute critical ischaemia, e.g. femoral embolism, although subcritical ischaemia, for example from plaque thrombosis will return a sound (Earnshaw 2001). Patients with bradycardia will have a weak triphasic sound and patients with tachycardia will show only a biphasic sound as the heart is beating too rapidly for reverse flow to occur. The amplitude of the waveform is not significant since it depends on the angle of the probe. Software may be used to further analyse the waveform, providing quantitative information including acceleration time, pulsatility and resistive indices.

Claudication distance

If the patient complains of intermittent claudication or if pedal pulses seem weak or absent, this test can be used to give an indication of the severity of the arterial occlusion. The patient is exercised, preferably on a treadmill for test standardisation, and the distance the patient walks before the onset of pain is noted. The treadmill incline should be between 0 and 10%, at a speed of 3–4 km/h, usually for 5 minutes (Laing & Greenhalgh 1986). Patients should not be asked to exercise if there is a history of angina, and it is recommended that a full resuscitation kit should always be present for any exercise test (see also exercise ABPI).

Ankle–brachial pressure index (ABPI/ABI)

The ABPI is also known as the ankle/arm index (AAI) and provides a good indication of the presence of ischaemia in the lower limb (see Box 6.4). The test has growing recognition as a health marker and screening high for cardiovascular disease (Heald et al 2006), particularly in high risk populations, for example smokers and people with diabetes. The quantitative outcome is also helpful because the drop below 1 is proportional to the extent of arterial narrowing, as well as an indicator of mortality (Leng et al 1996 ,Vogt et al 1993). A recent paper suggested the ABPI was more useful than pulse palpation when detecting early PAD disease (Collins et al 2006). The test is not without limitations, most notably the false elevation of ankle values as a consequence of arterial wall stiffness. Moreover, although the most common cut-off point indicating abnormality is <0.9, values denoting ischaemia range in the literature from 0.8 to 0.97 (Carter 1969, Criqui et al 1985, Ouriel et al 1982).

The ABPI is determined by recording the systolic pressure at the brachial artery and at one or both of the ankle level arteries (posterior tibial or dorsalis pedis). If the blood pressure is similar in the upper and lower limb, the ratio will be around 1, reflecting the absence of any significant narrowing in the

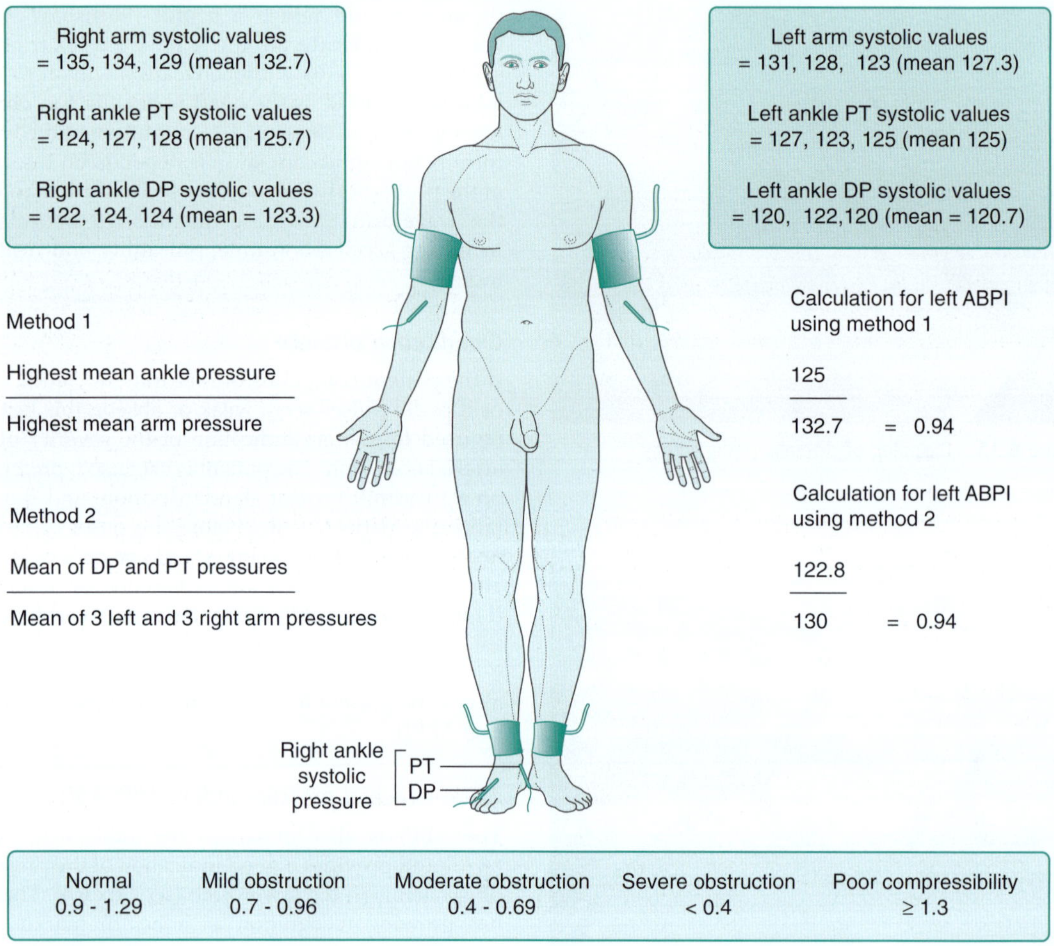

Figure 6.17 Calculation of the ABPI.

vascular tree. The ratio is formed by dividing the brachial value into the ankle value (Fig. 6.17). It has been demonstrated that the method of obtaining the brachial systolic pressure does not affect the ratio (Gardner & Montgomery 1998), so this may be taken by auscultation, for example as part of taking blood pressure, or by using Doppler sounds (Figs 6.15, 6.16), or by an automated oscillometric blood pressure device. A stethoscope cannot detect changes in small vessels, so Doppler equipment or oscillometric equipment are used for ankle arteries, but it must be noted that only systolic pressure is obtainable when using the Doppler probe (at ankle or arm levels). An advantage of using the Doppler equipment is the additional information from listening to the pulse characteristics.

The value obtained at the ankle will depend on the position of the patient. If the person is supine and the legs are at the same horizontal level as the heart the ratio should be 1.1–1.2 (Fronek et al 1973, Rutherford et al 1979), as there is higher resistance at the ankle arteries (Rutherford et al 1979). This is the optimum position, as no false elevation of ankle pressure will occur. However, it is not always practical for someone to lie flat. If the patient is sitting or standing, the pressure in the artery at the ankle will be greater than in the arm, because of the vertical column of blood between heart and ankle. As a rule of thumb the ankle systolic pressure will be 2 mmHg higher for every inch below the heart. Inter-observer and intra-observer repeatability studies have shown that variation as much as 0.2 (Fisher et al 1996) can be expected between readings, which must be taken into account when interpreting the results. Reliability can be optimised by experience and taking the mean of three readings.

Box 6.4 Taking an ABPI

- Advise the patient about the procedure and ensure they are comfortable and rested, lying supine where possible
- Place the arm cuff 2–3 cm above the elbow crease on the right arm*
- Obtain the systolic pressure at the brachial artery by any method, for example as part of taking blood pressure or using the Doppler (Fig. 6.18)
- For best practice take three times and repeat for left arm
- Ensure each value taken is written down
- Place the arm cuff around the ankle *or* use a thigh cuff if fit is tight, for example in obesity or severe oedema, 2–3 cm above the malleoli
- Place a small blob of coupling gel over the posterior tibial (Fig. 6.15) or dorsalis pedis (Fig. 6.16) artery (if only time for one, use the posterior tibial)
- Position the Doppler probe at approximately 45° against the flow and in line with the vessel (see Figs 6.15, 6.16).
- Obtain the best sound you can and listen for the waveform characteristics
- Inflate the cuff until the sound disappears*
- Slowly release the cuff and record the value of the first returning sound
- For best practice take three times and repeat for the dorsalis pedis artery
- Repeat for the other leg
- Perform calculations/use reference chart to obtain the ABPI for each leg

Pitfalls

- Using the wrong sized cuff
- Failing to maintain the probe directly over the artery (return of sound hard to detect)
- Not accounting for patient position
- Failure to record the method/equipment used, so subsequent changes could be misinterpreted

*If you have taken the brachial systolic first you know approximately the pressure at which the ankle vessel should collapse. If the sound continues as tourniquet pressure exceeds this, it may mean the vessel is non-compressible. There is no official upper limit, but if the sound is still present at pressures upwards of 220, further inflation is likely to be painful. Prior knowledge of the brachial systolic can help prevent painful cuff inflation.

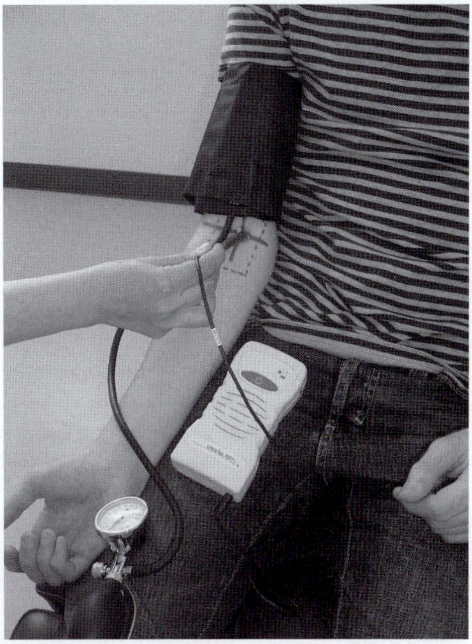

Figure 6.18 Brachial Doppler for ABPI.

IMAGES

It is considered best practice to take readings from both arms, but there is no consensus as to whether the highest reading is then used for the ratio, or if the left and right are added together and divided by two. A difference of greater than 20 mmHg between the two arms is clinically relevant, since this may indicate aortic regurgitation, or occlusive disease of the subclavian and/or brachiocephalic arteries. To obtain the ratio, two methods are recommended; the first is to use the highest of the two brachial systolic pressures and the highest of the PT or DP (TransAtlantic InterSociety Consensus (TASC) 2000) and the second is to use the average of the brachial pressures and the average of the ankle pressures (McDermott et al 2000). Calculations using both methods are shown in Figure 6.17.

Mild to moderate atherosclerotic change may not produce an abnormal resting ABPI, since an adequate collateral circulation may have developed (Carter 1972). A normal index in the presence of suspicious signs, symptoms or medical history should prompt an exercise test, where a drop in the ratio post-exercise is also a strong indicator of PAD and cardiovascular mortality (Harm et al 2006). This is not a routine test for the primary care setting. A standardised treadmill exercise regimen is used (see claudication distance) and the patient walks with the detached pneumatic cuffs around each ankle. In a healthy adult, unless exercise is severe, the index will show no change or will rise, but rapidly return to the resting value once exercise has stopped. In a person suffering from PVD, the ankle pressure will not rise and may fall, taking a long time to return to resting values. This is because at rest, if perfusion to the affected muscle group is suboptimal, the microvasculature will be maximally dilated. Exercising the limb will further decrease blood flow to the calf because vessels will dilate in the thigh, causing the pressure distal to the stenosis to fall still further. The pressure drop is proportional to the extent of the stenosis and ≥20% is considered significant (Henerici & Neuerburg-Heusler 1998). It may be misleading to re-record the brachial systolic pressure, as this is expected to increase with exercise, a result which will widen the gap between ankle and arm pressures. A normal result indicates an alternative cause should be sought for the signs/symptoms (Stoffers et al 1996).

If the patient cannot be exercised, the hyperaemic test can be used. A second occlusion cuff is placed around the thigh and inflated to just above the brachial systolic pressure for 5 minutes, although this may be limited in the presence of ischaemic pain. The cuff is released and the ankle pressure is immediately taken and repeated every 30 seconds for 3 minutes, for comparison to the pre-occlusion recordings. The proximal cuff halts the arterial supply as well as venous drainage, causing metabolites to accumulate. This has a vasodilatory effect on the blood vessels, so that in a healthy person on releasing the thigh cuff, blood will rush into the area, producing a temporary hyperaemia. This will cause a transient decrease of less than 20% of the pre-test value and will recover within 1 minute. If there is vascular disease, the fall will be >20% and will take 1–3 minutes to return to baseline.

A high ABPI does not exclude disease. Pressures may be overestimated by non-compressible vessels, which may manifest as a value within the normal range, but in the presence of signs/symptoms of arterial disease. The index obtained may be above 1.3, or the ankle value may be unobtainable, when the Doppler signal does not disappear because the pulse cannot collapse. Any of these scenarios indicate an alternative method of arterial supply evaluation must be found (see toe Doppler and pole test). It is worth remembering that the peroneal artery is usually spared from calcification. An elevated ABPI result should also prompt further investigations, since this finding is associated with increased mortality (Resnick et al 2004). The majority of the literature takes ≥1.3 to be the cut off for ABPI elevation, but there have been some indications this may rise still further to ≥1.4 (Vicente et al 2006).

Pole test

If severe ischaemia is suspected, but a high ABPI is obtained due to calcification (or no value can be obtained), the pole test can be used to calculate the ABPI (Smith et al 1994). The pole test is a variation on Buerger's test using a handheld Doppler machine. With the patient supine, the suspect pedal artery is located by auscultation and the affected leg raised until the pulse signal can no longer be heard. A 'pole' or suitable measuring device is used to measure the vertical distance between the couch/heart and this point is noted. The value in centimetres is multiplied by 0.735, which gives the absolute ankle systolic pressure, or supplies the ankle reading for use in the ABPI (Sumner 1989). Calcification will have no effect on this reading, but the method is limited to those patients with pressures less than 60 mmHg (Smith et al 1994) and for those with the flexibility required for leg elevation.

Segmental pressures

Pressure recordings at ankle level have been expressed in absolute terms to reflect the extent of compromise. Values of below 35 mmHg in non-diabetics (Raines et al 1976) and below 50 mmHg in the diabetic population (Larsson et al 1993) are associated with tissue ischaemia and inability to heal. Absolute systolic pressures may be taken at varying anatomical levels to help localise a stenosis. A drop of >30 mmHg detected below the occlusion is considered significant (Nicholson et al 1993). An appropriate sized cuff is inflated at key sites, namely upper thigh, lower thigh, upper calf and ankle and the pressure at which the Doppler signal returns (typically at one of the pedal vessels) is recorded. Note that upper thigh pressures should normally exceed brachial pressure. Each value may be used in the ABPI ratio, to compare with overall changes.

Toe Doppler pressures/toe brachial index

Medial arterial calcification (MAC) is not thought to affect digital arteries and therefore this test may replace the ABPI for those who are known to have medial calcification (Brooks et al 2001). Discovery of MAC is usually by an ABPI >1.3 or visible ankle/foot arteries as an incidental finding on plain radiograph. Pulsatile flow in the digit is detected via oximetry, or using a small Doppler probe (8 MHz). Care must be taken to check skin temperature (should not be <27°C) and to warm as required, since local vasoconstriction may alter the result. Normal toe pressures are 10–15 mmHg below arm systolic pressure. A 2.5–7 cm cuff is placed around the proximal great toe and connected to a sphygmomanometer. A small probe is used gently over the digital artery to detect a signal and the cuff is inflated until the sound is ablated. The cuff is slowly released until the sound is once again detected, which is taken as the systolic pressure. A mean of three values should be used. The final value is used as if it were the ankle pressure, with the arm systolic pressure divided into it to give the toe/arm ratio (Samuelsson et al 1996). Ischaemic changes are associated with pressures below 30–50 mmHg (Henerici & Neueburg-Heusler 1998) and in one study, major amputation was associated with a value of 13 mmHg (Varatharajan et al 2006).

Blood tests

There is no specific test for PAD, but vascular events are associated with atherogenic findings, such as dyslipidaemia and diabetes, which should always be tested for. Levels of inflammatory markers, such as C-reactive protein, are elevated in vascular inflammation and the atherosclerotic process (Aso et al 2004). The high risk of a thrombophilic tendency (Vig et al 2006) is pertinent and blood profiles should be checked accordingly. Elevation of the serum levels of amino acid homocysteine (linked to vitamin B deficiencies) is considered a risk factor for development of atheroma and venous thrombosis, possibly from endothelial injury. In one study, of 150 patients with symptomatic PVD, 37.5% had hyperhomocysteinaemia (Vig et al 2006).

Hospital and laboratory tests

If an ischaemic limb has been identified, further investigation may be required to assess:

- the risk of tissue breakdown
- the prognosis for ulcer healing
- suitability for reconstructive surgery
- the level at which amputations should be performed.

Macrocirculation

- Duplex ultrasound
  This combines B mode ultrasound and Doppler to give both an image of the artery under investigation and the flow within that artery. It takes time and requires expertise, but using Doppler and pulse-generated run-off (PGR) a complete non-invasive assessment of the lower limb can be achieved, which reduces the need for contrast angiography.

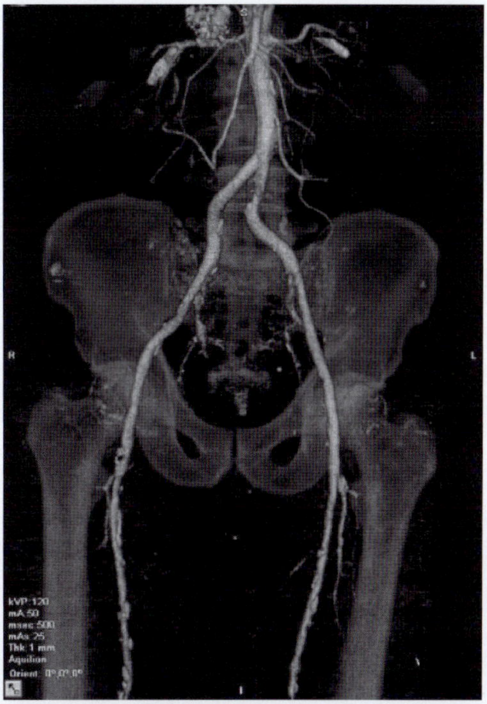

Figure 6.19 CT arteriogram.

- Angiography (arteriography) (Fig. 6.19)
  At present this procedure, especially using intra-arterial digital subtraction angiography, remains the gold standard for imaging the arterial supply of the lower limb. A needle is inserted into the femoral artery and a radio-opaque dye is injected just proximal to the occlusion. It can be used to locate occlusions and stenotic vessels and to determine whether a collateral circulation has been established. It helps to determine the most appropriate revascularisation procedure and, if a bypass procedure is to be performed, the site of the distal anastomosis. It is also used to predict the prognosis for limb salvage and graft patency. Intra-operatively, the angiogram enables the surgeon to have an accurate picture of distal run-off. It carries more risks than non-invasive procedures, which are likely to replace it as technology improves.
- Magnetic resonance angiography
  Good images of blood vessels can be obtained without the need for contrast material, although

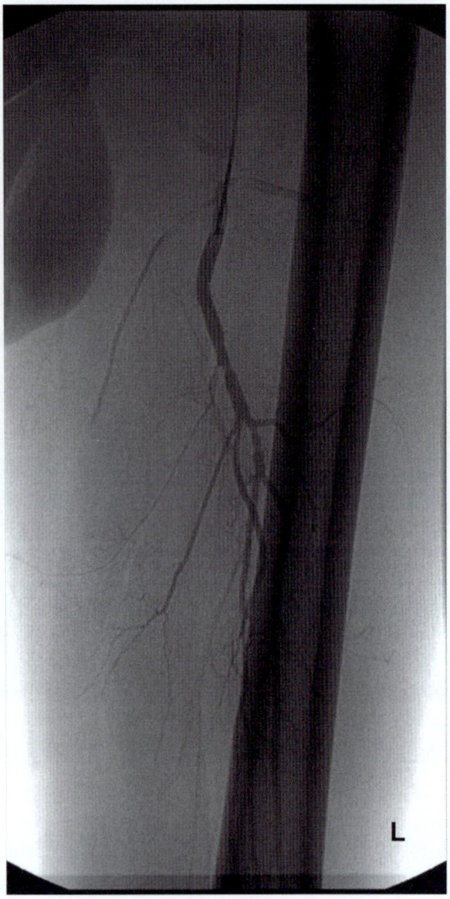

Figure 6.20 CT angiography.

gadolinium can be introduced to enhance the image. Blood flow, as well as the blood vessel can be visualised. The technique is expensive.

- CT arteriogram
  Precise three-dimensional imaging of blood vessels of all sizes, luminal changes and location and extent of calcification are seen with this test. It provides excellent detail (Fig. 6.20), although ionising radiation is a disadvantage. Contrast material is injected into the vein, which carries less risk than catheterising an artery.
- Venous occlusion plethysmography
  This is a non-invasive method for the measurement of blood flow in a limb, predominantly used for research. The technique can also quantify peripheral vascular responses in sympathetically mediated reflexes. Changes in blood volume can also be measured by strain gauge or infra-red (photo) plethysmography.

Microcirculation

- Transcutaneous oxygen tension ($TcPO_2$)
  The skin is heated to dilate the capillaries and the oxygen which diffuses to the surface of the skin equilibrates with an electrolyte solution held in a small chamber on the skin. The partial pressure of oxygen in the solution is measured by an electrode which screws into the chamber. This value reflects the difference between oxygen supply and consumption in the local tissues. It is a useful indicator of the tissue perfusion adjacent to a non-healing wound. Healing is expected above 40 mmHg, 20–30 mmHg is a grey area in which prognosis is uncertain, and below 20 mmHg, healing is unlikely (Oishi et al 1988). This is not a routine test but can be used as a predictor of healing or required level of amputation and to establish the success of angioplasty. Limitations include the time taken to perform the tests and concerns about repeatability (Rosfors et al 1994).
- Capillary microscopy (capillaroscopy)
  With the patient in a sitting position, the capillaries of the pedal nail fold can be examined, using an oil immersion microscope under a strong light. The nutritive capillaries are distinct and well filled with blood in a person with no arterial disease but, as ischaemia progresses, the capillaries become hazy and less distinct. The number of capillaries per millimetre can be measured and morphological and functional changes, for example, microhaemorrhage observed. This can be used to determine functional disturbances of the microcirculation, usually for investigations into chronic diseases, for example rheumatoid arthritis. New techniques for examining the capillary bed include spectral imaging techniques which harness the absorption of haemoglobin under polarised light, allowing examination of the microcirculation in areas other than the skin.
- Laser Doppler flowmetry
  This measures the movement of red blood cells in cutaneous vessels, utilising the Doppler shift principle as light frequencies change when they are reflected by moving objects. Disturbances of the microvasculature can be detected by measuring localised skin perfusion. The use of 'challenges', such as the administration of vasoactive substances can be applied to evaluate vasomotor activity. The technique can be helpful in situations when toes Doppler is impractical and it has been shown to correlate well with toe Doppler pressures (Tsai et al 2000). Arbitrary units of

measurement, for example blood perfusion units can be a disadvantage, since blood flow is not being measured directly in real units. Moreover, only a small volume of skin is used for measurements.

Venous disease

Venous problems may arise in the superficial, communicating and/or deep veins. Venous disease refers to any condition adversely affecting tissue drainage and venous return to the heart. It is more common in women, with one factor being increased venous pressures during pregnancy. A high body mass index is also relevant, as is age (Heit et al 2001). Clinical manifestations are frequently in the lower limb, as a consequence of gravitational forces. Drainage from the capillary bed and blood flow is managed by a system of drainage from superficial vessels to deep, with superficial veins above the muscle layer in the superficial fascia, deep veins in the skeletal muscle and communicating (perforating) veins linking the two systems. All the veins have one-way valves, preventing retrograde flow. Prolonged standing and/or weakness of valve structures can lead to valve incompetence, pooling of blood and accumulation of interstitial tissue fluid, leading to conditions such as vessel wall thrombosis and varicose veins.

There are three main pathological processes affecting veins, which can be interlinked:

- Weakness of vein walls or valves
- Inflammation of the vein wall and superficial thrombosis (thrombophlebitis)
- Deep vein thrombosis.

The vein wall may become dilated, sometimes because of genetic weakness, or as a consequence of valve inefficiency and increased hydrostatic forces. Laxity in the vessel wall will in any case deter effective closure of the valve leaflets. The valve itself can be weak or rarely congenitally absent and can sustain permanent damage and chronic leakage from thrombotic episodes.

The second condition is often referred to as phlebitis, which affects superficial or communicating veins. Trauma is a common cause, following wounds, insect bites or intravenous catheters. Increased gravitational pressure, such as during pregnancy or prolonged immobility cause blood to pool and encourage thrombosis in superficial and deep veins. Phlebitis is more common in the presence of varicose veins and saphenous veins are most frequently involved. This may occur in isolation, but also may be associated with deep vein thrombosis and pulmonary embolism (Beatty et al 2002, Heit 2006, van Weert et al 2006), which should be considered while clerking and examining the patient. Further, it may be a sign of systemic disease, for example malignancy (Unno et al 2002).

A major cause of venous disease and chronic venous insufficiency is deep vein thrombosis and its sequelae. Clot formation on the valve pocket may go unrecognised (high rates at post-mortum with no clinical history), or may cause sudden death or permanent valve damage. The clinical incidence of deep vein thrombosis is at least 1 in 1000 Europeans, with recurrence rates of 30% (Heit 2006). Acute complications can be fatal, namely pulmonary embolism, when a fragment of the thrombotic material breaks away, travels through the veins into the right side of the heart and into the lung. Here it may cause a dead space and sudden death, or ongoing chest pathology. Propagation is more likely from thrombi in veins proximal to the knee, but calf level thrombosis can be clinically significant (Fulbrick & Becker 1988). A 'post-phlebitic' syndrome may arise in the ensuring 20 years which reflects sustained venous hypertension from valvular reflux and/or venous obstruction. A spectrum of clinical conditions arise, including varicose veins, venous eczema, oedema, skin thickening and ulceration, all of which may adversely affect quality of life and mobility.

Genetic defects relevant to vein disease include structural weaknesses of vein structures, but also a predisposition to clotting. Familial thrombosis has been linked to deficiencies in the clotting and fibrinolytic cascades (resistance to activated protein C (factor V Leiden), antithrombin deficit) and elevation of levels of the procoagulant proteins, namely factors II, VIII, IX and XI and fibrinogen.

History and risk factors

Medical and symptomatic history is important, since venous problems can arise from serious underlying conditions, such as pelvic obstructions and deep vein thrombosis. As varicose veins and recurrent deep vein thromboses tend to have a familial predisposition, it is important to question family history. Varicose veins may be part of the post-thrombotic syndrome (Case history 6.3) but do not necessarily indicate previous deep vein thrombosis. Childbearing and particularly multiple pregnancies increase the likelihood of venous disease. Risks for venous ulcers include age, multiple pregnancies, obesity, previous varicose ulcers and socioeconomic factors

Case history 6.3

A 59-year-old solicitor of Sri Lankan origin presented to the clinic with an ulcer of 12 months' duration over the right medial malleolus. The past medical history revealed a deep vein thrombosis while recuperating from a major abdominal operation when she was 20 years old. The thrombosis had been treated effectively at the time but the patient had noticed some 20 years later her right leg beginning to ache and feel heavy after prolonged standing, with varicose veins appearing in the lower leg. Both legs had been oedematous before this occurred. In her early 40s, the skin around the area had become discoloured and itchy. She has hypertension and a family history of strokes. She was taking co-amilozide 2.5/25 mg od, ramipril 2.5 mg od and quinine 200 mg at night. She has three grown up daughters. She has never smoked and drinks occasionally. She grew up in Sri Lanka and visits annually.

The history of the presenting complaint was itchy skin prior to the ulcer occurring and the medial ankle had been knocked, causing a wound. Symptomatic history was of 'bursting' pain in both legs which worsened on standing for long periods and was relieved by elevation of the legs. She had no symptoms of paraesthesia and could walk for 'miles' before the onset of the ulcer. The wound has never been infected.

Examination of the lower limbs was remarkable for pitting oedema left leg and non-pitting oedema right leg. Both legs displayed varicose veins, haemosiderosis and atrophie blanche, with varicose eczema in the distal third of the right limb. The distal aspects on both legs and feet looked scaly and the skin was thickened and indurated with a 'woody' texture. The skin on both limbs was warm and all pulses were within normal limits. Blood pressure was 150/93 mmHg. The ulcer was protected with a padded dressing and the ABPI in both legs was 1.1. The Doppler signal from the right popliteal vein in the popliteal fossa indicated venous reflux.

The differential diagnosis of the oedematous limbs could be venous hypertension, with the right leg known to have had deep vein thrombosis. However, the left leg may also have sustained an asymptomatic deep vein thrombosis, still producing a state of chronic valve reflux. Furthermore, there may have been recurrence of deep vein thrombosis in the right leg, worsening the valve function. Another possibility would be filariasis, since this is prevalent in Sri Lanka. Infection with lymph filarial worms can produce chronic lymph obstruction, scaly skin and non-pitting oedema. However, long-standing venous congestion could also have caused this in the right leg.

The arterial supply was found to be adequate and the diagnosis seemed to be venous ulceration, as a result of post-thrombotic complications. Further lymphatic examination would be appropriate if filarial worms are included in the diagnosis. Given the satisfactory ABPI results and the palpable pulses, compression bandaging could be of benefit to effect healing. Duplex studies or venography may be necessary to further characterise the nature of the obstruction.

such as low income. Factors leading to thrombosis are given by Virchow's triad (Box 6.5).

Symptoms

Uncomplicated varicose veins may be asymptomatic, but present a cosmetic problem to many women. Where superficial veins are affected by phlebitis, the vein and surrounding area will be tender with erythema or cellulitis. If thrombophlebitis is present the vein will be palpable as a linear, indurated cord and is usually associated with tenderness, erythema and warmth.

The onset of deep vein thrombosis can be asymptomatic or cause severe pain, tenderness and warmth in the calf. Oedema (usually pitting) causes the affected limb to enlarge. Measured at the widest point of the calf or thigh, a difference ≥2 cm between limbs is considered a significant, but non-specific finding. Deep vein thrombosis begins with clinical suspicion and eliciting risk factors, but diagnosis involves the D-dimer blood test and vein imaging

Box 6.5 Factors encouraging thrombosis

Virchow's triad:

- stasis, for example post-operative immobility
- hypercoagulability, for example high fibrinogen levels, dehydration
- injury to the endothelium, for example vein injury following surgery

(Wells et al 2006). A ruptured popliteal cyst, as sometimes occurs in patients with rheumatoid arthritis, can produce similar symptoms, as may cellulitis.

Pain and discomfort are frequently associated with venous morbidities and are due to oedematous constriction (tightness, aching, heavy or 'restless legs'), skin changes (such as thickening), irregularity of collagen and fat deposition (lipodermatosclerosis), infection (such as recurrent cellulitis), and scarring (see atrophie blanche and ulcers). Varicose eczema and ulcers can also be painful.

The term venous claudication is sometimes used for pain arising from deficient venous drainage. It can be described as bursting pain or cramps and since these may be initiated by exercise, symptoms must be differentiated from arterial claudication.

Observations and signs

Hosiery

The wearing of elastic or support stockings or bandages suggests some problem with venous drainage. The extra compression provided by the stocking aids venous blood flow and reduces peripheral oedema.

Colour

A study on 5247 people found the most common sign of venous disease to be telangiectases and varicosities (Chiesa et al 2005). Callejas & Manasanch (2002) found this to present second only to oedema as the most frequent finding. Telangiectases (visibly dilated microvasculature) present as either blue protruding (venule) or red non-protruding (arteriole) ramifications from underlying vessels (Fig. 6.21). This sign does indicate venous problems (Pascarella & Schmid Schönbein 2005), even in the absence of varicose veins, since the reflux may be originating from the deep veins (Krnic et al 2005).

Mottled bluish/purple discoloration may appear in the lower third of the lower limb. This is due to stagnation of blood in the veins from poor drainage. Atrophie blanche refers to white patches on the skin around the ankles, which occurs due to strangled microcirculation and leads to fibrotic and sclerotic changes in the skin (Fig. 6.22).

Brown iron complexes of haemosiderin may be deposited in the tissues. This results from persistently increased hydrostatic pressure, which encourages blood components to escape. The chronic leakage of red blood cells and decomposition in the tissues causes brown staining, as macrophages take up the pigment. The dermal haemosiderin accumulation appears as dark brown patches, often speckled, but large areas may be densely pigmented (Fig. 6.23). Differential diagnoses from haemosiderosis are sunburn and erythema ab igne, a condition common in elderly people, but usually forming a distinctive reticular pattern. Also necrobiosis lipoidica diabeticorum, a condition associated with diabetes, produces yellowish patches on the shins which turn brown.

Temperature

In venous insufficiency the skin often feels warm (Kelechi et al 2003), possibly as a result of venous dilation. The presence of local inflammation/infection should be assessed. Cellulitis, general malaise, a rise in core temperature and a portal of entry will be strong indicators of the presence of infection.

Varicose veins

These may be due to incompetent valves in the superficial or communicating veins alone, or as a consequence of deep vein thrombosis. Back pressure due to an obstruction in the deep veins will

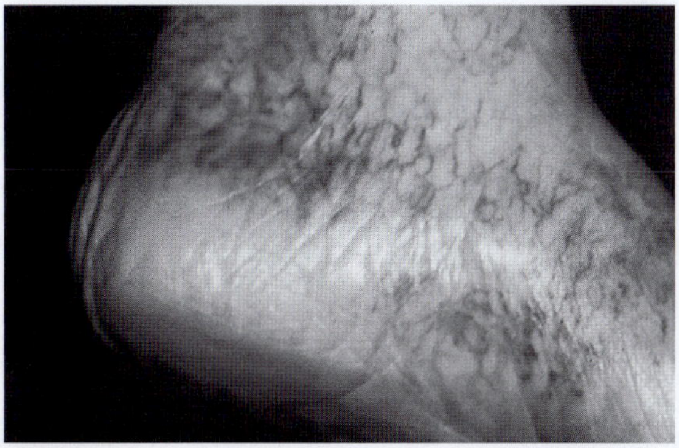

Figure 6.21 Telangiectasia.

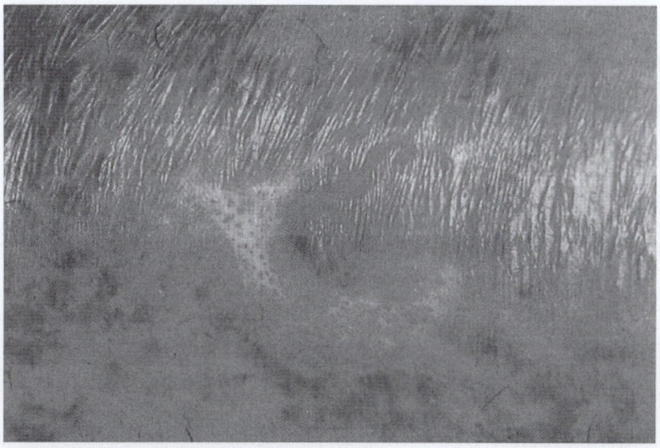

Figure 6.22 Atrophie blanche.

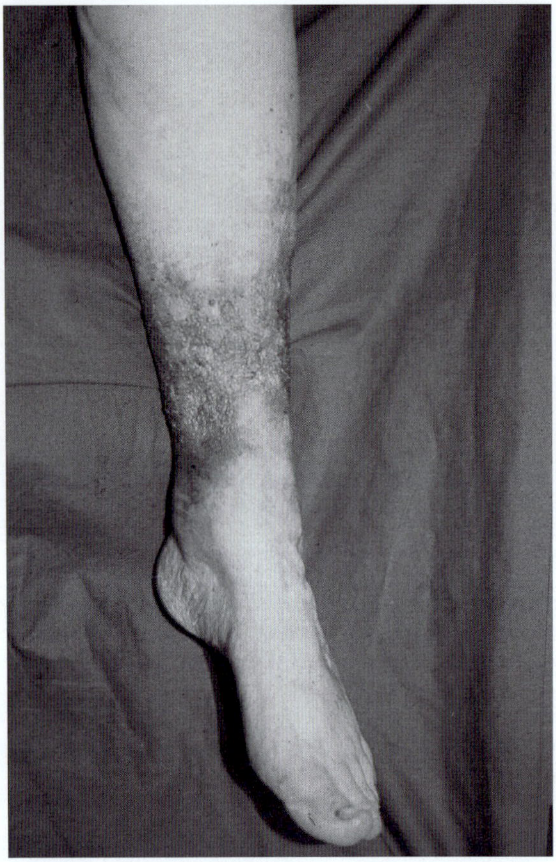

Figure 6.23 Haemosiderosis.

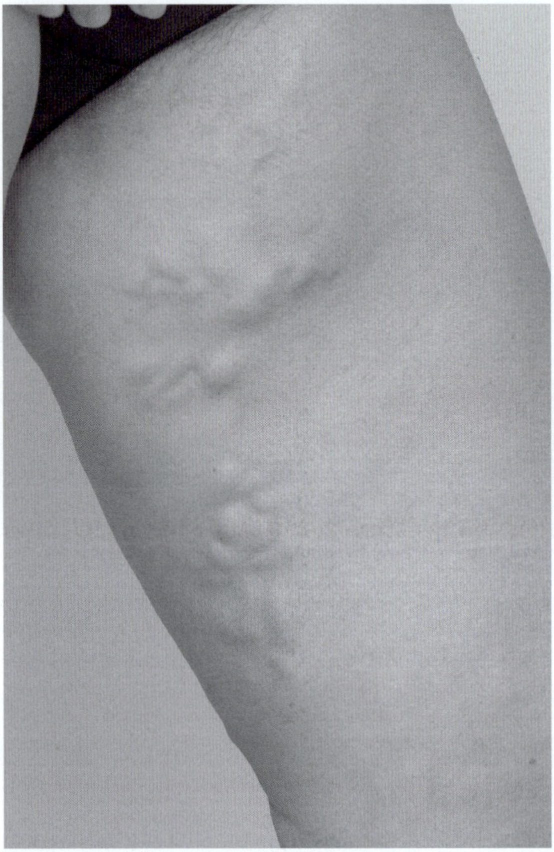

Figure 6.24 Varicose veins.

accumulate through the communicating veins to the superficial veins. This causes the superficial veins to become incompetent and forward flow of blood is deficient. These veins are very extensible, with non-uniform areas of weakness, and have little support in the superficial tissues. Therefore, they bulge unevenly due to the pressure of blood, giving the knotted appearance of varicose veins. Varicosities are especially apparent on standing (Fig. 6.24).

Tissue viability

Poor drainage results in the accumulation of waste products, which are detrimental to tissue viability. Trophic skin changes are most associated with age, varicose veins and pitting oedema (Carpentier et al 2004).The skin may eventually become indurated. The appearance is hard and leathery, with loss of skin mobility over deeper structures. If the stasis is a consequence of DVT, atrophy, venous (gravitational) eczema and venous ulcers may result.

Dermatological conditions

Venous incompetence is often marked by dermatological changes.

Varicose or venous eczema

This is also known as stasis eczema. Signs of discoloration and pigmentation, scaly and lichenified skin, in the presence of oedema, haemosiderosis (Fig. 6.23) and atrophie blanche suggest a diagnosis of varicose eczema (Fig. 6.23). The area can be pruritic and scratching may lead to the development of ulcers. Patients with gravitational eczema often find that they become sensitised to topical antibiotics and to preservatives in other topical medicaments and bandages.

Lipodermatosclerosis

The abnormal separation of endothelial cells in a state of elevated venous pressure allows chronic extravasation of fluid from the veins, as well as poor uptake of deoxygenated blood at the venule end of the capillary bed. As the pores in the stressed vessel wall expand over time, large proteins such as fibrinogen can escape and so can red blood cells. Fibrinogen undergoes chemical change in the soft tissues to form fibrin, which coats local structures, including the microvasculature. The fibrotic changes in the skin produce hardening and adhesions in the dermis, affecting normal adipose deposition and local perfusion. A current hypothesis offers a link between such changes and venous ulceration. It is proposed that this subcutaneous sclerosis combined with leaky vessels can 'trap' leucocytes which release inflammatory mediators and proteolytic enzymes causing skin breakdown (Saito et al 2001, Coleridge Smith 2002). Growth factors may be prevented from travelling through the damaged tissues to support healing (Trent et al 2005).

Venous or 'varicose' ulcers

Despite this being the most common form of leg ulcer, the pathophysiology remains poorly characterised. These account for up to 85% of all leg ulcers (Simon et al 2004), are more common in women than men and have a higher prevalence among elderly people (Fowkes et al 2001). It is important to note that a 'venous ulcer' may not have a pure etiology. Moffatt and colleagues (2004) found that co-morbid conditions, such as diabetes, lymphoedema and rheumatoid arthritis were present in 35% of cases.

The venous ulcer is generally found in the lower one-third of the leg (gaiter area), typically around the malleoli. Ulcers may spread around the leg (Fig. 6.25). Venous ulcers are associated with the post-thrombotic syndrome (Walker et al 2003), but are rarely a consequence of superficial varicosities. They are usually shallow with irregular borders and have either a granulating or slightly sloughy base unless infected. Exudate is moderate to heavy and the surrounding skin can show typical venous changes, namely hyperpigmentation, eczema and sclerosis. In one study, cellulitis and trauma were found to be the most frequent ulcer triggers, with less common initiation from factors including dermatitis and pruritus (Shai & Halevy 2005). Venous ulcers can be painful (Charles 2002, Nemeth et al 2004), although they are not recognised to cause the severe pain associated with ischaemic ulcers. Bacterial infection can complicate long-standing ulcers, which may become malodorous. A heavy bioburden from bacterial colonisation may also delay healing (Ebright 2005).

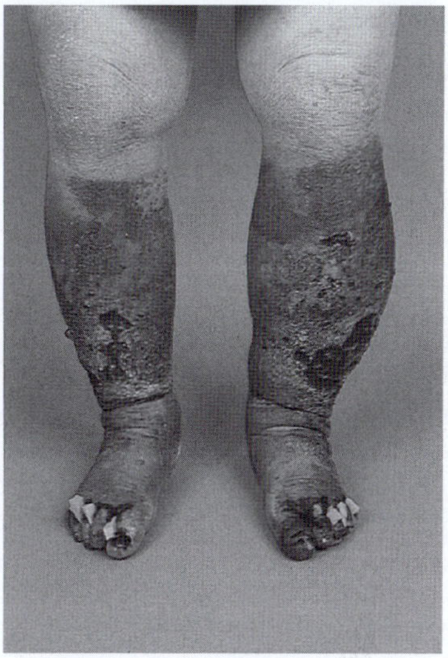

Figure 6.25 Venous ulceration.

IMAGES

These ulcers are notoriously indolent. It is not unusual for a patient to have a venous ulcer for many years which, despite much attention, refuses to heal (see Case history 6.3). Previous theories of tissue hypoxia preventing healing have been replaced by findings of abnormal cellular processes and, in particular, abnormal inflammatory mechanisms. Premature ageing of fibroblasts under conditions of venous hypertension has been found and may be important to impaired healing and repair (Stanley et al 2005). Histological studies have revealed increased matrix metalloproteinases, supporting the theory of unrestrained enzymatic activity inhibiting repair (Norgauer et al 2002). The role of activated leucocytes has already been outlined under dermatological changes.

Adequate compression is important to assist healing, but prior assessment of limb perfusion is essential. Non-healing has been linked to poor arterial circulation and previous deep vein thrombosis (Treiman et al 2001), as well as a duration of over 3 months and a size greater than 10 cm (Meaume et al 2005). Rarely, malignant change, for example squamous cell carcinoma may occur after many years (Smith et al 2001) and relevant signs should be checked, for example rolled edges and a hyperplastic base (Marjolin's ulcer). Large indentations, scar tissue and localised brown pigmentation may be evident where an ulcer has healed.

Venous gangrene

Extensive thrombosis affecting peripheral veins can cause severe tissue hypoxia because venous outflow is obstructed, thus arterial inflow is also halted. This is rare.

Oedema

Oedema may be associated with venous problems, occurring as part of the sequelae to deep vein thrombosis. The increased hydrostatic pressure causes leakage of tissue fluid, so that oedema results. The accumulation of interstitial fluid places constant stresses on the lymph drainage, which ultimately cannot cope with returning the excessive fluid. In advanced cases, the oedema clearly alters the shape of the lower limb, with loss of the normal ankle and even calf curvatures. If swelling is focal, consider inflammatory and/or infectious causes. In early or mild venous disease, more discrete oedema may be observed by examining the contours of the normally sharp edges of the malleoli, which appear blurred. Over time, the plasma proteins, including fibrinogen, are deposited in the subcutaneous tissues and the odema becomes organised, whereupon it cannot be squeezed by digital pressure and becomes non-pitting.

Leg shape

Patients with chronic venous ulceration and oedema may develop characteristic 'champagne/inverted bottle' legs. The ankle area becomes narrowed and hardened, but the calf is wider. This is often associated with lipodermatosclerosis, haemosiderosis and ulceration.

Clinical tests

In cases of superficial vein incompetence, clinical examination and Doppler tests are often sufficient to identify the site of reflux. Further investigations will depend on the history of the problem, the severity of symptoms and the type of management considered appropriate. Indications for duplex scanning or venography include suspicion of deep vein thrombosis (usually in the presence of an elevated D-dimer result), severe or recurrent varicose veins and skin changes, such as venous eczema, haemosiderosis or ulceration.

Pitting/non-pitting oedema

Digital pressure is firmly applied to the area for a period of 3–5 seconds. If an imprint of the fingers remains, the oedema is described as pitting.

Trendelenburg's test: To assist mapping of the faulty segment, the patient lies supine with their leg raised to establish venous drainage. This is maintained by placing four fingers firmly into the medial thigh at the saphenofemoral junction and asking the patient to stand. If the varicosities do not refill, but fill immediately when the finger pressure is released, the incompetence is located at the saphenofemoral junction. If the veins fill independently of the pressure applied, the faulty valve is located distally.

Doppler applications

In contrast with the pulsating sounds of arteries, veins give a non-pulsatile, continuous, low-pitched sound, like wind sighing down a chimney, because of the effects of respiration on the flow of venous blood in the thorax. However, if there is excessive fluid in the lower limbs, as in congestive heart failure, the veins may give a pulsatile sound. Doppler auscultation can be used to test for valvular incompetence as follows.

With the patient standing, the Doppler probe is placed over the vein suspected of incompetence. This is determined by the distribution of the varicose veins, so will be at the saphenofemoral junction for the long saphenous and in the popliteal fossa for the short saphenous vein. The calf is squeezed and after 1–2 seconds released. Two sharp sounds should be heard. The first sound is forward flow towards the probe as the vein is squeezed and the second sound is reverse flow due to gravity on release of the pressure. If there is no sound on compression this indicates a blockage between site of compression and probe. If the second sound is not abrupt, but continues and fades away, it suggests leakage of blood through the valves. This test should *not* be performed if deep vein thrombosis is suspected.

Blood tests

The D-dimer test is highly specific and can be used to rule in or exclude deep vein thrombosis when there is clinical suspicion (Wells et al 2006). Venous blood is analysed for particles formed from fibrinolysis, which is increased during deep vein thrombosis and also in any hypercoagulable state, for example infection, malignancy or recent surgery. Cut-off values for test results vary depending on the analysis method.

Hospital tests

Venous angiography

A radiopaque dye is injected into the affected vein to show valvular incompetence and the presence of an obstruction.

Duplex ultrasound

High-frequency sound waves are used (i) to obtain a picture of the veins (a B-mode image) and (ii) to determine the velocity and direction of flow within the vein (spectral analysis). Images reveal whether the veins are essentially normal or whether the valves are allowing reflux.

Plethysmography

Venous pressures and filling times may be measured by a range of methods, including impedance or air plethysmography, venous occlusion, phleborheoplethysmography and mercury strain-gauge plethysmography. Such techniques have been superseded by duplex and venography, but are still used for research.

Lymphatic drainage

The lymphatic vessels play an important part in draining tissue fluid and returning the lymph via the thoracic duct, to the heart. If lymphatic drainage is adversely affected, oedema (lymphoedema) results. A survey in 2006 found this to be rare in the UK and Ireland, with less than 10 cases per annum presenting to the consultants surveyed in the report. The majority of cases were primary lymphoedema and the rest presented with malignancy related lymph damage (Tiwari et al 2006).

Medical and family history

The history is key, since the majority of diagnoses of lymphoedema are made clinically. A swollen leg(s) has a range of causes including deep vein thrombosis, ruptured Baker's cyst, malignancy, trauma (for example ruptured Achilles tendon), pregnancy and lipoedema. A history of permanent oedema, usually confined to the lower limbs, suggests primary lymphoedema, especially if there is a family history of the disease, as one form is an autosomal dominant condition (Milroy's disease). Onset is either early in life (lymphoedema praecox) or after the age of about 35 years (lymphoedema tarda). It affects females more than males. Unlike venous oedema, once it is organised, it will not be alleviated by leg elevation.

Case history 6.4

A 40-year-old Caucasian man attended clinic complaining of difficulty in undertaking routine footcare of the left foot. An assessment of the vascular status revealed that the left leg was considerably larger than the right and the skin was thickened, dry and coarse. The nails on the left were very thickened, distorted and discoloured. Examination of the left leg showed the presence of non-pitting oedema. The patient said the left leg had become very swollen and the skin thickened and dry after an operation on his groin.

The medical history revealed that the patient had had testicular cancer. This had been treated by surgical removal of the testicles and radiotherapy. His problems with the left leg had resulted after the course of radiotherapy.

A diagnosis of secondary lymphoedema was made. It is likely that the radiotherapy damaged the left-side inguinal lymph nodes and, as a result, lymphatic drainage of the left leg was adversely affected, resulting in lymphoedema.

In contrast, secondary lymphoedema will arise as a result of some trauma to the lymphatic system, such as obstruction, for example from tropical infection (Case history 6.4) or damage due to radiotherapy, malignant disease, surgery, or trauma such as ankle fracture or severe sprain. A key differential diagnosis is that of lipoedema, an abnormal accumulation of fat predominantly in the legs, which can encourage lymphoedema. It occurs almost exclusively in women and usually spares the feet.

Observation

Oedema

In primary lymphoedema the oedema begins as a soft, pitting form but progresses to tissue sclerosis with increasing turgor, non-pitting oedema and hyperkeratosis. The condition can be unilateral or bilateral. Secondary lymphoedema is usually unilateral and considerable fibrosis may occur.

Tissue viability

Stagnant tissue fluid will interfere with diffusion of gases and nutrients and removal of waste products and, as a result, impair tissue viability. It may be associated with troublesome cellulitis and usually results in thickening and scaling of the skin, which can lead to an 'elephantiasis' appearance, that is an oedematous leg with skin that resembles elephant skin.

Lymphangitis and lymphadenitis

As the majority of tissue fluid normally drains into the lymphatic system, it follows that any infection present in the tissues, as indicated by the presence of cellulitis, will also drain into the lymph vessels unless dealt with by the inflammatory response at the site of infection. The presence of infection in the lymphatic vessels causes local inflammation, seen as red streaks following the course of the vessel and is called lymphangitis. Should the infection reach the lymph nodes/glands into which the lymph vessels drain, they will become tender and swollen (lymphadenitis). If not effectively treated, microorganisms will travel and multiply in the bloodstream (bacteraemia) and finally cause widespread systemic infection (septicaemia/blood poisoning).

Yellow nail syndrome

The nail appears yellow in colour, thickened but smooth and there is an increase in lateral curvature. The rate of growth of the nail is reduced. The condition is associated with primary and chronic lymphoedema and it has been proposed the discoloration is from persistent protein leakage. This sign must be fully investigated, since there are also associations with conditions such as lymphoma.

Clinical tests

It is not usual to carry out any clinical tests for lymphoedema apart from those which will distinguish it from other types of oedema, such as whether it is pitting or non-pitting, and Stemmer's sign (see below).

Stemmer's sign

Primary lymphoedema can cause thickening of the skin fold at the base of the second digit (finger or toe). Inability to lift the skin when the dorsal surface is grasped is a positive sign of lymphoedema and helps exclude lipoedema. If negative, the sign does not exclude primary lymphoedema.

Hospital tests

Duplex imaging can be used for lymph vessels. Lymph nodes and lymph drainage can be evaluated by taking lymphoscintigraphy. Angiography for lymphatic vessels (lymphangiography) can be carried out in the same manner as for venography. In primary lymphoedema X-rays may show hypoplasia of the lymphatic system, with the lymphatic channels appearing scanty and spidery. Full blood counts and biochemical markers may help support the diagnosis.

Summary

A systematic approach to vascular assessment is essential, as well as appropriate interpretation of the results, which means factoring in age, medical health, extent of impact on the person's life and prognosis. Indications for referral are:

- signs of critical ischaemia, that is tissue necrosis, ulcers or gangrene
- infection
- claudication or rest pain
- suspicion of deep vein thrombosis
- skin changes related to any circulatory abnormality.

If the presentation is acute, that is suspicion of deep vein thrombosis, femoral embolism, or infected gangrene, a patient should be sent to the hospital for assessment. Referrals are usually made to a general practitioner and it is important to communicate the reasons for concern. It is insufficient to refer simply with an abnormal ABPI result, or the absence of one pulse. Items for inclusion must be relevant medical, family and social history, for example smoking, symptoms, for example claudication at 180 m, and the context. For example, this patient would benefit from a cardiovascular health check up or lifestyle advice or that further investigations may be necessary as suspicion of femoropopliteal stenoses.

Box 6.6 Key investigations and findings for assessment of peripheral circulation

- Thorough patient clerking
- Symptomatic history
- Absence of one or more pedal pulses
- ABPI <0.9 (false negatives in diabetic population)
- Intermittent claudication or rest pain
- One or more positive leg elevation tests
- A difference in temperature between the two lower limbs of 2°C or more
- Oedema (venous or lymphoedema)
- Skin or soft tissue changes related to circulatory malfunction
- History or presence of ulceration

This chapter has emphasised an assessment process by which practitioners can establish a diagnosis of vascular pathology. Case studies have been included to illustrate the presentations of vascular problems. Good history taking and physical examination greatly assist the diagnosis of PAD, but rely on a combination of accurate measurements and appropriate questioning. Key areas are summarised in Box 6.6.

References

Aboyans V, Criqui M H, Denenberg J O et al 2006 Risk factors for progression of peripheral arterial disease in large and small vessels. Circulation 113:2623–2629

Aksoy D Y, Gürlek A, Cetinkaya Y et al 2004 Change in the amputation profile in diabetic foot in a tertiary reference center: efficacy of team working. Experimental Clinical Endocrinology Diabetes 112:526–530

Albert M A, Glynn R J, Ridker P M 2003 Alcohol consumption and plasma concentration of C-reactive protein. Circulation 107:443–447

Andreozzi G M, Martini R 2004 The fate of the claudicant limb. European Heart Journal 4:B41–45

Aso Y, Okumura K, Inoue T et al 2004 Results of blood inflammatory markers are associated more strongly with toe-brachial index than with ankle-brachial index in patients with type 2 diabetes. Diabetes Care 27:1381–1386

Barnhorst D A, Barner H B 1968 Prevalence of congenitally absent pedal pulses. New England Journal Medicine 278:264–265

Barnoya J, Glantz S A 2005 Cardiovascular effects of secondhand smoke: nearly as large as smoking. Circulation 111:2684–2698

Beard J D 2000 ABC of arterial and venous disease. Chronic lower limb ischaemia. British Medical Journal 320:854–857

Beatty J, Fitridge R, Benveniste G et al 2002 Acute superficial venous thrombophlebitis: does emergency surgery have a role? International Angiology 21:93–95

Bhatt D L, Steg P G, Ohman E M et al 2006 International prevalence, recognition, and treatment of cardiovascular risk factors in outpatients with atherothrombosis. Journal of the American Medical Association 295:180–189

Boyko E J, Ahroni J H, Davignon D et al 1997 Diagnostic utility of the history and physical examination for peripheral vascular disease among patients with diabetes mellitus. Journal of Clinical Epidemiology 50:659–668

Braunwald E 2001 Heart disease: a textbook of cardiovascular medicine, 6th edn. W B Saunders, Philadelphia

Brooks B, Dean R, Patel S et al 2001 TBI or not TBI: that is the question. Is it better to measure toe pressure than ankle pressure in diabetic patients? Diabetic Medicine 18:528–532

Buckenham T 2003 Angioplasty for intermittent claudication. Has the balloon finally burst? New Zealand Medical Journal 116(1168):U304

Callejas J M, Manasanch J 2002 Epidemiology of chronic venous insufficiency of the lower limbs in the primary care setting. International Angiology 23:154–163

Campbell W B, Ridler B M F, Szymanska T H 1998 Current management of acute leg ischaemia: results of an audit by the vascular surgical society Great Britain and Ireland. British Journal of Surgery 85:1498–1503

Carpentier P H, Maricq H R, Biro C 2004 Prevalence, risk factors, and clinical patterns of chronic venous disorders of lower limbs: a population-based study in France. Journal of Vascular Surgery 40:650–659

Carter S A 1969 Clinical measurement of systolic pressures in limbs with arterial occlusive disease. Journal of the American Medical Association 207:1869–1874

Carter S A 1972 Response of ankle systolic pressure to leg exercise in mild or questionable arterial disease. New England Journal of Medicine 16:148–153

Chantelau E, Lee K M, Jungblut R 1997 Distal arterial occlusive disease in diabetes is related to medial arterial calcification. Experimental and Clinical Endocrinology and Diabetes 105(Suppl 2):11–13

Charles H 2002 Venous leg ulcer pain and its characteristics. Journal of Tissue Viability 12:154–158

Chiesa R, Marone E M, Limoni C et al 2005 Chronic venous insufficiency in Italy: the 24-cities cohort study. European Journal of Vascular and Endovascular Surgery 30:422–429

Christensen J H, Freundlich M, Jacobsen B A, et al 1989 Clinical relevance of pedal pulse palpation in patients suspected of peripheral arterial insufficiency. Journal of Internal Medicine 226:95–99

Coleridge Smith P D 2002 Deleterious effects of white cells in the course of skin damage in CVI. International Angiology 21(2 Suppl 1):26–32

Collins T C, Suarez-Almazor M, Peterson N J 2006 An absent pulse is not sensitive for the early detection of peripheral arterial disease. Family Medicine 38:38–42

Criqui M H, Fronek A, Klauber M R et al 1985 The sensitivity, specificity, and predictive value of traditional clinical evaluation of peripheral arterial disease: results from noninvasive testing in a defined population. Circulation 71:516–522

Criqui M H, Langer R D, Fronek A et al 1992 Mortality over a period of 10 years in patients with peripheral arterial disease. New England Journal Medicine 326:381–386

Dormandy J, Mahir M, Ascady G et al 1989 Fate of the patient with chronic leg ischaemia. Journal of Cardiovascular Surgery 30:50–57

Dumville J C, Lee A J, Smith F B et al 2004 The health-related quality of life of people with peripheral arterial disease in the community: the Edinburgh Artery Study. British Journal of General Practice 54:826–831

Earnshaw J J 2001 Demography and etiology of acute leg ischemia. Seminars in Vascular Surgery 14:86–92

Eason S L, Petersen N J, Suarez-Almazor M et al 2005 Diabetes mellitus, smoking, and the risk for asymptomatic peripheral arterial disease: whom should we screen? Journal of the American Board of Family Practice 18:355–361

Ebright J R 2005 Microbiology of chronic leg and pressure ulcers: clinical significance and implications for treatment. Nursing Clinics of North America 40:207–216

Edmonds M E, Morrison N, Laws J W 1982 Medial arterial calcification and diabetic neuropathy. British Medical Journal (Clinical and Research Edition) 284(6320):928–930

Edmonds M E 2000 Medial arterial calcification and diabetes mellitus. Zeitschrift für Kardiologie 89(Suppl 2):101–104

Elliott R, McGrath LT 1994 Calcification of the human thoracic aorta during aging. Calcified Tissue International 54:268–273

Falk E, Shah P K, Fuster V 1995 Coronary plaque disruption. Circulation 92:657–671

Faries P L, LoGerfo F W, Hook S C et al 2001 The impact of diabetes on arterial reconstructions for multilevel arterial occlusive disease. American Journal of Surgery 181:251–255

Fawcett R S, Linford S, Stulberg D L 2004 Nail abnormalities: clues to systemic disease. American Family Physician 69:1417–1424

Fisher C M, Burnett A, Makeham V et al 1996 Variation in measurement of ankle-brachial pressure index in routine clinical practice. Journal of Vascular Surgery 24:871–875

Fisicaro M 2003 Why are cardiologists to be concerned about obliterating arterial disease of the lower leg? Italian Heart Journal Supplement 4:306–318

Fornengo P, Bosio A, Epifani G et al 2006 Prevalence of silent myocardial ischaemia in new-onset middle-aged type 2 diabetic patients without other cardiovascular risk factors. Diabetic Medicine 23:775–779

Forst T, Pfutzner A, Kann P et al 1995 Association between diabetic-autonomic-C-fibre-neuropathy and medial wall calcification and the significance in the outcome of trophic foot lesions. Experimental and Clinical Endocrinology and Diabetes 103:94–98

Fowkes F G, Evans C J, Lee A J 2001 Prevalence and risk factors of chronic venous insufficiency. Angiology 52(Suppl 1):S5–15

Fowkes F G, Housley E, Cawood E H et al 1991 Edinburgh Artery Study: prevalence of asymptomatic and symptomatic peripheral arterial disease in the general population. International Journal of Epidemiology 20:384–392

Fronek A, Johnson K H, Dilley R B et al 1973 Non-invasive physiologic tests in the diagnosis and characterization of peripheral arterial occlusive disease. American Journal of Surgery 126:205

Fulbrick J T, Becker D L 1988 Calf deep venous thrombosis: a wolf in sheep's clothing? Archives of Internal Medicine 148:2131–2138

Gardner A W, Montgomery P S 1998 Comparison of three blood pressure methods used for determining ankle/brachial index in patients with intermittent claudication. Angiology 49:723–728

Gilbey S G, Walters H, Edmonds M E et al 1989 Vascular calcification, autonomic neuropathy, and peripheral blood flow in patients with diabetic nephropathy. Diabetic Medicine 6:37–42

Grazuleviciene R, Azaraviciene A, Dulskiene V et al 2002 Social status, psychological stress and myocardial infarction risk among 35–64-year-old women. Medicina (Kaunas) 38:659–665

Greenland P, LaBree L, Azen S P et al 2004 Coronary artery calcium score combined with Framingham score for risk prediction in asymptomatic individuals. Journal of the American Medical Association 291:210–215

Halperin J L 2002 Evaluation of patients with peripheral vascular disease. Thrombosis Research 106: V303–311

Harm H H, Feringa H, Jeroen J J et al 2006 The long-term prognostic value of the resting and postexercise ankle-brachial index. Archives of Internal Medicine 166:529–535

Heald C L, Fowkes F G, Murray G D et al 2006 The Ankle Brachial Index Collaboration. Risk of mortality and cardiovascular disease associated with the ankle-brachial index: systematic review. Atherosclerosis 189(1):61–69

Heit J A 2006 The epidemiology of venous thromboembolism in the community: implications for prevention and management. Journal of Thrombosis and Thrombolysis 21:23–29

Heit J A, Rooke T W, Silverstein M D 2001 Trends in the incidence of venous stasis syndrome and venous ulcer: a 25-year population-based study. Journal of Vascular Surgery 33:1022–1027

Henerici M, Neueburg-Heusler D 1998 Vascular diagnosis with ultrasound. Thieme, New York

Hiatt W R, Hoag S, Hamman R F 1995 Effect of diagnostic criteria on the prevalence of peripheral arterial disease: the San Luis Valley diabetes study. Circulation 91:1472–1479

Hirsch A T, Criqui M H, Treat-Jacobson D et al 2001 Peripheral arterial disease detection, awareness, and treatment in primary care. Journal of the American Medical Association 286:1317–1324

Hobbs F D 2003 Cardiovascular disease and lipids. Issues and evidence for the management of dyslipidaemia in primary care. European Journal of General Practice 9:16–24

Hobbs S D, Wilmink A B, Bradbury A W 2003 Ethnicity and peripheral arterial disease. European Journal of Vascular and Endovascular Surgery 25:505–512

Huntleigh Diagnostics 1999 Library of sounds-support booklet for audio cassette. Huntleigh Diagnostics, Cardiff, pp 5–21

Insall R L, Davies R J, Pront W G 1989 Significance of Buerger's test in the assessment of lower limb ischaenia. Journal of the Royal Society of Medicine 82(12):729–31

Johnston K W, Demorais D, Colapinto R F 1989 Difficulty in assessing the seventy of aorto–iliac disease by clinical and arteriographic methods. Angiology 32:609–614

Kallio M, Forsblom C, Groop P H et al 2003 Development of new peripheral arterial occlusive disease in patients with type 2 diabetes during a mean follow-up of 11 years. Diabetes Care 26:1241–1245

Kelechi T J, Haight B K, Herman J 2003 Skin temperature and chronic venous insufficiency. Journal of Wound, Ostomy, and Continence Nursing 30:17–24

Khan N A, Rahim S A, Anand S S et al 2006 Does the clinical examination predict lower extremity peripheral arterial disease? Journal of the American Medical Association 295:536–46

Krnic A, Vucic N, Sucic Z 2005 Correlation of perforating vein incompetence with extent of great saphenous insufficiency: cross sectional study. Croatian Medical Journal 46:245–251

Kroger K, Stewen C, Santosa F 2003 Toe pressure measurements compared to ankle artery pressure measurements. Angiology 54:39–44

Kroger K, Ose C, Rudofsky G et al 2002 Symptoms in individuals with small cutaneous veins. Vascular Medicine 7:13–17

Laing S, Greenhalgh R M 1986 Treadmill testing in the assessment of peripheral arterial disease. International Angiology 5:249–252

Lange S, Trampisch H J, Haberl R et al 2005 Excess 1-year cardiovascular risk in elderly primary care patients with a low ankle-brachial index (ABI) and high homocysteine level. Atherosclerosis 178:351–357

Larsson J, Apelqvist J, Castenfors J et al 1993 Distal blood pressure as a predictor for the amputation in diabetic patients with a foot ulcer. Foot and Ankle International 14:247–253

Lawson I R, Ingman S R, Masih Y et al 1980 Reliability of palpation of pedal pulses as ascertained by the kappa statistic. Journal of the American Geriatric Society 28:300–303

Leibson C L, Ransom J E, Olson W et al 2004 Peripheral arterial disease, diabetes, and mortality. Diabetes Care 27:2843–2849

Leng G C, Fowkes F G R 1992 The Edinburgh claudication questionnaire: an improved version of the WHO/Rose questionnaire for use in epidemiological surveys. Journal of Clinical Epidemiology 45:1101–1109

Leng G C, Fowkes F G R, Lee A J et al 1996 Use of ankle brachial pressure index to predict cardiovascular events and death: a cohort study. BMJ 313:1440–1444

Leskinen Y, Salenius J P, Lehtim K I et al 2002 The prevalence of peripheral arterial disease and medial arterial calcification in patients with chronic renal failure: requirements for diagnostics. American Journal of Kidney Disease 40:472–479

Libby P 2001 Current concepts of the pathogenesis of the acute coronary syndromes. Circulation 104:365–372

McAlpine R R, Morris A D, Emslie-Smith A et al 2005 The annual incidence of diabetic complications in a population of patients with Type 1 and Type 2 diabetes. Diabetic Medicine 22:348–352

McDaniel M D, Cronenwett J L 1989 Basic data related to the natural history of intermittent claudication. Annals of Vascular Surgery 3:273–277

McDermott M M, Criqui M H, Liu K et al 2000 Lower ankle/brachial index, as calculated by averaging the dorsalis pedis and posterior tibial arterial pressures, and association with leg functioning in peripheral arterial disease. Journal of Vascular Surgery 32:1164–1171

McGee S R, Boyko E J 1998 Physical examination and chronic lower-extremity ischemia. Archives of Internal Medicine 158:1357–1364

Meaume S, Couilliet D, Vin F 2005 Prognostic factors for venous ulcer healing in a non-selected population of ambulatory patients. Journal of Wound Care 14:31–34

Moffatt C J, Franks P J, Doherty D C et al 2004 Prevalence of leg ulceration in a London population. Quarterly Journal of Medicine 297:431–437

Morrison H 1933 A study of the dorsalis pedis and posterior tibial pulses in one thousand individuals without symptoms of circulatory affections of the extremities. New England Journal Medicine 208:438–440

Mukamal K J, Jadhav P P, D'Agostino R B et al 2001 Alcohol consumption and hemostatic factors: analysis of the Framingham Offspring cohort. Circulation 104:1367–1373

Mukamal K J, Jensen M K, Grønbaek M et al 2005 Drinking frequency, mediating biomarkers, and risk of myocardial infarction in women and men. Circulation 112:1406–1413

Murphie P 2001a Macrovascular disease aetiology and diabetic foot ulceration. Journal of Wound Care 10:103–107

Murphie P 2001b Microvascular disease aetiology in diabetic foot ulceration. Journal of Wound Care 10:159–162

Myers K A, Scott D F, Devine T J et al 1987 Palpation of the femoral and popliteal pulses: a study of the accuracy as assessed by agreement between multiple observers. European Journal of Vascular Surgery 1:245–249

Nardone D A, Roth K M, Mazur D J et al 1990 Usefulness of physical examination in detecting the presence or absence of anemia. Archives of Internal Medicine 150:201–204

Nemeth K A, Harrison M B, Graham I D 2004 Understanding venous leg ulcer pain: results of a longitudinal study. Ostomy/Wound Management 50:34–46

Newby D E, McLeod A L, Uren N G et al 2001 Impaired coronary tissue plasminogen activator release is associated with coronary atherosclerosis and cigarette smoking: direct link between endothelial dysfunction and atherothrombosis. Circulation 103:1936–1941

Newman A B, Sutton-Tyrrell K, Vogt M T et al 1993 Morbidity and mortality in hypertensive adults with a low ankle/arm index. Journal of the American Medical Association 270:487–489

Newman A B, Naydeck B L, Sutton-Tyrrell K et al 2001 The role of comorbidity in the assessment of intermittent claudication in older adults. Journal of Clinical Epidemiology 54:294–300

National Institute for Health and Clinical Excellence 2006 Management of hypertension in adults in primary care. Clinical guideline 34. NICE, London

Nicholson M L, Byrne R L, Steele G A et al 1993 Predictive value of bruits and Doppler pressure measurements in detecting lower limb arterial stenosis. European Journal of Vascular Surgery 7:59–62

Niskanen L, Siitonen O, Suhonen M et al 1994 Medial artery calcification predicts cardiovascular mortality in patients with NIDDM. Diabetes Care 17:1252–1256

Norgauer J, Hildenbrand T, Idzko M 2002 Elevated expression of extracellular matrix metalloproteinase inducer (CD147) and membrane-type matrix metalloproteinases in venous leg ulcers. British Journal Dermatology 147:1180–1188

Nuzzaci G, Giuliano G, Righi D et al 1984 A study of the semeiological reliability of dorsalis pedis artery and posterior tibial artery in the diagnosis of lower limb arterial occlusive disease. Angiology 35:767–772

O'Brien D P, Walsh T N, Given H F 1990 The warm knee sign-an evaluation. European Journal of Vascular Surgery 4:531–534

O'Rourke R A, Brundage B H, Froelicher V F et al 2000 American College of Cardiology/American Heart Association Expert Consensus document on electron-beam computed tomography for the diagnosis and prognosis of coronary artery disease. Circulation 102:126–140

Oishi C S, Fronek A, Golbranson F L 1988 The role of non-invasive vascular studies in determining levels of amputation. Journal of Bone and Joint Surgery (Am) 70:1520–1530

Ouriel K, McDonnell A E, Metz C E et al 1982 Critical evaluation of stress testing in the diagnosis of peripheral vascular disease. Surgery 91:686–693

Otsuka R, Watanabe H, Hirata K et al 2001 Acute effects of passive smoking on the coronary circulation in healthy young adults. Journal of the American Medical Association 286:436–441

Paraskevas N, Ayari R, Malikov S et al 2006 'Pole test' measurements in critical leg ischaemia. European Journal of Vascular and Endovascular Surgery. 31:253–257

Pascarella L, Schmid Schönbein G W 2005 Causes of telangiectasias, reticular veins, and varicose veins. Seminars in Vascular Surgery 18:2–4

Raines, J K, Darling, R C, Buth, J et al 1976 Vascular laboratory criterial for the management of peripheral vascular disease of the lower extremities. Surgery 79:21

Resnick H E, Lindsay R S, McDermott M M et al 2004 Relationship of high and low ankle brachial index to all-cause and cardiovascular disease mortality: the Strong Heart Study. Circulation 109:733–739

Robertson G S, Ristic C D, Bullen B R 1990 The incidence of congenitally absent foot pulses. Annals of the Royal College of Surgeons of England 72:99–100

Rosfors S, Celsing F, Eriksson M 1994 Transcutaneous oxygen pressure measurements in patients with intermittent claudication. Clinical Physiology 14:385–391

Rutherford R B, Lowenstein D H, Klein M F 1979 Combining segmental systolic pressures and plethysmography to diagnose arterial occlusive disease of the legs. American Journal of Surgery 138:211–218

Saarinen J, Suominen V, Heikkinen M et al 2005 The profile of leg symptoms, clinical disability and reflux in legs with previously operated varicose disease. Scandinavian Journal Surgery 94:51–55

Sackett D L, Rennie D 1992 A primer on the precision and accuracy of the clinical examination. Journal of the American Medical Association 267:2638–2644

Saito S, Trovato M J, You R et al 2001 Role of matrix metalloproteinases 1, 2, and 9 and tissue inhibitor of matrix metalloproteinase-1 in chronic venous insufficiency. Journal of Vascular Surgery 34:930–938

Samuelsson P, Blohmé G, Fowelin J et al 1996 A new non-invasive method using pulse oximetry for the assessment of arterial toe pressure. Clinical Physiology 16:463–467

Shai A, Halevy S 2005 Direct triggers for ulceration in patients with venous insufficiency. International Journal of Dermatology 44:1006–1009

Simon D A, Dix F P, McCollum C N 2004 Management of venous leg ulcers. British Medical Journal 328(7452):1358–1362

Sims A J, Reay C A, Bousfield D R et al 2005 Low-cost oscillometric non-invasive blood pressure monitors: device repeatability and device differences. Physiology Measurements 26:441–445

Smith J, Mello L F, Nogueira Neto N C et al 2001 Malignancy in chronic ulcers and scars of the leg (Marjolin's ulcer): a study of 21 patients. Skeletal Radiology 30:331–337

Smith F C T, Shearman C P, Simms M H et al 1994 Falsely elevated ankle pressures in severe leg ischaemia: the pole test – an alternative approach. European Journal of Vascular Surgery 8:408–412

Stanley A C, Fernandez N N, Lounsbury K M et al 2005 Pressure-induced cellular senescence: a mechanism linking venous hypertension to venous ulcers. Journal of Surgical Research 124:112–117

Steptoe A, Feldman P J, Kunz S et al 2002 Stress responsivity and socioeconomic status: a mechanism for increased cardiovascular disease risk? European Heart Journal 23:1757–1763

Stoffers H E, Kester A D, Kaiser V et al 1996 The diagnostic value of the measurement of the ankle brachial systolic pressure index in primary health care. Journal of Clinical Epidemiology 49:1401–1405

Sumner D S 1989 Noninvasive assessment of peripheral arterial disease. In: Rutherford R B (ed.) Vascular surgery. W B Saunders, London, pp 61–111

Sumner D S 1998 Non-invasive assessment of peripheral arterial occlusive disease. In: Rutherford K S (ed.) Vascular surgery, 3rd edn. W B Saunders, London, pp 41–60

Takahashi O, Shimbo T, Rahman M 2006 Validation of the auscultatory method for diagnosing peripheral arterial disease. Journal of Family Practice 23:10–14

Tiwari A, Myint F, Hamilton G 2006 Management of lower limb lymphoedema in the United Kingdom. European Journal of Vascular and Endovascular Surgery 31:311–315

TransAtlantic InterSociety Consensus (TASC) 2000. Management of peripheral arterial disease (PAD). European Journal of Vascular and Endovascular Surgery 19(Suppl A):Si-xxviii, S1–250

Treiman G S, Copland S, McNamara R M et al 2001 Factors influencing ulcer healing in patients with combined arterial and venous insufficiency. Journal of Vascular Surgery 33:1158–1164

Trent J T, Falabella A, Eaglstein W H et al 2005 Venous ulcers: pathophysiology and treatment options. Ostomy/Wound Management 51:38–54

Tsai F W, Tulsyan N, Jones D N et al 2000 Skin perfusion pressure of the foot is a good substitute for toe pressure in the assessment of limb ischemia. Journal of Vascular Surgery 32:32–36

Tsuchiya M,Asada A, Kasahara E et al 2002 Smoking a single cigarette rapidly reduces combined concentrations of nitrate and nitrite and concentrations of antioxidants in plasma. Circulation 105:1155–1157

Unno N, Mitsuoka H, Uchiyama T et al 2002 Superficial thrombophlebitis of the lower limbs in patients with varicose veins. Surgery Today 32:397–401

van der Feen C, Neijens F S, Kanters S D et al 2002 Angiographic distribution of lower extremity atherosclerosis in patients with and without diabetes. Diabetic Medicine 19:366–370

van Weert H, Dolan G, Wichers I et al 2006 Spontaneous superficial venous thrombophlebitis: does it increase risk for thromboembolism? A historic follow-up study in primary care. Journal of Family Practice 55:52–57

Varatharajan N, Pillay S, Hitos K et al 2006 Implications of low great toe pressures in clinical practice. Australia and New Zealand Journal Surgery 76:218–221

Vicente I, Lahoz C, Taboada M et al 2006 Ankle-brachial index in patients with diabetes mellitus: prevalence and risk factors. Revista Clínica Española 206: 225–229

Vig S, Chitolie A, Bevan D et al 2006 The prevalence of thrombophilia in patients with symptomatic peripheral vascular disease. British Journal of Surgery 93:577–581

Vogt M T, Cauley J A, Newman A B 1993 Decreased ankle/arm blood pressure index and mortality in elderly women. Journal of the American Medical Association 270:465

Walker N, Rodgers A, Birchall N et al 2003 Leg ulceration as a long-term complication of deep vein thrombosis. Journal Vascular Surgery 38:1331–1335

Watkins P J, Edmonds M E 1983 Sympathetic nerve failure in diabetes. Diabetologia 25:73–77

Wattanakit K, Folsom A R, Selvin E et al 2005 Risk factors for peripheral arterial disease incidence in persons with diabetes: the atherosclerosis risk in communities (ARIC) Study. Atherosclerosis 180:389–397

Wells P S, Owen C, Doucette S et al 2006 Does this patient have deep vein thrombosis? Journal of the American Medical Association 295:199–207

Williams D T, Harding K G, Price P 2005 An evaluation of the efficacy of methods used in screening for lower-limb arterial disease in diabetes. Diabetes Care 28:2206–2210

Woods B O 1991 Clinical examination of the peripheral vasculature. Cardiology Clinics 9:413–427

Zweiffler A J 1965 Significance of knee skin temperature in ischaemic legs. Archives of Internal Medicine 115:151–154

Further reading

Altenkamper H, Eldenburg M, Altenkauper H et al 2003 A colour atlas of venous disease. Manson Publishing

Frykberg R G 1991 The high risk food in diabetes mellitus. Churchill Livingstone, Edinburgh

Levick J R 2003 An introduction to cardiovascular physiology. Hodder Arnold, London

Merli G, Weitz H H, Carabasi A R 2003 Peripheral vascular disorders. Saunders, Edinburgh

Walker W E 1991 A colour atlas of peripheral vascular disease. Wolfe Medical, London

CHAPTER

7

Neurological assessment

M C Spruce

Indicates video of assessment on DVD

Chapter contents

Introduction

The purpose of this chapter is to enable the practitioner to detect the presence of neurological alteration or abnormal function, appreciate its clinical impact and construct an appropriate management plan. To be able to do this you will need to link clinical features to the organisation of the nervous system. Evaluating the medical history and its relationship to clinical neurophysiology will enable the practitioner to match relevant assessment techniques to presenting features.

The chapter is organised to provide the practitioner with a logical and systematic approach to assessing clinically relevant aspects of the sensory, motor and autonomic nervous system. At the end of key sections, the principles discussed are applied to a series of case studies, assisted by a step-by-step aide-memoire.

The pneumonic, **CIGAR©**, has been developed to produce a systematic approach to key areas within the neurological assessment, allowing the practitioner to link clinical signs to altered physiology and relevant assessments. CIGAR will be used through out this chapter:

- **C**linical signs
- **I**n-depth medical history
- **G**eneral physiology
- **A**ssessments/tests
- **R**eferral and risk status.

Why and when to undertake a neurological assessment

Neurological conditions are a primary cause of altered lower limb function, potentially leading to deformity, ulceration and in severe situations, amputation (Table 7.1). Consequently, a neurological assessment is a vital tool to determine the risk status, treatment and appropriate management for **all** individuals.

Table 7.1 Neurological conditions that may affect the lower limb

Condition	*Description*
Cerebral vascular accident (CVA) (stroke)	Due to haemorrhage, embolus or thrombosis of the cerebral arteries
Parkinsonism	Degeneration of dopaminergic receptors. Usually idiopathic but can be drug induced
Friedreich's ataxia	One of a group of hereditary syndromes affecting the cerebellum. Inheritance is autosomal recessive. Onset in childhood, death usually around 40 years
Multiple sclerosis	Patchy demyelination of the CNS. Shows relapses and remissions. Onset 20+
Poliomyelitis	Virus that affects lower motor neurones (LMNs)
Syringomyelia	Progressive destruction of the spinal cord due to blockage of central canal, e.g. tumour
Tabes dorsalis	Occurs with tertiary stage syphilis
Spina bifida	Defective closure of vertebral column. Congenital
Motor neurone disease	Degeneration of both upper motor neurones (UMNs) and LMNs. No sensory loss. Onset usually 40 and 60 years. Death usually due to respiratory infection. Idiopathic
Subacute combined degeneration of the spinal cord	Due to lack of vitamin B_{12}. Usually seen in pernicious anaemia. Affects both sensory and motor tracts in the spinal cord. See UMN signs, sensory and proprioceptive deficit. Reversible if detected in time
Charcot–Marie–Tooth disease/ peroneal muscle atrophy/ hereditary motor–sensory neuropathy	Affects peroneal nerve, predominantly motor with variable sensory deficit. Commonest inherited neuropathy. Usually autosomal dominant. Onset in teens, slowly worsens
Guillain–Barré syndrome	Post-viral autoimmune response, rapid onset, potentially fatal from respiratory failure. Predominantly motor effects, with muscle weakness and paralysis, but some sensory loss; 80% of patients show full recovery. Also chronic relapsing form
Neurofibromatosis	Autosomal dominant condition that leads to tumours of nerves and compression of spinal cord
Peripheral neuropathy	Occurs due to a variety of causes, e.g. alcoholism, injury, diabetes mellitus
Myasthenia gravis	Autoimmune disease that affects the neuromuscular junction and leads to severe fatigue and weakness/paralysis
Myopathies	Range of relatively rare diseases affecting muscle only. May be inherited or acquired. Symptoms similar to LMN diseases but no fasciculation

To achieve this, the practitioner needs to link pertinent information from an assessment to possible underlying causes or abnormal responses. Indeed, the practitioner needs to think much like a clinical detective, allowing a diagnosis to be made based on a sound understanding of physiology, rather than matching the 'evidence' to a potential culprit. This allows the diagnosis to be clinically meaningful, for example, rubor and heat in the diabetic foot need not be dismissed as cardinal signs of infection. On the contrary, increased vasodilation due to autonomic dysfunction may in fact indicate Charcot's foot. Hence, it is imperative that the clinician appreciates all potential diagnoses, and is capable, through a process of discriminatory assessment, to match physiology to pathology. In the above example, infection would remain a prime suspect, allowing appropriate intervention to save the individual from likely ulceration and amputation.

The National Institute of Health and Clinical Excellence (NICE; www.nice.org.uk) has produced guidelines stating that all individuals with diabetes mellitus should receive annual neurological screening. In addition, elderly patients may require further neurological monitoring, given that studies by Mold et al (2004) found that 26% of healthy individuals between 65 and 75 years displayed altered neurological status. The reported incidence in the ≥85 years age group was increased to 54%. Accordingly, although all new patients require an initial assessment, high-risk groups should receive a full review twice yearly under ideal circumstances.

Relevant information gained from the assessment should be shared with appropriate members of the multi-disciplinary team, but more importantly, with the patient (facilitating empowerment). As with any aspect of patient assessment the aim is not merely to gather information, but to *act* upon it.

Clinical overview of the function and organisation of the nervous system

Function

The primary function of the nervous system is to permit rapid communication between the collection of cells and tissues which constitute our bodies. This allows them to function as an organised whole, within acceptable limits (homeostasis). While the nervous system offers rapid communication, its effects last for only a short period of time. Therefore, it needs to work alongside the generally slower acting endocrine system, the effects of which are longer lasting.

Organisation of the nervous system

The nervous system can be organised on the basis of either its anatomical location (central and peripheral) or its function (somatic and autonomic) (see Fig. 7.1). However, while these classifications exist independently in text books, in reality, they function as a coordinated whole. For example, when learning to drive, we know that the clutch and accelerator are important, but only when they are in the correct combination will the car move effectively.

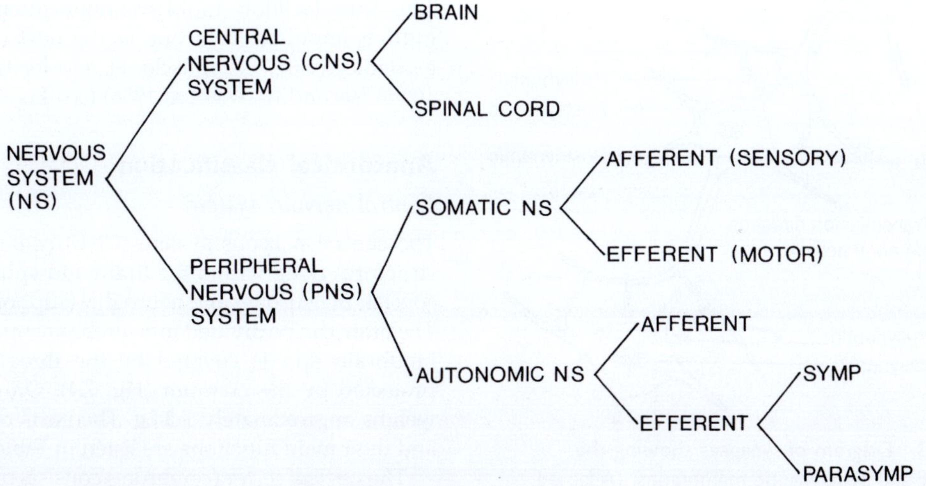

Figure 7.1 Flow diagram of the organisation of the nervous system.

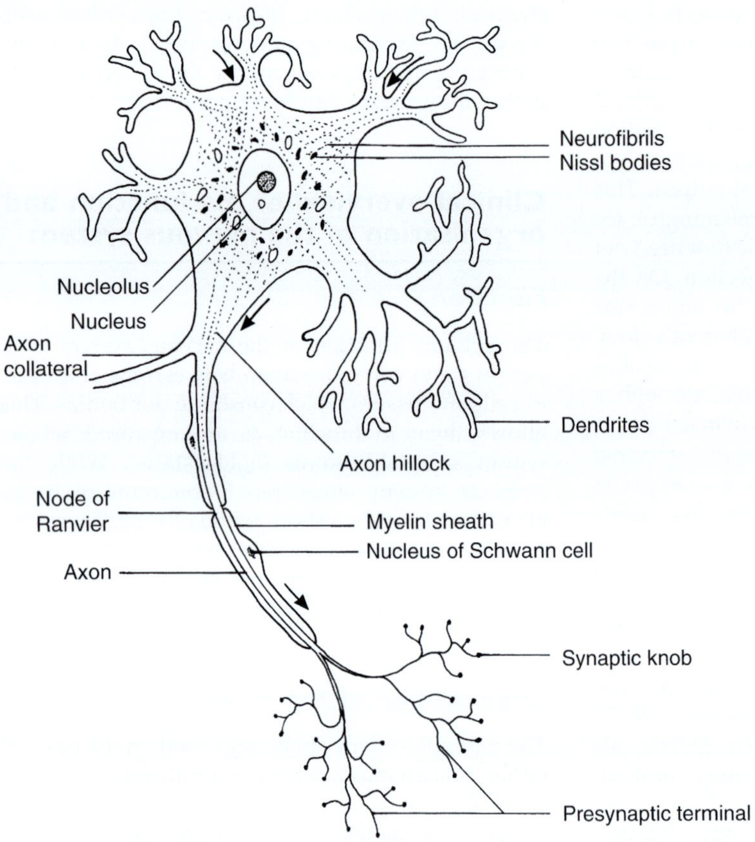

Figure 7.2 A single neurone (not to scale) has four parts: cell body, dendrites, axon, presynaptic terminals. Note that in the CNS some neurones may have no axons.

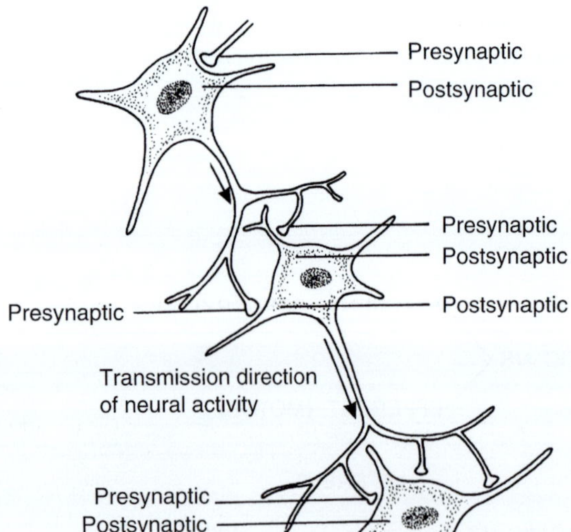

Figure 7.3 Diagram of synapses showing the presynaptic and postsynaptic membranes. (Adapted from Vander et al 1998.)

Building blocks of the nervous system

When conducting an assessment, it is important to know what one is assessing. Neurones are one of the primary building blocks of the nervous system (Fig. 7.2). They facilitate rapid communication by transmitting impulses from one to the next or to other excitable tissue, i.e. muscle, at a velocity of up to 100 m/second (Bawa et al 1984) (see Fig. 7.3).

Anatomical classification

Central nervous system

The central nervous system (CNS) contains all the structures lying within the **brain** and **spinal cord**. It consists of neurones and neuroglial (supporting) cells. The brain can be divided into forebrain, midbrain and hindbrain and is covered by the three meninges, protected by the cranium (Fig. 7.4). On average, it weighs approximately 1.3 kg. The parts of the brain and their main functions are listed in Table 7.2.

The *cerebral cortex* (cerebrum) consists of two hemispheres (right and left) and is principally associated

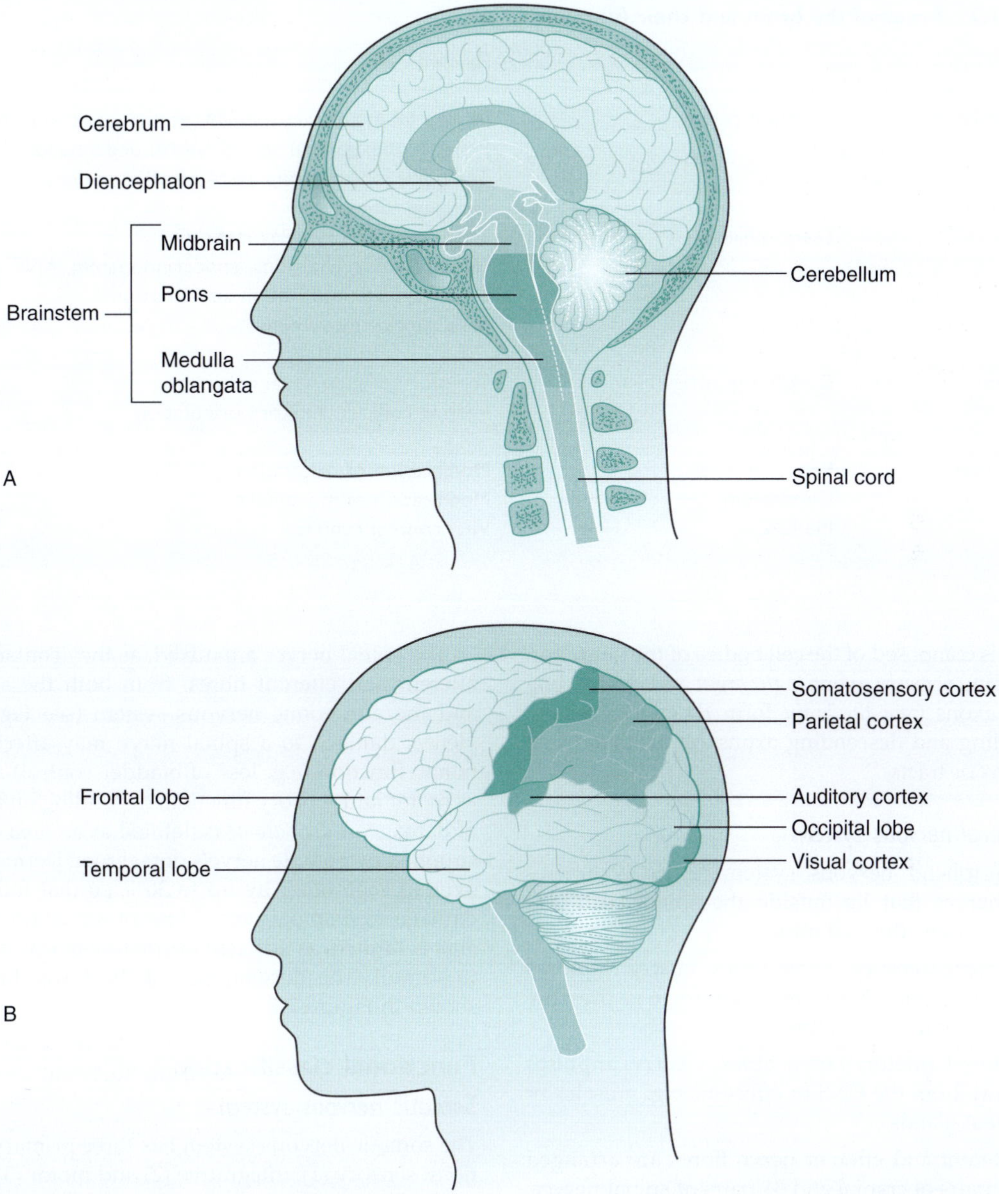

Figure 7.4 The brain **A** Anatomy of the brain **B** Position of the lobes and cortex. (Adapted from Vander et al 1998.)

with sensory perception and voluntary motor activity, the somatosensory cortex (see Fig. 7.4). Damage to this area following a cerebrovascular accident (CVA), can result in features classically associated with this condition, i.e. spasticity, altered sensation and speech. The cortex is highly convoluted, which increases its surface area and, therefore, the number of neurones it contains – an estimated $10^{2783000}$ synapses! The *cerebellum* consists of two hemispheres which are primarily composed of the anterior and posterior lobes and is a vital centre for the coordination of voluntary movement, posture and balance. Hence, an ataxic (uncoordinated) gait may be an indicator of a lesion to the cerebellum.

The spinal cord is enclosed in the 32 vertebrae of the spinal column (Fig. 7.5). In cross-section, it is composed of a grey centre, similar in shape to the letter H with a white outer area (Fig. 7.6A). The grey

Table 7.2 Areas of the brain and their function

Area		*Function*
Forebrain	Cerebral cortex	Frontal lobe: abstract thought, conscious action, speech Parietal lobe: general senses, verbal understanding Temporal lobe: hearing, taste, smell, emotions Occipital lobe: vision
	Diencephalon	Thalamus: sensory relay station Hypothalamus: emotions, endocrine system, ANS Limbic system: motivation and emotions Basal ganglia: movement
Midbrain	Corpora quadrigemina	Superior colliculi: visual orientation Inferior colliculi: auditory orientation
Hindbrain	Pons Cerebellum Medulla	Modification of respiration Modification of movement Vital control centres

matter is composed of the cell bodies of the neurones. Ascending sensory axons *to the brain* and descending motor axons *from the brain* form the white matter. Ascending and descending axons are arranged into columns or tracts.

Peripheral nervous system

The peripheral nervous system (PNS) comprises those nerves that lie outside the spinal cord and brain. It can be divided into:

- afferent (sensory) nerve fibres – carry impulses towards the CNS from receptors, e.g. pressure and vibration receptors
- efferent (motor) nerve fibres – carry impulses away from the CNS to effectors, e.g. muscles or sweat glands.

The afferent and efferent nerve fibres are arranged into 12 pairs of cranial and 31 pairs of spinal nerves. The spinal nerves emerge from the spinal cord as two roots, a dorsal (posterior) and a ventral (anterior) root, which join to form the peripheral mixed spinal nerve (Fig. 7.6A). The dorsal root ganglion contains the cell bodies of afferent (sensory) fibres. Incoming sensory information to the spinal cord is transmitted along an afferent neurone in a mixed nerve, into the dorsal root and enters the dorsal horn of the spinal cord, where it synapses with either an internuncial or motor neurone (Fig. 7.6B). The ventral root contains mainly efferent (motor) fibres, the cell bodies lying within the ventral and lateral horns of the spinal grey matter (Fig. 7.6A).

The spinal nerves are mixed, as they contain both afferent and efferent fibres, from both the somatic and the autonomic nervous system (see Fig 7.6B). Hence, damage to a spinal nerve may affect autonomic function (e.g. loss of bladder control) as well as motor and sensory function, depending on the site of damage. A *dermatome* is defined as an area of skin supplied by a single nerve's dorsal root. Dermatomes overlap each other by up to 30%, so that following damage to a spinal nerve, loss of sensation in that area is limited, as adjacent dermatomes will respond to stimuli. The dermatomes of the lower limb are shown in **Figure 7.7**.

Functional classification

Somatic nervous system

The somatic nervous system has three primary functions: sensory (1), integrative (2) and motor (3), all of which are active at a conscious level. To demonstrate their role, let us consider the painful act of stepping on a sharp object:

1. Sensory – afferent nerves detect changes (stimuli) in the external environment and its relation with the body.
   Stepping barefoot onto a drawing pin triggers a pain response.
2. Integrative – interprets and stores sensory information within the central nervous system (CNS).
   The pain response will be recognised and processed.

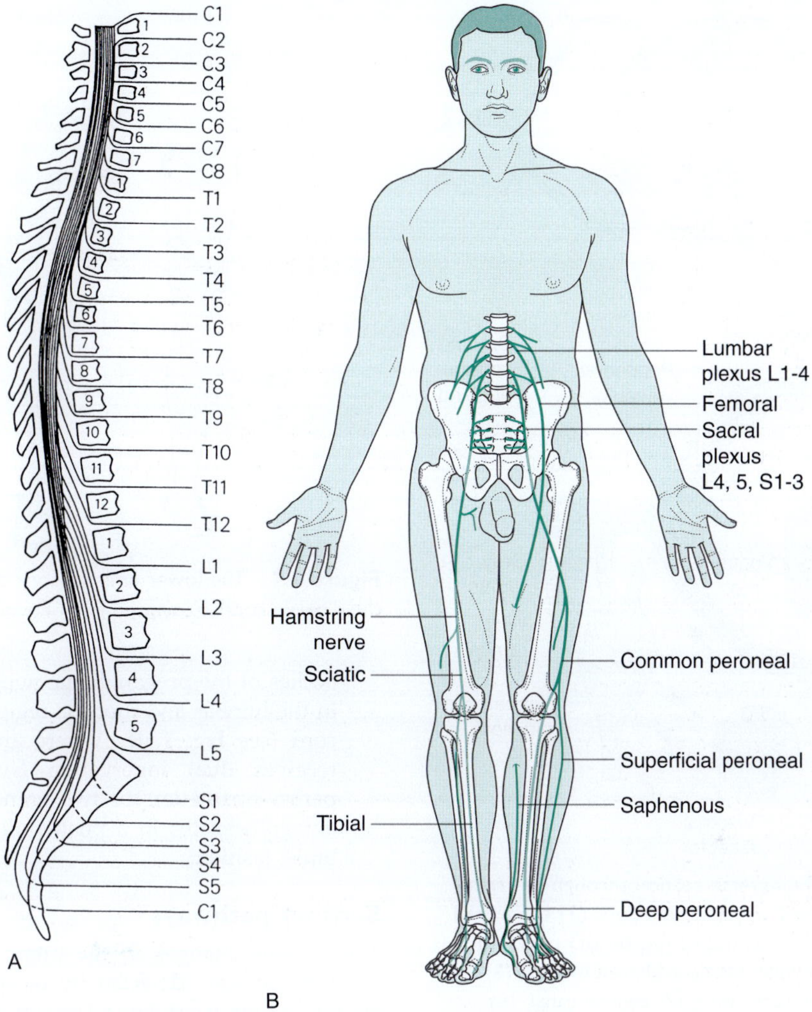

Figure 7.5 The spinal cord **A** Relationship of vertebrae to spinal cord segments (reproduced from Matthews & Arnold 1991, with permission) **B** Organisation of the lumbar and sacral plexi and innervation of the lower limb. (Adapted from McClintic 1980.)

3. Motor – efferent nerves produce a response, muscle contraction or glandular secretion.
   Muscle contraction produced causing the foot to be rapidly withdrawn.

Note: the receptors detect changes in the external environment and the effectors bring about movement of the skeleton through muscular (motor) response.

Autonomic nervous system

The autonomic nervous system (ANS) innervates and regulates the body's internal organs and environment. While reading this book, you may not be aware of the partial pressure of oxygen in your arterial blood or the relaxing wall of your bladder. However, it is the ANS, which is responsible for regulating the status of our internal organs and performing complex reflex activities at a subconscious level.

The afferent neurones of the ANS travel with those of the somatic system, although the receptors are situated in internal organs, i.e. baroreceptors of the carotid sinus. The efferent branches of the ANS differ from those in the somatic system, as there are two neurones (preganglionic and postganglionic) in each pathway. The first cell body lies within the CNS, with the second in the autonomic ganglia outside. The efferent outflow is divided into the sympathetic

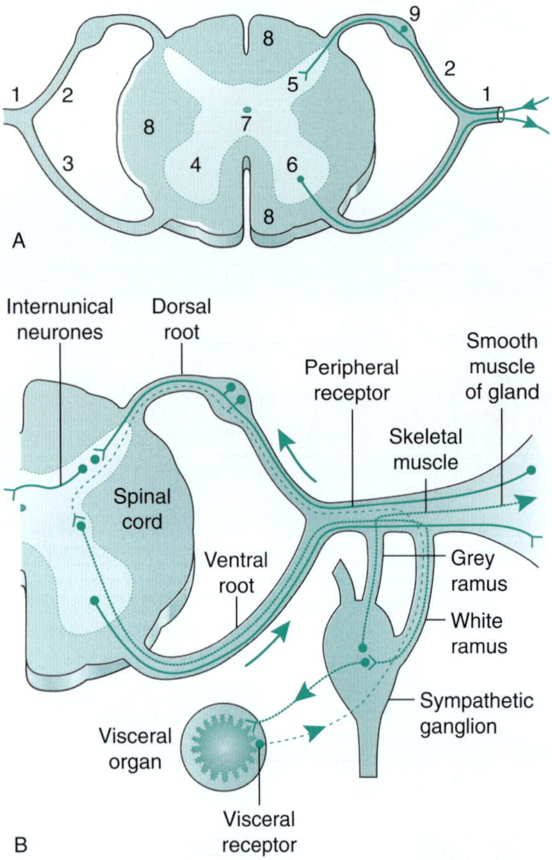

Figure 7.6 **A** Transverse section through the spinal cord showing mixed spinal nerve roots: (1) the paired mixed spinal nerves; (2) dorsal (posterior) root; (3) ventral (anterior) root; (4) central grey matter; (5) dorsal horn; (6) ventral horn; (7) central canal; (8) surrounding white matter; and (9) dorsal root ganglion **B** Connection between sensory and motor neurones and the spinal cord. (Adapted from McClintic 1980.)

and parasympathetic systems (Fig. 7.8):

- Parasympathetic nervous system
  This is the efferent part of the autonomic nervous system, which is associated with 'resting and digesting' activities, i.e. increased food digestion, absorption and production of insulin. The cell bodies of the preganglionic neurones are situated in the brain stem and sacral region of the spinal cord (craniosacral outflow). The postganglionic cell bodies are found in ganglia close to or within the effector organ.
- Sympathetic nervous system
  This is the efferent branch of the autonomic nervous system, which prepares the body for action – the fight or flight response. The cell bodies of the preganglionic neurones are found in the lumbar and thoracic regions of the spinal cord (see Fig. 7.5B). Where an effector organ receives dual innervation (sympathetic and parasympathetic), the two branches usually act antagonistically, in a push–pull or accelerator–brake fashion.

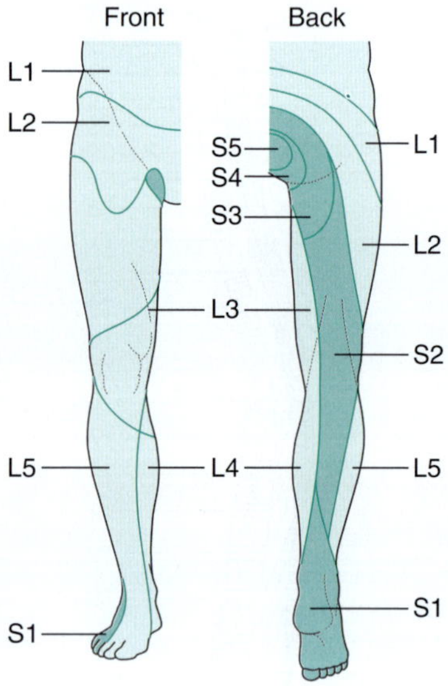

Figure 7.7 The lower limb sensory dermatomes and their nerve roots. (Adapted from Epstein et al 1992.)

Sensory pathways

The various changes in the internal and external environments are detected by receptors. Receptors are found within specialised organs, such as the rods and cones of the eye, and are also distributed throughout the body, for example the pain receptors of the skin and gut. Receptors within the specialised organs contribute to the complex senses of sight, hearing, taste and smell. Exteroceptors in the skin detect pressure, touch, temperature, pain and position sense in relation to the external environment. They are termed somatic receptors (Table 7.3). These receptors and their associated pathways form an integral part of the neurological assessment.

Interoceptors detect stimuli in the body's internal environment that do not usually reach consciousness. They communicate with subconscious levels of the brain. Baroreceptors located in the walls of arteries and veins are a classic example of interoceptors; they monitor internal changes in blood pressure. Receptors in the muscles, tendons and joints registering position, sense, tension and degree of stretch are called proprioceptors. They send impulses both to

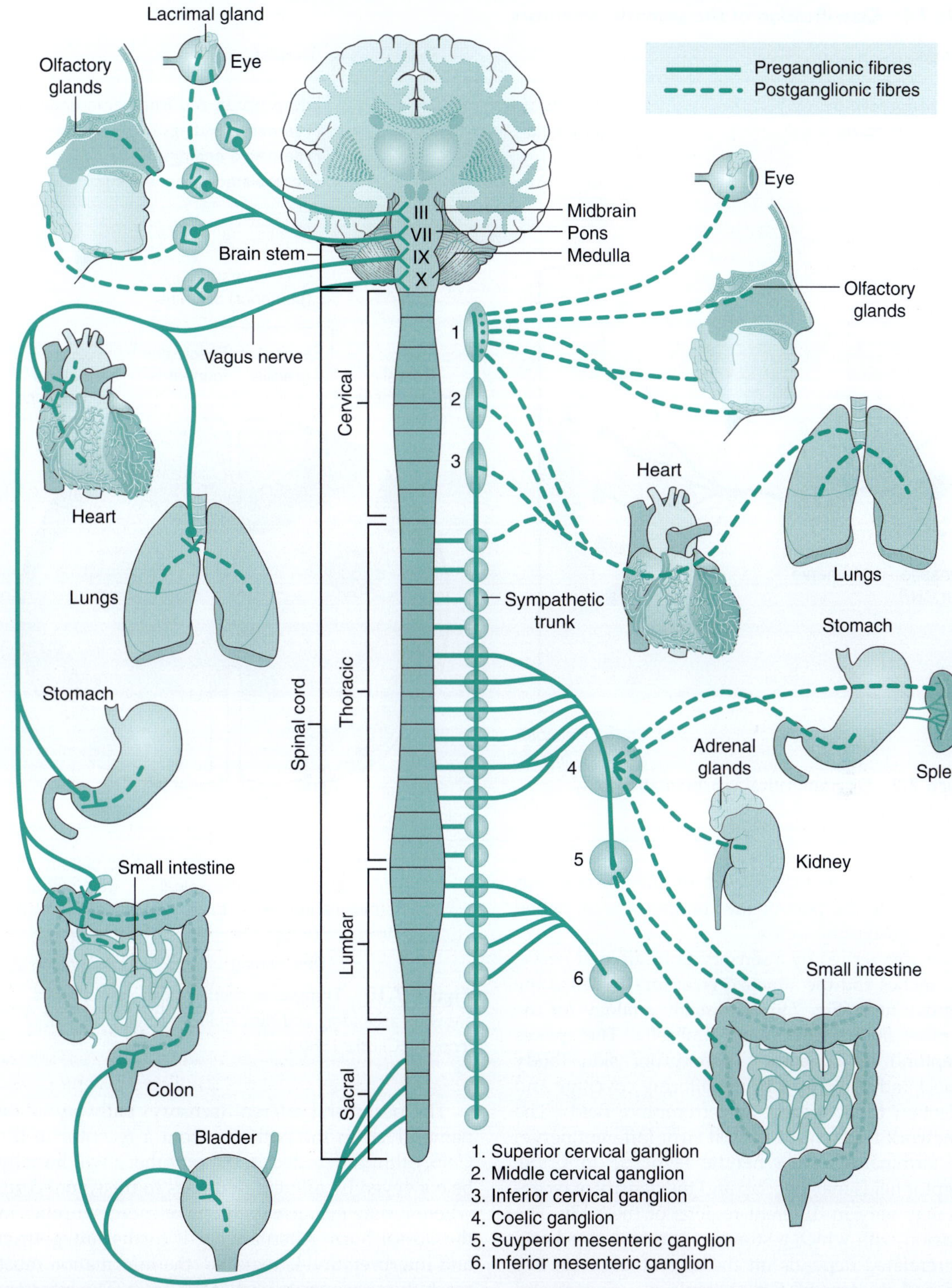

Figure 7.8 Autonomic outflow. (Adapted from Vander et al 1998.)

Table 7.3 Classification of the somatic receptors

Category	*Sense*	*Receptor*
Mechanoreceptor	Touch, pressure	Encapsulated and free nerve endings
Thermoreceptor	Warmth, cold	Free nerve endings
Nociceptor	Pain	Free nerve endings
Proprioceptor	Position	Encapsulated nerve endings

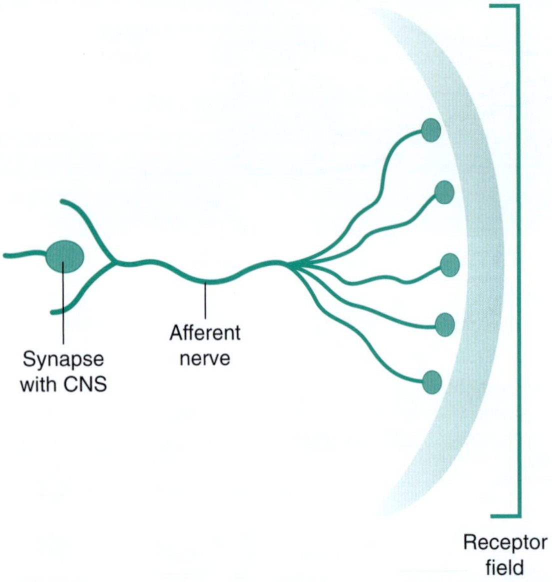

Figure 7.9 Diagrammatical representation of a sensory unit.

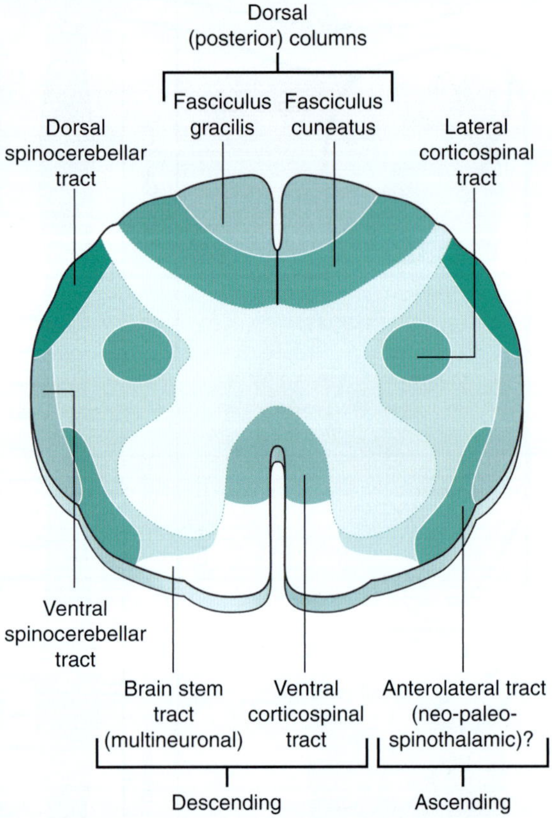

Figure 7.10 Transverse section of the spinal cord showing ascending and descending pathway. (Adapted from McClintic 1980.)

the cerebellum, which is part of the unconscious brain, and to the part of the conscious brain called the somatosensory cortex.

The area served by a sensory unit (afferent nerve, its branches and the attached receptors) is called the receptive field (Fig. 7.9). A possible analogy for the receptive field is that of an umbrella. The spokes (receptors) lie beneath a waterproof skin (body tissues) and make up a frame offering coverage and protection for a specific area (receptive field). The framework feeds into a central strut (afferent nerve) and terminates at the handle (synapse to CNS). Receptor fields may overlap and the density of receptors may vary in different regions of the body. The precision with which a stimulus can be located and differentiated depends on the size of the receptive field and its density. For example our fingers and thumbs are very good at detecting stimuli from the external environment as the receptive fields in them are small and dense.

The peripheral afferent (sensory) pathway is the name given to the pathway from a receptor to the CNS. Stimuli detected in the periphery will initially be conveyed by afferent neurones to the spinal cord, where it may synapse with one or more neurones in the dorsal horn. Alternatively, if further integration and interpretation is required, the information must reach the appropriate part of the brain. The information travels to these higher centres in ascending tracts or columns of the white matter of the spinal cord (Fig. 7.10).

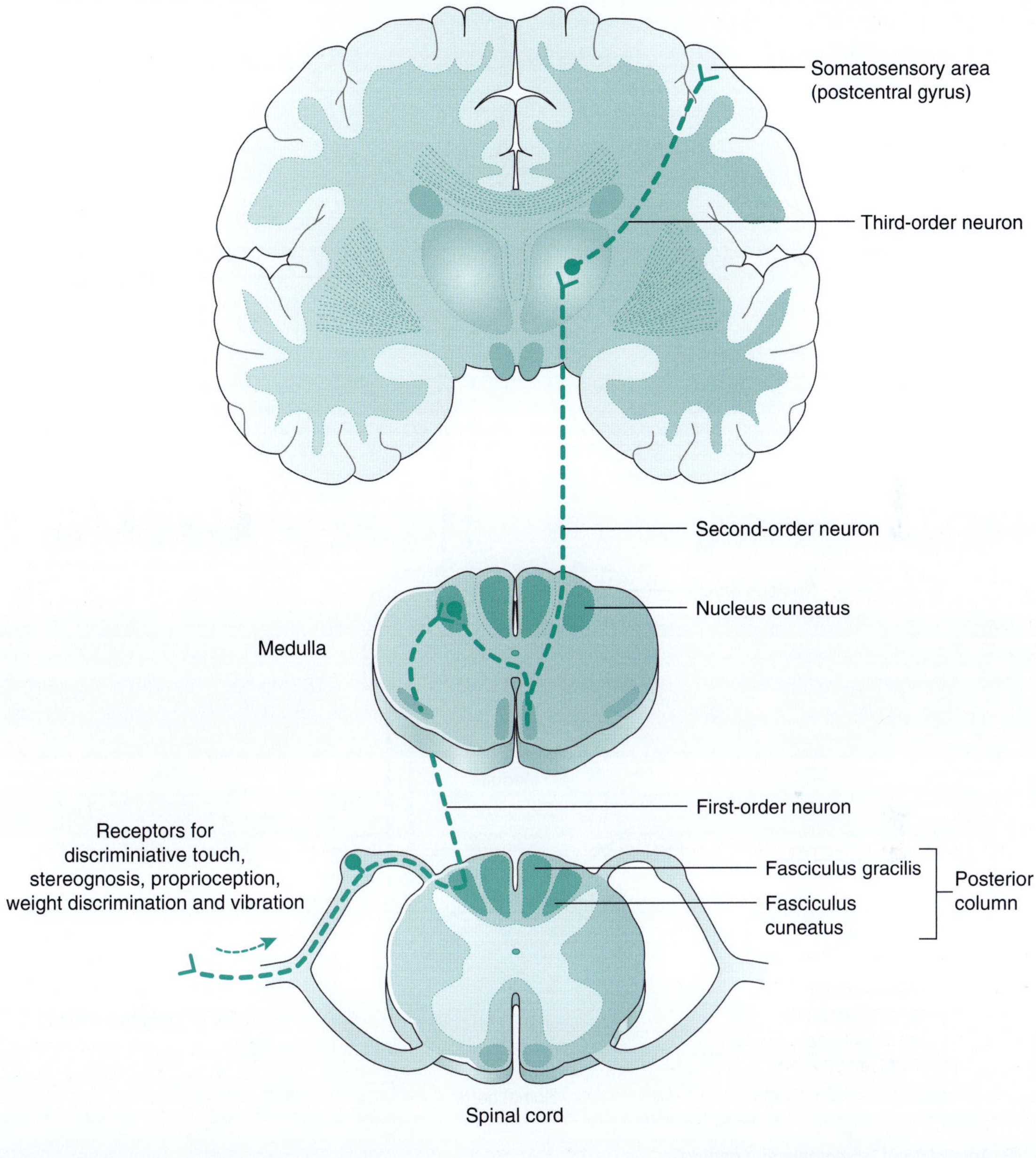

Figure 7.11 The spinothalamic tract showing first, second and third order neurones.

There are two main ascending tracts (Budd 1984):

- Dorsal columns
- Spinothalamic/anterolateral.

Most of the tracts are named according to their origin and destination, i.e. the spinothalamic tract, carrying pain information, runs from the spinal cord up to the thalamus, an important sensory relay station in the brain. The ascending tracts from receptor to sensory cortex involve three neurone links (Fig. 7.11):

1. First-order neurons – convey impulses from the receptors to spinal cord or brain stem
2. Second-order neurons – convey impulses from the spinal cord and brain stem to thalamus

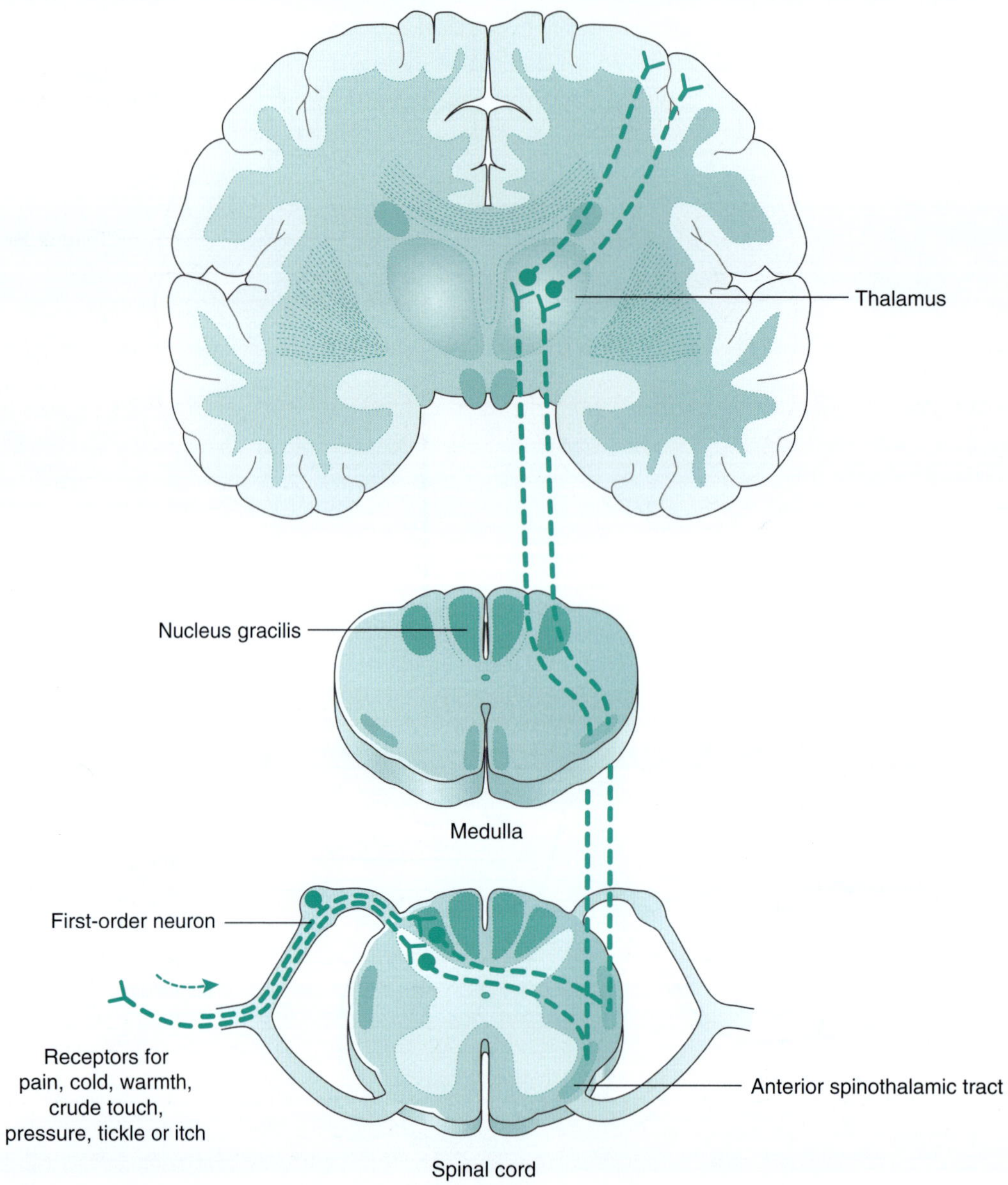

B. Anterolateral (spinothalamic) pathway

Figure 7.11 *Continued.*

3. Third-order neurons – convey impulses from the thalamus to the somatosensory cortex, resulting in conscious perception.

The information carried by the three-neurone link is simultaneously transmitted to the cerebellum and brain stem (unconscious) by off-shoots (collaterals).

The ascending tracts and their function are given in Figure 7.11.

The majority of ascending tracts cross over to the opposite (contralateral) side of entry, either in the spinal cord or in the brain stem, synapsing with areas of the thalamus before continuing to the conscious sensory cortex. Neurological damage to the spinal

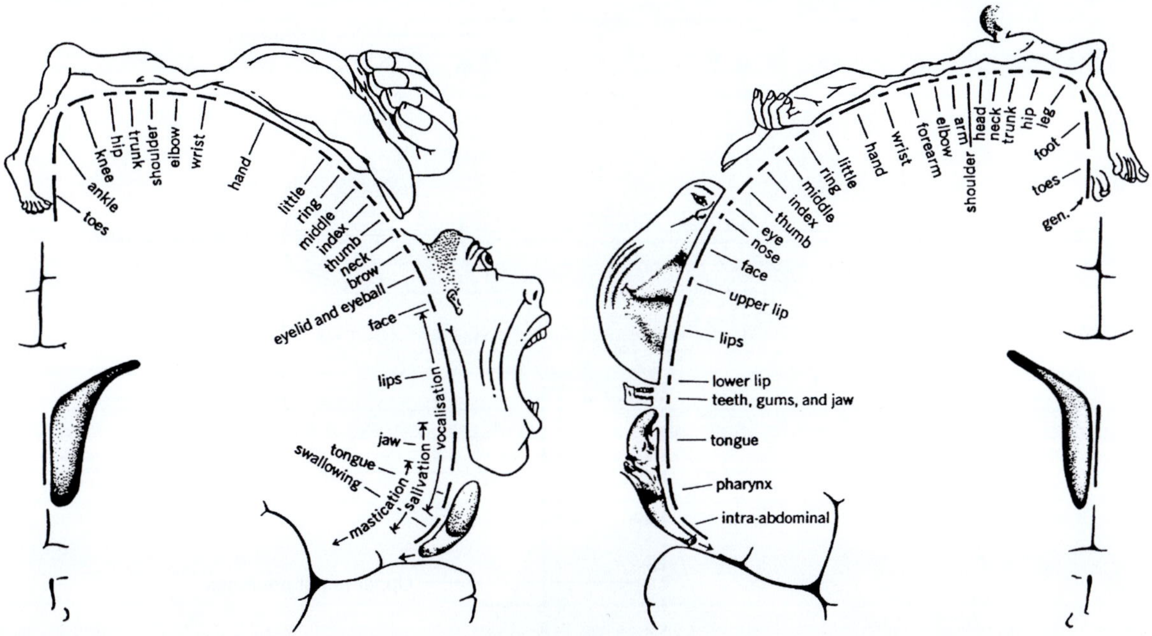

A B

Figure 7.12 Diagram illustrating the somatotopic organisation of (**A**) the motor and (**B**) the sensory cortices. The left half of the body is represented by the right hemisphere of the brain and the right half of the body by the left hemisphere. (Reproduced from Wilson 1990, with permission.)

cord may produce numbness on either the contralateral side, if the site of damage is before the tracts cross, or the ipsilateral (same) side, if the site of damage occurs after the tracts have crossed. The organisation continues in the brain, allowing specific areas of the cortex to receive the information from the various parts of the body (Fig. 7.12). This is called somatotopic organisation. This arrangement explains why a stroke/CVA affecting a particular part of the sensory cortex produces numbness or paraesthesia in a particular part of the body on the opposite (contralateral) side.

Motor pathways

Just as all conscious stimuli are interpreted in the cortex, so all conscious actions originate there. The whole area is known as the sensorimotor cortex; one part is called the primary motor cortex and initiates conscious action (Fig. 7.12B). Damage to this region affects particular actions on the contralateral (opposite) side of the body. Close to this area is the premotor cortex, which is involved in the planning of actions. Since the actions produced by these neurones are the conscious movements of the body, the muscles involved will be skeletal and the neurones part of the somatic motor system.

Neurones in the brain, responsible for initiating commands, are called upper motor neurones (UMNs). They do not send impulses directly to the muscles, but exert their influence via neurones in the ventral (anterior) horn of the spinal cord and are called lower motor neurones (LMNs). LMNs send impulses to the skeletal muscles via their axons, forming the peripheral efferent pathways within spinal nerves.

The descending pathways from brain to spinal cord can be divided into two main tracts: the rapid corticospinal tract and the slower multineuronal tract (Fig. 7.13).

The corticospinal (lateral and anterior) tract is mainly responsible for the skilled movements of small, distal limb muscles, such as those used in dexterity. Most of the fibres, but not all, cross over in the brain stem and descend in the white matter of the spinal cord. The corticospinal tract forms a rough pyramid shape as it passes through the brain stem, hence is termed the pyramidal tract. Its location within the spinal cord can be seen in Figure 7.10.

The multineuronal tract (extra pyramidal) mainly influence the large, proximal limb muscles and the axial muscles of posture, having a predominantly inhibitory effect on the ventral horn cells (Fig 7.13). Consequently, damage to UMNs can lead to loss of the inhibition or 'damping down' effect on the LMNs,

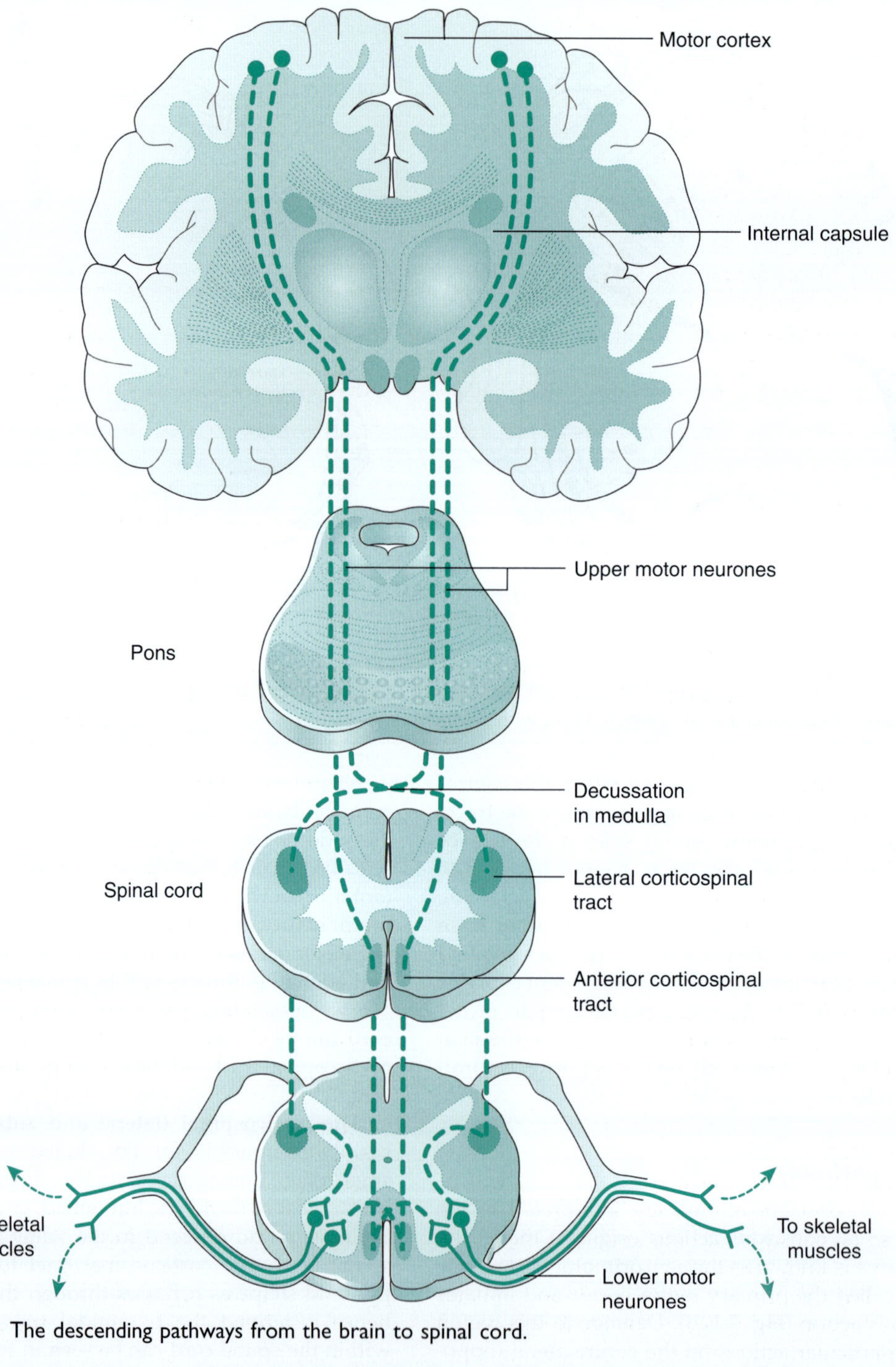

Figure 7.13 The descending pathways from the brain to spinal cord.

producing 'hyper-reflexia' or an exaggerated patellar reflex response. They are also responsible for the anti-gravity reflexes, which keep our knees extended and head erect, so maintaining upright posture. Although influenced by UMNs, the tracts are only recognisable as separate pathways, emerging from the brain stem to travel through the spinal cord as the vestibulospinal, tectospinal and reticulospinal tracts.

The division of the descending tracts is not clear cut, as they demonstrate redundancy, there being much overlap and interaction between the two. Other areas of the brain also have strong modifying influences, such as the cerebellum and the basal ganglia.

Cerebellum

The actions of the cerebellum are unconscious and very important in postural reflexes. The cerebellum has no direct descending pathways to the spinal cord. Instead, it has a rich afferent input and sends modifying influences to the sensorimotor cortex, the reticular formation and the brain-stem nuclei. Thus, symptoms of cerebellar defects may be due to lesions in the ascending spinocerebellar tracts, in the cerebellum itself or efferent pathways going to other parts of the brain.

The cerebellum receives all information about positional sense. Spinocerebellar tracts carry proprioceptive information from muscles, tendons, joints and cutaneous pressure receptors. The cerebral cortex gives information about the determined actions and communicates this to the cerebellum. These data are integrated and compared with the information on intended actions received from the cerebral cortex. Modifying influences are subsequently sent back to the motor cortex and brain stem, so that descending instructions to the LMNs can be altered where necessary.

Basal ganglia

At present, the precise functions of the basal ganglia in movement are unknown, but they are thought to enable abstract thought (ideas) to be converted into voluntary action (Ganong 1991, p 200). Like the cerebellum, they function at an unconscious level and have no direct pathway to LMNs, but influence the sensorimotor cortex and the descending reticular formation. As the main action of the basal ganglia is on the descending extrapyramidal tracts, they have become known as the 'extrapyramidal system' and conditions affecting them are referred to as extrapyramidal syndromes, most significant among them being parkinsonism.

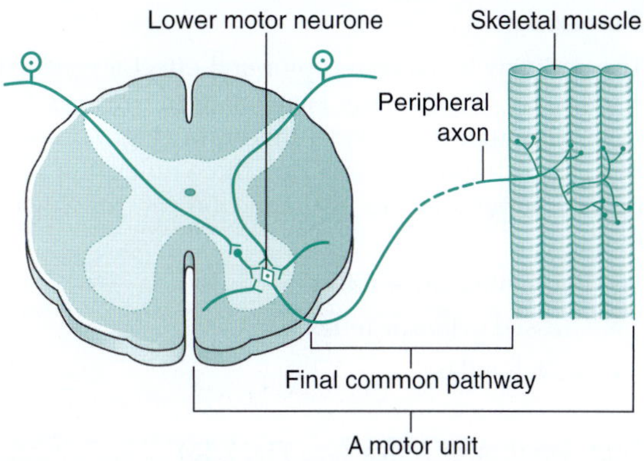

Figure 7.14 The final common pathway of a motor unit.

The final common pathway of conscious action is excitation of an LMN in the ventral (anterior) horn of the spinal cord and passage of an impulse along its axon in the spinal nerve to the skeletal muscle (Fig. 7.14). A single LMN can be subject to many simultaneous excitatory and inhibitory influences from many neurones, approximately 10000–15000 synapses. If the sum of these influences is excitatory, the LMN will be stimulated to discharge an impulse along its axon, causing the skeletal muscle to contract.

Reflexes

Reflex actions are automatic responses to particular stimuli and form the basis of much of our behaviour, from the simple knee jerk to driving a car. They are also very important in posture, balance and gait. Reflexes can be inborn (inherited, innate, instinctive) or acquired (learned). Examples of the former are eye blink, pupil dilation/constriction, pain withdrawal and sweat secretion. Examples of the latter are swimming, walking, driving or even debriding callus! We may be aware of some, while others may never reach consciousness.

In all cases, the pathway allows the body to respond rapidly to a given stimulus. Generally, inborn reflexes produce stereotypical responses, usually protective or those essential to posture and balance. Acquired reflexes are more complex, involving the conscious cortex and many different effectors, so that the response is more easily modified. As an example, try standing upright and leaning backwards as far as you can. What happens to your arms and knees? Can you prevent their movement? Now, compare this to the ease with which you can change from a walking to a running gait.

Reflex arcs

The pathway between receptor and effector is called a reflex arc, has five key elements and involves the CNS, although not always the brain (Fig. 7.15 and Box 7.1). Additionally, there are three reflexes of particular importance to the function of the lower limb:

- Pain withdrawal reflex
- Crossed extensor reflex
- Stretch reflex.

Pain withdrawal reflex (see Fig. 7.16)

1. Injured cells release local chemical mediators that sensitise the nociceptors.
2. Proportional to the damage done, impulses are transmitted along the afferent pathways to the CNS (in this case, the spinal cord).
3. The afferent neurone activates internuncial neurones in multiple segments (point of entry, ascending and descending) of the spinal cord.
4. Efferent neurones (LMNs) transmit impulses from the CNS to the skeletal muscles (effectors).
5. The neurotransmitter, acetylcholine, is released by the efferent neurones and combines with receptors at the motor endplate on the muscle fibres, causing muscle contraction and withdrawal.

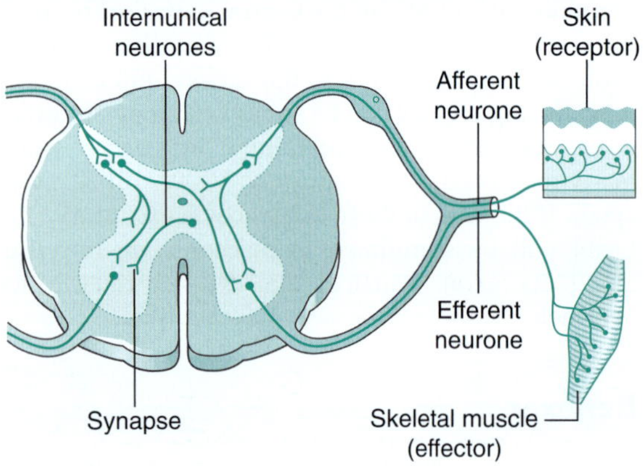

Figure 7.15 The reflex arc. (Reproduced from McClintic 1980, with permission.)

Box 7.1 Essential elements of a reflex arc

1. A detector to detect the change (stimulus) in either the internal or external environment
2. Afferent neurones that send the information into the CNS along the afferent pathways
3. An integrating centre to match the appropriate response to the stimulus. This will be in the brain or spinal cord. Different parts of the CNS communicate with one another via ascending and descending pathways
4. Efferent neurones that carry instructions from the CNS via efferent pathways to the effectors (skeletal, smooth or cardiac muscle or gland)
5. An effector to carry out the necessary response

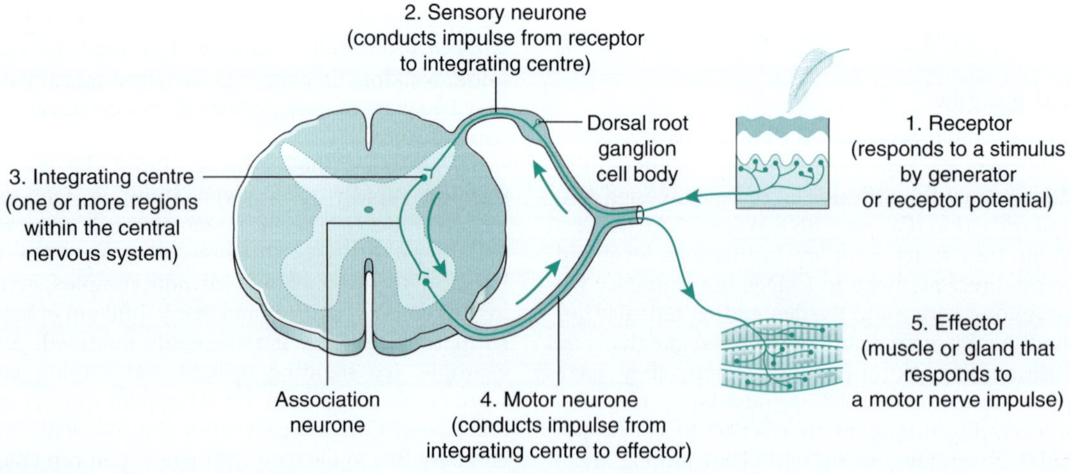

 Figure 7.16 The pain withdrawal arc.

The presence of more than one synapse in the reflex arc means that the arc is described as polysynaptic. The reflex is ipsilateral, as sensory (afferent) input and motor (efferent) output both occur on the same side of the spinal cord.

Crossed extensor reflex (see Fig. 7.17)

This reflex is often superimposed on the pain withdrawal reflex and is a postural reflex, enabling an injured lower limb to be withdrawn, while the remaining limb bears weight:

1. A painful stimulus triggers the nociceptors (pain receptors).
2. Afferent neurones transmit impulses to the CNS.
3. The afferent neurones activate both ipsilateral and contralateral internuncial neurones within the spinal cord, at several levels.
4. Many efferent neurones (LMNs) become excited and their antagonists inhibited. This ensures that the flexors of the injured limb contract while the extensors relax, whereas in the contralateral limb the flexors are inhibited and the extensors contract to provide a rigid support.
5. Acetylcholine is released by the efferent neurones at the motor endplate causing muscle contraction.

The crossed extensor reflex is polysynaptic and contralateral. This reflex occurs not only when a lower limb is injured, but during normal gait, as one limb is in the swing phase and the other is weightbearing.

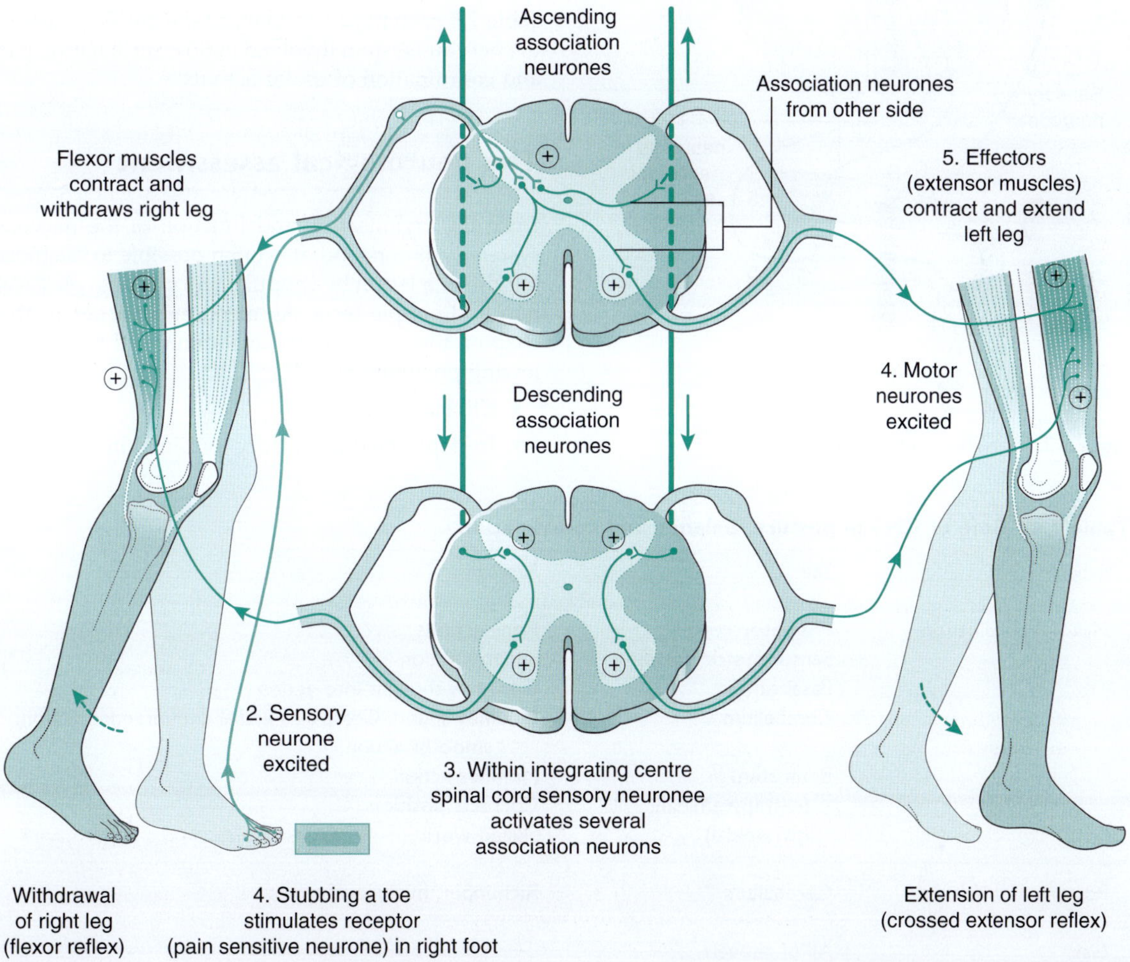

Figure 7.17 The crossed extensor reflex.

Stretch reflex (see Fig. 7.18)

This is a very important reflex for all motor activity, especially when new actions are being learned. It can be demonstrated by the patellar and Achilles tendon reflexes and supplies the cerebellum with information about the state of contraction in muscle:

1. Striking the tendon with the patella hammer causes stretching of the muscle and activates specialised receptors (muscle spindles).
2. The stretched muscle spindles generate impulses which travel along the neurone towards the CNS.
3. The neurone enters the spinal cord and synapses directly with a motor (efferent) neurone in the anterior horn and an inhibitory internuncial neurone.
4. The excited efferent neurone (LMN) transmits the impulse from the CNS along its axon to the stretched extensor skeletal muscle fibres. The inhibitory internuncial neurone inhibits the antagonistic (flexor) muscles.
5. Acetylcholine is released by the efferent neurones and the extensor muscle contracts, while the flexor muscles relax, relieving the detected stretch.

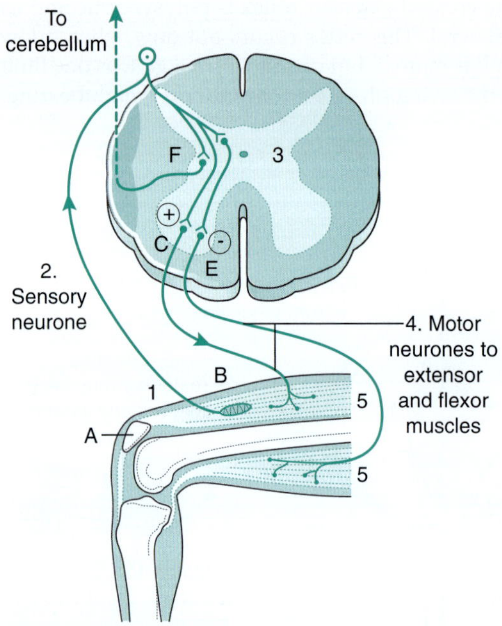

Figure 7.18 The stretch reflex.

Coordination and posture

Table 7.4 presents a summary of the various parts of the nervous system involved in posture, balance, gait and coordination of motor activity.

The neurological assessment

Once the organisation and function of the nervous system is understood, it is often possible to diagnose the site of a lesion by careful history taking, observation and simple tests. As mentioned earlier in this chapter, this process can be summarised by the following pneumonic:

- Clinical signs
- In-depth medical history (outlined in Ch. 5)

Table 7.4 Role of CNS in posture, balance and coordination

Action	*Site*	*Function*
Motor coordination	Premotor cortex	Plans actions
	Sensorimotor cortex	Initiates action
	Basal ganglia	Converts thought into action
	Cerebellum	Modifies action. Compares actual and intended action, smooths action
	Brain stem	Modifies action
	(extrapyramidal)	Corrects position
	(pyramidal)	Skilled work
Posture and balance	Cerebellum	Rich input, miniprogrammes
Gait	All of above	

- **G**eneral physiology
- **A**ssessments/tests
- **R**eferral and risk status.

Clinical signs

The patient should be observed while walking, sitting and speaking, as well as while performing particular tasks. A change in the level of consciousness, inability to follow simple instructions and deficits in voluntary movement or sensation, including the presence of pain, all provide important clues. Important points to note are listed in Box 7.2

In-depth medical history

It is important to undertake a thorough medical and social history (Ch. 5). In particular, the following should be borne in mind. Onset and duration may provide vital clues as to the cause of a problem. For example, Guillain–Barré syndrome has a sudden, postviral onset.

The history of the problem and the type of onset may help reach the diagnosis. For example, pain, numbness, a sensation of heaviness or a 'pins and needles' sensation in the arm could be due to compression of nerve roots in the spine, as seen in cervical spondylosis, or an attack of angina pectoris. With angina the sensation is likely to be spasmodic and associated with exercise or some other stress while in the case of cervical spondylosis it would be of a more continuous nature.

A history of frequent falls with no loss of consciousness suggests a lesion in one of the areas of the brain dealing with balance and posture, such as the cerebellum or basal ganglia. Such episodes can be seen in patients with Parkinson's disease or in multiple sclerosis (Table 7.5). Where loss of consciousness

Box 7.2 Seven-point observation examination

- Distribution and modalities affected – unilateral or bilateral
- Movement – weakness or paralysis
- Muscles or movement affected
- Muscle tone and bulk
- Sensation – paraesthesia or anaesthesia
- Deformity – cavoid foot type often associated with UMN damage
- Tremor

Table 7.5 Common neurological conditions associated with falls

Condition	*Clinical features affecting the lower limb*
Parkinson's disease	Shuffling and narrow based gait with small rapid steps. Loss of arm swing with difficulty initiating movement and turning quickly. Rigidity of leg extensors. A backward step may be taken to prevent falling when stopping
Peripheral sensory neuropathy	Protective 'withdrawal' to pain response may be lost. Broad-based, high stepping, stamping gait and increased plantar pressures due to a loss of proprioception and sensory input. Darkness or removal of other sensory information exacerbates this condition, i.e. Romberg's test (ask patient to close their eyes and note if they become unstable)
Distal weakness	Damage to LMN can lead to limb being lifted up or over objects, i.e. lifting limb onto treatment couch. Foot drop and foot slap may occur, if the ankle dorsiflexors are impaired (particularly tibialis anterior). A waddling gait may develop and there is difficulty in rising from a seated position
Cerebellar ataxia	A broad-based, unstable, tremulous gait often described as a 'drunken' stagger. Gait often leans towards the affected cerebellar side. Falls tend to occur backwards or sideways
Spasticity	Associated with CVAs and UMN lesions. Extension of the hip and knee with a plantarflexed inverted foot leading to a limb length discrepancy. Toe box and lateral border of shoes become scuffed. Usually unilateral presentation with a circumductory gait for affected limb.

has occurred, the period of unconsciousness and the age of the patient should be taken into account prior to diagnosis. The presence of a severe headache is an important sign, since, although it often has a completely benign cause, it may also indicate a more serious event, e.g. brain tumour or subarachnoid haemorrhage or the less sinister migraine or tension headache. Consequently, it is vital that the onset, nature and duration of the 'headache' should be established.

General physiology

The causes of neurological disorders are many and can be classified as follows:

- Heredity, e.g. Huntington's chorea, peroneal muscular atrophy, Friedreich's ataxia, malignant hyperpyrexia
- Developmental defect, e.g. spina bifida, syringomyelia
- Trauma, e.g. severing of the spinal cord or a peripheral nerve, concussion
- Ischaemia, e.g. stroke, cerebral haemorrhage
- Compression, e.g. tumour of the cerebellum, Morton's neuroma, common peroneal nerve palsy
- Infection, e.g. human immunodeficiency virus (HIV) infection, Creutzfeldt–Jakob disease, herpes zoster (shingles), Guillain–Barré syndrome, lepromatous neuropathy
- Autoimmune, e.g. myasthenia gravis, polymyositis, possibly multiple sclerosis
- Nutritional/metabolic, e.g. Korsakoff's psychosis, subacute combined degeneration of the spinal cord, diabetic neuropathy
- Iatrogenic, e.g. tight plaster cast causing nerve palsy, drug-induced myopathies (lithium, high-dose steroids, etc.)
- Idiopathic, e.g. Parkinson's disease, motor neurone disease, non-familial Alzheimer's disease.

The effects of any lesion in the nervous system will depend on the area involved. For example, occlusion of the posterior cerebral artery, which feeds the occipital lobe of the brain (striate cortex), may result in visual disturbances, while occlusion of a cerebellar artery may elicit ataxia and an occlusion of the vasa nervosum of a peripheral nerve may effect a 'glove and stocking' paraesthesia. Nerve function deficit is called neuropathy and is classified according to the numbers and types of nerves involved and the site of the lesion (Table 7.6).

Table 7.6 Classification of neuropathies

Type of neuropathy	*Description*
Mononeuropathy	Abnormality of a single nerve
Mononeuritis multiplex	Asymmetrical abnormality of several individual nerves
Radiculopathy	Abnormality of a nerve root
Polyneuropathy	Widespread, symmetrical abnormality of many nerves, usually characterised as sensory/motor/autonomic 'glove and stocking' distribution

Assessment

The assessment process involves a general overview of neurological function followed by assessment of:

- levels of consciousness
- sensory function
- motor function (to include muscles)
- posture and coordination
- autonomic function.

Many neurological conditions present with multiple signs and symptoms because more than one part of the nervous system is affected. It is important to bear this in mind when assessing each of the above parts, ensuring that all the information is viewed contextually to facilitate a definitive diagnosis. For example, multiple (disseminating) sclerosis is a progressive disease affecting the CNS, where repeated patchy demyelination of nerve sheaths occurs, leading initially to a temporary and later, permanent loss of function. The nerve axons most often affected are the optic nerves – the optic nerve is considered an outgrowth from the CNS rather than a peripheral nerve. Multiple sclerosis along with Parkinson's disease is the second most common disease to affect the CNS, after strokes (Wilkinson 1993, p 135). Similarly, neurological disturbances in the lower spinal cord can be betrayed via blurring of vision (diplopia), unsteady gait, weakness in the lower limbs, lower limb sensory loss and/or disturbances of micturition.

The type of pain and its distribution can help to establish whether the problem affects a nerve pathway or is referred via entrapment of a spinal nerve. Patients should be asked, if their limbs feel weak or sluggish (paresis): a slow, progressive onset of muscular weakness suggests muscular dystrophy, whereas an acute onset suggests a demyelinating disease. Alternatively, a burning, lancinating pain with allodynia (normal touch stimuli perceived as painful) indicates a neuropathic origin, such as painful peripheral diabetic neuropathy.

Social habits

Smoking and alcohol consumption should be noted. Smoking is a risk factor for certain conditions, such as atherosclerosis and therefore, CVAs. Chronic alcoholism can affect both motor coordination and memory (Korsakoff's psychosis). Indeed, the actual cause is an alcohol-induced thiamine deficiency, which damages the limbic system (Wilkinson 1993, pp 49–50). Such patients appear alert and fully conscious, but recent memory of time and place is severely impaired. The patient denies any loss of memory and frequently attempts to disguise the deficit by confabulation. Similarly, indications of a lifestyle consistent with a risk of contracting HIV infection, such as intravenous drug misuse, may explain neurological deficit; the infection can produce a progressive encephalopathy.

Gender

Some conditions occur much more frequently in one sex than the other. For example, myasthenia gravis affects females more than males, whereas Duchenne's muscular dystrophy, which is an X chromosome linked disease, is seen much more in males.

Age

There is a general slowing in the passage of impulses throughout the nervous system with age, as shown by nerve conduction tests. Defective sensory perception is present in around 20% of people over the age of 65 years (Ch. 16). In fact, the likelihood of neurological abnormalities increases with advancing years. Moreover, many conditions affecting the nervous system have typical onsets at particular ages. For example, shingles (herpes zoster), parkinsonism and CVAs are all associated with the over-60 age group, whereas Charcot–Marie–Tooth disease usually manifests in the 20, and in some forms of spina bifida effects are observed from birth. However, where two or more systemic conditions coexist, the picture may be altered – for example, patients with diabetes mellitus or sickle cell anaemia can be predisposed to earlier onset of CVAs. Coexisting chronic disease can also be helpful in diagnosing the cause – for example, atherosclerosis and hypertension are major risk factors for strokes (McLeod & Lance 1989 pp 210–211, Primatesta et al 2000).

Risk and referral

Following the neurological assessment, all tests must be considered holistically to ensure maximum validity. Patients displaying any significant loss of sensory, motor or autonomic neuropathy should be considered as being at increased risk of developing lower-limb complications. The NICE guidelines on the management and referral process for footcare in individuals with diabetes mellitus should be adhered to. A clinical staging tool for the 'at-risk' diabetic foot has been development by Edmonds & Foster (2005) (Table 7.7).

Table 7.7 Staging the diabetic foot

Stage	*Clinical presentation*
1 Normal	Foot not at risk. No neuropathy ischaemia, swelling, callus or deformity present
2 High risk	Patient has developed one or more risk factors for ulceration: neuroischaemic or neuropathic foot
3 Ulcerated	Foot has a skin breakdown. Usually an ulcer, but some minor injuries cuts, splits, blisters or grazes are also included, given their tendency to develop into ulceration
4 Infected	Ulceration has developed infection with the presence of cellulitis
5 Necrotic	Necrosis has occurred. In the neuropathic foot, infection is the primary cause; in the neuroischaemic foot, infection is normally the key reason for tissue destruction, although ischaemia exacerbates it
6 Unsalvageable	Foot cannot be saved and major amputation is required

Assessment of the level of consciousness

The cerebral cortex and the reticular formation of the brain stem are the two areas of the brain most concerned with maintaining consciousness. The general level of the patient's awareness, ability to answer questions and follow instructions can all give indications of the level of consciousness.

Clinical signs

Transient ischaemic attacks (TIAs) may be accompanied by disorders of speech (dysphasia), vision, movement (dyskinesia) or swallowing (dysphagia), depending on the area of brain involved. However, a full recovery is usual. CVAs can result in neurological deficits similar to those seen in TIAs, but are often permanent, though partial or total recovery is possible depending on the extent and site of damage to the brain. Epileptic attacks can involve the whole brain (global) and result in a brief loss of consciousness (petit mal), which may not show any other symptoms or may last much longer, being accompanied by tonic-clonic jerks (grand mal). Such an attack is often preceded by an 'aura' and the patient may cry out. Attacks can also be focal, as in a Jacksonian attack, which affects only the primary motor cortex and in which, different parts of the body show jerks as the attack spreads over the motor cortex. An age-specific study by Wallace et al (1998) demonstrated that the prevalence of epilepsy in the UK is increasing in the 65 years and over age group.

A hypoglycaemic state associated with diabetes mellitus, particularly through altered insulin regime, can lead to symptoms ranging from drowsiness to confusion, with possible aggressive behaviour and potentially, loss of consciousness or coma. Consequently, it is vital that these symptoms are recognised quickly and the patient receives prompt treatment. Altered levels of consciousness are described in Table 7.8.

In-depth medical history

Any history of loss of consciousness should always be questioned further to try to establish whether the cause was:

- a simple faint
- a TIA or full-blown stroke
- an epileptic episode
- a metabolic disorder, such as a hypoglycaemic coma.

Table 7.8 Assessment of the level of consciousness

Level	*Observable effects*
Alert wakefulness	Patient is fully aware of environment and self and responds to stimuli
Confusion	Patient shows lack of attentiveness, cannot concentrate and has impaired memory
Delirium	Patient is anxious, excited, agitated and may be hallucinating
Lethargy	Patient is drowsy but responds to verbal stimuli
Stupor	Patients is unconscious but responds to pain
Coma	Patient cannot be roused

Simple faints (syncope) are always due to a temporary interruption of blood supply to the brain, which is rapidly restored by placing the patient in the prostrate position. This may be caused by:

- benign causes, such as emotional shock, causing vasovagal syncope
- autonomic neuropathy, if the fainting episode is associated with a change to an upright posture
- serious event, such as haemorrhage or anaphylactic shock.

General physiology

Strokes are the result of prolonged/permanent interruption of the blood supply to the brain and are the most common condition to affect the CNS. TIAs are a temporary interruption in the vascular supply to the brain and like strokes, usually occur in the older person (60+ years). Both strokes and TIAs are primarily caused (80% of cases) by thrombosis resulting from atheromatous plaques in cerebral vessels, haemorrhage effecting the remainder (McLeod & Lance 1989, p 282). TIAs usually last from 1 to 30 minutes and always for less than 24 hours.

Epileptic attacks can occur at any age and are due to unusual electrical activity in the cortex, which could be caused by a lesion or a tumour. Alteration to glycaemic control in individuals with diabetes mellitus can result from increases to insulin or oral hypoglycaemic medications, emotional stress and the presence of infection. Consequently, these factors should be considered prior to treating the patient.

Assessment

In the clinic, the following can be used to establish the level of consciousness:

- the patient's response to a question and answer schedule
- whether the patient can follow simple instructions
- the patient's response to stimuli.

Dementia should also be considered, when assessing the patient. While this does not specifically affect consciousness, it does impair memory, intellect and personality and will have a profound influence on patient management. Table 7.9 outlines some causes of dementia.

Risk and referral

The patient should be referred to their GP if they show a mild altered level of consciousness. If the altered level of consciousness is severe immediate medical assistance may need to be sought. The underlying systemic causes of a loss of consciousness, i.e. CVA, diabetes mellitus, may greatly influence the risk status, treatment and subsequent management planning for the individual.

The following is a summary of possible test protocols after referral:

- **Oculoplethysmography** – This is a non-invasive test to detect carotid lesions.
- **Duplex Doppler ultrasound** – This technique uses sound waves of 4–8 MHz. Duplex Doppler may reveal stenosis or occlusion of the carotid arteries, a possible cause of CVA or TIA, and is often used prior to an angiogram.
- **Angiography** – Interarterial angiography with injection of a radiopaque dye into the suspected artery will show atherosclerotic plaques in cerebral vessels.
- **Brain scans** – Computed tomography (CT) or magnetic resonance imaging (MRI) can be used to confirm TIAs, full-blown CVAs, neoplastic mass, multiple sclerosis lesions, or epileptic foci.
- **Electroencephalogram** – This traces the electrical activity of the cortex, as measured by scalp electrodes. EEGs are normally used to confirm a clinical diagnosis and locate the focus of epilepsy.
- **Lumbar punctures** – A hollow needle is inserted into the spinal canal through the intervertebral space between L3 and L4 or L4–5 to withdraw cerebrospinal fluid. This is analysed for micro-organisms, glucose levels, protein levels, blood cell types and concentration, and hydrostatic pressure.
- **Myelography** – This test is usually combined with MRI or CT investigations. A radiopaque dye is introduced into the subarachnoid space via a lumbar puncture. It is used to diagnose tumours of the spinal cord, diseases of the intervertebral disc space, bony abnormalities and spondylotic lesions of the vertebral column.

Laboratory tests

DNA testing is primarily used to detect mutant genes, while other biochemical tests locate faulty enzymes to assist the diagnosis of hereditary metabolic diseases, which affect the CNS: Huntington's chorea, familial Alzheimer's disease, Tay–Sach disease, Charcot–Marie–Tooth disease and inherited myopathies, such as McArdle's syndrome.

Table 7.9 Conditions associated with dementia

Vascular	Cerebrovascular disease Cranial arteritis
Infection	Encephalitis of any cause Syphilis
Degenerative	Alzheimer's disease Lewy body dementia Huntington's disease Parkinson's disease
Endocrine	Hypothyroidism Hypocalcaemia
Toxic	Alcohol Exposure to heavy metals (lead) and chemicals
Vitamin deficiency	B_{12} Thiamin
Traumatic	Post head injury

Assessment of lower limb sensory function

It is important that the sensory system is intact, for a person to respond to their external and internal environment. Failure to respond, especially to noxious stimuli, can lead to serious pathological changes and may possibly be life-threatening. Indeed, seminal work by Boulton (1998) has demonstrated that careful sensory assessment permits the best form of wound healing, namely, preventing its occurrence in the first instance! Some patients may actually be unaware of sensory loss; hence, it is essential that the practitioner assesses the sensory system and communicates any untoward findings to the individual. An appropriate management strategy can be designed with the patient's participation, facilitating empowerment, while reducing risk of future complications.

Table 7.10 Distribution resulting from damage to sensory tracts

Distribution	*Site affected*
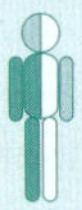	Thalamic Sensory loss opposite side
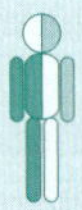	Midbrain stem Contralateral sensory loss below face and ipsilateral loss to face
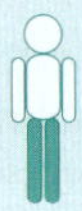	Transverse thoracic spinal cord Loss of all sensory input below site of damage
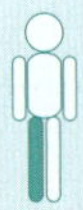	Dorsal column Vibration, light touch and proprioception loss
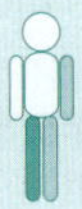	Unilateral cord lesion (Brown–Séquard) Contralateral pain and temperature loss with ipsilateral weakness and dorsal column loss below lesion
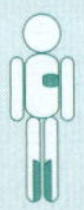	Individual sensory roots affected Distribution may vary dependent upon aetiology, i.e. compression or shingles
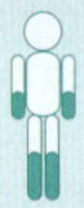	Polyneuropathy (peripheral nerves) Sensory loss (pain, temperature, vibration and light touch)

Clinical signs

Damage to the ascending tracts in the spinal cord will produce either ipsilateral or contralateral effects, depending on the site of the lesion in relation to the point of crossover (see Table 7.10).

The exact effect of peripheral nerve damage depends on the site and the nature of the damage, since this dictates the repair process involved (see Table 7.11).

In-depth medical history

The nature and distribution of any sensory deficit can be an important aid in diagnosing the underlying cause. This may take the form of complete anaesthesia (total lack of sensation) or paraesthesia (an altered sensation). Examples of paraesthesia include pins and needles, burning, pricking, shooting pain and dull ache. Patients should be asked, if they experience any abnormal sensations and moreover, if they have a history of foot ulceration.

Phantom limb

An unusual phenomenon arising from amputation of a limb is that of 'phantom limb', where the patient

Table 7.11 Classification of nerve damage

Type	*Damage*
Neurapraxia	Mild trauma or compression causing local demyelination and leading to temporary loss of function. Full recovery within days or weeks
Axonotmesis	Crush injuries causing degeneration of axon and myelin sheath (wallerian degeneration). Neurolemma sheaths intact and reinnervated
Neurotmesis	Whole nerve axon severed. Surgical repair needed to ensure reinnervation of distal trunk

has the very real sensation of the amputated limb still being present. The most unpleasant effect is the sensation of pain, which is said to occur in 70% of amputees (Melzack 1992). The traditional explanation, that this is due to the growth of neuromas in the nerve stumps and their generated impulses cannot be the entire explanation, since cutting the afferent pathways from such nerves does not abolish the pain. Melzack has suggested that the phantom sensations are due to learned circuits in the brain, capable of generating impulses in the absence of sensory inputs.

Referred pain

Injury to the viscera often produces pain in a somatic structure some distance away. This is called referred pain. For example, a myocardial infarction can produce pain in the left arm, as both the heart and the skin of the left arm have developed from the same dermatomal segment. However, the exact mechanism is still not clearly understood, although both convergence and facilitation are thought to have a role (Ganong 1991, pp 132–133). Damage to a spinal nerve may result in referred pain experienced around the heel; this occurs, if there is damage to S1.

Neuropathic pain

Diabetes mellitus and post-herpetic are systemic conditions associated with the development of neuropathic pain. The condition is extremely disabling and painful and is frequently described as a burning or lancinating pain with normal touch sensation being perceived as painful (allodynia). While the aetiology of this condition is not fully understood, alteration to spinal cord sensitivity (spinal wind-up) and inappropriate nerve repair (spinal re-wiring) are both considered to be play key roles in this condition (Spruce et al 2003). A detailed history of the pain can indicate if neuropathic mechanisms are likely to be involved, thus allowing a differential diagnosis. Table 7.12 shows the modified LANSS (Leeds Assessment of Neuropathic Symptoms and Signs) assessment tool.

General physiology

Conditions, which may cause sensory deficits, are outlined in Box 7.3. The most important area of the brain for somatic sensory perception is the parietal cortex (see Fig. 7.12). Any damage to this area, whatever the cause, will produce a contralateral sensory deficit in the appropriate part of the body. Damage to the occipital lobe (striate cortex) will produce visual disturbances. The most common cause of such neurological deficits is an occlusion or haemorrhage of one of the cerebral arteries (MacDonald et al 2000).

Box 7.3 Causes of sensory deficits

- Diabetes mellitus
- Subacute combined degeneration of the spinal cord (vitamin B_{12} deficiency)
- Congential absence of particular sensory neurones
- Spina bifida
- Syringomyelia
- Tabes dorsalis
- Nerve inujuries
- Guillain–Barré syndrome
- Multiple sclerosis
- Cord compression/lesion, e.g. tumour (Brown–Séquard syndrome)
- Chronic alcoholism

Assessment

Assessment involves checking whether sensory units are functioning normally and, if not, the extent of damage and the possible cause. Sensory deficits may arise as a result of damage to:

- parietal cortex
- ascending pathways
- receptors.

Simple apparatus is all that is needed to undertake an assessment of sensory function (see Table 7.13).

Proposed sensory testing protocol:

1. Observe patient's gait and coordination (walking to or sitting in treatment area).
2. Explain the purpose of testing and nature of equipment to be used (many think a monofilament is a needle).
3. Demonstrate the test to patient, usually on the back of their hand (ensure the patient can feel the stimulus, i.e. upper limb neuropathy. If not, move proximally).
4. Ask the patient to close their eyes (results may be unduly influenced by observing the test).
5. Conduct test starting distally and working proximally. Randomise order of testing sites, where appropriate, to reduce bias.
6. Use forced-answer questions, where possible, help to eliminate observer influence, e.g. 'Which

Table 7.12 Modified LANSS assessment tool

Question	***Score***	
Would you describe our pain as strange, unpleasant sensations in your skin, e.g. pricking, tingling, pins and needles?	No 0	Yes 5
Does the skin in the painful areas look different from normal, e.g. mottled, more red/pink?	No 0	Yes 5
Is the skin in the affected area abnormally sensitive to touch?	No 0	Yes 3
Does your pain come on suddenly in bursts for no apparent reason when you're still, e.g. like electric shocks, bursting or jumping sensations?	No 0	Yes 2
Do you feel that the skin temperature in the painful area has changed abnormally, e.g. hot or burning?	No 0	Yes 1
Testing		
Lightly stroke cotton wool across the non-painful and then painful area. If normal sensations are experienced in the non-painful site, but painful or unpleasant sensations are experienced in the painful area, allodynia is present	No 0	Allodynia 5
Neurotip applied to painful and non-painful sites	Equal (both areas) (in painful area only) 0	Altered 3
Scoring		
Questionnaire subtotal Sensory testing subtotal Total (maximum 24)		
<12 means neuropathic mechanisms are **unlikely** to be involved. >12 means neuropathic mechanisms are **likely** to be involved.		

is cooler/warmer/vibrating, etc., number 1 or number 2?'

7. Repeat test three times on each site. If two or three answers are affirmative (per site), the patient is not considered to have a clinical sensory deficit in that modality. Ensure the testing site is appropriate to the selected assessment.
8. Record the information accurately supported with digital images, if relevant (change of colour associated with neuropathic pain).
9. Communicate your findings back to the patient, remembering to avoid technical jargon.

The results of each test should state the extent of any neuropathy, e.g. 'loss of vibration perception from toes to ankles' to aid monitoring of the deficit. If a mononeuropathy is suspected, e.g. anterior tibial damage contributing to foot drop, the dermatomes innervated by that nerve should be investigated. A deficit may not always be due to pathological causes: factors such as overlying callus render the skin less sensitive and the normal slowing of conduction rates with ageing will further result in reduced sensation.

Testing large-diameter fibres

- Light touch
  Either cotton wool or a fine brush can be used for this test. However, it should be noted that

Table 7.13 Sensory testing

Test	*Equipment**	*Fibre type and pathway in spinal cord*
Light touch	Cottonwool/brush/monofilament	A-beta fibres
Two-point discrimination	Dividers, two orange sticks	Ipsilateral dorsal column
Vibration (pressure)	Tuning fork/neurothesiometer	
Temperature	Warm and cold test tubes/dissimilar metals	A-delta and C fibres Contralateral (anterolateral columns)
Sharp pain/pinprick	Neurotips	
Proprioception	Dorsi/plantarflexion of hallux	A-alpha fibres Ipsilateral dorsal columns

*All the methods are acceptable, only tests using 10 g monofilaments, tuning fork and neurothesiometers/biothesiometers have been evaluated for validity and repeatability for predicting ulceration in a diabetic population.

this test is rarely used in normal clinical neurological screening. The nerves being tested are large-diameter A-beta fibres which ascend in the dorsal columns, transmitting light touch perception. The receptors (Meissner's corpuscles) lie in the superficial dermis. The skin of the foot is stroked lightly with a wisp of cotton wool or brush. The patient may incorrectly distinguish between the lesser toes in this test, but this is normal and is due to the particular innervation of the lesser digits.

- Two-point discrimination
  Blunt-ended orange sticks or the two points of a pair of dividers can be used for this test, providing the points of the dividers have been blunted to avoid accidental skin penetration. The nerves being tested are again the large-diameter A-beta fibres, but here, the density of the touch receptor field is being assessed. The plantar surface of the foot is usually tested. The patient is asked, with eyes shut, to state how many points can be felt when the tips of a compass lightly press the skin surface simultaneously. The distance between the tips of the compass that allows the patient to detect two points rather than one should be noted. Usually the distance on the foot of a healthy young adult is 2 cm. It will increase with age and if the skin is calloused. Additionally, conditions which lead to soft tissue stiffening, i.e. glycosylation in diabetes mellitus can cause an altered response. The receptors responsible for identifying two-point discrimination are also essential for stereognosis – the ability to recognise objects by touch – very important for readers of Braille. However, the clinical usefulness of this test for the majority of patients as a predictive marker for neurological complications remains subjective.
- Pressure
  The 10 g monofilament is used for this test. The first monofilament for detecting neuropathy was the Semmes–Weinstein monofilament produced by the Hansen's Disease Center, USA. In theory, this monofilament buckles when a force of 10 g is applied. Ever since, a wide variety of monofilaments have been produced, all purported to buckle at the same force – 10 g. However, McGill et al (1998) and Booth & Young (2000) studied 10 g monofilaments from a range of manufacturers and found inconsistencies in their deforming pressures. However, the clinical relevance of this variation has yet to be determined. Booth & Young (2000) also showed that all monofilaments degrade with use and recommended a 24-hour rest period between repeated use of a single monofilament to allow for recovery. At the time of publication, researchers at the University of Southampton are developing a wholly new device, which counters all the previously identified limitations of the monofilament.

A range of monofilaments of different diameters and buckling forces are also available, but these are more useful for research purposes, rather than for routine screening. In view of its small size, low cost and ability in detecting large-fibre neuropathy, the monofilament is considered one of the most useful tools a clinician can possess and is recommended by the International Diabetes Federation, the World Health Organization European St Vincent Declaration and the International Working Group on the diabetic foot (International Consensus on the Diabetic Foot 1999) and NICE guidelines (2004; see www.nice.org.uk).

The nerve fibres being tested are once more those belonging to the A-beta group. The receptors are encapsulated and lie in the dermis, but are slow adaptors and so detect constant pressure rather than vibration. Both touch and pressure receptors can respond to applied pressure and are capable of discriminating the amount of force used. Light touch will stimulate a small area of nerve endings and increasing pressure will recruit more and more receptors. Precisely when the stimulus becomes pressure, rather than touch and whether a different receptor is actually involved, is not clear, so the stimulus is sometimes referred to as the 'touch-pressure sensation'.

The monofilament is applied at right angles to the skin surface with just enough pressure to deform the filament into a 'C' shape. Testing sites are the metatarsal heads (1, 3 and 5) the plantar aspect of the heel and dorsum of the foot. Testing sites indicate areas at increased risk from ulceration due to raised plantar pressures in diabetes mellitus, thus dermatomes are not tested. Care should be taken not to slide the filament or brush the skin. It should be held in that position for 2 seconds, the patient having been asked to state when and where pressure from the 10 g monofilament is felt at various points, with eyes shut. Inability to detect the 10 g monofilament at >1 more sites (per foot) is taken to indicate neuropathy of large fibres.

- Vibration

Either a simple 128 Hz tuning fork or a graduated Rydel–Seiffer version can be used. The nerve fibres being tested are again large-diameter A-beta fibres, sensitive to pressure; the deeply placed pacinian corpuscles are particularly sensitive to rapidly changing pressures or vibrations.

The vibrating tuning fork is placed on the skin above a bony prominence such as the apex of the hallux, malleolus or the first metatarsophalangeal joint (MTPJ). It is important to ask the patients to describe exactly what and where they feel the stimulus, as most patients will be able to feel pressure, but not necessarily any vibratory sensation. Most patients describe the vibratory sensation as a 'buzzing' higher up the limb, but not at the site tested, indicating distal damage. The Rydel–Seiffer tuning fork is an attempt to produce a semiquantitative result to enable comparisons to be made with other patients and on different occasions. It has detachable clamps which can be moved to different positions on the prongs, to alter the vibrating frequency from 64 Hz to 128 Hz. As the prongs vibrate, the apex of a cone drawn on the clamps, upright or inverted, will appear to move vertically up or down a scale from 1 to 8. The position of this cone is noted when the patients confirm that the vibration sensation stops. At 128 Hz, the apex should reach at least halfway along the scale, i.e. to the number 4, depending on which cone is being observed. If vibration sensation is lost before this point is reached, the patient is said to have a vibratory perception deficit. A recent study by Miranda-Palma et al (2005) indicated that the 128 Hz tuning fork shows greater sensitivity for predicting diabetic foot ulceration than other available clinical testing. However, this may reflect reliability deficits previously discussed in relation to the 10 g monofilament testing.

Neurothesiometers provide an alternative method of assessing vibration. The neurothesiometer is basically a vibrator that delivers impulse energy of increasing strength, measured in volts per micrometre. The mains-operated version, the biothesiometer, has been superseded by the battery-operated neurothesiometer, to meet health and safety requirements. Cassella et al (2000) recommended that rather than using a pistol grip with the apparatus, the head of the tool should rest in the palm of the operator's hand, while being applied to the patient. Only in this way, with no extraneous pressure being applied, could truly reproducible vibratory perception thresholds (VPTs) be determined.

The neurothesiometer is positioned at the tip of the hallux (most distal point) and the strength of the vibrations is increased, until the patient can detect a 'buzzing' sensation in the hallux. This reading is called the VPT and values of over 25 V are taken to indicate a significantly increased risk ulceration due to peripheral neuropathy. The measurement should be repeated three times and the average value taken. Using data from

392 patients with diabetes mellitus, Coppini et al (2000) found that a VPT score based on comparison with an age-related norm, showed overall better sensitivity in identifying patients with subclinical neuropathy; this measurement protocol facilitating the regular monitoring of a diabetic population. Of note, a VPT score >15.1 has been suggested to indicate increased risk of developing diabetic foot complications, as vibration is considered to be one of the first modalities to be affected.

Testing small-diameter fibres

- Temperature

  Two test tubes filled with warm and cool water are preferable to immersing saline sachets in cool and warm water, which quickly lose their temperature differences. Metal rods cooled or warmed in water can also be used. Thermotips, a small cylinder made of two metals with dissimilar conductivities is easier to transport and use.

  The test validates the integrity of the warm and cold temperature receptors that feed into the anterior part of the anterolateral columns. The nerve fibres involved are narrow diameter A-delta and C fibres. Warmth receptors operate in the range of 30–43°C, while cold receptors operate in the range of 35–20°C (Vander et al 1998). Temperatures above 43°C or below 20°C will trigger pain receptors. The skin temperature is usually a few degrees cooler than that of core temperature, i.e. between 30°C and 35°C, though a greater difference may exist in extremes of environment. The temperature of the warm water should be above 35°C and that of the cold water below 30°C. Again, with eyes closed, the patient is asked to state which they find the water cooler/warmer from the tubes presented.

- Pain

  Disposable Neurotips (Owen Mumford) are advised for this test. Neurotips have a sharp and a blunt end, but the sharp end cannot pierce the skin. Spring-loaded devices, which are designed to deliver a stimulus at a force of 40 g, are thought to be the safest and most reliable way of testing for pinprick sensitivity (Wareham et al 1997). The use of the sharp end of a patella hammer is not advisable, as it may be sharp enough to penetrate the skin and is non-disposable. A hypodermic syringe should not be used under any circumstances.

  The test demonstrates the integrity of the sharp pain pathway, which begins with free nerve endings in the dermis. A-delta fibres travel into the spinal cord and synapse in the dorsal horn. The postsynaptic fibres cross to the contralateral anterolateral columns, which travel up to the brain.

  Using disposable Neurotips and with the patient's eyes closed, the patient is asked to state which is sharper, the first or second sensation. The two ends should be presented in random sequence to avoid correct guessing by the anxious-to-please patient. Neuropathy does not always mean an absence of pain, as observed in diabetic patients with neuropathy, who can experience a period of intense pain (Boulton 2000). The development of pain in a previously insensate diabetic foot should also be investigated, as it can be an indicator of deep infection.

  NICE annual screening guidelines advocate the use of the 10 g monofilament and vibration detection testing to identify those individuals at an increased risk of developing ulceration. Thus, it is paramount that these tests are not done in isolation. There is a body of evidence to suggest that additional subclinical signs of neuropathy may exist, which can indicate an increased risk of complications. Indeed, Winkler et al (2000) have reported the existence of a subgroup of type 1 diabetic neuropathy patients who have autonomic symptoms severe enough to warrant treatment (severe bladder or gastroparesis, orthostatic hypotension and diabetic diarrhoea), with relatively preserved large-fibre sensory modalities, such as vibration and touch-pressure sensation.

  The association between a loss of vibration and 10 g monofilament detection and foot complications in patients without diabetes cannot be directly applied. A study by Nakayama et al (1998) on rats showed that small-diameter, unmyelinated nerve fibres decrease in number with ageing, whereas larger-diameter fibres maintain both conduction ability and population. In the absence of solid evidence to the contrary, it would seem advisable to carry out sensory testing on both small and large fibres. Indeed, any testing is better than none and research studies have shown that a range of sensory tests may be used to calculate a neuropathy disability score (NDS). For further discussion of peripheral neuropathy assessment in patients with diabetes mellitus, see Boulton et al 1998, Young & Matthews (1998) and Chapter 18.

- Referred pain
  Entrapment of a spinal nerve may lead to paraesthesia, pain and weakness of muscles in the lower limb. Normally, when pressure is applied to a site of pain, the pain becomes worse. However, with referred pain, the level stays roughly the same. A suspected entrapment of the sciatic nerve usually leads to pain, when the affected leg is raised as the patient is lying in a supine position.

Risk and referral

The primary clinical importance of an altered sensory response (sensory neuropathy) is that it greatly elevates the risk status of the patient (Fig. 7.19). This applies to all individuals, but appears to offer the greatest scope for complications in the diabetic population. A flow diagram has been developed by NICE detailing the diabetic foot (type 2) care pathway (www.nice.org.uk).

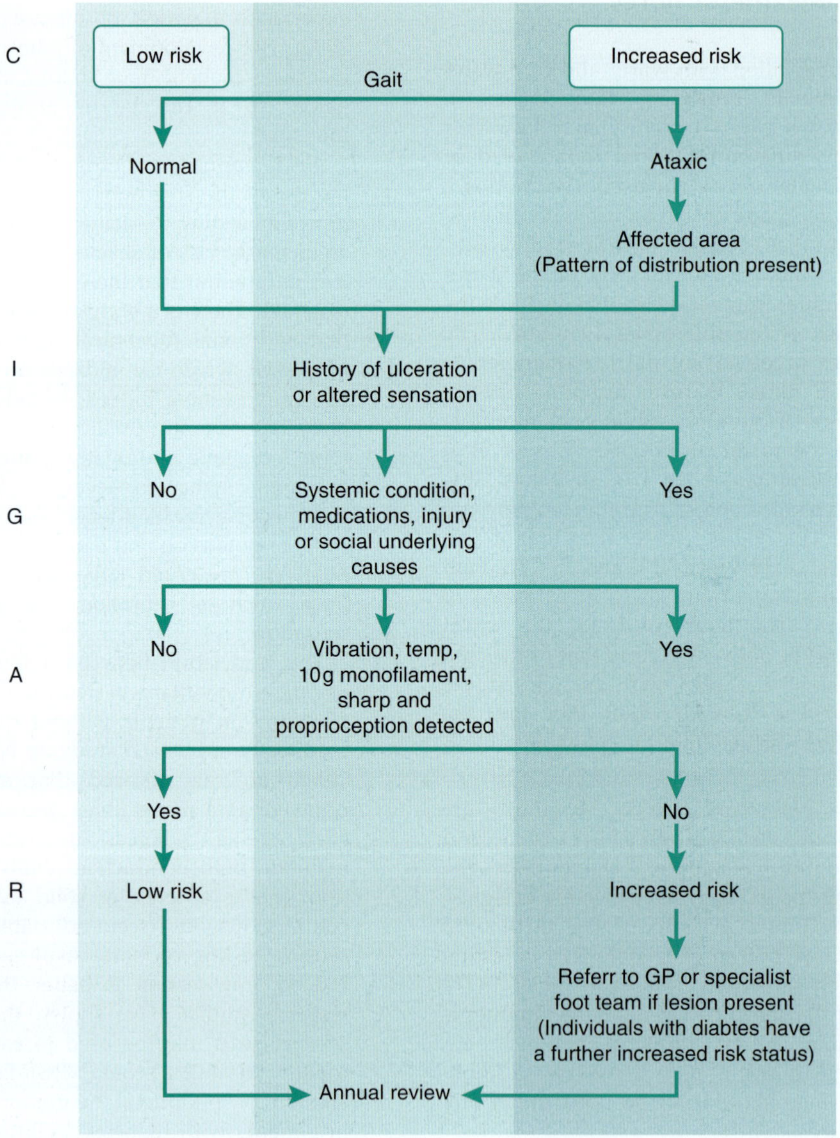

Figure 7.19 Aide-memoire for risk status.

Although a range of hospital-based tests can be done, i.e. nerve conduction velocity and biopsies, these may not be directly available to the practitioner. Consequently, all suspected abnormalities must be communicated to the patient's general practitioner (GP) and/or the relevant specialist foot team (including the multi-disciplinary team).

Assessment of lower limb motor function

If the motor system is functioning normally, muscles should display a resting tone, show good muscle power on active contraction and be able to move against resistance (Ch. 10). Lower limb motor dysfunction can occur as a result of damage to upper motor neurones, lower motor neurones, peripheral nerves or muscles. Assessment of the motor system involves testing both upper and lower motor neurones. The clinical pneumonic, **CIGAR©**, will be applied to upper and lower motor neurones lesions assessment individually.

Upper motor neurone lesions

Clinical signs damage to the corticospinal neurones and tracts will result in contralateral loss of skilled movements. Lack of movement will, in turn, eventually lead to a form of muscle atrophy, known as disuse atrophy. Damage to the multineuronal pathway causes release of inhibition on the LMNs in the spinal cord, especially those which innervate the antigravity muscles, producing the effect most commonly associated with UMN lesions, that of spasticity or stiffness in the limbs.

Gait

Observation of the patient's gait is an important part of the assessment for UMN lesions. In the lower limb, the effect is extension at the hip and knee, with plantarflexion and inversion of the foot. If the effect is unilateral, the person is described as hemiplegic. The inability to flex the knee and hip leads to a circumductory gait, with the lateral border of the forefoot and toes often scraping the ground. If both sides are affected, the person is paraplegic and the gait is described as a scissors gait, with the knees adducted and feet abducted. Walking aids such as Zimmer frames are therefore essential.

Box 7.4 Conditions associated with UMN signs

- Cerebral palsy due to anoxia at birth
- Cerebral vascular accidents
- Brain injury
- Friedreich's ataxia
- Spinal injury
- Brain or spinal tumours
- Amyotrophic lateral sclerosis (motor neurone disease)
- Vitamin B_{12} deficiency
- Multiple (disseminated) sclerosis
- Later stages of syringomyelia

In-depth medical history

Communication with the patient during this element of the assessment may reveal a reduction in level of consciousness, alteration to speech patterns or cognitive function, which may indicate a UMN lesion. CVAs are the most common cause of UMN events in the UK. Box 7.4 outlines other conditions associated with UMN signs.

General physiology

UMN lesions occur due to damage anywhere between the cortex and L1 in the spinal cord. Since the spinal cord ends at level L1, lesions below this level will not produce UMN signs. Although a specific area of the frontal lobes (precentral gyrus) is designated the primary motor cortex (see Fig. 7.12), many neurones from other areas of the cortex are also involved in planning and initiating conscious movement and thus, can be termed UMNs. This includes neurones of both descending tracts. Damage to the descending tracts will produce the same effects as damage to the neurones themselves.

Assessment

The lower limb reflexes, patellar and Achilles, should show a normal response. Reflex pathways involve both an afferent and an efferent component and, therefore, a deficit in either component would be expected to have an observable effect on the response, as would abnormal influences by higher centres on the LMN. Reflex responses can be graded as follows

(Fuller 1993, p 135):

- 3+ = clonus
- 2+ = increased*
- 1+ = normal
- ± = obtainable with reinforcement
- 0 = absent.

*Values of 2 and above suggest UMN lesions:

- The patellar reflex

This tests the integrity of the spinal reflex pathway (L3, L4) and demonstrates descending influences on the ventral horn cell. It is important that the limb being tested is as relaxed as possible. The patient should sit sideways on the examination couch with the feet clearing the ground. The practitioner can gently push the leg to be tested, which should swing freely in response. A gentle tap on the patellar tendon with the hammer should elicit a knee jerk. If the leg is not relaxed, the patient should clasp both hands around the other knee and pull (Jendrassik manoeuvre). This releases spinal influence and allows the leg to relax. The test should be undertaken on both legs:

- Achilles reflex
  This tests the spinal reflex pathway (S1, S2). The response is best elicited, if the foot of the patient is slightly dorsiflexed. By applying gentle pressure to the plantar surface of the forefoot with one hand and tapping Achilles tendon, pressure is maintained. The patient can either sit on a couch, with legs extended and the limb being tested crossed over the other, or kneel on a chair, with the foot to be tested hanging slightly over the edge of the chair. In a healthy young adult, the forefoot will gently plantarflex. In an elderly person, no visible movement may be seen, but a very slight plantarflexion will be felt against the practitioner's hand.
- Exaggerated reflex responses
  Due to the reduced inhibition by the multineuronal tracts, the alpha LMNs responsible for the contraction of extrafusal fibres are hyperexcited. This results in exaggerated patellar and ankle tendon reflexes and clonus – increased rhythmic contractions elicited at the ankle or patella by causing brisk stretch of the muscles. More than three contractions as a result of testing the patellar or Achilles reflex is indicative of UMN damage (Fuller 1993, p 135).
- Clasp-knife spasticity
  The affected limb will be initially stiff to passive stretch, but if gentle stretch is continued, the limb may suddenly relax, rather like the opening of a clasp-knife. This is due to a length-dependent inhibition of the stretch reflex (Fig. 7.18).
- Plantar reflex
  Damage to the corticospinal neurones or their axons has another effect that is clinically detectable, namely the plantar reflex or Babinski's sign. It has been suggested that the abnormal reflex, a dorsiflexing big toe, is due to release of a spinal inhibitory reflex (Van Gijn 1975). The plantar surface of the foot is stroked firmly and briskly from the posterolateral border of the heel to the hallux, as shown in **Figure 7.20**. The **normal** response is a slight **plantarflexion** of the hallux and lesser toes, although no response may also be observed, especially in the elderly, where the sensory pathway may be affected. In patients with corticospinal tract dysfunction, the hallux will extend (dorsiflexion of the hallux) and the lesser toes may fan out. This is the extensor response, sometimes referred to as positive

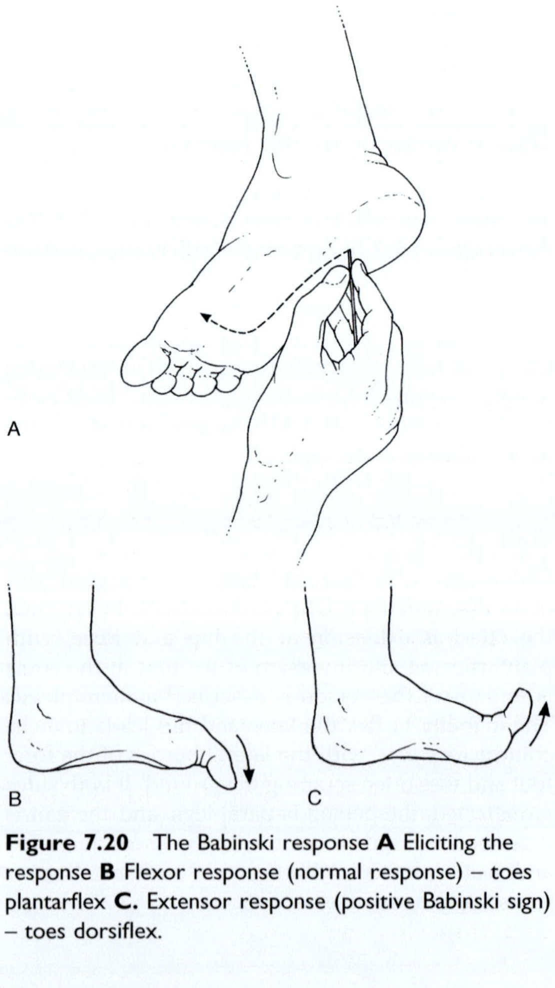

Figure 7.20 The Babinski response **A** Eliciting the response **B** Flexor response (normal response) – toes plantarflex **C.** Extensor response (positive Babinski sign) – toes dorsiflex.

Babinski's response. However, the normal response does not become established until the person has learned to walk, hence an extensor response is quite normal in babies. It is important not to rely only on this test for the diagnosis of UMN lesions, as it is easy to elicit a pain withdrawal response, which may appear similar to an extensor response. The rest of the clinical picture should also suggest UMN lesions.

- Muscle tone
  Due to the release of spinal inhibition in UMN conditions, the LMNs will be in a hyperexcited state and, thus, firing more frequently. This will result in greater muscle 'tone' and the affected muscle will feel very firm or tense.

Any condition, which causes damage to the UMNs or their descending tracts can produce UMN signs. If the cortex is affected, the effects will occur on the contralateral side of the body, and if the lesion is in the spinal cord, the effects will be on the same side, below the level of the lesion (Case history 7.1).

Risk and referral

The use of tests to diagnose UMN lesions will vary according to the suspected cause. For example, brain scans are indicated, if a CVA is suspected, whereas an X-ray, a CT scan or an MRI would be used if a tumour of the spine were involved. Individuals with UMN damage will display a moderately increased risk status, which may be further elevated by an underlying systemic cause, i.e. CVA in a diabetic individual. Any suspected change in UMN neurological status should be communicated immediately to the patient's GP, in appropriate terms. However, referral to physio- and occupational therapists and a wider multi-disciplinary team may represent the keystone for the rehabilitation of these individuals.

Case history 7.1

A 70-year-old Caucasian woman presented to the clinic complaining of excessive wear on the lateral border of the left shoe and a corn on the dorsum of the fifth toe. The patient walked with a stick and had a slow, circumducted gait; the left arm was held in a flexed position.

Neurological assessment revealed normal tendon reflexes and muscle power in the right leg but exaggerated tendon reflexes and an extensor plantar response (positive Babinski's sign), clonic spasm of the muscles and signs of muscle atrophy in the left leg.

Diagnosis: History taking revealed the patient had a major CVA, which had affected the right cortex. The clinical features were consistent with the history. Fortunately for the patient she was right-handed so her speech was not affected and she was still able to feed herself and write.

Lower motor neurone lesions

Clinical signs

As the LMN cell body, its efferent fibres, the neuromuscular junction and the 10–600 skeletal muscle fibres it innervates, all act as a coordinated whole, damage to any part of this motor unit will produce similar effects of weakness (paresis), complete loss of function (paralysis) and/or reduced/absent reflexes. Myopathies will also produce weakness or paralysis, even if the LMN remains intact.

In contrast to UMN lesions, which affect particular movements, LMN lesions and myopathies affect particular muscles (Case history 7.2). For example, if the

Case history 7.2

A 52-year-old Caucasian woman presented to the clinic with plantar callus and fissuring, which had arisen following plantar fasciotomy to correct 'clubbed feet'. The patient stated that she had been born with normal feet, but by the time she was 6 years old she could not run or jump properly and by the time she was an adolescent her feet had become high-arched and inverted.

She had noticed a gradual weakness in her arms and legs and on one occasion, when 41 years old, she had almost dropped a baby while working as a nursing auxiliary. This incident had caused her to be sent for a neurological examination which revealed slowed motor nerve conduction velocities. She had a recent history of several falls, with her ankle 'going over'. She also complained of aching joints in the feet, knees and hips. Her 27-year-old son was similarly affected.

Neurological examination showed all sensory perception except vibration to be normal, but reflexes were absent. Muscle power was reduced in all limbs and muscle wasting of hands, feet and calf muscles was noted. Orthopaedic examination showed reduced dorsiflexion and eversion, with a pes-cavus-type foot and high-stepping gait.

Diagnosis: The patient had Charcot–Marie–Tooth disease, also known as peroneal muscle atrophy. It is an inherited peripheral neuropathy and exists in more than one form, the two most common forms being autosomal dominant.

tibialis anterior nerve is affected, the anterior tibial muscle is unable to control deceleration of dorsiflexion at the ankle in gait, producing a characteristic slapping gait, so increasing plantar pressures (Root et al 1977).

In-depth medical history

Diseases principally affecting the muscles are called myopathies, but this can be confusing, as often lesions in the LMN have given rise to atrophy of the muscle. Therefore, assessment of all parts of the motor unit are considered in this section. For classification of myopathies, see Table 7.14.

General physiology

LMNs or their spinal nerves exit at all segments of the spinal cord, hence LMN symptoms can be seen following damage to any segment from C1 to S5.

Table 7.14 Classification of myopathies

Classification	*Descriptor*
Inherited	Muscular dystrophies (at present untreatable) Duchenne's – X-linked recessive condition. Commonest and most serious of the inherited dystrophies. Affects males, females are carriers. Onset before age 10 years. Weakness in proximal and girdle muscles of lower limb first, later upper limbs also. Hypertrophy and later fatty infiltration (pseudohypertrophy) of calf muscles. Cardiac muscle also affected. See elevated levels of serum phosphokinase. Death from respiratory failure usual between 20 and 30 years Becker's – X-linked recessive condition. A more benign variety of the above Dystrophia myotonica – autosomal dominant condition. Gene located on chromosome 19. Insidious onset, usually between 20 and 50 years, but can be present earlier. Progressive weakness and wasting of distal as well as proximal limb muscles, facial and sternomastoids. Cardiomyopathy, cataracts and frontal baldness also common. Myotonia is failure of muscle to relax immediately after contraction. Patient cannot open hand quickly after making a fist. Faulty gene leads to defective chloride ion transport, resulting in membrane hyperexcitability facio-scapulo-humeral-autosomal dominant condition – benign, often asymptomatic. Wasting and weakness of facial, scapular and humeral muscles mean patient has difficulty in whistling, heavy lifting, etc., as well as scapula in abnormal position. Limb girdle – variable inheritance (may be treatable, depending on cause). Several causes: specific biochemical defect, benign form of motor neurone disease, polymyositis, hormonal and metabolic disease
Biochemical defect	McArdle's syndrome. Abnormality of glycogen metabolism due to deficiency of muscle phosphorylase. Patient suffers from fatigue, cramps and muscle spasm Malignant hyperpyrexia. No muscle wastage or weakness. Symptoms occur during or immediately after administration of a general anaesthetic, especially if halothane or the muscle relaxant suxamethonium chloride is given. Defect in calcium metabolism gives rise to prolonged muscle contraction, in turn raising body temperature. Fatal in 50% of cases
Acquired inflammatory	Polymyositis-autoimmune disease. Infiltration of monocytes and muscle necrosis. Weakness of proximal limb, trunk and neck muscles. Patient has difficulty raising hands above head, getting up out of low chairs and bath. May be associated pain on muscular exertion Dermatomyositis. As above, with additional involvement of skin of face and hands, with erythematous rash
Non-inflammatory	Secondary to high-dose steroids and thyrotoxicosis. These are the most usual causes, but can also be associated with alcoholism, Cushing's disease, Addison's disease, acromegaly, osteomalacia and malignancy. See weakness of proximal limb muscles and shoulder girdle. Trunk may also be involved

Box 7.5 Conditions associated with LMN symptoms

- Poliomyelitis
- Diabetes mellitus
- Motor neurone disease
- Syringomyelia
- Vitamin B_{12} deficiency
- Cord compression/lesion/trauma
- Spina bifida
- Charcot–Marie–Tooth disease

However, due to the anatomy of the spinal cord, any damage to the cord from L2 will only result in an LMN lesion. It is possible to see a combination of UMN and LMN symptoms, if the lesion is between C1 and L1, e.g. syringomyelia. The conditions leading to LMN lesions are listed in Box 7.5.

The clinical severity of weakness (paresis) or flaccid paralysis depends on the site and extent of damage. The sites of damage may involve:

- LMN, e.g. poliomyelitis virus (Case history 7.3)
- peripheral axon, e.g. diabetes mellitus
- neuromuscular junction, e.g. destruction of cholinergic receptors of the skeletal muscle as in myasthenia gravis.

Case history 7.3

A 54-year-old Caucasian man first presented to the clinic complaining of corns and callus under the metatarsal heads of both feet. He was unable to bend down to cut his toe nails.

A vascular assessment revealed weak pulses in both feet, with the right foot being cold. A neurological assessment revealed diminished reflexes in the right leg and absence of vibration sense in the right foot. Two-point discrimination was 2 cm in the left foot and 10 cm in the right foot. Orthopaedic examination showed a leg length discrepancy of 2.5 cm, the right leg being the shorter and having developed a functional equinus at the ankle. Muscle wastage was apparent in the lower limb of the right side. The patient walked with a limp.

Diagnosis: The signs and symptoms are all consistent with poliomyelitis. The patient had contracted the virus when a child. The LMNs of the right side of the spinal cord at the level of the lumbar plexi had been affected.

Nerve impulses are essential to the health of the muscle, thus deficiencies lead to a more rapid atrophy of muscle, skin and other soft tissue than seen in UMN lesions. This is known as denervation atrophy. In addition, the denervated muscle becomes highly sensitive to very small amounts of neurotransmitter (acetylcholine), possibly due to upregulation of receptors. This results in a quivering of the muscle (fasciculation), seen on an electromyogram as fibrillation. Note: this effect will not be seen if the lesion is in the muscle itself.

Assessment

- Muscle power
  Muscle power can be graded according to the Medical Research Council scale (Fuller 1993, p 107) as follows:
  - 5 = normal power
  - 4+ = submaximal movement against resistance
  - 4 = moderate movement against resistance
  - 4– = slight movement against resistance
  - 3 = moves against gravity, but not resistance
  - 2 = moves with gravity eliminated
  - 1 = flicker
  - 0 = no movement.

  A reduced strength of contraction suggests paresis or paralysis
- Fatigability
  If the site of the lesion is the neuromuscular junction, the muscle will show a sliding decrease in response or fatigability, as seen in myasthenia gravis. The acetylcholine receptors are destroyed in an autoimmune attack and, although the first quanta of neurotransmitter can diffuse to remaining receptors, subsequent release of neurotransmitter is less likely to make contact, so that the response fades. The muscle cells are able to replace the receptors, but the autoimmune attack will invariably strike again, in the same or different muscles.
- Muscle tone
  In the skeletal muscles of a healthy person, there will always be some motor units firing, which means that the muscle will feel firm. This is referred to as the 'tone' of the muscle. In LMN or muscle damage, the muscle will feel flabby, due to lack of tone.

- Patellar and Achilles tendon reflexes
  Reflexes will be weak or absent, because of interruption of the final common pathway. A single reduced or absent reflex suggests mononeuropathy or radiculopathy. A reduction or absence of all lower limb reflexes suggests polyradiculopathy, cauda equina lesions, peripheral polyneuropathy or a myopathy. In the latter, there will be no sensory deficit. Values of below 1 suggest LMN lesions, peripheral sensory nerve or muscle damage.

Risk and referral

Any alteration to individuals' neurological status must be considered as a contributory factor to elevated risk status. However, all neurological testing must be taken in context and never viewed in isolation. Consequently, to determine the clinical risk, information from sensory testing, vascular status, gait/foot pressure analysis, tissue vitality and medical history must be considered holistically. Referral to the patient's GP should always be considered if abnormal findings are reported. In addition, alteration to muscle bulk and symmetry should be recorded in the patient's notes with pictorial (digital images) evidence, thus allowing effective evaluation of treatment and pathological progression. Furthermore, such digital information may be shared with the GP and multi-disciplinary team for an enhanced management strategy, providing all the relevant consent and data protection legislation are observed.

Referral for tests vary according to the suspected cause, for example, if diabetic polyneuropathy is suspected, the diagnosis should be confirmed by a combination of sensory testing and fasting blood glucose measurements, in accordance with the World Health Organization criteria. Referral to the relevant GP would be the primary pathway in this case. However, if the patient required immediate specialist treatment, referral to the diabetes department within secondary care could be considered. In this instance, hospital testing will include the following:

- Nerve conduction velocity
  This compares the affected side with established norms, e.g. diagnosis for tarsal tunnel syndrome (Galardi et al 1994). Alternatively, axonal degeneration can be determined, as seen in polyneuropathies of diabetes mellitus, alcoholism, nerve entrapment, Friedreich's ataxia and toxicity due to heavy metals (Zouri et al 1998). Charcot–Marie–Tooth disease is interesting, as two subtypes have been identified: HMSN type I, which shows primarily segmental demyelination, and HMSN type II, which shows mainly axonal degeneration (McLeod & Lance 1989).
- Electromyography
  This uses a needle electrode inserted into the muscle to show the electrical activity of the muscle in response to an electrical stimulus. Abnormal results are detected in dysfunction of motor nerves, neuromuscular junction lesions and in myopathies (Matthews & Arnold 1991). Electromyography is the only means of electrophysiological testing for myopathies.
- Nerve and muscle biopsies
  Histological examination of nerve and muscle tissue will show structural abnormalities, while biochemical tests will detect enzyme dysfunction, e.g. in distinguishing Duchenne's muscular dystrophy from the treatable connective tissue disease of polymyositis, which also shows muscle weakness and atrophy of limb girdles.

The differences between UMN and LMN lesions are summarised in Table 7.15.

Assessment of coordination and proprioception function

The receptors in the muscles, joints and tendons all feed positional information to the cerebellum and cortex. In turn, the cerebellum and the cortex bring about vital postural reflexes, necessary for accurate movement. The basal ganglia also play an important part in the coordination of movement. Accordingly, damage to these parts of the nervous system may have an effect on both gait and coordination. Conditions that may affect coordination and proprioception function are listed in Table 7.16.

Clinical signs

Careful observation of motor activity can give an indication of a deficit in posture, balance or coordination; for example, a stamping gait may be due to loss of proprioception, as in tabes dorsalis, where the ascending tracts in the dorsal columns degenerate. The patient will not know where their body is in space and so lifts the legs much higher than necessary to clear the ground. Similarly, the patient will also be unaware of when their foot is about to make ground contact and thus, stamps it down. This has the advantage of stimulating pressure receptors

Table 7.15 Differences between UMN and LMN lesions

Test	*Clinical signs of UMN lesions*	*Clinical signs of LMN lesions*
Patella reflex and Achilles	Exaggerated response	Loss or diminished
Plantar (Babinski's) response	Dorsiflexion of hallux and fanning of lesser toes	Plantar flexion of hallux and lesser toes – normal response
Abdominal reflex	Lost	Normal
Electrical excitability of muscle	Normal	Fasciculation (fibrillation seen on EMG)
Muscle bulk (observation and measurement)	Muscle wasting over a period of time due to lack of use	Rapidly wasting due to lack of innervation
Muscle power	Clasp knife spasticity	Reduced resistance to exerted pressure
Muscle tone	Increased in muscle tone (clonus and spasticity)	Flaccid muscles (lack of tone)
Gait	Extension of the hip and knee with inversion and plantarflexion of the foot, circumductory gait – hemiplegic or paraplegic	Weakness (paresis) or complete loss of function (paralysis) requiring calipers or walking aids may be required
Distribution	Whole limb affected	Certain muscle groups affected, depending upon site of damage; deformity due to contracture of antagonists

UMN, upper motor neurone; LMN, lower motor neurone.

proximally, as vibrations from the foot travel up the leg and so provide much needed information to the brain.

Dysarthria

Cerebellar dysfunction affects the speech muscles and produces a scanning speech, with inappropriate syllabic stress and volume.

Dysdiadochokinesia

Actions are no longer smooth, continuous movements, but are broken down into their component parts, producing clumsy, jerky actions.

Tremor

Associated with cerebellar defect, due to the dysfunction of the stretch reflex and/or is an intention tremor, i.e. one which increases in amplitude, as the person tries to carry out any tasks with the affected limb. The tremor disappears at rest. Tremors may have a physiological or neurological cause; consequently, the appearance, disappearance and nature of the tremor should be noted.

Gait

If balance is upset, the patient will feel unsteady and adopt a wide-based gait. As voluntary movement is also affected, the gait will be clumsy or staggering, as if drunk. Such gait is described as ataxic. The patient may complain of deviating to one side, which suggests the dysfunction is limited to one hemisphere.

In-depth medical history

Parkinson's disease

This is the commonest extrapyramidal disease and is due to depletion of dopaminergic neurones in the

Table 7.16 Conditions that may result in poor coordination

Part	*Conditions*
Cerebellum	Tumour Multiple sclerosis Arnold–Chiari malformation Friedreich's ataxia Other hereditary spinocerebellar ataxias Hypothyroidism Repeated head trauma as in boxing
Basal ganglia	Parkinsonism Huntington's chorea Wilson's disease Sydenham's chorea
Ascending pathways	Subacute combined degeneration of the spinal cord Guillain–Barré syndrome Tabes dorsalis Alcoholism

substantia nigra, which project to the caudate nucleus. The most troublesome effect is hypo/bradykinesia, which results in the patient having great difficulty initiating or stopping movement (Case history 7.4). Rest tremor and rigidity are also features. If the hand is affected, the tremor may cause the patient to move both the index finger and thumb in a 'pill-rolling' movement. The patient may show a 'mask-like' face and speak in a soft voice. Micrographia (small handwriting) is also a characteristic.

General physiology

Cerebellum

The cerebellum has modifying influences on the UMNs in the cortex and on brain-stem nuclei. It receives rich proprioceptive information and adjusts the activity of the UMNs to ensure that the actual action and intended action are matched. The cerebellum is essential for smooth, accurate movement, posture and balance. Dysfunction of the cerebellum or of its afferent and efferent tracts, produces characteristic effects that are easily observable.

Basal ganglia

Although the basal ganglia also have a modifying role on voluntary movement, the effects of their dysfunction is quite different from that of the cerebellum. Damage to the basal ganglia produces either a poverty of movement (hypo/bradykinesia), as seen in Parkinson's disease, or jerky writhing movements (choreoathetosis), as seen in the inherited disease of Huntington's chorea (Case history 7.5), or the benign

Case history 7.4

A 65-year-old Caucasian woman presented to the clinic requesting nail care. On examination her nails were long, thickened and mycotic and a variety of dorsal, apical and interdigital lesions were present.

The patient could appreciate temperature, light touch and pressure and reflexes were normal, but she was very confused and nervous, so that communication was difficult. A full orthopaedic assessment could not be carried out because of the patient's inability to relax her legs and feet. Ankle dorsiflexion was limited and the feet adopted a varus position. Most of the toes showed retraction deformities. Movements were hypokinetic and gait was stooped and shuffling. There was a minor rest tremor in the right arm.

Diagnosis: The symptoms are consistent with Parkinson's disease. This is a progressive idiopathic condition which gradually affects all limbs. Mental confusion/dementia is not always present.

The antigravity muscles are affected, producing a stooped posture with knees flexed, so that the patient's centre of gravity is no longer over the base of gait. This causes the festination seen in a gait, when the patient has to move more and more quickly to avoid falling forward. Moreover, the gait tends to be shuffling, with poor heel-ground contact – 'marche à petits pas'. The tendon reflexes, however, are unaffected. There may be a general resistance to passive stretch, described as 'lead-pipe rigidity'. It may show a superimposed intermittent release of the resistance, producing a series of jerks, the so-called 'cog-wheel' effect.

In a patient with Parkinson's disease, there is no habituation with the glabellar tap reflex. The glabellar tap reflex involves the practitioner gently, slowly and repeatedly, tapping the forehead of the patient between the eyes. In a healthy person, the first tap or two will elicit the eye-blink reflex, but this will rapidly habituate. The frequency of the tremor may be measured via hospital tests, but usually the above clinical tests and a positive response to drug therapy will be sufficient to confirm the diagnosis of Parkinson's disease.

Case history 7.5

A 30-year-old Caucasian man attended the clinic complaining of sore corns. Enquiry revealed that he had learning disabilities. Examination showed warm, hyperhidrotic feet with a poor skin condition and fibrous lesions on the plantar aspect of the feet. The left foot had marked pes cavus deformity. The gait revealed limping and shuffling with excessive arm movement to maintain balance.

Over the next few years further mental and physical deterioration became apparent. The patient's brother was similarly affected and so apparently had been their father.

Diagnosis: A diagnosis of Huntington's chorea was made. This disease is inherited as an autosomal condition with complete penetration and late onset, and is characterised by progressive chorea and dementia.

and brief effects of Sydenham's chorea, associated with rheumatic fever.

Assessment

Proprioception in joints

To test proprioception distally, the practitioner holds the sides of the hallux between forefinger and thumb. While the patient's eyes are shut, the toe is moved up and down and the patient should be able to state the final position of the toe. The sides of the hallux are held rather than the dorsal and plantar surfaces, to avoid additional pressure information being generated. This information travels from receptors in joints in the largest-diameter, fastest nerve fibres of the A-alpha class into the spinal cord, up to the cerebellum in the ipsilateral spinocerebellar tracts and to the conscious cortex in the dorsal columns. A positive result shows that the pathway to the cortex is intact. An inability to give the correct responses would be seen in conditions, such as tabes dorsalis.

Romberg's sign

This test can be used to confirm proprioceptive disturbance in the dorsal columns or peripheral nerves (Fuller 1993, pp 41–42). Patients are observed standing with feet together and eyes open and then closed. If patients cannot maintain their balance with their eyes open, this suggests either a cerebellar or a vestibular defect and if a patient rocks backwards and forwards with eyes open, a cerebellar defect could be the cause. In such cases, this is not positive Romberg's sign and Romberg's test cannot be performed. Closing the eyes will deprive the patients of visual information, so that the brain has to rely on proprioceptive input; if this is not being transmitted, the patients will sway and find it difficult to keep balance. The practitioner must be ready to catch the patient. Positive Romberg's sign could be due to cord compression, tabes dorsalis, vitamin B_{12} deficiency or degenerative spinal cord disease.

Nystagmus

These are rapid eye movements due to vestibular dysfunction and can be elicited, by asking the patient to make a sudden rapid head movement. Its presence indicates a cerebellar lesion.

Heel–shin test

The patient is asked to slide the heel of one leg straight down the shin of the other. Patients with cerebellar dysfunction often cannot to do this because of lack of coordination, and their heel will follow a wavy path down the other leg.

Heel–toe test

The patient is asked to walk in a straight line heel to toe. Patients with cerebellar dysfunction will stagger about the midline, but it must be remembered that there are many other causes of an unsteady gait, especially in elderly people.

Finger–nose test

The patient is asked to stand comfortably and then, with eyes shut and one arm outstretched, to bring their fingertip to the nose. Repeat for the other arm. Cerebellar dysfunction will cause the patient to overshoot (hypermetria) or undershoot (hypometria) and miss the nose.

Muscle tone

This will be generally reduced in the affected limbs.

Tendon reflexes

These may be unusually sustained, because of the oscillations of an abnormal stretch reflex, but should not be exaggerated. Occasionally, a weak response can be seen in cerebellar syndromes.

Risk and referral

While the sensory pathways are not directly affected, the cerebellum coordinates and modifies the motor

Table 7.17 Aide-memoire for tests for poor coordination

Head	Nystagmus. Rapid eye movements elicited by asking the patient to make a sudden rapid head movement Finger–nose test. Cerebellar dysfunction will cause the patient to overshoot (hypermetria) or undershoot (hypometria)
Shoulders	Romberg's sign. The practitioner must be ready to catch the patient (or support at shoulders). A positive Romberg's sign could be due to cord compression, tabes dorsalis, vitamin B_{12} deficiency or degenerative spinal cord disease
Knees and Toes	Heel–shin test. Patients with cerebellar dysfunction are often unable to do this and the heel will follow a wavy path down the other leg Tendon reflexes. These may be unusually sustained, but not be exaggerated. Occasionally, a weak response can be seen in cerebellar syndromes Heel–toe test. Patients with cerebellar dysfunction will stagger about the midline, but remember that there are many other causes of an unsteady gait in the elderly

response to the sensory stimulus. Consequently, individuals with cerebellar lesions may be at an increased risk from fall. Alternatively, injury may result from an uncoordinated motor response, i.e. burn, resulting from spilt hot drink or increased plantar pressures from a stamping gait.

Table 7.17 provides an aid memoire for assessment of patients with poor coordination.

Assessment of autonomic function

Autonomic nerves innervate the viscera and internal structures, such as blood vessels, since they enable the nervous system to maintain homeostasis (see Fig. 7.8). Medical history may reveal abnormalities of bowel and bladder function.

Clinical signs

There will be various signs suggestive of autonomic neuropathy, such as abnormal sudomotor responses in the skin and abnormal cardiovascular responses in the heart and peripheral blood vessels (Faris 1991). Sudomotor neuropathy usually leads to an absence of sweating and a dry skin, although it may produce hyperhidrosis. Vasomotor neuropathy usually produces a warm red skin and an absence of vasoconstriction in response to cold, although it may occasionally produce a prolonged vasoconstriction. Sustained vasoconstriction will promote hypertension, a factor which has been significantly linked with the development of atherosclerosis, vessel disease and renal failure. Alternatively, it may lead to postural hypotension. Arteriovenous shunting may also be manifested in the diabetic neuropathic foot, causing distended veins over the dorsum of the ankle (Cameron et al 2001). Neuropathy of nerves to the cardiac pacemaker tissue may lead to failure of the heart to respond appropriately to the demands of the body, e.g. an absence of tachycardia in response to exercise. Key clinical signs are:

- dry skin (absence of sweating)
- macerated, hyperhidrotic skin (increased sweating)
- warm red skin (vasomotor neuropathy)
- distended veins over the dorsum of ankle (arteriovenous shunting)
- hypertension (vasomotor neuropathy)
- postural hypotension (vasomotor neuropathy)
- increased bradycardia (slowing of the heart rate).

In-depth medical history

It is important that injury or interruption to the spinal cord or nerves is recorded, as damage to these sites can affect the sympathetic or parasympathetic nervous systems. Systemic conditions, such as diabetes mellitus, multiple sclerosis, polio and motor neurone disease can have significant impact on autonomic responses and should be immediately reported, given their role as key risk indicators for potential autonomic dysfunction.

General physiology

The condition commonly associated with autonomic neuropathy is diabetes mellitus, where the foot will often appear red and feel dry and warm, described by Edmonds (2004) as the classic neuropathic foot. There may be co-existent neuropathy of other small fibres, such as pain and temperature fibres (A-delta and C), as well as large-fibre (A-alpha and A-beta) involvement, giving rise to the picture of a typical neuropathic foot (Ch. 18). Less common conditions exhibiting autonomic neuropathy are Guillain–Barré syndrome, amyloidosis and congenital autonomic failure. It should be remembered that other conditions, such as infection and anaemia and certain drugs, such as beta-blockers, can also affect the cardiovascular system and thereby, give a false-positive result.

Assessment

Currently, there is a lack of clinical tests for the clinician to perform, despite the potential serious nature of autonomic dysfunction.

Sweat response

There is only one clinically non-invasive assessment technique for this modality – the Neuropad. The device has been validated in studies examining the autonomic responses of individuals with diabetic neuropathy (Papanas et al 2005). The small plaster-like device is applied to the plantar aspect of the first metatarsal for a few minutes, if the Neuropad changes colour, the sweat response is present. However, the Neuropad is not sensitive to autonomic dysfunction, which may produce hyperhidrosis. Consequently, observation of clinical signs and a good in-depth medical history remain invaluable assessment tools for autonomic function.

Risk and referral

If autonomic dysfunction is suspected, the patient will show a mild-to-moderate increased risk status, particularly if vasomotor and sudomotor alteration is reducing tissue vitality. However, if this is further complicated by an underlying systemic condition, i.e. diabetes mellitus, the risk level will potentially be further elevated. It is also important that observed changes, i.e. dry skin are not automatically linked to autonomic neuropathy, as this may be due to a range of non-pathological causes. An understanding of the basic physiology of the autonomic nervous system will also allow the practitioner to identify the patient with a history of hypertension as being at an increased risk of developing peripheral vascular disease and associated complications. Referral for the following tests can be requested.

Heart rate

The pulse is taken while the patient is in a supine position and repeated when an upright posture is adopted. The normal response is an increase in heart rate of greater than 11 beats per minute. A loss of response suggests parasympathetic abnormality.

Blood pressure

Repeat the above test measuring blood pressure in the two positions. The systolic blood pressure should fall on standing, by approximately 30 mmHg and the diastolic pressure by about 15 mmHg. An increased drop suggests sympathetic abnormality. Failure of the cardiovascular system to compensate for postural effects can lead to postural syncope.

Table 7.18 Conditions that affect more than one part of the nervous system

Condition	*Parts affected*
Diabetes mellitus	Sensory, motor (LMN) and autonomic
Motor neurone disease	LMN and UMN
Spina bifida	LMN and sensory
Syringomyelia	Sensory, LMN and UMN
Vitamin B_{12} deficiency	Sensory, LMN and UMN
Multiple sclerosis	Sensory and UMN
Cord compression/ lesion	Sensory, LMN and UMN
Guillain–Barré syndrome	LMN, sensory and autonomic
Charcot–Marie–Tooth disease	Mainly LMN but possible sensory
Nerve injuries	Depends upon site, may result in LMN, UMN, sensory or autonomic

Valsalva's manoeuvre

Valsalva's manoeuvres is not advisable, if there is evidence of proliferative retinopathy. The patient is asked to take a deep breath and exhale against a closed glottis for 10–15 seconds and then breathe normally. The pulse rate is taken during Valsalva's manoeuvre and on release. Heart rate should increase during the manoeuvre and fall on release. No increase during the manoeuvre suggests sympathetic abnormality and no decrease on release suggests parasympathetic abnormality. These tests reveal abnormal responses of the baroreceptor reflex, which implicates defects in innervation of the cardiac pacemaker tissue, rather than peripheral autonomic neuropathy, for which there are no clinical tests.

Summary

This chapter has considered the assessment of the various components on the nervous system. However, as stated earlier, it is important to remember that a number of conditions may affect more than one part. By means of assistance, those conditions capable of effecting damage to more than one part of the nervous system are summarised in Table 7.18. Above all, it is essential that all aspects of the nervous system are assessed, so as to allow the practitioner the fullest picture of neurological function (Case history 7.6). Table 7.19 summarises the neurological signs and symptoms. Table 7.20 provides an aide-memoire for neurological assessment.

Case history 7.6

A 47-year-old Caucasian man was referred to the clinic with a small ulcer beneath his right heel since 6 months. He had visited Nigeria when he was 29 years of age, where he had contracted schistosomiasis with resultant paraparesis from his lower abdomen downwards. Since then he had had repeated ulceration of both feet. The present ulcer was covered with dense callus which when debrided revealed a lesion 15 mm in diameter and 8 mm deep. Its border was surrounded by macerated callus.

A vascular assessment showed no remarkable features, all tests indicating a good blood supply to the foot. The neurological assessment revealed absent reflexes, lack of appreciation of all senses and constant 'pins and needles' sensation around his hips and legs. The skin of the feet was dry. The patient used a walking stick to support his right leg and walked with an abductory gait to achieve ground clearance as the right foot could not dorsiflex. The right leg showed wasting of the triceps surae.

Diagnosis: A diagnosis was made of neuropathic ulcer associated with peripheral sensory, motor and autonomic neuropathy due to damage in the spinal cord caused by the parasitic blood fluke *Schistosoma haematobium.*

Table 7.19 Summary of neurological signs and symptoms

Feature	*Site of lesion*	*Possible disease*	*Possible pattern*
Apraxic gait Aphasia, speech defects Visual defects	UMN (hemisphere)	Stroke Head injury Hydrocephalus	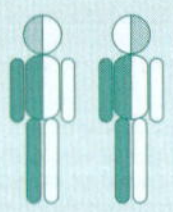
Progressive focal deficit epilepsy	UMN (head)	Tumour, ischaemic stroke, previous intracranial disease	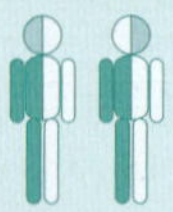
Increased tone and reflexes Weak arm extensors Weak leg flexors	UMN (head/spinal cord) Neck, cervical region	Stroke Cerebral palsy Neck injury Multiple sclerosis	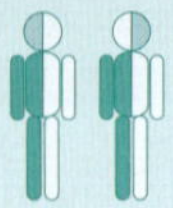

Table 7.19 *Continued*

Feature	*Site of lesion*	*Possible disease*	*Possible pattern*
Hypo/bradykinesia Festinating gait Lead pipe/cog-wheel rigidity Rest tremor	Basal ganglia	Parkinson's disease	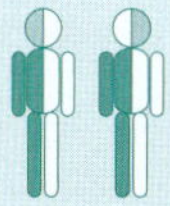
Choreoathetotic movements	Basal ganglia	Huntington's chorea Sydenham's chorea (rare)	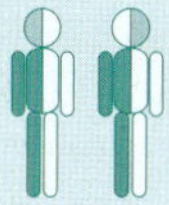
Nystagmus Dysarthria Cranial nerve palsies	Brain stem	Multiple sclerosis Syringomyelia	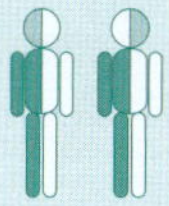
Nystagmus Dysarthria Scanning speech Diminished pendular reflexes Intention tremor Ataxic gait Loss of proprioception Dysdiadochokinesia (clonus)	Cerebellum Spinal cord	Friedreich's ataxia Stroke Tumour Vitamin B_{12} deficiency Syringomyelia Spina bifida	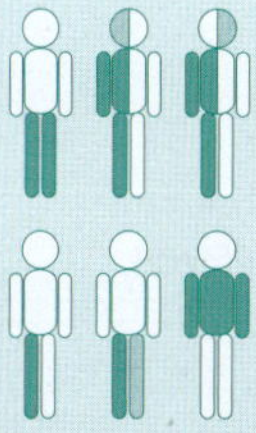
Diminished tendon reflexes Loss of proprioception Paresis/paralysis Pain Paraesthesia/anaesthesia Arteriovenous shunting Loss of sweat response	LMN (spinal cord/nerve roots/axons) Spinal nerves (autonomic nervous system)	Diabetes mellitus Poliomyelitis Chronic alcoholism Rheumatoid arthritis Guillain–Barré syndrome Charcot–Marie–Tooth disease Vitamin deficiencies (B1, B6, B12) Tumour Disc protrusion Trauma	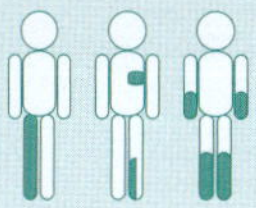
Progressive fatigability and weakness	Neuromuscular junction	Myasthenia gravis	
Proximal limb muscle weakness and wasting, but no sensory loss and no fasciculation	Muscle	Myopathies	

UMN, upper motor neurone; LMN, lower motor neurone.

Table 7.20 Aide-memoire

Clinical signs	Seven-point observation: distribution, weakness, muscles or actions affected, muscle tone and bulk, sensation, deformity and tremor
In-depth medical history	Onset, duration, falls, consciousness, headaches, peripheral neuropathy or CNS damage
General physiology	Heredity, developmental, trauma, ischaemia, compression, infection, autoimmune, nutritional/metabolic, iatrogenic and idiopathic
Assessment	Consciousness, sensory, motor, autonomic function, posture and coordination, social, gender and age
Risk and referral	Reduction in peripheral nerve function increases risk status significantly. High-risk groups include those individuals with neuropathy, reduced/altered immune response, vascular disease, deformity, impaired wound healing and diabetes mellitus

References

Bawa P, Binder M D, Ruenzel P et al 1984 Recruitment order of motoneurones in stretch reflexes is highly correlated with their axonal conduction velocity. Journal of Neurophysiology 52:3410–3420

Booth J, Young M 2000 Testing the reliability of 10 g monofilaments. Diabetic Medicine 17:S74

Boulton, A J M 1998 Lowering the risk of neuropathy, foot ulcers and amputations. Diabetic Medicine 15(Suppl 4): S57–S59

Boulton A J M (ed) 2000 The pathway to ulceration. In: Boulton A J M, Connor H, Cavanagh P R (eds) The foot in diabetes, 3rd edn. J Wiley, Chichester, p 22

Boulton A J M, Gries F A, Jervell J A 1998 Guidelines for the diagnosis and outpatient management of diabetic peripheral neuropathy. Diabetic Medicine 15:508–514

Budd K 1984 Pain. Update postgraduate centre series. Update, Guildford

Cameron N E, Cotter M A 2001 Diabetes causes an early reduction in autonomic ganglion blood flow in rats. Journal of Diabetes and its Complications 15(4):198–202

Cassella J P, Ashford R L, Kavanagh-Sharp V 2000 Effect of applied pressure in the determination of vibration sensitivity using the neurothesiometer. The Foot 10:27–30

Coppini D V, Weng C, Young P J et al 2000 The 'VPT score' – a useful predictor of neuropathy in diabetic patients. Diabetic Medicine 17:488–490

Edmonds M E 2004 The diabetic foot 2003. Diabetes Metabolism Research Reviews 20(S1):S9–S12

Edmonds M, Foster A 2005 Ulcer-free survival in diabetic foot patients. Diabetic Medicine 22(10):1293–1294

Epstein O, Perkin G, de Bono D et al 1992 Clinical examination. Gower Medical, London

Faris I 1991 The management of the diabetic foot. Churchill Livingstone, Edinburgh

Fuller G 1993 Neurological examination made easy. Churchill Livingstone, Edinburgh

Galardi G, Amadio S, Maderna L et al 1994 Electrophysiologic studies in tarsal tunnel syndrome – diagnostic reliability of motor distal latency, mixed nerve and sensory nerve conduction studies. American Journal of Physical Medicine and Rehabilitation 73:193–198

Ganong W 1991 Reviews of medical physiology, 15th edn. Lange, London

International Consensus on the Diabetic Foot 1999 International Working Group on the Diabetic Foot, p 32

Kalter-Leibovici O, Yosipovitch G, Gabbay U et al 2001 Factor analysis of thermal and vibration thresholds in young patients with Type 1 diabetes mellitus. Diabetic Medicine 18:213–217

MacDonald B, Cockerell O, Sander J et al 2000 The incidence and lifetime prevalence of neurological disorders in a prospective community-based study in the UK. Brain 123:665–676

McClintic J R 1980 Basic anatomy and physiology of the human body. John Wiley, New York

McGill M, Molyneaux L, Yue D K 1998 Use of the Semmes-Weinstein 5.07/10 gram monofilament: the long and the short of it. Diabetic Medicine 15:615–617

McLeod J, Lance J 1989 Introductory neurology, 2nd edn. Blackwell Science, Oxford

Matthews P, Arnold D 1991 (eds) Diagnostic tests in neurology. Churchill Livingstone, Edinburgh

Melzack R 1992 Phantom limbs. Scientific American, April: 90

Miranda-Palma B, Sosenko J M, Bowker J H et al 2005 A comparison of the monofilament with other testing modalities for foot ulcer susceptibility. Diabetes Research and Clinical Practice 70(1):8–12

Mold J W, Vesley S K, Keyl B A et al 2004 The prevalence, predictors and consequences of peripheral sensory neuropathy in older patients. Journal of the American Board of Family Medicine 17:309–318

Nakayama H, Noda K, Hotta H et al 1998 Effects of ageing on numbers, size and conduction velocities of myelinated and unmyelinated fibers of the pelvic nerve in rats. Journal of the Autonomic Nervous System 69:148–155

Papanas N, Papatheodorou K, Papazoglou D et al 2005 Reproducibility of the new indicator test for Sudomotor function (Neuropad®) in patients with type 2 diabetes. Clinical Endocrinology and Diabetes 113(10):577–581

Primatesta P, Bost L, Poulter N R 2000 Blood pressure levels and hypertension status among ethnic groups in England. Journal of Human Hypertension 14(2):143–148

Root M L, Orien W P, Weed J H 1977 Normal and abnormal function of the foot. Clinical biomechanics – volume 2. Clinical Biomechanics Corporation, Los Angeles, p 254

Spruce M C, Potter J, Coppini D V 2003 The pathogenesis and management of painful diabetic neuropathy: a review. Diabetic Medicine 20(2):88–94

Vander A J, Sherman J H, Luciano D S 1998 Human physiology, 7th edn. McGraw Hill, New York, pp 238–239

Van Gijn J 1975 The Babinski response: stimulus and effector. Journal of Neurology, Neurosurgery and Psychology 38:180–186

Wallace H, Shorvon S, Tallis R 1998 Age-specific incidence and prevalence rates of treated epilepsy in an unselected population of 2,052,922 and age specific fertility rates of women with epilepsy. Lancet 352(9145):1970–1973

Wareham A, Rayman A, Rayman G 1997 Pin-prick sensory thresholds in detecting risk of neuropathic ulceration. Diabetic Medicine 14:S32

Wilkinson I M S 1993 Essential neurology. 2nd edn. Blackwell Science, Oxford

Wilson K J W 1990 Ross & Wilson Anatomy and physiology in health and illness. 7th edn. Churchill Livingstone, Edinburgh

Winkler A S, Ejskaer N, Edmonds M et al 2000 Dissociated sensory loss in diabetic autonomic neuropathy. Diabetic Medicine 17:457–462

Young M, Matthews C 1998 Neuropathy screening: can we achieve our ideals? The Diabetic Foot 1:22–25

Zouri M, Feki M, Hamida C B et al 1998 Electrophysiology and nerve biopsy: comparative study in Friedreich's ataxia and Friedreich's ataxia phenotype with vitamin E deficiency. Neuromuscular Disorders 8:416–425

Further reading

Berkow R (ed) 2000 The Merck manual. Merck Sharp & Dohme Research Laboratories, New Jersey

Fuller G 1993 Neurological examination made easy. Churchill Livingstone, Edinburgh

Joel A, DeLisa J B (eds) 1993 Electrodiagnostic evaluation of the peripheral nervous system. In: rehabilitation medicine: principles and practice, 2nd edn. Lippincott, Philadelphia

Kandel E, Jessel T, Schwartz J 1991 The principles of neural science. Elsevier, New York

Wilkinson I M S 1998 Essential neurology, 2nd edn. Blackwell Science, Oxford

CHAPTER

8

Dermatological assessment

I Bristow, R Turner

Chapter contents

Introduction

Dermatology is the study of the skin and its disorders. More than just an inert barrier, the integument is a highly active organ with an important role in physiology and homeostasis. There are over 5000 recognised skin disorders in existence but the largest percentage of skin disease is due to a handful of conditions, which may range from the trivial (i.e. minor bruising) to life-threatening (i.e. malignant melanoma). Most skin diseases do not have a significant mortality, although they cause significant morbidity and have a substantial effect on the quality of life of patients (Harlow et al 1998). Typically, skin disorders affect individuals in a number of ways (the four Ds):

- Discomfort: itching and pain
- Disability: foot ulceration, hand eczema
- Disfigurement: scarring or rashes
- Death: skin cancers.

Approach to the patient

The key to a good dermatological assessment is, firstly, a thorough history. This provides essential information and initiates an understanding of the patient as a person, the environment and an appreciation of the psychological aspects to the skin disease. The second stage is examination of the skin (with investigations when required). The skin is an easily accessible structure, but it is frequently difficult for non-dermatologists to examine and record their findings. Therefore, a basic orderly approach is required if a successful outcome is to be achieved.

Psychological aspects of skin disease

The skin defines who we are and how we are perceived to be. It is on our appearance we are judged by others (Lawton 2000). One only has to see the amount of time and money invested in changing or enhancing our appearance to appreciate how important the skin and its appendages are. A common mistake of students when faced with a patient with widespread skin disease is to remain at a distance, avoiding any physical contact. Skin diseases are subconsciously often perceived as nasty, dirty or infectious.

As a practitioner, preconceptions need to be overcome if the patient is to be reassured that they are in the care of an empathetic, understanding professional. It should be remembered that the problems of the skin patient may be more than skin deep, even with conditions that are perceived by the practitioner to be trivial. Many patients with most common skin disorders, such as psoriasis and eczema, have a quality of life that is similar to the quality of life of patients with other chronic diseases such as rheumatoid arthritis, cancer and heart disease. Often, the extent of the skin disease is not correlated with the sufferer's well-being (Jayaprakasam et al 2002) and many conditions may be aggravated by psychological stress, such as atopic dermatitis, psoriasis and lichen planus. It should also be borne in mind that often just acknowledgement and discussion of the wider problems with a patient, in a sensitive and empathetic manner, is an important aspect of the assessment.

The purpose of assessment

The assessment procedure is at the heart of the diagnostic and treatment process. From a patient's perspective assessment is seen as the reaching of a diagnosis and arriving at a decision on the most suitable form of treatment, i.e. what it is and what can be done about it. Most patients' fears regarding skin disease revolve around issues such as 'Is it catching?' and 'Will it get better?'. All the information gathered during the assessment will help to inform and reassure the patient accordingly.

The difficulty is that, to the untrained eye, many skin diseases appear similar. The second challenge is deciding whether the skin disease is part of an underlying systemic condition; therefore, the importance of the whole assessment process cannot be overstressed.

Many underlying conditions may be reflected in the condition of the skin and nails. For example, clubbing of the nails is a feature often associated with smoking and lung disease. Recurrent ulceration and infection of the foot is a common diagnostic marker in diabetes mellitus. Recognising such features will improve the likelihood of a successful diagnosis and treatment plan.

How common is skin disease?

Reliable data are difficult to obtain but skin disorders are thought to affect around a quarter of the population, with only a small percentage seeking professional help. Typically, 10–20% of a general practitioner's annual workload involves skin disorders (Office of Population Census and Surveys 1991–1992), and podiatrists also spend a significant amount of time treating skin conditions (e.g. hyperkeratosis, nail disorders and wounds). The most common disorders that affect the lower limb (Gawkrodger 2002) are:

- fungal and other skin infections
- dermatitis/eczema
- psoriasis
- warts
- tumours (benign and malignant).

Skin structure and function

The skin (or integument) is the largest organ system and covers around 1.8 m^2. The skin is much more than just an inert wrapping, it is a highly active organ that fulfils many functions (Table 8.1) which are determined by its structure. The skin comprises three layers: an epithelium (epidermis) and a connective tissue matrix (the dermis) firmly bound together at the dermo-epidermal junction (Fig. 8.1); below the dermis lies the subcutaneous (fat) layer.

Across the whole body surface, there are considerable regional variations in the skin's structure, which in turn dictates its specific properties. These local variations may then influence the microclimate and, therefore, the pattern of organisms. Such variation may also account for the typical distribution of skin disease.

Epidermis

The epidermis (Fig. 8.2) is an avascular structure, relying on the diffusion of materials across the dermo-epidermal junction for nutrients and waste disposal. It is principally composed of keratinocytes

Table 8.1 Functions of the skin

Function	*Specific property*
Barrier properties	Physical: thermal/mechanical/ radiation Chemical: irritants/allergens/water loss Microbiological: infections/ infestations
Sense organ	Touch/vibration/pressure/temperature Nociception
Other	Thermoregulation and assistance in maintaining blood pressure Vitamin D and cholesterol production

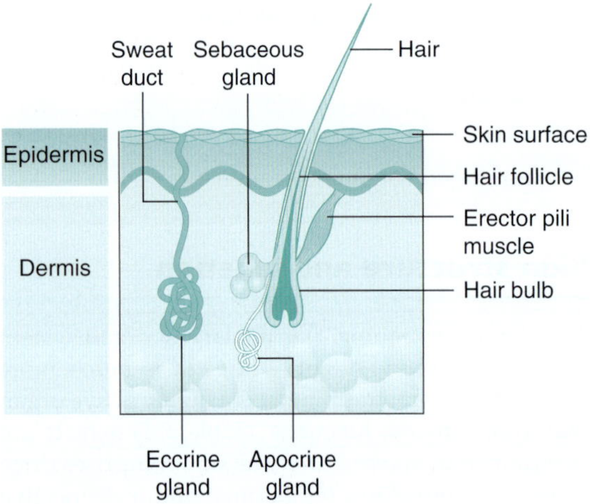

Figure 8.1 Normal skin (not to scale) showing epidermis and dermis and the skin appendages, excluding nail.

(corneocytes), which make up approximately 80% of the cells, as well as melanocytes, Merkel's discs and Langerhans' cells. Appendages of the epidermis include the nails, sweat glands and sebaceous glands (Fig. 8.1).

The epidermis ranges in thickness from around 0.4 mm to 1.5 mm, depending on the anatomical location; it is divided into four layers.

Basal layer (stratum germinativum)

For the most part, the basal layer consists of a single, undulating layer of cuboidal keratinocytes.

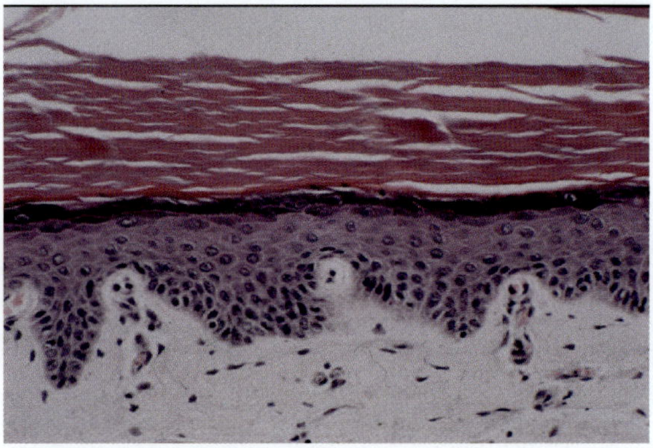

Figure 8.2 The epidermis.

The cells within this layer are firmly attached to the dermo-epidermal junction (DEJ) by tonofilaments which arise from the cytoplasm of the cells linking into the hemidesmosomes anchored into the DEJ (Venning 2000). These mitotically active cells generate the cells of the more superficial layers of the epidermis.

Scattered throughout this layer are specialist cells known as melanocytes. In sun-exposed areas (e.g. the face) they may have a ratio of 1 in 4, whereas on unexposed areas such as the plantar surface of the foot their numbers may decrease to 1 in 30. These cells are well developed in the epidermis of humans as we have a relatively hairless integument. Melanocytes are dendritic cells which produce the pigment melanin in specialist organelles known as melanosomes. These melanin granules then pass along the dendritic processes of the cell and are distributed evenly to adjacent keratinocytes. The melanin forms a protective cap over the cell nucleus, its function being to limit the amount of harmful ultraviolet radiation reaching the DNA within the nucleus. In addition, melanin and its hormonal pathways has a wider role in modulating inflammation within the skin (Eves et al 2006). The amount of melanin produced across various races is roughly equal; however, in darker skins the melanin granules are much more dense and less susceptible to degradation as they ascend through the epidermis.

Merkel's cells are specialised nerve endings of unknown origin, possibly a modified keratinocyte (McKee 1996) found in the basal layer. Their function is thought to be the perception of light touch. They are typically only found in specific regions of the skin, being numerous on the volar (pulp) surfaces of the fingers and toes, in the nail beds and the dorsum of the foot.

Prickle cell layer (stratum spinosum)

The new cells generated by the active basal layer pass into the stratum spinosum. Here they become more polyhedral in shape. Internally, large numbers of keratin filaments (tonofilaments) surround the nucleus, whereas externally the cells have abundant spinous processes. These are desmosomes, bonding adjacent cells together, and are an important component of the epidermis, as they resist mechanical stress. In the upper part of this layer are the first lamellar granules. These secretory organelles contain many substances such as glycoproteins, phospholipids, sterols and lipases. The granules are responsible for the barrier function found higher in the epidermis (Ishida-Yamamoto et al 2007).

Langerhans' cells make up about 8% of the epidermis and are particularly found in the stratum spinosum. They are derived from bone marrow and are dendritic in structure, forming no apposition with the cells around them. Functionally, these cells are outposts of the immune system in the epidermis, recognising and presenting antigens to sensitised T lymphocytes and they have an important role in hypersensitivity and allergic reactions. Patients with specific skin diseases may have reduced numbers of Langerhans' cells.

Granular layer (stratum granulosum)

By the time the ascending cells have reached the granular layer they are much more flattened in appearance and are packed with keratohyalin granules. These granules are primarily composed of proteins and various types of keratins. As the cells move up towards the next layer of the epidermis the lamellar granules migrate to and fuse with the cell membrane, expelling their contents into the intercellular space. The ejected lipid material is then organised into sheets at the junction with the stratum corneum. This forms a hydrophobic barrier (an almost watertight seal) along the junction of the two layers. In eczematous plaques, this process of extrusion is often reduced, leading to increased water loss through the epidermis and resultant fissuring (Cork 1997).

Horny layer (stratum corneum)

As the cell becomes cornified it loses a percentage of its water content and has a very flattened appearance with around 15–20 layers of keratinocytes. The remaining intracellular water accumulates, acting as a plasticiser with intracellular keratin, and causes the cell to swell. This improves the barrier seal to the epidermis and prevents fissuring of the skin under normal tensile forces (Cork 1997). Cells at this level begin the little understood pre-programmed cell death with most of the intracellular material undergoing breakdown, leaving just the keratin and protein matrix within these now cornified cells.

Remnants of organelles and melanin pigment may be present within the stratum corneum. Normally, cells in this layer have lost their nucleus, but it may remain in incompletely keratinised cells (parakeratosis). The deeper cells in this layer are densely packed and so this area is often referred to as the stratum compactum (originally called the stratum lucidum).

As cells ascend the stratum they continue to change. Modifications to the lipid membranes of the keratinocytes reduce adhesion, and so cells become less densely packed. There is also degradation of desmosomes, which further weakens cellular adhesions until the cells ascend to a level where desquamation is likely – the stratum disjunctum.

The skin as a barrier

The whole process of cell generation, maturation and degradation strives to create an effective barrier from water loss and from invading organisms, allergens or irritants. Many mechanisms are in place to help fulfil this function. However, the main threats to this barrier include trauma (scratching, etc.), desiccation and hydration. Drying of the epidermis, central to many skin diseases, causes keratinocytes to shrivel and lose apposition, leading to fissuring, while excessive hydration strips the lipid barrier from the epidermis.

Control of the keratinisation process

The epidermis can be considered an active organ, constantly generating keratinocytes in the basal layer which, in a period of 28–70 days, ascend through the superior layers, and undergo a cycle of maturation, keratinisation and desquamation. Regulation of this process is complex, but local factors within the epidermis, dermis and other tissues can modulate the rate of proliferation (e.g. inflammatory mediators in the dermis, tissue growth factors, fibroblasts, vitamin A derivatives). Disease processes may also disturb the normal equilibrium. Psoriasis often accelerates epidermal transit time to as little as 5 days, whereas skin carcinomas may trigger an uncontrolled proliferation of cell growth within the epidermis.

Dermo-epidermal junction

The dermo-epidermal junction (DEJ) is the point at which the dermis meets the epidermis. The DEJ is a basement membrane divided into a number of layers, crossed by a complex of filaments, keratins and proteins that form an anchoring surface between the dermis and epidermis. In areas of greater mechanical stress, to enhance adhesion the dermis makes regular finger-like folds into the overlying epidermis, known as dermal papillae. These are complemented by protrusions from the epidermis into the dermis, known as rete pegs or epidermal ridges. This undulation serves to increase the surface area of attachment and is a major feature of the plantar surface of the foot, where mechanical stresses can be high. Pathologically, the DEJ is the site of many pathologies and this can lead to loss of adhesion and the development of blistering diseases (e.g. epidermolysis bullosa, dermatitis herpetiformis).

Dermis

Below the dermo-epidermal junction lies the dermis. This consists essentially of dense fibroelastic connective tissues in a gel-like base (ground substance) which contains glycosaminoglycans. Collagen strands provide tensile strength, with elasticity afforded by interwoven elastic fibres that make this a pliable tissue. Accommodated within the dermis are the skin appendages, macrophages, fibroblasts and the neurovascular network.

The thin, upper layer or papillary dermis contains most of the blood and lymphatic vessels, whereas the less vascular, deep reticular layer, is much more dense with collagen and elastic fibres. Cells of the immune system, i.e. T lymphocytes and mast cells, are present in the dermis.

Subcutaneous layer

The dermis is separated from the fascia by the subcutaneous (fat) layer. This is a layer of fat cells rich in nerves, blood vessels and lymphatics. Its main function is to provide thermal insulation and physical protection. To this end, it is well developed across the plantar surface, particularly across the metatarsal heads and heels where it may be up to 18 mm thick. Attached to the underlying fascia, plantar fat is divided into vertical chambers by dividing fibrous septae, which act as an effective shock absorption system.

Blood supply and lymphatics

The main blood supply to the skin arises from a network (or plexus) of vessels located in the subcutaneous layer. At this lowest level, branches supply eccrine sweat glands located deep in the reticular dermis. Vessels ascend and fan out to form a second plexus in the mid-dermis. Arterioles from this level supply hair follicles and their associated structures. Other vessels ascend further to form a third plexus in the papillary dermis.

From the papillary plexus, single capillaries loop upwards into the dermal papillae. These tiny vessels loop and descend to drain into venules within the papillary plexus and then descend further into the deeper dermis, eventually reconnecting with the subcutaneous blood vessels. Within the foot, the sole contains the most densely organised network of capillaries in the skin (Pasyk et al 1989), which correlates well with the thickness of the overlying epidermis. It has no thermoregulatory role.

Lymph vessels are found throughout the dermis. Within the papillary dermis, highly distensible lymphatic end bulbs drain intercellular fluids and smaller particles. These empty into larger vessels, which descend to the lymphatics in the subcutaneous layer. Ryan (1995) suggests that their function is key to maintaining turgidity, which is vital to retain mechanical resilience in the skin, requiring a fine balance between supply and drainage, as dehydration and oedema can lead to a reduction in skin stiffness and deformation in the structure of collagen and elastic fibres.

Skin appendages

Hair follicles and sebaceous glands

Hair follicles and their associated sebaceous glands are found on the lower limb, sparing the plantar surface. Compared with sebaceous glands in other areas of the skin (i.e. face, chest), these glands are relatively inactive.

Sweat glands

Sweat glands exist in two forms. The larger apocrine glands are exclusively associated with the hair follicle in the groin and axillae, whereas the smaller eccrine gland is a simple coiled structure located in the reticular dermis with an opening directly onto the epidermis. Stimulated primarily by the sympathetic branch of the autonomic system, sweat glands are an important mechanism for thermoregulation, mainly above waist level (Ryan 1995). They are most numerous on the palms and soles. Under normal circumstances a small, steady flow of sweat is produced, which is thought to aid grip. This function is further enhanced on the palms and soles by the presence of dermatoglyphics. These skin creases, present at birth, are a result of the unique arrangement of collagen fibres in the dermis and are more prominent on the weightbearing surfaces of the foot (pulp of the toes, heel and metatarsal area) and palmar area (fingerprints). Not only do they act like the tread on a tyre in conjunction with the small amounts of sweat, but within these areas, there is a dense and highly organised neural network in the underlying dermis (Montagna 1960) which provides a rich tactile perception necessary to protect the integrity of the foot.

History and examination of the skin

Dermatological assessment consists of three parts:

- history taking
- clinical examination
- common investigations and tests.

It is often tempting when assessing the skin to leap straight to examination without resorting to the standard clinical practice of history taking followed by examination. Although this approach may give a correct diagnosis in experienced hands, often, to those new to dermatology, this will lead to an incorrect or incomplete conclusion. However, a brief initial examination may help to direct questioning for the history.

History taking

Ideally, conduct the consultation in a private environment, with sufficient time to allow the patient to talk freely. You should expect to spend most of the consultation listening, only using questions to direct the history. It is important to ask patients what they think is the cause of the problem, as they are often correct. Starting the consultation by asking: 'How may I help you?' or 'Tell me about your problem' is beneficial. It lets patients know that they may talk and that there is willingness to listen, thus setting them at ease. However, certain facts are necessary to make a diagnosis and, if these are not offered, they should be asked for directly.

Duration of the problem

The duration of a disease is essential to know. Whether the disease is constant, deteriorating or fluctuating or whether there are periods of relapse and remission is useful. Acute or self-limiting conditions are usually inflammatory or infective (i.e. fungal infections), whereas chronic or progressive symptoms may be an indication of a more serious disease. Stressful events may give a remitting and relapsing pattern, particularly with psoriasis, eczema and lichen planus.

Relieving or exacerbating factors

Ask the patient if anything helps the problem or makes it worse. Many conditions improve in sunlight, for example psoriasis, whereas others are made worse, for example lupus erythematosus.

Relationships to physical agents

Find out whether light, heat or cold plays a part in the problem. Is the problem associated with any particular activity? Has injury played a part in the problem? Has there been exposure to chemical or plant material?

Treatment

This is one of the most essential questions. Alongside their usual medications, often patients will have tried to treat the problem themselves and will have bought over-the-counter medications, preparations from health shops or perhaps borrowed a prescribed medication from a friend or family member. They may also have tried cosmetic preparations that they do not consider relevant. It is often helpful to ask them to bring in everything they put on the skin. In some instances the true appearance of the skin lesion may be altered or masked by previously applied medicaments. For example, a steroid cream applied to a fungal infection will dramatically increase the spread of the eruption.

Past medical history

It is important to elicit any history of skin diseases, in particular psoriasis, eczema and skin cancer; all these conditions are pertinent to the lower leg and foot. Other salient conditions include information regarding a history of allergy, through either occupation or domestic exposure (e.g. epoxy resins from work or Elastoplast at home). Internal medical conditions may also be relevant, as many may manifest themselves in the skin. For example, dermatitis herpetiformis is a blistering disorder that is commonly associated with coeliac disease, a gluten intolerance affecting the gut.

Occupation

Many occupations expose the skin to irritants and allergens. A patient may need to wear a particular garment or item of footwear as part of their job and that may be causing the problem. It may be that other members of the workforce are similarly affected. Outdoor workers or workers who are exposed to wet or cold will also have problems particular to them;

for instance, skin cancer is higher in those with outdoor occupations.

Social history

It is useful to know who is at home with the patient as they may be able to help with the treatment. Alcohol consumption is relevant to a number of skin conditions, particularly psoriasis. Enquiries about smoking should be made when considering circulatory problems. Smoking can have significant effects on the skin and is associated with hypersensitive corns on the plantar surface.

Family history

A number of skin conditions run in families, for example palmoplantar keratoderma. Recessively inherited diseases may skip generations, so information is required about distant relations too.

Recognising the norm in the assessment of skin is essential. Normal variations are seen due to race and the normal ageing process. Any given population will include a significant range of skin colours. Lesions that appear red or brown on white skin, for example often appear black or purple on pigmented skin and mild redness may be masked completely. In addition, some conditions have a distinct racial predisposition (e.g. melanoma in Caucasians). However, across all races, normal skin will not be different from surrounding skin and will feel smooth.

As the skin ages, it appears more translucent with irregular pigmentation. Thinning of the skin occurs at all levels, including the subcutaneous layer, which may be evident on the plantar area of the foot. Natural turgidity and elasticity seen in younger individuals is lost. Pinching of the skin results in 'tenting', as the skin fails to return to its natural shape. As a result of decreased sweat and sebum production, the normal skin surface barrier is compromised and so is more prone to the effects of drying and irritation. A reduced immune response as the numbers of lymphocytes and Langerhans' cells decrease, potentially leaving the skin more open to infection and malignant change. Also, any inflammation that occurs as a result of decreased immune surveillance tends to be dampened down; hence, signs of inflammation may seem less acute. With ageing, the nails may reduce their rate of growth and often become thicker and slightly yellow in colour.

Clinical examination

Clinical examination of the skin uses a variety of senses. Sight is obviously the most important, but touch and smell are also valuable. Many trainees unused to dermatological assessment will shy away from touching the skin. This is clearly a natural reaction, but must be overcome in order to assess the area fully. Observation is an important stage in examination and it is important to follow a particular pattern:

- General distribution (localised, widespread or regional)
- Individual lesion morphology
- Assessment of other structures
- Assessment of the nails
- Assessment of the sweat glands.

General distribution

When a widespread eruption is suspected, it is important to look and ask about all of the skin. Patients may often be reluctant to discuss other areas or simply not connect them to the current condition. For example, scalp psoriasis can mimic dandruff. A patient concerned with scaly plaques on the knees may not connect the two, particularly if they have had dandruff for some time. Many disorders have a typical pattern or predilection for specific sites, although it should be remembered that patterns could occasionally vary from the norm. Eczema has a common pattern – affecting the flexor surfaces of the arms and legs along with the face. Symmetry of the eruption should also be recorded as this usually denotes an endogenous condition. Table 8.2 gives examples of the distribution patterns of various dermatoses.

Table 8.2 Common patterns of skin disorders

Condition	*Typical distribution pattern*
Atopic eczema	Antecubital and popliteal fossa, face, neck, hands
Contact dermatitis	Hands, face, feet
Psoriasis	Extensor surfaces of knees and elbows, scalp, back, nails
Lichen planus	Flexor surfaces of wrist, ankles, oral cavity, genitalia
Erythema nodosum	Anterior surfaces of shins

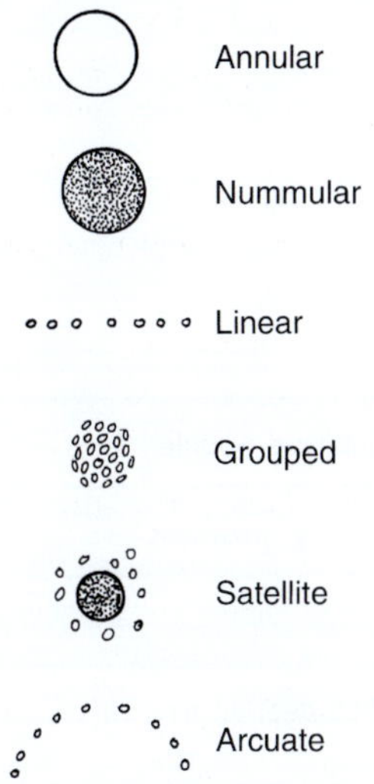

Figure 8.3 The various configurations of lesion patterns.

Individual lesion morphology

Individual lesions should be assessed. A magnifying glass is useful along with good lighting. Initially it is important, if there is more than one lesion, to describe the arrangement (Fig. 8.3). This can include:

- annular (ring-like), e.g. psoriasis, lichen planus, granuloma annulare
- nummular (round, coin-like), e.g. nummular eczema
- discoid (disc-like), e.g. eczema, psoriasis
- reticulate (net-like), i.e. livedo reticularis
- arcuate (curved), e.g. contact dermatitis
- grouped, e.g. insect bites, dermatitis herpetiformis
- Koebner's phenomenon, e.g. warts, psoriasis (Fig. 8.4), lichen planus, molluscum contagiosum.

Note that some disorders may have several configurations. Koebner's phenomenon is when skin lesions of a specific disease appear following trauma at a site which was previously unaffected. The edge of the lesion should also be inspected. Is it discrete or ill-defined? For example, psoriasis and fungal infections have much more marked, well-defined edges than eczema. Surface contour should also be noted (Fig. 8.5).

Colour

To interpret the skin colour of lesions, good lighting is essential, as temperature and dependency will modify appearances. Rashes or lesions that are pink, purple or red will be due to blood. If the blood is within vessels gentle pressure will whiten or blanch the lesions – this is erythema, and can be viewed best through a glass slide or tumbler. If it is not possible to blanch the lesion, this may be due to extravasation (loss of blood constituents into the skin) or pigmentation due to melanin.

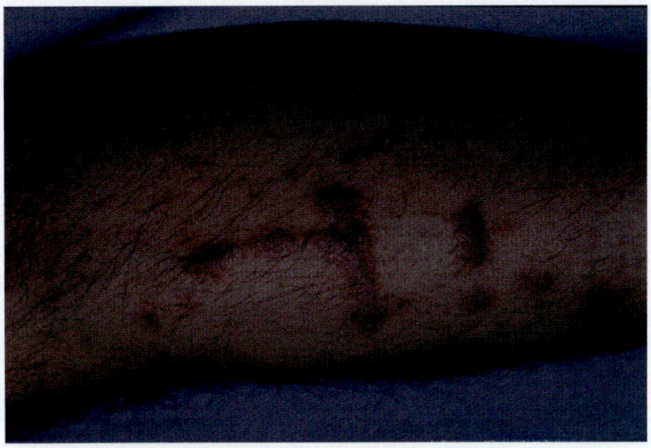

Figure 8.4 Psoriasis.

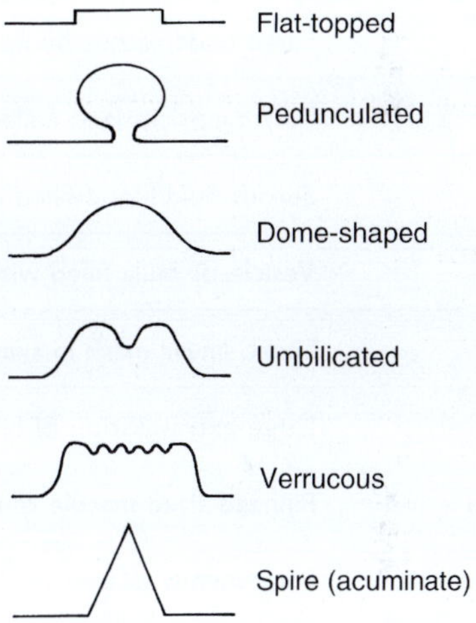

Figure 8.5 The different surface contours of lesions.

Touch

It is possible to determine surface changes in texture and whether the skin disease relates only to the surface of the skin or whether it relates to the structures beneath. Light touch is required to perceive superficial changes (i.e. texture of a surface lesion), whereas progressively deeper pressure will reflect changes to the lower structures in the dermis and

Table 8.3 Primary skin lesions

Term	*Description and example*
Erythema	Redness, often due to inflammatory response
Macule	Flat, differently coloured, e.g. freckles, vitiligo
Papule	Palpable, solid bump in skin, e.g. lichen planus
Nodule	Palpable, deeper mass than a papule, e.g. ganglion, rheumatoid nodule
Plaque	Elevated, disc-shaped area of skin over 1 cm in diameter, e.g. psoriasis
Tumour	Large mass over 2 cm in diameter, e.g. lipoma
Cyst	Subdermal, fluid-filled fibrous swelling, loosely attached to deeper structures, e.g. dermal cyst
Weal	Large oedematous bump, e.g. insect bite
Vesicle	Tiny, pinprick-sized collection of fluid, e.g. mycosis, pompholyx
Bulla	Serous fluid/blood-filled intraepidermal or dermoepidermal sac, e.g. bullous pemphigoid
Pustule	Vesicle or bulla filled with pus, e.g. acne, pustular psoriasis
Burrow	Short, linear mark in skin visible with magnifying lens, e.g. scabies
Ecchymosis	Large extravasation of blood into the tissues, i.e. bruising
Petechia	Pinhead-sized macule caused by blood seeping into skin
Telangiectasia	Permanently dilated small cutaneous blood vessels

subcutaneous layers. Oedema feels flocculent under the fingers. Typical surface changes include a soft moist texture due to excessive sweating or a dry and roughened texture due to a lack of sweating, that is anhidrosis. Deeper lesions may be described as hard, nodular, mobile, soft, etc.

Odour

Skin odour is a neglected aspect of skin examination but is useful. Colonisations of pseudomonas, staphylococcus or diphtheroids have distinctive smells (microbiology may help to confirm this) as do odours associated with excessive sweating (bromhidrosis) and incontinence.

When examining individual lesions, clear descriptions using well-recognised terms are essential. This allows good communication between health professionals. In dermatology, there are many descriptive terms: some obvious, others less so. Familiarity with this terminology will ensure good inter-professional communication. Skin lesions can be classified as primary or secondary. Primary lesions arise due to the initial effects of a condition; secondary lesions evolve from or as a complication of primary lesions. The distinction between primary and secondary is not always clear; some lesions can be classed as primary or secondary (Tables 8.3, 8.4). Some of the more common terms used in assessing the surface of the skin are described below.

Scaly

Normally the skin sheds skin cells individually or in small clumps. This is imperceptible to the eye. If the skin is weathered or diseased, skin shedding becomes abnormal, the clumps of skin become larger and appear as flakes or scales. These scales may be small,

Table 8.4 Secondary skin lesions

Term	*Description and example*
Scale	Flake of skin, e.g. mycosis, psoriasis
Crust	Scab, dried serous exudates, e.g. acute eczema
Excoriation	Scratch marks, e.g. pruritus
Fissure	Crack in dry or moist skin
Necrosis	Non-viable tissue
Ulcer	Loss of epidermis; may extend through the dermis to deeper tissue, e.g. venous ulcer
Scar	Fibrous tissue production post-healing
Keloid	Excessive production of fibrous tissue post-healing
Striae	Lines in skin that do not have normal skin tone, e.g. striae tensa in pregnancy, Cushing's disease
Purpura	Purplish lesions which do not blanche under pressure, e.g. vitamin C deficiency
Urticaria	'Nettle rash', e.g. drug eruption, allergy, heat
Lichenification	Patchy 'toughening' of skin, e.g. chronic eczema
Haematoma	Blood-filled blister
Sinus	Channel that allows the escape of pus or fluid from tissues

as in the dryness (xerosis) of atopic eczema, or large, as in ichthyosis. Scratching the surface of skin is helpful as it accentuates scaling and may help with diagnosis. Psoriasis will demonstrate pinpoint bleeding when scratched and the scaling will become more pronounced (Auspitz's sign).

Crusting and exudation

When the skin is injured or infected, it bleeds, oozes serum or discharges pus. This is an exudate; it dries to form a crust, which is distinguished from scale by clinical appearance and history. While avoiding hurting the patient, try to remove the crust as this often obscures the true pathology. Crusting is a common feature in eczema.

Hyperkeratosis and lichenification

If keratin is abnormal, it forms thickened areas as shedding fails. These can be localised, appearing as horns on the skin and usually reflect a viral or neoplastic process. Sometimes the surface can be papillomatous (warty). The areas of thickening can be more diffuse, e.g. chronic plantar eczema or corns. Such areas are less flexible and will often crack, forming deep fissures. Lichenification is a reaction of the skin to chronic rubbing or scratching and involves the whole epidermis. The affected area of skin thickens and the skin markings become more pronounced. It is a common feature of atopic eczema and usually occurs on the flexures.

Excoriations, erosions and ulcers

Excoriation means scratch and is usually a feature of itching or, less commonly, pain. It may represent underlying skin pathology such as scabies or eczema or indicate disease elsewhere, e.g. renal or hepatic failure. Erosions are partial-thickness breaks in the surface of the skin caused by physical injury including excoriation or where blisters have broken. An ulcer is an area of full-thickness skin loss, usually covered by exudate or crust.

Atrophic

The surface of the skin is depressed and blood vessels are visible beneath. It may be due to atrophy of the epidermis or dermis. The skin is often pale and wrinkled.

Macules and patches

These are localised impalpable areas of colour change: macules are less than 1 cm in diameter and patches are greater than 1 cm.

Papules, plaques and nodules

A papule is any lesion less than 1 cm in diameter that rises above the surface of the skin. A nodule is larger than 1 cm in diameter, but otherwise similar to a papule, and usually due to pathology within the dermis. A plaque is a raised lesion that is wider than it is thick and often represents epidermal pathology.

Vesicles, bullae, pustules and abscesses

Small blisters less than 1 cm are called vesicles. Blisters larger than 1 cm are called bullae. Pus-filled vesicles or bullae are pustules, large pustules are abscesses.

Weal

These are transient papular or plaque-like swellings of the skin due to dermal oedema and frequently seen in urticaria.

Scars

These can be macules, papules or plaques and are a feature of repair following dermal injury. A glossary of terms can be found in Tables 8.3 and 8.4.

Assessment of other structures

When examining the skin, other structures such as the nails, hair and mucous membranes may add clues to the diagnosis. For example, lichen planus commonly causes lesions in the mouth; this may be an important finding in differentially diagnosing it from other conditions such as eczema and psoriasis. Palpation of the lymph nodes is important in patients with suspected skin malignancy.

Assessment of the nail

The nails should be inspected as part of the main dermatological assessment. The nail has evolved as a rigid structure to improve dexterity but in the foot the nail is purely a protective plate overlying the deeper structures and acting as a counter pressure to the volar tissues (Baran et al 2003). The nail unit (Fig. 8.6) is well provided with a rich neurovascular supply and, as a result, is sensitive to internal changes, often manifesting these subtle changes in the nail structure. External factors too, such as trauma, can modify nail shape. Therefore, a proper footwear assessment should be undertaken, to complete the clinical picture, when looking for reasons for changes in nail shape, colour, etc. A glossary of the main terms used to describe nail changes can be found in Table 8.5.

Key aspects of examination include assessment of the following factors.

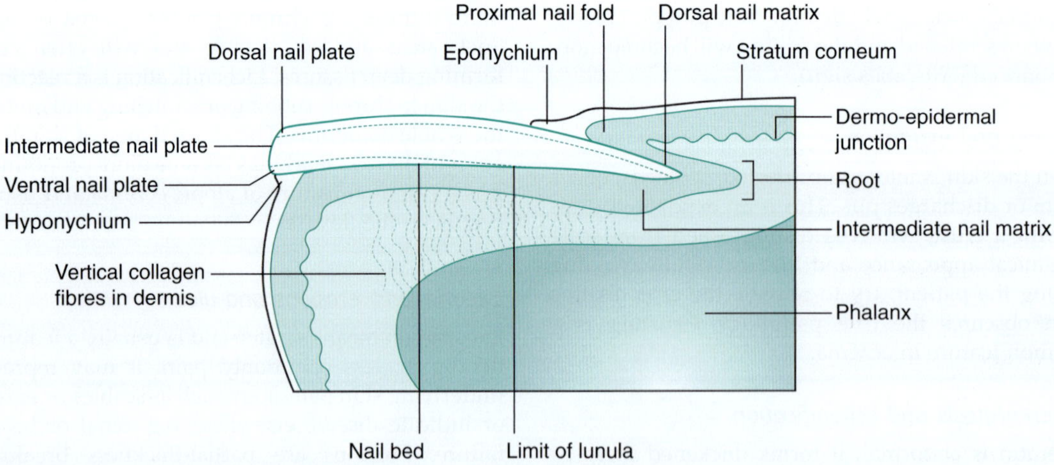

Figure 8.6 Structure and anatomy of the nail.

Table 8.5 Glossary of nail conditions

Condition	*Definition*
Onychauxis	Thickening of the nail plate, usually due to trauma
Onychogryphosis	Thickened nail with a distortion in the direction of growth
Onycholysis	Separation of the nail from the nail bed, distal to proximal
Onychomadesis	Separation of the nail from the nail bed, proximal to distal
Onychocryptosis	Ingrowing toe nail
Involution	An inward curvature of the lateral or medial edges of the nail plate, towards the nail bed
Splinter haemorrhage	Longitudinal, plum-coloured linear haemorrhages (around 2 mm in length) under the nail plate
Paronychia	Inflammation of the tissues surrounding the nails
Onychomycosis	Fungal infection of the nail plate
Chromonychia	Abnormal coloration of the nail tissue
Koilonychia	Transverse and longitudinal concave nail dystrophy which gives a spoon-shaped appearance
Clubbing	Increased longitudinal curvature of the nail plate with enlargement of the pulp of the digit
Beau's lines	Transverse ridging of the nail plate seen as the result of a temporary cessation of nail growth

Pattern of affected nails

It is important to always assess finger nails as well as toe nails and note any findings. Often finger nails may show changes more readily (i.e. clubbing). Where only one or two nails are affected, or one foot, local causes should be suspected, whereas nail changes in all digits in both feet and hands suggests a systemic or internal cause. On the foot, the length or the position of the toes may give clues to local nail abnormalities. Typically, the longest toe may show nail changes as a result of interaction with footwear.

Rate of nail growth

There is great variation between individuals in the rate of nail growth. The average rate for a finger nail is 0.1 mm/day (or 3 mm/month), whereas toe nails grow at a half to a third of this rate (Zaias 1980). Consequently, a normal finger nail will grow completely in about 6 months, whereas a toe nail will take 12–18 months. Such information is useful to determine the approximate time of events, for example the time of trauma to a nail, the likely clearance time of a haematoma. Most systemic disorders lead to a decline in the rate of nail growth but a few may have the opposite effect (psoriasis, hyperthyroidism, nail trauma and drugs).

Shape of the nail plate

The breadth of the nail matrix and length of the nail bed normally dictate the shape of the nail plate (finger nails being rectangular and toe nails, quadrangular). The contour of the underlying phalanx, and toe position, may modify this. The most commonly occurring nail shape alteration in the toe nail is transverse over-curvature or involution (pincer

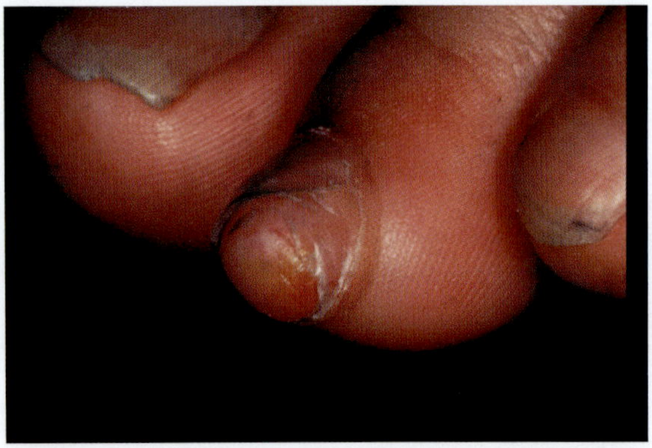

Figure 8.7 Subungual exostosis affecting the second toe.

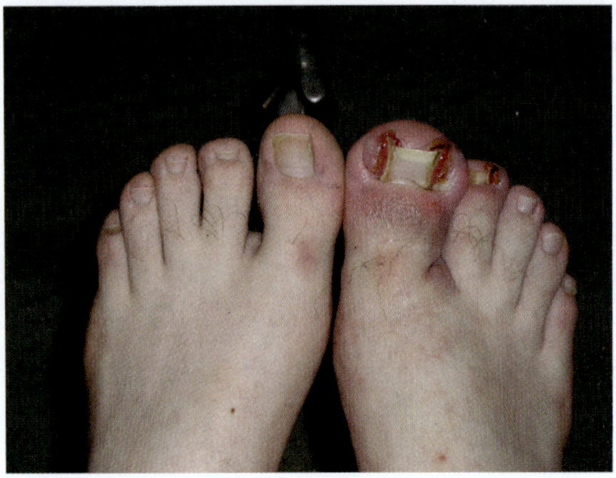

Figure 8.8 Onychocryptosis.

nail). This is typically seen in the nail plate of the hallux and is often accompanied by pain when direct pressure is applied to the nail. If there is an underlying subungual exostosis (Fig. 8.7), lifting of the distal nail plate occurs, often accompanied by pain. Frequently seen in young adults, a lateral X-ray will differentiate between this and other causes of painful nails such as onychocryptosis (Fig. 8.8) or abnormal involution of the nail plate sometimes referred to as pincer nail (Fig. 8.9). Internal causes of nail shape alterations include koilonychia (spooning) and clubbing, and their causes are listed in Table 8.6.

Colour of the nail plate and bed

Changes in nail colour (chromonychia) may arise as a result of external or internal factors. Finger nails, in particular, are vulnerable to occupational causes such as chemical agents. Colour change can occur on the surface of the nail, within the nail plate itself or below in the underlying nail bed or lunula. A powerful pen torch or laser pointer shone in the pulp of the digit, through the nail plate, can help to isolate the source. Table 8.7 lists the more common causes of chromonychia. Splinter haemorrhages are plum-coloured streaks of about 3–4 mm seen running longitudinally under the nail plate. These are the result of extravasation of blood between the nail bed and plate. Typically they are caused by trauma, though, if the majority of nails are affected, disorders such as rheumatoid disease, vasculitis or skin diseases (psoriasis and eczema) should be suspected.

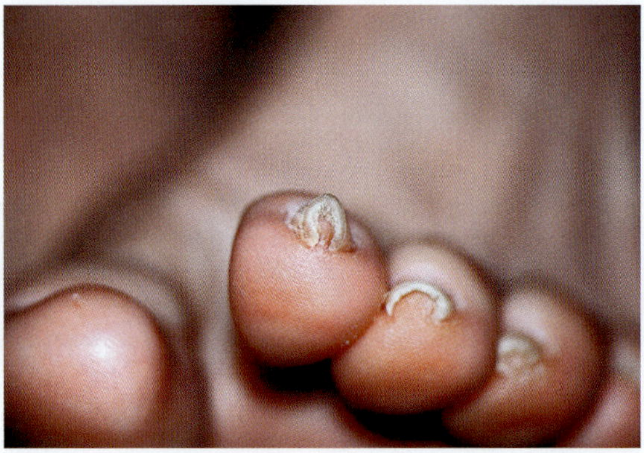

Figure 8.9 Pincer nail.

Surface texture

The surface of the nail is normally smooth but changes may occur. Subtle longitudinal lines may arise with age or as a result of minor trauma, although specific diseases may accentuate their appearance (rheumatoid arthritis, peripheral vascular disease and lichen planus). Solitary lines or ridges may signify a tumour within the matrix or be the result of a previous paronychial infection. Transverse lines are common in the hallux as a result of repeated minor trauma from footwear. When transverse lines affect the majority of nails simultaneously they are known as Beau's lines and may represent a sudden period of illness. By noting their distance from the cuticle, a rough calculation can be made as to the time of the illness. Pits are small erosions in the nail found on the surface of the nail plate. When only a few nails are affected it is considered a variant of normal but multiple nail involvement is seen in a number of skin diseases such as psoriasis, lichen planus, eczema and alopecia.

Table 8.6 Causes of nail spooning and clubbing

Koilonychia (spooning)	*Clubbing*
Idiopathic	Idiopathic
Hereditary	Hereditary
Iron deficiency anaemias Insulin-dependent diabetes Physiologically thin nails Psoriasis	Lung disease: bronchiectasis lung cancers abscess lung infections fibrotic lung disease emphysema asthma in childhood
Alopecia Lichen planus Raynaud's disease	Cardiovascular disease: congestive heart failure subacute bacterial endocarditis myxoid tumours congenital heart disease
Scleroderma/systemic sclerosis Renal transplant Thyroid disease	Alimentary disease: ulcerative colitis Crohn's disease gut cancers
Acromegaly Occupational (immersion in oils, acid and alkali)	Endocrine: active hepatitis auto-immune thyroiditis acromegaly Other: polycythaemia cirrhosis malnutrition

Loosening or shedding of the nails

Onycholysis is the detachment of the nail from the bed in a distal to proximal fashion, whereas onychomadesis occurs in the opposite direction. The aetiology for both conditions is similar (Table 8.8), but it is most frequently the result of trauma, particularly overzealous nail care or fungal infection. The loosened area is usually white, although in some disorders the area may adopt a different colour. Onychomadesis is the less common of the two conditions. Proximal detachment occurs most frequently due to acute bacterial infection of the proximal nail fold or an acute skin eruption affecting the nail bed such as a blister or psoriatic plaque.

Nail thickness

Thickening of the nail (onychauxis) is probably the most commonly observed toe nail condition. Long-term trauma to the nail plate can lead to hypertrophy of the nail, often with a brown discoloration. Typically, the condition affects the hallux or longest toe as a result of footwear interaction. Other conditions such as fungal infections, psoriasis and lichen planus may also lead to onychauxis. Onychogryphosis is a more severe thickening of the nail plate often with gross deformity and a deviation in the direction of nail growth. Pachyonychia congenita is a rare inherited disorder hallmarked by congenital thickening of the nail plate.

Table 8.7 Causes of nail discoloration (chromonychia)

Discoloration	*Cause*
Nail bed	
Brown	Idiopathic, subungual wart
White	Anaemia, cirrhosis, renal disease
Green	Pseudomonas infection, blistering diseases
Yellow	Subungual corn, wart or exostosis, jaundice
Brown/black	Haematoma
Lunula	
Red	Congestive heart failure, alopecia
Brown/black	Haematoma, melanoma, melanonychia
Nail plate	
White	Onychomycosis, trauma, onycholysis
Yellow	Nicotine or urine staining, yellow nail syndrome, jaundice
Brown	Mycotic infection, onychauxis, onychogryphosis, shoes dyes, melanoma

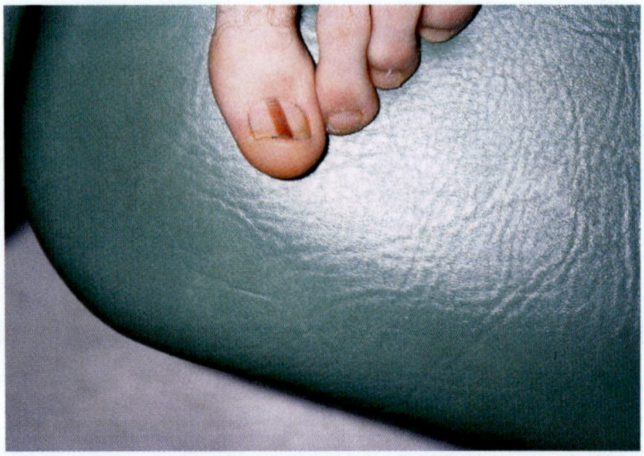

Figure 8.10 Melanonychia.

Periungual changes

The periungual tissues seal the nail unit from damage but may show disease themselves. These tissues may be breached by inappropriate nail care or prolonged immersion, for example in water and chemicals, leading to infection or chemical irritation and thus paronychia. Acute paronychia is more commonly

Table 8.8 Causes of nail shedding

Level of separation	*Cause*
Onycholysis	Trauma (nail surgery, nail picking) Peripheral vascular disease Psoriasis Rheumatoid arthritis Subungual tumours Eczema
Onychomadesis	Nail matrix infection or inflammation Subungual blistering Drugs

associated with infection (Fig. 8.11), whereas the chronic variety is often confined to the hands, most often as a result of irritant reactions. Other periungual conditions include tumours:

- Periungual warts (Fig. 8.12) – usually asymptomatic, easily diagnosed by their appearance.
- Corns/callus – found within the nail sulci – may lead to pain on compression of the nail plate. Nail edges may be thickened or involuted.
- Subungual exostosis – diagnosed by X-ray, may lead to lifting of the nail plate.
- Fibromas – associated with tuberous sclerosis.
- Malignant tumours – basal cell carcinoma, squamous cell carcinoma, subungual melanoma.
- Glomus tumours (Fig. 8.13) – cause extreme pain when exposed to slight trauma or changes in temperature, often visible by digital illumination.

Assessment of the sweat glands

Eccrine sweat glands are particularly numerous across the palms and soles. Normally these sweat glands play no part in thermoregulation; their activity is increased during mental stress and anxiety. When assessing sweat gland function, excessive local sweating usually has a local cause, whereas generalised sweating may have a more systemic cause. The two most common disorders are:

- anhidrosis – a lack of sweating
- hyperhidrosis – excessive sweat production.

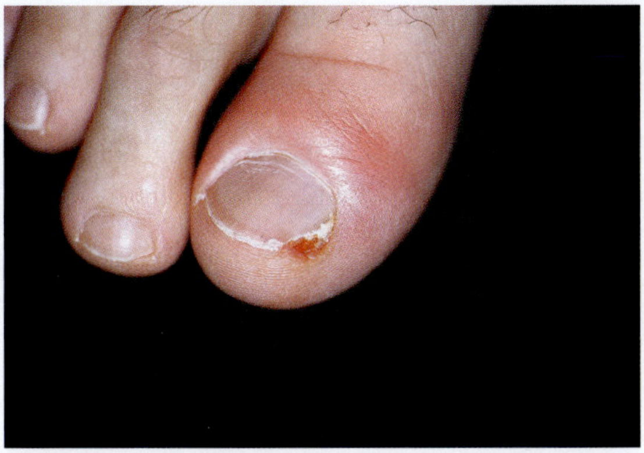

Figure 8.11 Paronychia.

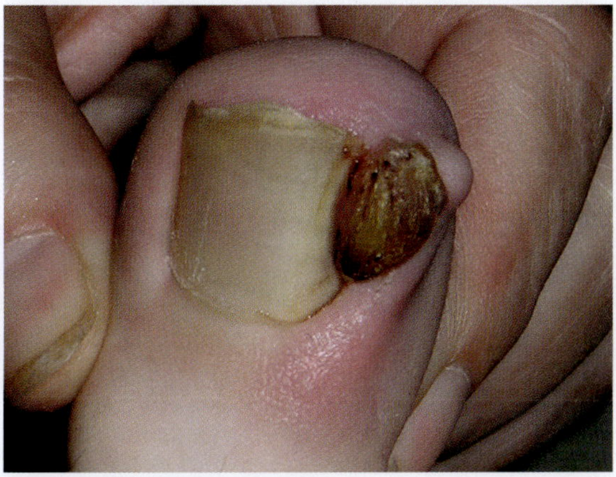

Figure 8.12 Periungual wart.

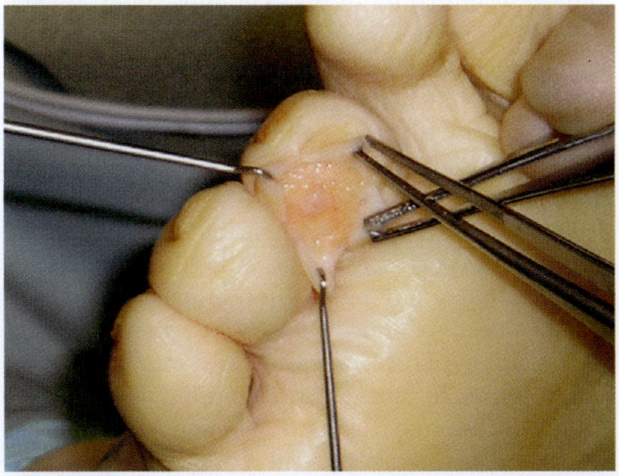

Figure 8.13 Glomus tumour (exposed during surgical excision).

The causes of each of these conditions are summarised in Table 8.9. When assessing sweating disorders it is pertinent to look for associated symptoms, for example concurrent tachycardia in the absence of

Table 8.9 Causes of sweating disorders

Cause	*Examples*
Anhidrosis	
Ageing	Sweat production decreases with age
Damage to neurological pathways	Autonomic neuropathy Diabetes mellitus Leprosy CNS disorders
Displacement of sweat ducts	
Dermatological lesions	Eczematous or psoriatic plaques Lichen planus Miliaria Lack or loss of sweat glands Damage/scarring to areas of skin Congenital lack of sweat glands (ectodermal dysplasia)
Hyperhidrosis	
Physiological	Normal in young adults Exercise Over-clothing or occlusive footwear Emotions or stress
Endocrine disorders	Hypoglycaemia Hyperthyroidism Acromegaly
Dermatological	Associated with palmoplantar keratoderma
Other	Drugs CNS disorders Cardiovascular disorders Respiratory failure Tumours

a fever may suggest thyrotoxicosis. An elevated temperature and lymphadenopathy may indicate infection.

Hyperhidrosis

When symmetrical, this condition is most commonly associated with young active individuals: it is usually physiological rather than pathological, with resolution occurring in the third decade. Sweat production may increase to such an extent that the skin becomes overhydrated and macerated, particularly if footwear/hosiery is occlusive. Moist fissures may develop, mostly interdigitally, along with blistering of the soles. At this stage secondary bacterial or fungal infection can occur, generating an unpleasant odour and even a brown discoloration to the skin (bromhidrosis).

Anhidrosis

Anhidrosis should be considered as a condition normally associated with ageing. In severe cases cracking and fissuring of the epidermis may occur, particularly around the heel. Deep fissuring may develop into the dermis with subsequent recurrent bleeding, a common feature with eczema.

Common tests and investigations

- Fungal assessment and other microbiology
- Histological assessment
- Patch testing.

Fungal assessment and other microbiology

Fungi thrive in the environmental conditions provided by the foot and are a major contributor to both primary and secondary disease. It is essential to have a high index of suspicion in any disease of the foot, particularly those that are scaly or blistering. Wood's light and mycology are the main methods of assessment in fungal disease.

Wood's light

This is filtered ultraviolet light, excluding the visible spectrum. Some fungi within the skin will fluoresce under Wood's light thus revealing subclinical infection and helping with diagnosis, but the fluorescence is not bright, so good blackout facilities are essential. Microsporum species are the main types detectable by this method (fluorescing green), but other pathogens also fluoresce, notably erythrasma (caused by *Propionibacterium minutissimum* and fluorescing coral pink).

Mycology

Fungal disease usually affects the most superficial aspects of the skin and so is easy to remove for assessment by scraping. A 15 blade is ideal to do this. After carefully scraping across the skin, the scale is collected either on a glass slide or onto a small piece of black paper. Where possible, if blisters are present, the whole roof should be removed. The undersurface of the blister is then scraped to remove the fungal debris onto a glass slide; the remaining skin is sent for culture. With nails, a clipping from the most proximal part of the affected nail is useful, along with any subungual debris. Potassium hydroxide (20%) when applied to the sample on the glass slide will render the sample transparent after 20 minutes or so, thus revealing the underlying fungal elements. The scrapings are then sent for expert examination and culture, after placing the sample onto folded black card. More than sufficient scrapings should be sent whenever possible to ensure a representative result.

Bacterial and viral culture

Infection with bacteria should be considered wherever inflammation or pus is present. A swab is taken by rubbing it onto the affected area; if the lesion is a blister or pustule, the surface should be broken first with a sterile needle. The swab is moistened with some of the culture medium when assessing dry lesions. Biopsy tissue can also be cultured. It is important that this does not dry out, so it is sent either in sterile water or within the culture medium of a swab. Viral specimens need a viral transport medium. Contact the microbiology lab before taking the sample, as some labs will take the specimens themselves.

Histological assessment

Clinical examination of the skin only allows a view of the surface morphology, whereas histopathology is an easy and valuable adjunct whenever diagnosis is in doubt. Under local anaesthesia, small suspicious lesions are usually excised in their entirety, whereas larger lesions need to have a carefully placed sample taken that includes both normal and abnormal skin. It is good practice to refer suspicious pigmented lesions for expert assessment rather than biopsy.

The three main biopsy techniques are punch, shave and ellipse. Punch biopsies are a simple method of obtaining tissue for histology which does not require much technical skill. The punch is similar to an apple core and comes in a range of sizes from 2 mm to 7 mm diameter. The punch will penetrate the skin to a maximum depth of 7 mm or 8 mm and so is useful for epidermal and superficial dermal pathology. Shave biopsies are a simple method of getting biopsy specimens, effective for assessing superficial skin disease using a razor or scalpel blade. Ellipse biopsy is useful for the removal of small lesions and for larger areas.

Patch testing

Allergic contact dermatitis is a common problem on the lower leg, particularly associated with footwear, medicated dressing and topical therapies. Patch testing assesses this by applying possible allergens to aluminium discs, which are placed onto the skin of the back and left in place for 48 hours. The discs are removed and the skin is assessed on the day and 2 days later. Positive reactions appear as red raised areas within the discs; sometimes the reactions can be very strong, resulting in erosions and blisters.

Recording of the assessment

At the end of the skin assessment it is important to ensure accurate recording of the history and examination to:

- ensure good record keeping
- act as a baseline, in case of any changes in the progression of a condition
- facilitate good communication with other medical professionals.

The use of colour photography and video equipment may also add objective, recorded evidence and allow the patient with poor mobility/eyesight to visualise and appreciate their skin problem.

Hyperkeratotic disorders

Hyperkeratosis is the term used to describe a thickening of the stratum corneum. In the foot, the most common causes are the mechanical forces of pressure, shear and friction acting on the epidermis, leading to corns and callus formation. However, other causes include skin diseases such as psoriasis, dermatitis or fungal infections and the less common palmoplantar keratodermas (PPK) (Table 8.10). Rarely, a sudden, acquired onset of symmetrical, plantar hyperkeratosis may indicate an internal malignancy.

Assessment of corns and callus

Corns and callus are a discrete form of hyperkeratosis distinct from the secondary lesions seen with other dermatological disorders. Callus plaques (callosities) are hard, dense, yellowish plaques of hyperkeratotic tissue usually found on the plantar surface of the foot, whereas corns appear as darker, harder, invaginated areas of hyperkeratosis present either alone or within a callus plaque.

Patients with calluses and/or corns complain of a number of symptoms, ranging from cosmetic irritation to severe pain affecting gait. Symptoms include a stabbing pain when walking, which may persist when resting or subside into a dull, soft tissue ache. Callus usually is reported as a stinging, burning sensation, which is worse just after the start of rest and on resuming weightbearing. An illustrative description of callus being like 'walking on stones' may be given. An erythematous 'halo' may be evident around either lesion type.

Calluses and corns appear to form in response to over-prolonged and excess mechanical stresses (such as intermittent pressure, shear and friction) from ground reaction forces on the foot and footwear during gait.

Corns and callus are always found on areas exposed to mechanical stress and often in a pattern which relates to the biomechanics of foot function. The few surveys undertaken into the incidence of callus and corn lesions on the foot are in general accordance as to their epidemiological features (Gillet 1973, Merriman et al 1986, Springett 1993, Whiting 1987). The commonest sites and lesions include (**Fig. 8.14**):

- diffuse callus beneath the third and fourth metatarsal heads
- callus solely beneath the second, first and fifth metatarsal heads
- dorsal corns on the fifth toes followed by the fourth, third and second
- interdigital lesions between the fourth/fifth toes followed by first/second and third/fourth toes.

Sex incidence ratio is between 1:2 and 1:4 male to female, with mode age of symptomatic onset between 40 and 70 years. The incidence decreases with reduced weightbearing and shoe wearing.

The site of the lesion, an indication of its severity, size, texture (hard and glassy or soft), duration and stimulators/exacerbators, for example a particular activity and/or pair of shoes, should be noted, along with colour differences and lesion contours, bulk, depth and width.

It is assumed that the maceration which appears as a milky yellow region under a callus plaque or corn is due to excess trauma and, as a result, water is squeezed from the viable layers of the epidermis into the lower keratinised layers of the stratum corneum. The features of maceration and extravasation may be considered as clinical indicators of marked mechanical stress (Fig. 8.15). Suitable management of these lesions is urgently required to prevent tissue breakdown and ulceration especially in the 'at-risk' foot (see Ch. 18).

Table 8.10 Causes of hyperkeratosis

Cause	*Clinical features*
Familial/inherited	
Palmoplantar keratoderma	Various types exist. Typically inherited forms begin in childhood
Ichthyosis	Many types. Characterised by dry, flaky skin affecting various parts of the body
Darier's disease	Palmoplantar hyperkeratosis may occur; usually lesions are punctate in form
Pachyonychia congenita	A disease characterised by thickened nails. Associated palmoplantar hyperkeratosis may occur
Acquired	
Palmoplantar keratoderma	Usually occurs in patients in their 20, in patterns described above
Keratoderma climactericum	Yellow/brown papules, which then coalesce to form thickened plaques across the soles of menopausal women. Fissuring is common
Reiter's disease	Red hyperkeratotic rash may occur on the soles called 'keratoderma blennorrhagica'. Difficult to distinguish from pustular psoriasis
Chronic dermatitis	Hyperkeratotic lesions may be observed accompanied by fissuring and crusting
Pustular psoriasis	Yellow/brown sterile pustules occur with hyperkeratosis of the palms and soles, typically in older patients
Syphilis	Distinctive copper pink papules may occur on the sole with hyperkeratosis
Lymphoedema	Dirty brown lesions may occur over oedematous areas of the foot and lower leg
Hypothyroidism	A mild hyperkeratosis may occur on the soles but resolves with treatment
Tinea pedis	Hyperkeratosis may occur as part of the eruption

Types of corn

Seed corns

The aetiology of seed corns is not clear. The empirically proposed association with tension stress has neither been proved nor disputed. These lesions appear similar in structure and biochemically to other mechanically induced hyperkeratoses. Unpublished work using high-powered liquid chromatography (HPLC) shows that they are not plugs of cholesterol as previously thought but, in common with other hyperkeratoses, have a high cholesterol content compared with normal plantar skin (O'Halloran 1990). Seed corns tend to occur at the margins of weightbearing areas of the plantar aspect of the foot either singly or as disperse clusters.

Hard corns

A hard corn (Fig. 8.16) appears as a darker patch within the epidermis, often with a callus covering. Texturally it is hard, glassy and dense when touched with a scalpel. When enucleated, a classic corn nucleus appears as a cone, although they may be any shape or multinucleated. Under greater trauma the contents of the papillary capillaries may be extruded into the epidermis as a brown-black stain (extravasation). A corn forming over a bursa may be associated

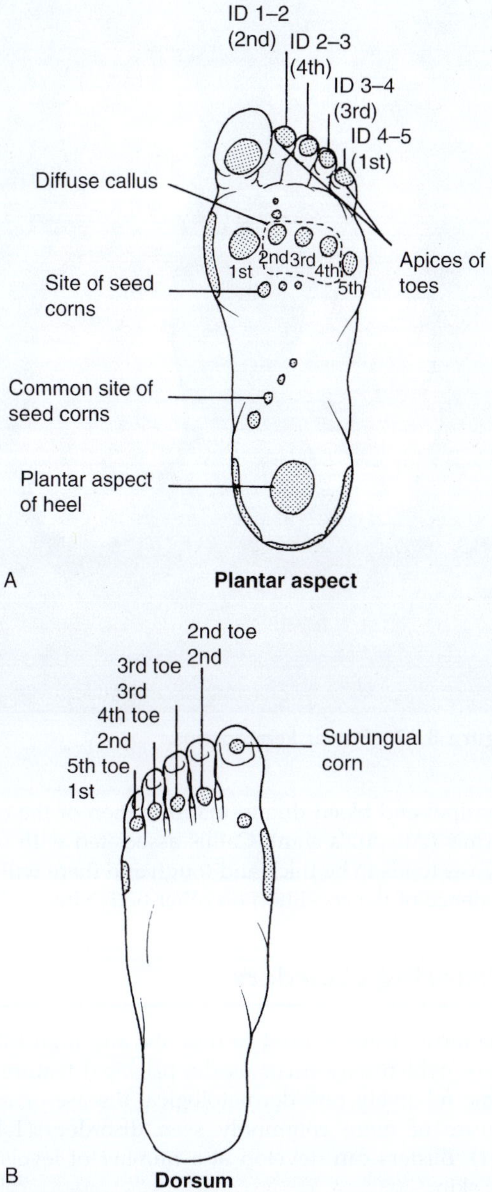

Figure 8.14 The common sites for corns and callus formation on the feet (Merriman et al 1987).

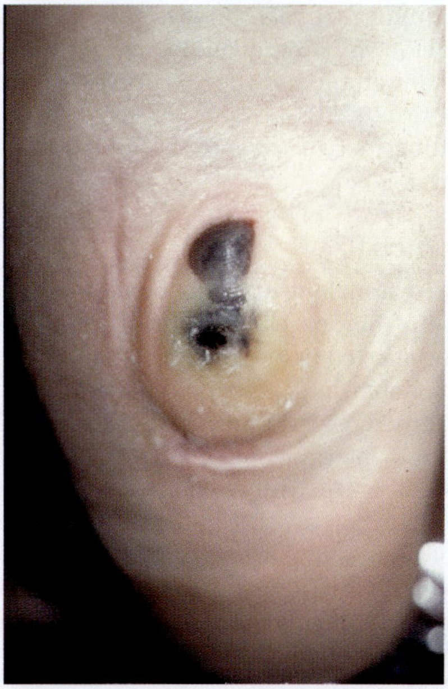

Figure 8.15 Extravasation within callus due to prolonged high pressure.

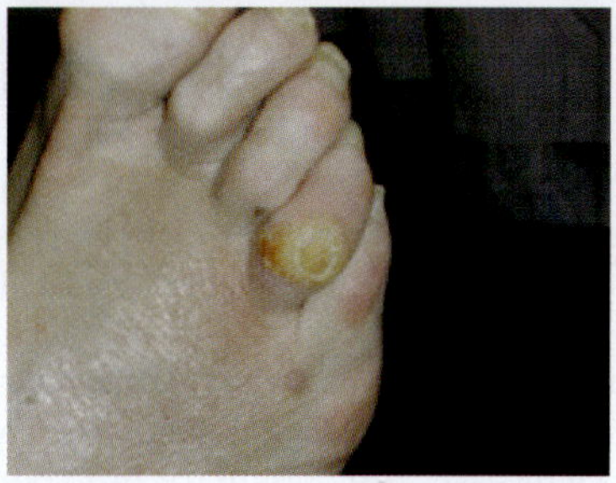

Figure 8.16 Dorsal hard corn.

with the formation of a sinus into the bursal sac; infection may result.

Vascular corns

When the skin is made translucent by application of water, alcohol or oil, clinical signs below the surface of the lesion become apparent. Intrusions of vascularised dermal tissue into the epidermis can be seen in vascular corns and, if cut, this vascular tissue bleeds profusely. These lesions usually occur at sites of excess mechanical stress, may have a relatively long history and may be painful on direct pressure. These features suggest that the lesion is a vascular corn rather than a foreign body or wart. Some practitioners make a distinction between vascular and neurovascular corns; others consider that they are one and the same.

Soft corns

Soft corns occur interdigitally and appear as soft, soggy epidermal masses (macerated tissue) which can easily blunt the scalpel blade. Pain is a frequent complaint. The condition appears to be caused by poorly fitting footwear, disease processes affecting the skeleton, for example rheumatoid arthritis, or biomechanical anomaly, for example excess pronation where the toe tissues are compressed and sheared in ill-fitting footwear, abnormal fourth or fifth ray function.

Fibrous corns

These arise from long-standing corns and involve the presence of fibrous tissue in the dermis below the corn. The affected tissues have an altered biomechanical behaviour: they appear more firmly attached to deeper structures than normal. Shear stresses occur at the tissue interface and, as this tissue cannot dissipate stress as efficiently as normal tissue, there may be a perpetuation of what appears to be chronic irritation of tissues, causing further fibrosis to develop. The precise aetiology of these lesions is not clear, although clinically there is a strong association of these lesions in patients who smoke.

Other causes of hyperkeratosis

The PPK are a complex group of relatively rare disorders which are difficult to classify. Historically, such conditions were named purely on clinical and histological appearance, which has led to a confusing array of nomenclature (Ratnavel & Griffiths 1997). The consistent feature within this group of diseases is hyperkeratosis of the palms and soles. Unlike normal callus, the amount is much increased with a rapid return rate following debridement. Typically, lesions bear no correlation to any weightbearing patterns. Palmar lesions may range from one or two minor patches to complete involvement. The majority of these diseases are hereditary but spontaneous cases can arise. Clinically, PPK may be categorised into one of four distinct patterns of disease:

- Diffuse PPK – diffuse hyperkeratosis across the palms and soles (usually sparing the arch) (Fig. 8.17)
- Focal PPK – discrete patches of hyperkeratosis with normal skin in between
- Punctate PPK – numerous punctate corn-like lesions spread across the palms and soles
- PPK with ectodermal dysplasia – PPK of any variety, with accompanying features of ectodermal abnormalities (e.g. hyperhidrosis, neurological or dental malformations).

Many other skin diseases may lead to the development of hyperkeratosis, which often takes on a different texture from the mechanically induced type. For example, in psoriasis the skin may flake off with

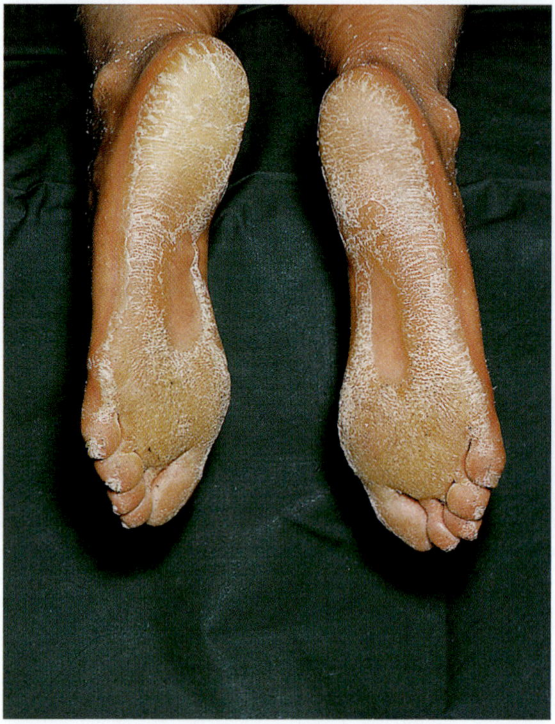

Figure 8.17 Plantar keratoderma.

a scalpel and bleed due to malformation of the epidermis (Auspitz's sign). Callus associated with ichthyosis tends to be thick and tough and there will be evidence of the condition on other body sites.

Blistering disorders

The term blister is used to describe any fluid-filled lesion which may occur as the principal feature of some relatively rare dermatological disease or as a feature of more commonly seen disorders (Table 8.11). Blisters can develop at a number of levels in the skin:

- Superficial – These blisters occur in the stratum corneum and are associated with infections, for example tinea pedis. Superficial blisters are more prone to rupture, leaving open erosions which may be complicated by secondary infection.
- Intraepidermal – These occur in the lower layers of the epidermis, usually the stratum spinosum, and are associated with, for example, acute eczema and viral vesicles.
- Subepidermal – These occur at the DEJ and are associated with, for example, epidermolysis bullosa.

Table 8.11 Main causes of blistering on the lower limb

Disorders with blistering	Disorders where blistering may as the principal feature or as a secondary feature
Epidermolysis bullosa	Friction – most common variety seen on the feet due to pressure and shearing forces
Bullous pemphigoid	Fungal and bacterial infections (e.g. tinea and erysipelas)
Pemphigus	Diabetes – an uncommon complication associated with hyperglycaemia
Dermatitis herpetiformis	Thermal injury (e.g. burns, cryosurgery) Eczema Erythema multiforme Severe sunburn/photosensitivity

Differential diagnosis requires a thorough history and examination (including information on concurrent illness, drug therapies and family history) along with the general pattern and distribution of the disease.

Family history is a key feature in epidermolysis bullosa (EB), an inherited group of disorders where the skin reacts to minor trauma by blistering; hence the feet are commonly involved. The spectrum of the disease ranges from EB simplex (minor blistering of the hands and feet with minimal scarring and little nail involvement) to a potentially lethal recessive dystrophic form (with more widespread blisters and scarring). As the disease is inherited, the onset is usually in childhood. Epidermolysis bullosa acquisita is an acquired form, akin to EB simplex, which usually affects middle-aged patients with a similar pattern.

Pemphigus is a relatively rare blistering disorder seen in middle age. Lesions tend to be intraepidermal (which rupture easily) and have an insidious onset often without a history of trauma. Unlike EB, pemphigus rarely affects the feet but oral lesions may be present. In both conditions, Nikolsky's sign may be present – the ability to raise a blister when firm finger pressure is applied across the affected skin.

Bullous pemphigoid (Fig. 8.18) is distinctive in that it usually affects people over 60 with large tense subepidermal blisters emerging on urticated skin, including the foot. Mucous membrane involvement is not a common feature.

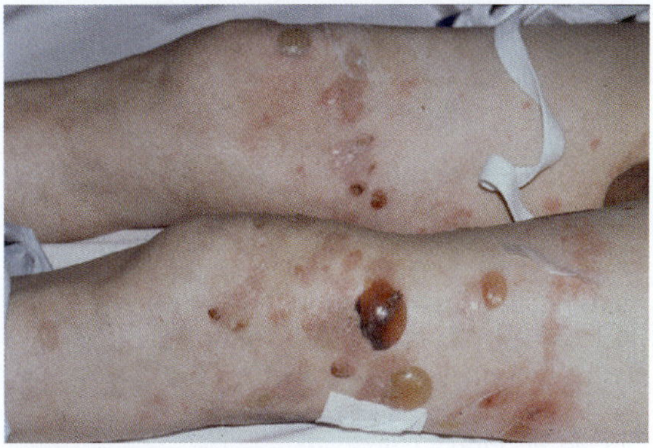

Figure 8.18 Bullous pemphigoid.

Typically seen on the extensor surfaces but rarely below the knees is dermatitis herpetiformis. Blisters are typically small and grouped, with the appearance of herpetic lesions. Pruritus is a common early symptom. Unlike pemphigus, oral lesions are not observed, but the majority of sufferers have also coeliac disease of the jejunum.

Inflammatory conditions of the skin

Eczema

Eczema is a descriptive term encompassing a wide variety of inflammatory diseases, many of which are pertinent to the lower limb. Clinical features vary greatly between each form of eczema and so are presented separately.

Subtypes of eczema

Atopic dermatitis

This increasingly common form of eczema presents at any age but is most common in childhood. Itch is the main symptom, with rash localised to the flexures. The itching and subsequent scratching can be severe. In some patients dryness and scaling is the major feature. Patients often have other allergic diseases such as hay fever or asthma. The signs are all manifestations of scratching and rubbing. First, the skin roughens and reddens; with continued scratching the skin becomes broken and later infected. The usual pathogen is *Staphylococcus aureus*, which produces golden weeping and crusted skin. Later, the skin thickens with accentuation of the normal skin folds (lichenification), with fissures developing where the skin is less flexible.

Asteatotic eczema

This is a common form of eczema usually seen in elderly people, especially those in institutional care. It results from low humidity, poor rinsing of soaps or detergents or over-vigorous washing. The usual symptom is soreness and itching, most frequently on the shins. The skin is scaly, pink and the surface broken in a crazy paving pattern.

Discoid eczema

Discoid eczema is a very localised form of eczema. It presents as multiple, isolated and coin-shaped lesions. Usually patients will complain of itching and, because of the shape of the lesions, assume they have a fungal infection. On examination, the lesions are red, scaly and superficially infected with golden crusting. Patients generally have dry skin or a previous history of eczema.

Lichen simplex

In this condition, patients usually complain of one or two itching patches. It frequently occurs on the medial aspect of the ankles and lateral calves. The itching may be very severe and keep the patient awake at night. The skin reacts to the scratching and rubbing by becoming thickened and lichenified (see above). Sometimes the lesions resemble plaques and other times nodules. The lesions are usually pink or brown and may be mistaken for lichen planus or psoriasis (see below).

Stasis dermatitis (venous eczema, gravitational eczema)

This form of eczema affects the lower legs. It usually occurs in patients with venous disease (previous varicose veins or deep venous thrombosis). Patients will complain of itching or soreness and may have a history of previous venous ulceration. The skin is red, scaly and weeping, usually in association with an ulcer or area of varicosity. The underlying skin may feel firm and be discoloured blue-brown with previous leakage of blood into the skin. Occasionally, the rash can spread beyond the areas of venous disease. One should always consider allergic contact dermatitis, as this is a common secondary feature.

Pompholyx

This is an acute eczema of the palms and soles. It is usually associated with a number of different forms of eczema elsewhere. As the plantar skin is so thick, instead of the skin weeping when it is inflamed, it forms small blisters under the skin instead. These can occasionally be mistaken for eczema elsewhere (Case history 8.1).

Case history 8.1

A 24-year-old health studies student presented in the late spring with a sudden outbreak of itchy, small blisters affecting her hands and feet. Her medical history was unremarkable and examination of her hands and feet revealed numerous small, fluid filled vesicles in a symmetrical distribution, which she reported as beginning on the inner aspects of the digits and spreading onto the palmar and plantar surfaces.

Diagnosis: The age of the patient, symmetry and characteristics of the eruption suggested a type of eczema known as pompholyx (or dyshidrotic eczema). Diagnosing the condition is fairly straight forward. Contact dermatitis may give rise to a similar eruption but is rarely seen on the plantar and palmar surfaces due to the skin thickness. Pustular psoriasis, which affects the palmar plantar areas may initially give rise to clear, fluid filled vesicles but these rapidly turn purulent and seldom itch but give rise to soreness. Pompholyx, most common in the 20–40-age group, is of unknown aetiology but can be provoked by hyperhidrosis, stress, warm weather, tinea infections and nickel allergies. On questioning, this patient had no history of nickel allergy but reported numerous bouts of tinea pedis interdigitally which she noticed more in the warmer weather. Examination of her webspaces and a fungal culture confirmed the presence of *Epidermophyton floccosum* – a common dermatophyte.

When managing pompholyx is it important to identify and treat factors which may trigger the eruption as well as the eczema itself. In this case, the use of a topical antifungal agent interdigitally along with a topical steroid to the affected areas was successful.

Psoriasis

This is a very common group of diseases. In its most usual form, it consists of well-defined, red plaques with loosely adherent silvery scale localised to the extensor surfaces. Two per cent of the population is affected and may present at any age but the second and third decades are the commonest. Scaly areas develop over weeks or months in the scalp, around the sacrum and umbilicus. The flexures and genitals may be affected. There are characteristic changes in the nails that are a useful aid to diagnosis: pitting and ridging. The nail may come away from the nail bed (onycholysis) and the undersurface of the nail can develop thick scaling. The damage is only transient. Arthritis is commonly associated with psoriasis and may take on a number of forms. Disease severity of the arthritis does not parallel the extent of the skin disease. Psoriasis and its variants commonly affect the lower legs.

Subtypes of psoriasis

Classic plaque psoriasis

This symmetrical rash affects the extensor surfaces of the skin. On the lower leg, the knees and shins are frequently involved and in this site may be thick and persistent, covering the whole shin. The plaques are variable in size, pink, red or purple and well demarcated. The scales are large and silver in colour and can be easily scraped away, revealing pinpoint bleeding. Usually nail changes will be evident on the toes.

Guttate psoriasis

This acute variant follows a streptococcal sore throat. Within a couple of weeks, small innumerable plaques of psoriasis cover the body. The rash tends to resolve with no treatment in 2–3 months. Occasionally it can be recurrent or go on to develop into classic plaque type.

Palmar plantar pustular psoriasis

This variant (Fig. 8.19) occurs primarily in middle-aged, female smokers. It is characterised by pustules on the palms and soles, with or without classic disease elsewhere. The pustules initially are creamy coloured; as they mature, they turn brown; finally, the roof falls away, leaving a scaly depression. They are commonly mistaken for fungal or bacterial disease but culture of the pustule is always sterile. A single digit may be all that is involved; in this form, the nail may be destroyed permanently. Smoking cessation does not help the rash (Case history 8.2).

Generalised pustular psoriasis and erythroderma

Occasionally, psoriasis may be pustular on the body. In this form, it is widespread, of acute onset, often with systemic upset. Lakes of pus can develop on the skin which later scale. Patients usually have a previous history of psoriasis. Occasionally, psoriasis can be so widespread it affects the whole body. With this, there is loss of normal skin function (barrier against infection, heat and water loss) and patients can become very ill (death is not unknown, usually due to coexisting conditions). This is called erythroderma.

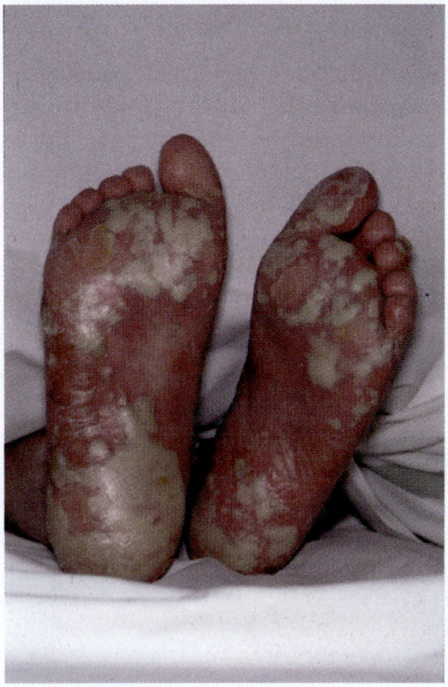

Figure 8.19 Plantar pustular psoriasis.

Case history 8.2

A 63-year-old cleaner requested a consultation for her irritable soles. The problem began 2 years earlier on her left foot with crops of pus filled blisters that were sore rather than itchy. The pustules had dried up leaving brown patches that then peeled away. More recently her right foot had been involved in a similar way and over the past week she had noted similar problems on her palms. Her general practitioner had treated her for both fungal disease and also tried penicillin with little effect. She was otherwise in reasonable health apart from arthritis in her spine. She was a smoker and consumed 40 units of alcohol per week. On examination she had multiple small pus filled blisters on her palms and soles, there were some areas that had dried up and appeared blood stained. Many areas were peeling off. Bacterial swabs of the pustules were negative.

Diagnosis: In view of the unusual appearance and extend of the problem she was referred to the dermatologist who made a diagnosis of palmar plantar pustular psoriasis.

Vasculitis

This condition frequently presents on the lower legs. The rash may have been precipitated by a new medication or an infection or another inflammatory medical condition. Clinically, there is inflammation within the blood vessels that results in leakage of blood into the surrounding skin. Lesions do not blanch. Early lesions are raised, red and itchy. Later, the skin may blister or ulcerate. Occasionally, the rash may be very extensive; commonly, it is modified by areas of pressure and may be accentuated around the shoe or sock line. Apart from ulceration, skin involvement is usually only a minor problem. Generalised involvement is sometimes a problem, with inflammation of vessels occurring in the gut, joints and kidneys that occasionally may result in renal failure or, rarely, death.

Lichen planus

Lichen planus (LP, **Fig. 8.20**) is a common inflammatory condition that frequently affects the lower leg. The main presenting symptom is itch and rash. The itch is often very severe; patients tend to rub more than scratch, as sometimes the rash is tender. The rash may be very widespread, appearing characteristically on the wrists, shins and sometimes diffusely on the body. The mouth is often sore; the genital mucosae can be involved. Scalp involvement may lead to permanent hair loss. The nails are also involved. The clinical appearances are typical. The rash consists of multiple flat-topped, polygonal papules that have a shiny surface. The colour is pale pink through to violet and sometimes brown. Resolving lesions often leave marked persistent pigmentation. Nail involvement produces pits on the nail surface; later, the nail thins and becomes abnormal, sometimes resulting in destruction of the nails. Inside the mouth, LP can appear as white lacy streaks on the mucosa to blisters to ulcers. On the lower leg, LP can become very thick (hypertrophic). LP frequently develops in areas of skin injury (koebnerisation), leading to bizarre linear forms of the rash. LP of the soles is less distinct, but the symptoms are similar and usually associated with more typical rash elsewhere. Lichen planus is usually relatively short-lived (1–2 years), but hypertrophic disease may become chronic.

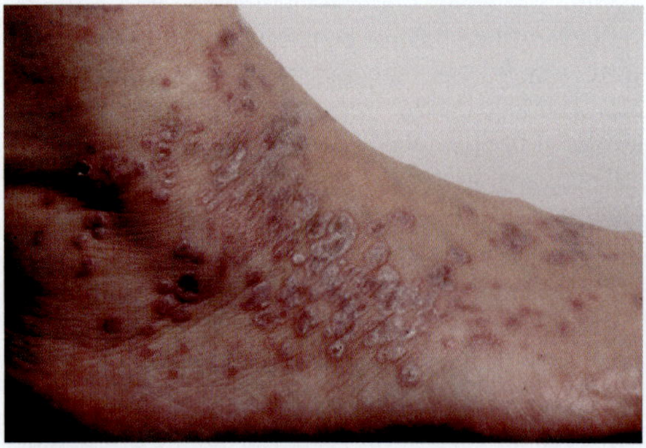

Figure 8.20 Lichen planus.

Granuloma annulare

Frequently misdiagnosed as tinea, this eruption is an idiopathic disorder that predominantly affects people under 30 (particularly children). Starting as a single red papule, it spreads concentrically (up to several centimetres in some cases), becoming concave in the centre with a pink papular edge. The lesions, which can be single or multiple, occur most commonly on the hand. They also occur on the foot and shins. Unlike tinea, the lesion is rarely scaly and does not itch. Diagnosis is confirmed by biopsy. The condition may be rarely associated with diabetes mellitus. Necrobiosis lipoidica may resemble this lesion but tends to have a yellowish hue.

Necrobiosis lipoidica

Necrobiosis lipoidica (**Fig. 8.21**) occurs on the shin and is commonly seen in patients with diabetes. Patients may be asymptomatic or complain of rash or ulceration. The lesions start as red patches, which enlarge, the centre becomes depressed and the skin yellows. Blood vessels may be visible traversing the patch. Occasionally, lesions ulcerate. Sometimes the rash may precede the diagnosis of diabetes or rarely may be the presenting feature. There are often multiple lesions.

Other inflammatory conditions

Sunburn

Exposure to sunlight (UVB radiation) will lead to an erythema after a latent period of 1–3 hours, depending on the amount of exposure. Excessive exposure can lead to desquamation (peeling) and, in the long term, can increase the risk of malignant changes in the skin.

Chilblains (perniosis)

This is a familial vasospastic response to prolonged exposure to cold. Typically, lesions begin on the apices of the toes, fingers and occasionally the ears. In women, lesions may appear in the region just above the footwear line where the ankle is only covered by thin hosiery (submalleolar perniosis). The chilblain begins as an erythema, turning into a purple, swollen lesion that may itch and burn. Ulceration of lesions is not uncommon.

Erythrocyanosis

A relatively common disorder, erythrocyanosis commonly affects young, overweight women, particularly those working in a cold environment. Exposure to cold invokes a vasospastic response, resulting in a purple-red discoloration in the buttock, thigh and shin area accompanied by a burning sensation.

Erythema multiforme

This skin disorder is characterised by symmetrical, concentric 'target' lesions occurring on the hands, feet and limbs. Individual lesions may have a blistered bluish-red centre with a more vivid surrounding erythema. Involvement of the genital, oral and conjunctival areas is not uncommon and appears in the more severe form of the disease known as Stevens–Johnson syndrome. The causes are diverse, but 50% of cases are idiopathic: known causes include drug eruptions and viral and streptococcal infections. Differential diagnosis should include other causes of blistering and fungal infections. Negative fungal culture and the symmetry of the eruption should establish the diagnosis.

Allergies and drug reactions

Allergic contact dermatitis

Typically, allergic contact dermatitis (Fig. 8.22) occurs as a result of the skin becoming sensitised to a specific allergen (a type IV hypersensitivity reaction), so that subsequent exposure to the allergen produces an acute reaction of erythema, weeping and blistering at the point of contact.

The site of the reaction depends on the area of skin exposed to the allergen. Sensitisation is more rapid on thin or moist skin; hence, reactions are most commonly seen on the face and antecubital fossa. Due to its thickness, the plantar surface of the foot rarely becomes involved. Shoe line eruptions tend to be seen on the margins where the skin becomes thinner towards the dorsum. The popliteal fossa is also an area of thinner skin and, occasionally, may show reactions to, for example the dyes used in nylon tights.

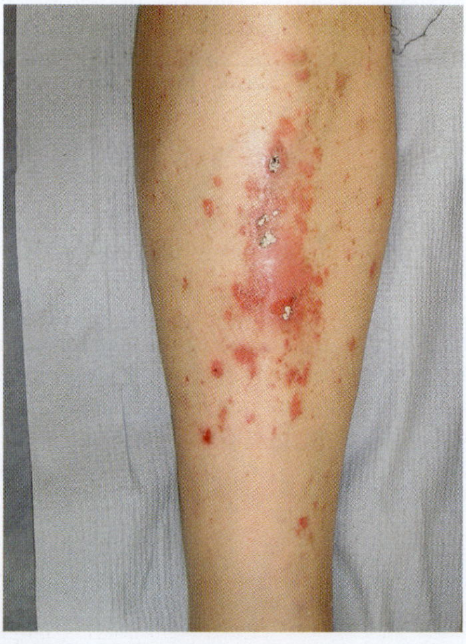

Figure 8.21 Necrobiosis lipoidica.

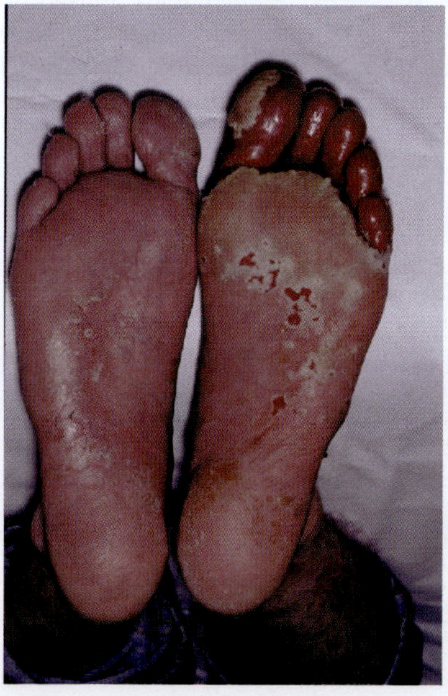

Figure 8.22 Acute contact dermatitis.

Table 8.12 Common causes of allergies in the lower limb

Location	*Common allergen*
Thigh (pocket area)	Phosphorus sesquisulphate (matches)
Popliteal fossa	Dyes in nylon tights
Foot and ankle	Venous leg ulcer treatments Chromates (leather tanning) Adhesives (epoxy resins) Metals (nickel in buckles) Medicaments, especially those containing lanolin and parabens

The common allergens affecting the lower limb are listed in Table 8.12. It is important to recognise that sensitised T cells may spread from the contact site and provoke eczematous type lesions elsewhere on the body. When the cause of the reaction is not apparent, patch testing should be undertaken to identify the causative agent (Case history 8.3).

Juvenile plantar dermatosis

Juvenile plantar dermatosis is thought to be a variant of contact dermatitis. The condition arises in schoolchildren as a scaly, erythematous, glazed eruption, typically affecting the forefoot and plantar surfaces of the toes, sparing the interdigital areas. Fissuring may accompany the condition. Differential diagnoses include tinea infection, psoriasis, contact dermatitis and adverse drug reaction. The symmetry and glazed appearance of the condition, along with the patient's age, are usually enough to make the diagnosis. With a contact dermatitis, a positive patch test would be obtained (Case history 8.4).

Drug reactions

Reactions to drugs may happen due to:

- a true allergic reaction to a drug (hypersensitivity)
- overdosage (toxic reaction)
- side effects of a drug
- alteration, by the drug, of the normal immune response.

The difficulty in differentiating the above factors is that, potentially, they can all mimic virtually any skin lesion. When a drug reaction is suspected, a thorough drug history is required (including any over-the-counter preparations the patient may be using). Most often the offending drugs are the ones taken in the past 2–3 weeks, although reactions are not uncommon in drugs taken safely for many years. Withdrawal from the drug usually results in resolution of the condition within a week or two. Drug reactions affecting the lower limb are rare.

Typical patterns of drug eruptions include:

- toxic erythema – generalised erythema accompanied by fever
- urticaria
- erythema multiforme
- vasculitis – typically seen as a painful purpura on the shins
- erythema nodosum.

Case history 8.3

A 44-year-old woman presented to her general practitioner with a short history of extreme irritation and swelling of her feet. The problem began after a holiday to Morocco and involved mainly the dorsum of both feet up to the ankle. Initially her symptoms had just been itching and scaling but in the past month the skin had broken down and was now continually weeping. She was otherwise in excellent health with no history of skin problems apart from minor irritation from cheap earrings. On examination there was widespread eczema with numerous areas of crusting, small blisters and erosions. Initial treatment was topical antiseptics (potassium permanganate), oral antibiotics and topical steroids (betamethasone valerate). She was advised to take time off work, keep her feet elevated and avoid any footwear. She responded quickly but unfortunately her symptoms recurred on return to work. She represented and felt it was her leather shoes she had bought on holiday that were the cause of her symptoms.

Diagnosis: A dermatology opinion was sought and she was shown subsequently to be allergic to cobalt and chromium by patch testing, metals that are used in the tanning process of leather. Differential diagnosis should be made from psoriasis and fungal infections. Depending on the point of exposure lesions may be symmetrical or asymmetrical with a well-defined edge. Fungal cultures and microscopy will typically be negative. Allergic dermatitis rarely affects children and elderly people, possibly due to a less vigilant cell-mediated immunity. With psoriasis, lesions should be present elsewhere and nail changes are likely.

Case history 8.4

An 8-year-old girl was referred to the podiatry clinic with dry, cracked feet. Her mother was concerned this was an eruption of her atopic eczema but unlike her usual eczema it had not responded to her prescribed steroid cream. Physical examination of the girl's feet revealed symmetrical, erythematous plaques with a 'glazed' appearance that involved the plantar metatarsal areas and the weightbearing surfaces of the toes. These areas were mildly tender to pressure but not painful. However, the skin showed superficial fissuring and was mildly thickened and on occasion they had cracked and bled. Other areas of the foot such as the dorsum, heel, arch and interdigital spaces were all unaffected. A negative fungal culture, combined with a symmetrical rash in a young child, ruled out the possibility of fungal infection while the failure to respond to a topical steroid suggested this was not a typical eczema.

Diagnosis: The classic glazed foot in a young child, which fails to respond to steroids suggested juvenile plantar dermatosis. The condition tends to occur in more active children and those with an atopic history. There is no one effective cure and it spontaneously resolves after 2–4 years. A patient's symptoms may be relieved with natural fibre socks and leather lined shoes, in addition to going barefoot as much as possible.

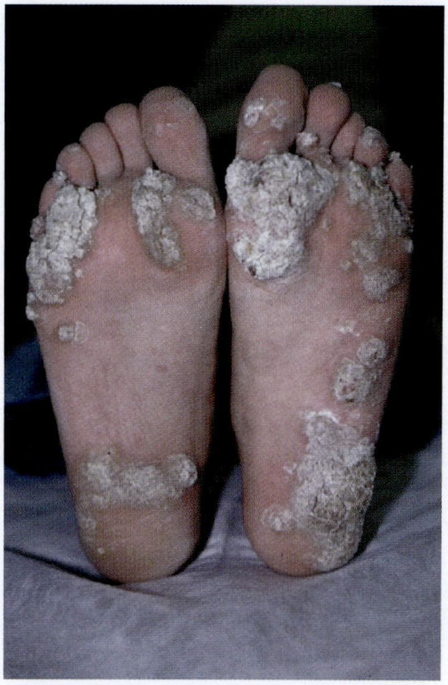

Figure 8.23 Extensive plantar warts in an immunosuppressed patient.

Infections of the skin

The surface of the skin is an effective barrier against most environmental agents, but through injury to the skin surface or when exposed to virulent organisms this barrier fails. The pattern of disease very much depends on the type of infection and so will be considered accordingly.

Viral

Verrucae

Verrucae (Fig. 8.23) are the predominant viral infection on the foot caused by infection of the skin with human papilloma virus (HPV). Around 5% of 16-year-olds will have warts at any one time (Williams et al 1991). The virus affects the stratum spinosum and causes hyperplasia and formation of a benign tumour. Typically, the plantar wart is found under a point of high pressure, for example the metatarsal heads or a bony prominence (Glover 1990). In its early stages it appears as a small, dark, translucent puncture mark in the skin. More mature lesions show thrombosed capillaries, a 'cauliflower-rough' surface and are painful when pinched. The patient may complain of increased discomfort on starting to walk after a period of rest, for example first thing in the morning. Different types of HPV cause different wart lesions, for example flat, genital or plantar.

Verrucae protrude above the level of the skin unless they occur on weightbearing surfaces. When they are found on weightbearing surfaces they protrude into the skin and, as a result, are more painful. Mosaic warts are made up of multiple, small, tightly packed individual warts and may not be painful, whereas plantar warts may be single or multiple and are usually painful. Occasionally, periungual warts may develop around the nail edge and lead to distortion of the nail plate.

Verrucae can usually be diagnosed from their clinical appearance; however, they can be confused with corns (particularly neurovascular or fibrous) and foreign bodies. Verrucae can occur on non-weightbearing and/or weightbearing areas of the foot, unlike corns and most foreign body injuries, which tend to occur solely on weightbearing areas. There may be multiple verrucae present, not only on the feet but also on the hands. Sideways pressure tends to cause a sharp pain, whereas corns and foreign bodies give rise to pain on direct pressure. Verrucae appear encapsulated and the skin striae are broken; corns do not appear encapsulated and the skin striae are not broken but pushed to one side. Any wart with an atypical appearance, particularly in elderly or immunosuppressed individuals, should be biopsied as, rarely, the lesion may undergo malignant change.

Molluscum contagiosum

This is a contagious infection (usually of children) which usually involves the trunk, but can affect the leg and foot. Infection with the causative poxvirus, usually by close contact, leads to a papular lesion, which may range in size from a pinhead to a pea. The hard, shiny pedunculated lesion has a central crater from which cheesy material may be expressed by pinching it. The uniqueness of this lesion makes the diagnosis straightforward.

Herpes zoster (shingles)

Shingles is a recrudescence of previous chicken pox, usually along a single dermatome. It can occur at any age, but most frequently in elderly or immunosuppressed individuals. It presents as a 1–3-day history of pain or burning in one limb followed by haemorrhagic blisters and later superficial ulcers. Pain may persist for many weeks and months.

Herpes simplex

Herpes simplex (cold sores) rarely affect the lower leg, although they may involve the thigh in rugby players (scrum pox) following infected oral exposure to an eroded area of skin on the sports field.

Bacterial

Bacterial superinfection, which is common particularly in the various forms of eczema, has been discussed earlier in this chapter. Primary bacterial infections (Fig. 8.24) are less common. In all these conditions, full investigation with bacterial swabs is essential.

Ecthyma

This infection affects the full thickness of the epidermis. The main pathogens are *Staphylococcus aureus* and *Streptococcus pyogenes*. The patient may have recently been to a humid climate or had an insect bite. It presents as a shallow ulcer with a thick, crusted top.

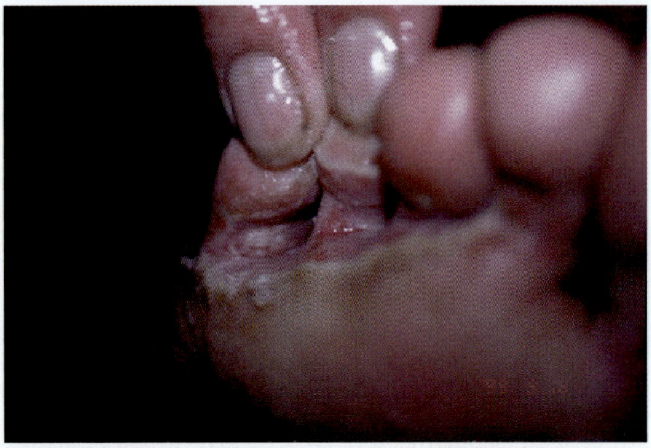

Figure 8.24 *Pseudomonas* infection affecting the interdigital area.

Cellulitis

Cellulitis or erysipelas is a serious infection usually of the lower leg caused most commonly by *Streptococcus pyogenes*. It presents as a flu-like illness that is rapidly followed by a painful red advancing area, usually on the lower leg. The affected area becomes swollen and the skin discoloured. The skin may even blister, necrose and ulcerate. Commonly, a 'portal of entry' is found such as tinea pedis (see below) or a fissured patch of eczema.

Pitted keratolysis

Bacterial overgrowths on the sole of the foot secrete proteolytic enzymes that produce multiple pits within the epidermis. The pathogens are microaerophilic diphtheroids. Pitted keratolysis (Fig. 8.25) is particularly common in patients with sweaty feet or who wear trainers. Usually it is asymptomatic, but sometimes the skin thins sufficiently to be tender. Odour is commonly offensive in such patients (Case history 8.5).

Erythrasma

This bacterial infection of creases and flexures occurs between the toes of the foot. It is commonly mistaken for tinea pedis. The pathogen is *Propionibacterium minutissimum*. The skin is usually macerated and red/brown in colour. Again, it has a strong odour and fluoresces coral pink in Wood's light.

Fungal

There are four patterns of fungal infection of the foot (tinea pedis). Asymmetry is a feature common to all subtypes. In all situations, scrapings are essential to

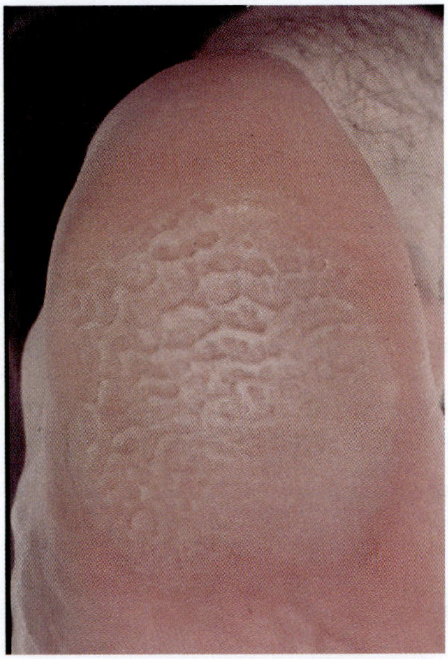

Figure 8.25 Pitted keratolysis of the heel.

Case history 8.5

A 40-year-old man was referred by his general practitioner with a long history of malodorous tender feet. The problem began in his early 20s, seeming to be worse in the summer but often got better when on holiday. He had not tried any specific treatment but had to wash his feet two or three times per day. On examination he was wearing trainers, which were damp with perspiration. His feet were strong smelling and had a macerated appearance on the soles. Over both heels were shallow erosions that had eaten into the keratin. A diagnosis of pitted keratolysis was made and the cause explained. He was advised to wear leather shoes which would allow better air circulation and recommended to keep his feet bare as much as possible. He was also offered topical antiperspirants (20% aluminium chloride) and a topical antibiotic (clindamycin). On review 3 months later he was much improved and found that he could keep his symptoms at bay just by not wearing shoes around the house.

fully assess for fungal disease. Interdigital scaling is the commonest form, usually presenting as itching and fissuring. This usually occurs between the third to the fifth toes where the skin is most macerated. The rash initially begins on one foot, only later

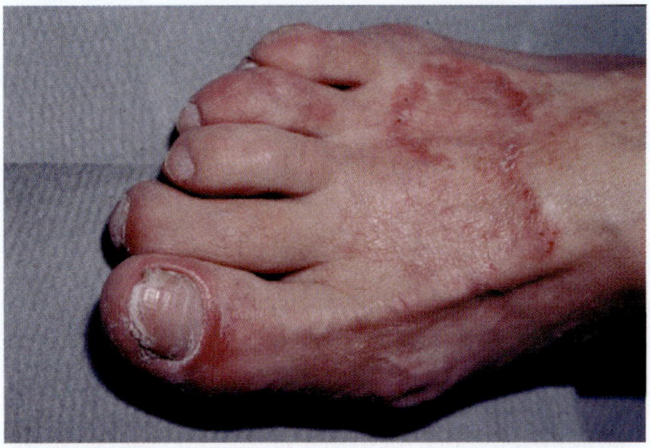

Figure 8.26 Tinea pedis affecting the dorsum of the foot.

extending to the other toes, nails and other foot. A variety of fungi and yeasts are implicated.

Extension onto the dorsa of the foot

In chronic disease, the fungus can spread onto the dorsa of the foot (Fig. 8.26), producing itchy scaly rings with an active edge. Fungal culture will help to differentiate this from discoid eczema. Typical causes include *Trichophyton rubrum* and less commonly *Epidermophyton floccosum*.

Blistering in the instep

The inflammatory reaction on the sole to fungus tends to produce blistering (*Trichophyton mentagrophytes*). It is usually unilateral. Removal of the blister roof will allow closer inspection and it may be sent for culture.

Moccasin foot

The soles of the foot can be generally involved with fungus (*Trichophyton rubrum*), producing thickened scaly feet. Often the disease affects both feet. The nails may also be involved. Most patients are unaware of the problem but will have a previous history of infection.

Onychomycosis

Tinea pedis may progress to the toe nails (onychomycosis), typically as a result of repeated trauma (e.g. from footwear). Infection may occur superficially on the nail plate or subungually invading under the hyponychium. Proximal subungual involvement occurs rarely in immunocompromised patients or following chronic paronychia. Total nail involvement and dystrophy may result (Case history 8. 6).

Case history 8.6

A 70-year-old retired secretary, presented at the podiatry clinic with problematic thickened nails which she had difficulty in managing. In addition the skin on her feet around the plantar surfaces and heels was found to be very dry, despite her best efforts with various emollients and moisturisers. On examination, her plantar skin was dry, with a dusty appearance, accentuated in the skin creases. A scraping was sent for mycology and was positive for the dermatophyte T rubrum.

Diagnosis: Tinea pedis. A large percentage of the elderly population have dermatophyte infection on their feet without significant symptoms. For many the condition is passed off as dry skin and treated as such. The plantar surface acts as a reservoir for the fungus and untreated it is able to spread to the nails, hands and other parts of the body. Patients presenting with toenail onychomycosis should be routinely checked for skin infection elsewhere on the foot.

Tinea incognito

Misdiagnosis of fungal infection is a problem as often the incorrect diagnosis made is eczema. The use of topical steroids to reduce inflammation consequently allows the unsuspected fungus to grow unchecked by the immune system. Patients present with a history of a persistent rash, usually on the foot, which fails to respond to steroid creams. The potency of the steroid used is often very high. The rash is red, ill-defined with nodules within, that when squeezed express pus. Scrapings confirm the presence of fungus.

Infestations and insect bites

Scabies

The mite *Sarcoptes scabiei* causes scabies. Itching is often severe despite sometimes having minimal evidence of infestation. Patients may describe itchy nodules or blisters. They will usually have family members presenting at the same time with itch. The signs are generally that of eczema but blisters and excoriations are more pronounced. The primary lesion is the burrow of the mite. It appears as a linear or serpiginous white line with scaly opening at one end and a minute grey or red dot at the other end (the mite). The mite may be extracted with a needle and examined using a microscope. Scabies should be suspected in any patient with a pronounced itch, and other sites of involvement (hands and trunk) should be sought.

Insect bites

A variety of insects will bite the skin, producing itch or painful nodules or blisters on the skin. The lower leg is commonly involved as it is often exposed (biting insects and fleas). Clues to suggest insect bite are grouped lesions, often along a sock or shoe line, and a history of presence of domestic animals or proximity to farms.

Larvae migrans

A variety of hookworms that are gut parasites in animals may find themselves in humans. Cats and dogs are the main carriers. The immature form of the parasite penetrates the skin and the larvae migrate under the skin to produce loops and tortuous tracks. Patients usually complain of itch and blistering, usually contracting the disease on beaches abroad but occasionally in the UK. The pattern of migration makes diagnosis easy. Fortunately, the disease is self-limiting.

Disorders of the subcutaneous tissue

The subcutaneous layer is a layer of primarily adipose (fat) tissue and covers most of the lower limb, particularly the thighs, anterior shins and plantar surface.

Atrophy

Atrophy is the most common disorder affecting the subcutaneous layer. It occurs most frequently as a result of ageing and trauma (e.g. heel pad atrophy in long-distance runners and the elderly) or as a result of granulomatous change (panniculitis) around injection sites (typically, diabetic patients using insulin injections). Affected skin becomes depressed and scarring may occur.

Painful piezogenic papules

On the plantar surface, around the heels, herniations of fat from the heel pad into the dermis may be evident on standing. As solitary or multiple nodules they may occasionally give rise to heel pain (Shelley & Rawnsley 1968), usually in middle-aged women.

Diagnosis is established based on pain resulting from direct pressure while standing, but when non-bearing, the lesion completely disappears.

Erythema nodosum

This is an uncommon eruption affecting the shins presenting as painful nodules on the shins and less commonly the thighs and forearms. The rash starts as painful areas that enlarge into hot, red nodules, which are acutely tender. These then resolve over a matter of weeks. The redness fades and takes on a bruised appearance. The condition is important, as it is often associated with other diseases such as sarcoidosis and a variety of infections.

Systemic disorders and the skin

The skin is an easily accessible structure and may often give clues regarding internal disease. Typical disorders which may affect the skin include connective tissue and endocrine diseases. Common systemic disorders and their effects on skin are summarised in Table 8.13.

Table 8.13 Systemic conditions and their associated skin changes

Condition	*Associated skin changes in the lower limb and foot*
Diabetes mellitus	Increased incidence of skin infections (fungal and bacterial), skin stiffening, ulceration (neurovascular), diabetic bullae, necrobiosis lipoidica, granuloma annulare
Lupus erythematosus	Erythematous scaly plaques with follicular plugging
Systemic lupus erythematosus	Periungual erythema, splinter haemorrhages, onycholysis and leuconychia. On the legs, erythromelalgia and erythema nodosum
Dermatomyositis	Periungual erythema with characteristic 'ragged cuticles'. Occasional calcification within the skin
Systemic sclerosis/ scleroderma	Tight waxy skin with later distal digital atrophy with calcinosis, ulceration and occasionally gangrene
Ehlers–Danlos syndrome	Fragile skin with frequent bruising, hypermobility, poor wound healing, typically showing large scars upon the knees
Rheumatoid arthritis	Skin atrophy, nodules, vasculitis with periungual infarcts, splinter haemorrhages and onycholysis with longitudinal ridging of the nails
Hyperthyroidism	Hyperhidrosis, clubbing, onycholysis, hyperpigmentation, pretibial myxoedema
Hypothyroidism	Anhidrosis, leuconychia, pruritus, palmar and plantar hyperkeratosis
Acromegaly	Hyperhidrosis, skin thickening, coarse hair
Hepatic disease	Clubbing, spider naevi and pruritus
Renal disease	Hyperpigmentation or skin yellowing, nail changes – half-and-half nails, onycholysis
Reiter's syndrome	Keratoderma blennorrhagica
Internal malignancy	Hyperpigmentation, palmoplantar keratoderma, secondary skin tumours, pruritus, nail clubbing, bullous eruptions

Pigmented lesions

Pigmented lesions represent a large part of general dermatological practice; this is also the case on the lower legs. Pigmented lesions arise as a result of a variety of processes, both neoplastic and inflammatory. Close attention to the clinical history and signs will allow distinction between most lesions.

Freckles or ephelis

These are probably the most common pigmented lesions seen on the skin. They are most common in those with fair skin who have been exposed to sunshine. Lesions are usually innumerable; they are visible but not palpable and the pigmentation within is usually evenly distributed and is generally slight. Darker freckles can also occur, particularly after prolonged or excessive sun exposure.

Lentigo

A lentigo is a lesion where there is an increase in the number of melanocytes within the skin, resulting in a pigmented patch. Lesions usually occur in older patients and usually arise on sun-exposed sites. Again, the lesion is visible and not palpable; it tends to be solitary and the pigmentation within it is usually light and always even.

Seborrhoeic warts

These are particularly common, developing with advancing age. They appear as well-defined, rough, warty, slightly raised lesions that have a stuck-on appearance. They usually occur on the trunk and proximal limbs but can arise on the lower leg. They do not develop on the sole. They are always benign but can become inflamed after minor trauma and may be mistaken for malignancy.

Pigmented naevi

Moles are collections of pigmented naevus cells (melanocytes) in the skin that contain the pigment melanin. The nature of moles will vary enormously depending on how many naevus cells are present, where in the skin they occupy and how pigmented they are: obviously, the greater number of naevus cells there are, the larger and more protuberant the lesion. Lesions that are close to the epidermal surface tend to be red/brown in colour; however, the further down the pigment is in the skin the bluer the colour becomes. In addition, the intensity of the colour will depend upon how much pigment is being produced. Moles are sometimes present at birth; their number increases during life, most commonly in the first two decades but can develop at any age. Moles may become larger and more pigmented with age and occasionally may regress. The clinical appearances of moles are infinitely variable, therefore making classification on macroscopic grounds alone almost impossible; however, they can be defined according to their microscopic appearances and knowledge of these patterns may be useful in the clinical setting.

Junctional naevi

Collections of melanocytes along the dermal-epidermal junction, junctional naevi are the usual type of mole for the sole of the foot. In this site the pigmentation usually follows the ridges and troughs on the epidermal markings. They are usually impalpable, the colour is red brown, and is symmetrical. They commonly occur in children and generally 'mature' by melanocytes falling away into the dermis, forming intradermal naevi. Here, the melanocytes have all fallen into the superficial dermis. Often, the naevus cells stop producing pigment and plump up. Clinically, the lesions are therefore protuberant and pale or skin-coloured. They may continue growing in adulthood. Compound naevi have both junctional and intradermal components and therefore share clinical features of both types of lesions.

Blue naevi

Melanocytes that have never reached the epidermis and instead have proliferated in the deeper dermis have a blue appearance. These often develop in later life, especially on sun-exposed sites, especially the dorsa of hands and feet and on the scalp. Blue naevi are small (less than 5 mm) and may be slightly raised. They can be differentiated from vascular malformations in that they do not blanch. They are almost always benign.

Malignant melanoma

In the assessment of pigmented lesions the potential diagnosis of melanoma (Fig. 8.27) should always be considered. There are a number of clinical symptoms and signs, which should alert you to the diagnosis (Table 8.14).

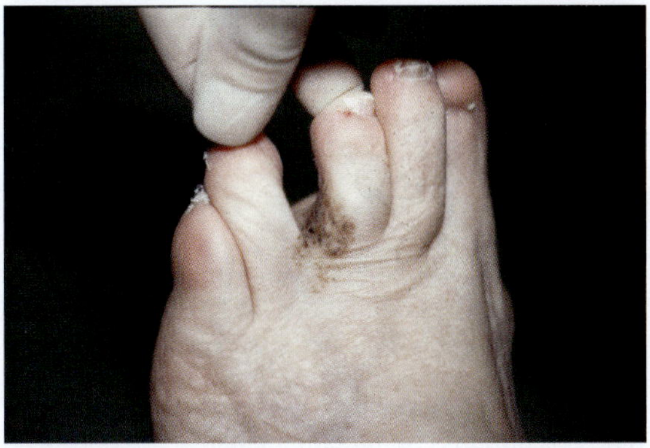

Figure 8.27 Interdigital melanoma.

Table 8.14 Pigmented lesion: suspicious signs and symptoms

Symptoms	*Signs*
Change in sensation	Loss of skin markings
Change in size	Irregular margins
Change in colour	Irregular pigmentation
Change in shape	Bleeding
Change in outline	Ulceration
New lesion	

Itching is an early and significant symptom that should be sought. Often, it may be the only presenting symptom, particularly where the melanoma is not in general view. There may be a change in the surface of the mole, skin creases may be lost, and hair follicles and pores may disappear. Almost always there will be an increase in the size, shape or thickness of the mole. This occurs over weeks and months and usually is asymmetrical. Colour will change within a mole; pigment can both increase and decrease within the same lesion. Also, as the melanocytes invade deeper into the skin, they may appear blue or even black. Rarely, melanoma may lose all pigmentation, making diagnosis very difficult clinically (although the patient may recall a pre-existing pigmented lesion). In advanced disease bleeding or ulceration of the surface of a melanoma may occur. The tumour can also spread by the time it is picked up; this may be clinically evident with tumours developing along the lines of lymphatic drainage (in transit metastasis), in the draining lymph nodes or at distant sites (for instance it may present as fits, weight loss or shortness of breath).

Case history 8.7

A 33-year-old Afro-Caribbean, presented with a 3-month history of a discoloured non-healing ulcer under his right great toe nail. The patient claimed that the nail had been injured during a game of football but instead of healing the area was getting worse. The nail was lifting off and beneath was an 8 mm moist erythematous nodule with a bluish grey discoloration in the surrounding nail bed. A biopsy was offered but the patient declined and was lost to follow-up. He presented again 6 months later with the nail totally destroyed, the pigmentation spreading onto the skin of both the proximal and distal nail folds. At this stage the patient underwent excision and grafting of the nail/nail bed. The lesion was confirmed to be an ulcerated subungual melanoma measuring 6 mm in thickness. Unfortunately 3 years later he died of metastasis to his lung, liver and brain.

Melanoma is very rare before puberty and usually occurs in large congenital moles. The majority of melanomas develop in later life, occurring in fair individuals on sun-exposed sites and most commonly in women on the lower legs. Melanoma may arise on the sun-protected sole of the foot and, as it is hidden from view, it usually presents late. Any unusual lesion on the foot should be suspected, particularly if there is pigmentation (Case history 8.7).

Skin tumours

Tumours of the skin need careful assessment, as there will be clues in both history and examination that will lead to accurate diagnosis. Most lesions will be benign, but a small proportion will be malignant (Table 8.15) and therefore life-threatening. Early referral of such lesions to a dermatologist can improve prognosis enormously. Points that should be sought in the history are, obviously, site of the lesion, how quickly it is growing, whether there are associated symptoms such as irritation or pain, or whether there are similar lesions elsewhere. Clinical signs that should be recorded are size, shape, surface, colour, outline, temperature and consistency. Dimensions should be recorded in the notes and, where possible, the lesion should be photographed.

Table 8.15 Principal tumours affecting the lower limb

Benign	*Malignant*
Dermatofibroma	Bowen's disease
Seborrhoeic wart	Basal cell carcinoma
Haemangioma	Squamous cell carcinoma
Lipoma	Melanoma
Clear cell acanthoma	Kaposi's sarcoma
Pyogenic granuloma	Porocarcinoma
Eccrine poroma	Metastasis
Glomus tumour	

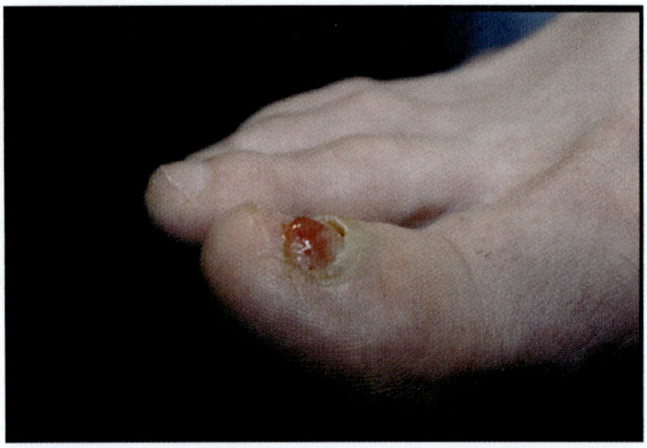

Figure 8.28 Pyogenic granuloma under the nail.

Benign tumours

Dermatofibroma

The lesions are very common, particularly on the lower leg. They are usually symptomless; often the patient is unaware that the lesion is even there. Sometimes they catch when the leg is scratched or shaved. They are felt as firm tethered nodules within the skin, sometimes with a slightly elevated surface. They often have a pigmented halo and for this reason may be mistaken for more sinister lesions. They are always benign.

Pyogenic granulomas

Pyogenic granulomas (Fig. 8.28) are common vascular proliferations that grow rapidly over a few days or weeks. They usually follow a minor injury. The surface is very easily broken and bleeding may be prolonged and frequent. In time, the lesion develops a surface epithelium that is more resilient, ultimately resembling a haemangioma.

Eccrine poroma

Eccrine poroma are benign tumours of the sweat duct that arise on the palms and soles, typically in the over-40 age group. They are pink or red, painless and usually 1–2 cm in diameter with a moist surface, surrounded by a moat-like depression. Occasionally, they can undergo malignant change.

Malignant lesions

Bowen's disease

Bowen's disease is squamous cell carcinoma confined to the epidermis only. It is a condition of the elderly, usually presenting as a well-defined, erythematous, scaly patch on the lower leg. When the scale is picked off the surface may bleed and weep. It occurs most commonly in women (suggesting a sun-related aetiology). The lesions are sometimes multiple. Left untreated they may persist for many years; however, sometimes this disease can progress on to true invasive squamous cell carcinoma.

Basal cell carcinoma

Basal cell carcinoma usually presents on the face but occasionally it occurs on the lower legs. Usually it presents as a fleshy nodule with a pearlescent appearance, having small blood vessels crossing the surface. Advanced lesions ulcerate and if neglected may become very large. Despite being locally destructive they do not metastasise. Occasionally, they remain superficial and indistinguishable from Bowen's disease.

Squamous cell carcinoma

Squamous cell carcinoma (SCC) is a common malignant tumour of the lower leg presenting as a lump or as a bleeding ulcer. The tumour grows over a period of weeks and months. In time the tumour becomes painful, particularly if it is invading bone or nerves. Usually it will develop on a background of sun damage but it is also associated with exposure to arsenic and aromatic hydrocarbons. Occasionally, it may develop with an old scar or leg ulcer; this should be considered, especially in ulcers that fail to heal with conventional measures or ulcers with fleshy or rolled edges. Metastasis generally tends to be a late

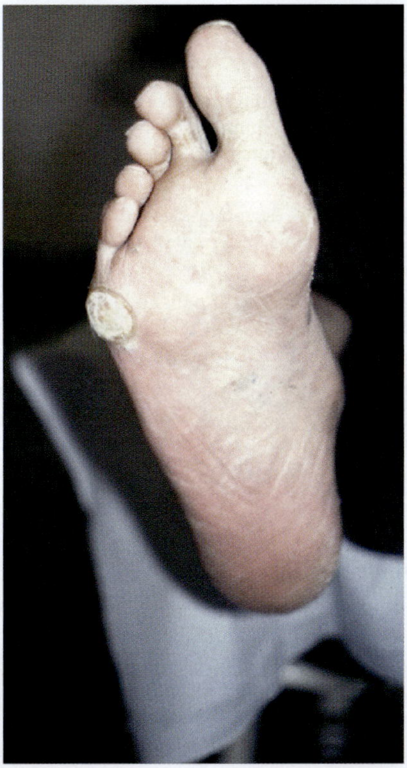

Figure 8.29 Metastatic lesion (secondary from a lung tumour).

event, usually to the regional lymph nodes. An SCC that arises on the foot may invade deeply with only minimal surface involvement, mimicking pressure or neuropathic ulcers. Often, in this site the tumour will have multiple sinuses that discharge offensive-smelling material.

Kaposi's sarcoma

This rare vascular tumour was described originally on the lower leg in males of eastern European extraction. It presents as blue-black or purple patches that later become plaques and nodules. Tumours range in diameter from 1 cm to 3 cm; they are usually multiple. Later lesions may involute or ulcerate. Oedema may become a problem. Kaposi's sarcoma is associated with human herpesvirus 8 and immunosuppression, notably human immunodeficiency virus (HIV) infection (Lebbe 1998).

Porocarcinoma

This rare sweat duct tumour often occurs on the lower leg. The history and clinical appearances are similar to SCC but the tumours are more likely to recur and metastasise.

Metastasis (Fig. 8.29)

Tumours of the lung, prostate, thyroid, kidneys and breast rarely spread to the skin. Usually when they do, it tends to be the scalp and upper body. However, tumours arising on the lower legs can metastasise to the draining lymph vessels and nodes, particularly melanoma and SCC. The tumours will usually appear as subcutaneous nodules; they may be large. They may be firm and may feel as if they are attached to related structures. The patient will usually have a history of previous tumours, but occasionally the metastasis may be the presenting feature.

Summary

Assessment of a patient's skin complaint requires careful accumulation of all of the pertinent factors related to the dermatological condition. A diagnosis is formulated from all the data gathered from the assessment and the practitioner's knowledge and clinical experience. Epidemiological data – information such as age and gender – may help. Information from observation, clinical tests and special investigations will also help to reduce the list of possible conditions. In most instances the diagnosis will become obvious, but on occasions it may not be possible to reach a definitive diagnosis. In this situation a provisional diagnosis should be made and the practitioner should treat the symptoms and observe the disease process to gain further insight of the condition. Occasionally, the effect of a treatment can be diagnostic in itself; for example a vesicular eruption that resolves with the use of an antifungal implies that the aetiology was mycotic. When a condition is diagnosed, the practitioner must decide what action is necessary based on available evidence.

References

Baran R, Dawber R P R, Tosti A et al 2003 A text atlas of nail disorders. Martin Dunitz, London

Cork M 1997 The importance of the skin barrier function. Journal of Dermatological Treatment 8:S7–13

Eves P, MacNeil S, Haycock J 2006 Alpha-melanocyte stimulating hormone, inflammation and human melanoma. Peptides 27:2444–2452

Gawkrodger D J 2002 An illustrated colour text of dermatology. Churchill Livingstone, London

Gillet du P 1973 Dorsal digital corns. Chiropodist July

Glover M G 1990 Plantar warts. Foot and Ankle 11(3):172–178

Harlow D, Poyner T, Findlay A et al 1998 High impairment of quality of life in adults with skin diseases in primary care. British Journal of Dermatology 139(Suppl 51):15

Ishida-Yamamoto A, Kishibe M, Takahashi H et al 2007 H RAB11 associated with lamellar granules. Journal of Investigative Dermatology 127(9):2166–1270

Jayaprakasam A, Darvay A, Osborne G et al 2002 Comparison of assessments of severity and quality of life in cutaneous disease. Clinical and Experimental Dermatology 27:306–308

Lawton S 2000 A quality of life for patients with skin disease. Skin Care Campaign Directory, London

Lebbe C 1998 Human herpesvirus 8 as the infectious cause of Kaposi sarcoma: evidence and involvement of cofactors. Archives of Dermatology 134(6):736–738

McKee P H 1996 Pathology of the skin with clinical correlations. Mosby-Wolfe, London

Merriman L, Griffiths C, Tollafield D 1986 Plantar lesion patterns. Chiropodist 42:145–148

Montagna W (ed) 1960 Advances in the biology of the skin: cutaneous innervation. Pergamon Press, Oxford

Office of Population Census and Surveys 1991–1992 Morbidity statistics from general practice. Fourth National Study 54:22

O'Halloran N 1990 A biochemical investigation into the cholesterol content of seed corns. BSc dissertation, University of Brighton

Pasyk K A, Thomas S V, Hassett C A et al 1989 Regional differences in the capillary density of the normal human dermis. Journal of Plastic and Reconstructive Surgery 83(6):939–945

Ratnavel R C, Griffiths W A D 1997 The inherited palmoplantar keratodermas. British Journal of Dermatology 137:485–490

Ryan T J 1995 Exchange and the mechanical properties of the skin: oncotic and hydrostatic forces control by blood supply and lymphatic drainage. Wound Repair and Regeneration 3:258–264

Shelley W B, Rawnsley H M 1968 Painful feet due to herniation of fat. Journal of the American Medical Association 205:308

Springett K P 1993 The influence of forces generated during gait on the clinical appearance and physical properties of skin callus. PhD thesis, University of Brighton

Venning V 2000 The dermo-epidermal junction: an important structure in dermatology. Dermatology in Practice 8(1):6–8

Whiting M F 1987 Survey of patients of large employer in SE England and Dept of Podiatry, University of Brighton. Unpublished, protected data

Williams H C, Potter A, Strachan D 1991 The descriptive epidemiology of warts in school children. British Journal of Dermatology 128:504–511

Zaias N 1980 The nail in health and disease. SP Medical, New York

Further reading

Baran R, Dawber R P R, Tosti A et al 1996 A text atlas of nail disorders. Martin Dunitz, London

Brodel R, Marchese-Johnson, S 2003 Warts diagnosis and management an evidence based approach. Martin Dunitz, London

Dawber R P R, Bristow I R, Turner W A 2000 A text atlas of podiatric dermatology. Martin Dunitz, London

Gupta l, Singh M 2004 Woods Lamp. Indian Journal of Dermatology, Venereology and Leprology 70:131–135

Harman R, Mathews C A N 1974 Painful piezogenic pedal papules. British Journal of Dermatology 90:573

Leung A K C, Chan P Y H, Choi M C K 1999 Hyperhidrosis. International Journal of Dermatology 38:561–567

Lewis-Jones S 2000 The psychological impact of skin disease. Nursing Times 96(27):2–4(suppl)

Litt J Z, Pawlak G P 1997 Drug eruption reference manual. Parthenon Publishing, London

Windsor A 2000 Sampling techniques. Nursing Times 96(27):12–13(suppl)

CHAPTER

9

Footwear assessment

W Tyrrell

Chapter contents

Introduction

Podiatrists and other healthcare professionals often condemn the footwear worn by patients. However, it is important to first consider just why the individual patient is wearing the shoes they have chosen. What are the criteria identified by the patient as being of significance in the choice of their footwear and what previous experience has affected their footwear selection? There is little doubt that footwear can be a mechanical and sometimes a chemical irritant to feet, but it can also be used as a therapy to reduce morbidity, and to improve foot health, mobility and quality of life.

Why do we wear shoes? The classic answer is 'protection'. In inclement conditions it is evident that footwear will provide a barrier against the cold and wet. In rough terrain soling will minimise trauma and the risk of damaging the integrity of skin. However, even when conditions are fair, we still wear shoes. Perhaps the major influences are not only climatic and not solely related to underfoot surfaces but also related to fashion, peer pressure and habit. In warmer climates, such as the Mediterranean regions, fishermen may be seen walking barefoot comfortably during the day, without sustaining damage to their feet, but then during the evening they may choose to wear shoes/sandals. Their feet develop a layer of physiological callus to provide a natural protection against walking on firm surfaces, but the shoes or sandals they chose to wear out of work form part of their social dress code. The clinician should determine the importance of footwear style to a patient's body image and take this into account when making footwear recommendations. The eventual footwear prescription derived in consultation with the patient may well be a compromise, but it should be a compromise that the patient will find acceptable and one which will minimise damage to foot health.

What do patients want from their footwear?

Patients may subconsciously use a list of preferential features which may include:

- Does the shoe suit me?
- Do I like the style?
- Do I like the colour?
- Is it what I want/need?
- Is it comfortable?
- Is the price right?

Before beginning to consider the suitability of the footwear presented by the patient we need to establish the type of footwear normally worn by the patient for the large part of the day and identify why they chose that particular style and material. It is also advisable to identify whether they have had any bad footwear experiences. For example have they been persuaded to buy 'sensible' footwear only to find that it was expensive and did not improve their foot comfort or their foot health? The purpose for which the footwear is to be used is significant and we should consider whether it is essentially designed to be smart or casual, for work or for a special occasions, regular use or a specific activity.

It is also useful to determine how a patient evaluates the fit of a shoe. They would probably consider a well-fitting shoe to be one which:

- does not hurt or slip
- seems to be long enough
- feels wide enough
- is comfortable and does not rub
- has a heel height they like.

The patient's perspective may be summarised in the word 'comfort'. Comfort is a term which relates to a lack of discomfort or pain and is directly related to sensitivity levels. It seems that in comparison with the hand, the foot has much lower sensitivity. Table 9.1 shows the differences in two-point discrimination at specific distances on sites on the hand and foot when monofilaments are applied (Goonetilleke & Luximon 2001).

Comfort may mean different things to different people. Is it the right feel? The absence of discomfort or pain? When patients like a particular footwear style and want to wear a favourite pair of shoes they can block the pain sensation. Feet and shoes are different shapes and when we put shoes onto our feet we are generally trying to fit an irregular shaped object into a more regularly shaped piece of footwear. However, if we try to replicate the actual individual foot shape into a shoe this will also give rise to problems as the foot undergoes changes in shape on weightbearing, with temperature change, impact, oedema and so on. For a shoe to fit, it ought to allow a certain 'feel' against the foot so that the wearer knows they have a shoe on their foot, but it should not cause any discomfort, pain or trauma. Neither should it require the foot to do any additional work in the form of gripping to make the shoe stay on the foot. The shoe should be secure at locations on the foot where deformations during gait will not be significantly large. Such positions will depend on shoe design and include: the grip around the heel, waist-girth, and the height of the shoe matching that at the midfoot. Forward movement of the foot should be restricted by a secure fastening across the instep.

Table 9.1 Sensitivity to Semmes–Weinstein monofilaments and two-point discrimination at points in the hand and foot

Site	*Touch sensitivity measured with Semmes–Weinstein monofilament (in mg)*	*Two point discrimination (in mm)*
Middle finger	6.8	2.5
Palm	20.1	11.5
Sole	35.9	22.5
Hallux	36.7	12.0

Parts of the shoe

Vamp

The vamp is the front section of the upper of the shoe. It can be made of one or more pieces of material. Sometimes several pieces of material are joined together to form a pattern. The seams and decoration can sometimes irritate the foot, especially bony prominences. In therapeutic footwear the vamp will usually be made of a single piece of leather with no seams. External decoration may be added including decorative aprons or stitching details but there will be only one continuous piece of material against the foot. In therapeutic footwear, the vamp is a common site for added depth, width or girth.

Toe puff (stiffener)

The toe puff is a stiffener between the vamp and the lining. It prevents the vamp collapsing and lifts it over the toes. Retail footwear often contains toe puffs which are extended proximally to cover part, or all, of the dorsal surface of the toes. Such toe puffs may exert pressure on the dorsal surface of clawed or hammered toes. Some footwear is made with toe puffs with additional strength, sometimes out of metal to give added strength and protection (e.g. industrial boots).

Tongue

The tongue is usually cut as an integral part of the vamp. It may or may not be padded. It is usually attached to the vamp only at its base, but it may also be made in 'bellows' form. In this form, the tongue material is part of the vamp, but it contains additional wings that are stitched to the quarters in a modified Gibson (Derby) construction (Fig. 9.1). This design allows for variable volume of the foot and so is useful for patients with foot and ankle oedema. A well-padded tongue is often important in patients with tarsometatarsal arthritis to reduce pressure over bony prominences.

Quarters

The quarters are preferably cut in one single piece of leather and contain a dart to meet the required shape at the back of the heel. More commonly, quarters are cut in two separate pieces which are sewn together at the centre back. It is important to avoid seams on the posterior aspect of the heel to prevent irritation of the soft tissues. The facings are also included as part of the quarters. In therapeutic footwear, quarters can be made with variable height or width dimensions to accommodate deformity such as a valgus heel or bony prominences around the ankle.

Heel counters

The heel counters are stiffeners which are included between the quarter and the lining at the back of the shoe. They help maintain the shape of the heel and prevent it from creasing down as the shoe is taken on and off and as the foot moves up and down during gait.

Heel counters may be extended medially, laterally, and proximally upwards from the ankles in boots. Heel counters provide stability and offer some control to the rear part of the foot during heel strike. Counters may also be made of extra strong material for additional reinforcement. Medial reinforcement is useful in pronatory syndromes and mid-foot

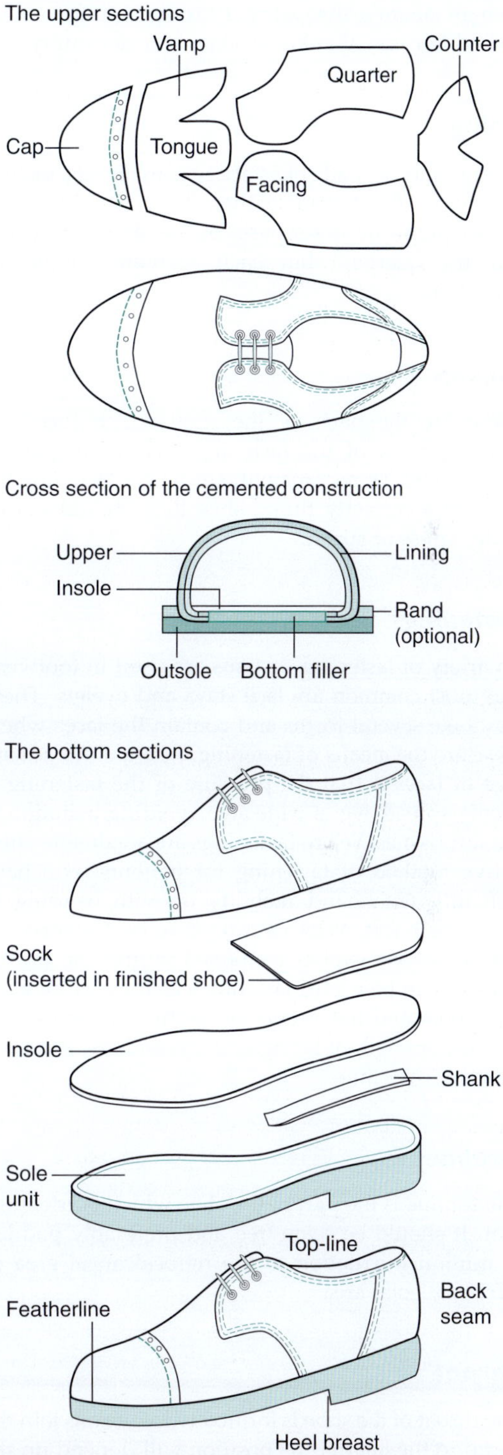

Figure 9.1 The parts of the shoe showing the components of a Gibson (Derby) style using a cemented (stuck-on) construction.

Charcot neuro-arthropathy. Proximal reinforcement is used in cases of ankle weakness or deformity.

Lining

Linings may be made of a variety of materials, including nylon, fleece and leather. They should reflect the shape of the main parts of the shoe (the vamp and the quarters) but each segment should be seam-free.

Facings

These are the parts of the shoe which form the meeting point of the fastenings. They are part of the quarters. They contain the means of fastening the shoe. In a correctly fitting shoe they should not be under stress or strain.

Fastenings

A variety of fastening systems are used in footwear. The most common are lace stays and eyelets. These may take several forms and contain the laces where these are the means of fastening the shoe. An advantage of laces is that the pressure of the fastening is evenly spread over a wide area avoiding irritation to the soft tissues. Velcro fastenings are a valuable alternative method of fastening for patients who have difficulty with hand mobility or with bending to reach their feet. Velcro straps may be fastened via D-rings or via eyelets contained within the facing. Buckles can be useful fastenings as long as they are functional and not purely decorative. They usually lack the strength of lacing systems and are often less effective over time.

Topline

The topline is the part of the shoe which borders the foot. It should be seam-free and preferably padded to minimize irritation to the retrocalcaneal area or infra-malleolar area.

Throat

The throat of the shoe is formed where seams join the vamp to the quarter. Its position will depend on the style of the shoe. A lower throat line where the vamp is shorter and the quarter longer will give a wider opening allowing easier foot placement into the shoe.

Innersole

The insole is the base of the inner aspect of the shoe. It may be covered by an inlay which contacts the plantar surface of the foot. (Note that what podiatrists understand by 'insole' is usually what shoe manufacturers refer to as 'inlay'.)

Outersole

This is the undersurface of the shoe which makes contact with the ground. It can be made of a variety of materials and textures. The texture determines the level of grip the shoe has on the walking surface.

Shank

Traditional shoe manufacturing methods include the use of a shank. This is a piece of metal that reinforces the waist of the shoe, maintains the relationship between the pitch of the heel and the forefoot and stops the shoe collapsing in the mid-foot. More modern constructions (e.g. Strobel) use resilient soling materials and do not use shanks.

Heel

This is the part of the shoe directly underneath the heel of the foot. The part of the heel nearest the ground which can be repaired is called the top-piece. The heel is usually pitched to a certain height, which is directly related to the toe spring or raised area under the toe part of the shoe.

Toe spring

This is the elevation of the front part of the shoe when the shoe is standing correctly on its treadline (which corresponds with the metatarsophalangeal joints). Toe spring facilitates walking action and compensates for any stiffness in the footwear (see Fig. 9.2).

The last

The last is the model form (Fig. 9.2) around which the shoe is made. Lasts are usually made of polyurethane, although wooden lasts may be used for high-quality, high-cost bespoke footwear.

Last measurements and sizing

The length of the last will equate with the finished length of the shoe that is made on it. The foot width and girth measurements are taken at several points.

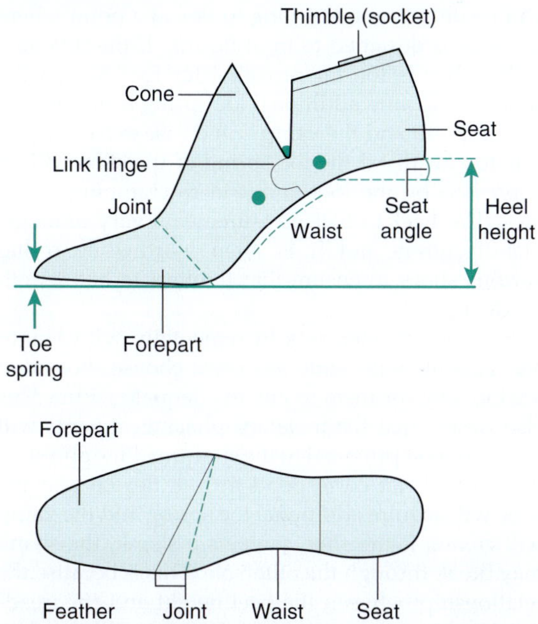

Figure 9.2 The last – the model on which the shoe is made.

The widest point on the last will equate with the width of the foot at the metatarsophalangeal joints. The width from medial to lateral across the plantar surface of the heel directly beneath the malleoli will also be transferred to the measurement at the corresponding point on the last. Girth measurements are taken at a minimum of five points on the foot to correspond with last dimensions. These points include the circumference of the foot at the metatarsophalangeal joints, the circumference of the foot immediately behind the metatarsal heads (known as the waist measurement), and the circumference of the foot at the instep – in the position of the cuneiform bones. Girth measurements will also be taken from the back of the heel at the plantar/retrocalcaneal border to the dorsal surface of the ankle joint and from the same point at the back of the heel to the point at which the instep girth was taken. These measurements are known as the short and long heel measurements, respectively (see Fig. 9.6B).

The recede

This is the part of the last which projects beyond the tip of the toes forming the contour of the front of the shoe. A tapering recede such as in pointed toe shoes increases the overall length of the shoe. In a poorly designed last the recede may encroach on the toes increasing pressure on the tips of the toes.

Treadline

This line corresponds with the position of the metatarsophalangeal joints and is the point at which the shoe will be designed to flex.

Toe spring

This describes the elevation of the under-surface of the last from the treadline forwards to the toes. It gives a slight rocker effect to the shoe. The amount of toe spring built into the last depends on shoe style, shoe construction method and sole thickness and heel height. Toe spring is designed to make walking in shoes easier. It compensates for the stiffness of the footwear and assists propulsion during gait. The more rigid the soling material the higher the elevation of the toe spring. The higher the heel height the lower the toe spring required.

The flare

This describes the curve or contour of the longitudinal bisection of the last. A last may be inflared, outflared or neutral. In order to describe the flare, a line which longitudinally bisects the heel of the last is carried forwards to the front of the last. The last is said to be inflared when the medial portion of the last across the treadline area is wider than that on the lateral side. The last is said to be outflared when the portion on the lateral side of the treadline is greater than that on the medial. When both sides are of equal width the last is said to have a neutral flare (Fig. 9.3).

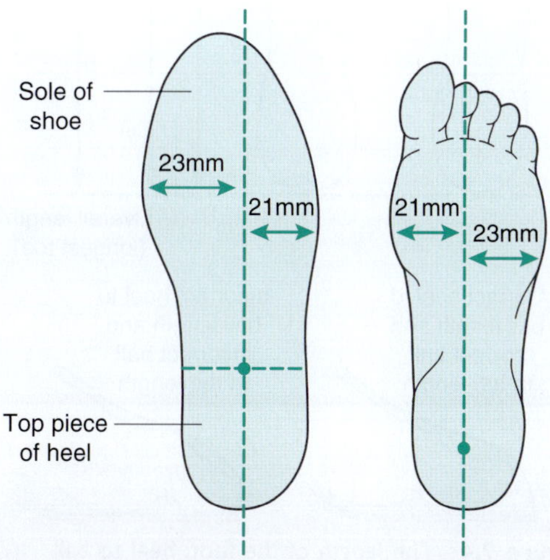

Figure 9.3 The flare of the last. The shoe will reflect this finished shape.

For reasons of cosmesis most lasts (and therefore most shoes) are inflared. Some orthopaedic shoes and trainers are of neutral flare. Few shoes are made with an outflare – on rare occasions shoes are made with an outflare to correct in-toeing in children.

The ideal shoe – the clinician's perspective

What to advise patients about footwear

The first and probably most evident feature is that footwear should fit the feet they are intended for. The length of the shoe should accommodate the longest part of the foot always remembering that digital formulae are not standard and that in some patients one or more of the lesser toes may be longer than the hallux. Length should then be subdivided into the length from the heel to the first metatarsophalangeal joint and the length from the first metatarsophalangeal joint to the toes (Fig. 9.4).

All feet are different and even if the overall shoe length is correct the treadline of the shoe may not correspond with the metatarsophalangeal joints. This will result in the foot trying to flex at a point where the shoe is designed to limit flexion. If the treadline of the shoe is too far proximal for foot flexion the shoe will acquire additional toe spring from the foot flexion point and the vamp will crease excessively. If it is too far distal the toe spring of the shoe will be depressed by the foot and lead to cramping of the toes. The heel to ball measurements vary amongst manufacturers and it is often worthwhile trying various shoes to ensure that the heel to ball length is adequate.

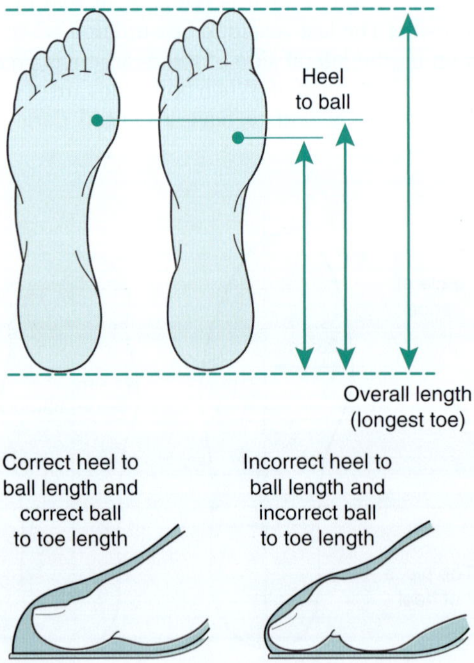

Figure 9.4 The length of the foot; heel to ball measurement.

Shoe width increases incrementally with length and patients with wide feet often choose shoes that are too long for them to obtain adequate width. This also means that the metatarsophalangeal joints will be positioned proximal to the shoe treadline and shoe flexion will not correspond to foot flexion and the shoe will acquire additional toe spring and the vamp will crease. If the shoe contains a shank, the shank may break through the outersole. This is because the relationship between the heel height and the treadline has been changed as the foot requires the shoe to flex in a more proximal position than it was designed to do (Fig. 9.5).

The shoe should be of correct width and girth at the metatarsal heads and of correct girth at the instep. Several other girth measurements need to be matched if the shoe is to fit properly (Fig. 9.6). The long heel measurement is perhaps one of the most important in obtaining a good fit and it dictates the positioning of the instep fastening. It is also necessary to remember that the shoe needs to change shape with the foot in gait. The time of the day when taking measurements is also important since normal daytime changes result in a 3% increase in foot volume (Janisse et al 1995) and vigorous exercise can cause an increase in foot volume by 8% (Merriman & Tollafield 1997). The shoe should be large enough to allow for changes in dimension as the day progresses and should also allow for changes in volume required by variation in hosiery, activity, or to accommodate dressings/padding where needed. If the patient needs to wear orthoses, the shoe needs to be able to accommodate them. The shoe should be of adequate width and depth and there should be no localised tight spots. The heel of the shoe should be broad based for stability on heel contact. There should be a functional fastening to hold the foot back in the shoe and to prevent impaction of the toes against the front of the shoe. The topline of the shoe should fit snugly and should not gape. It should not irritate the malleoli or Achilles tendon.

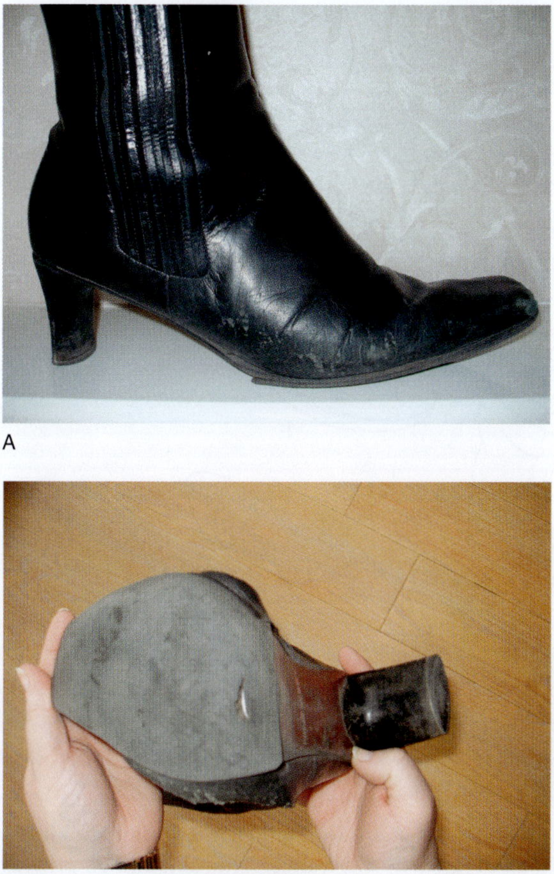

A

B

Figure 9.5 **A** A fashion boot which has acquired additional toe spring due to the foot flexion point being more proximal than the shoe treadline. **B** The shank has broken through the outersole of this shoe as a result of foot flexion taking place at a point proximal to the treadline of the shoe. The resultant relationship between the heel height and the treadline has been altered by foot function.

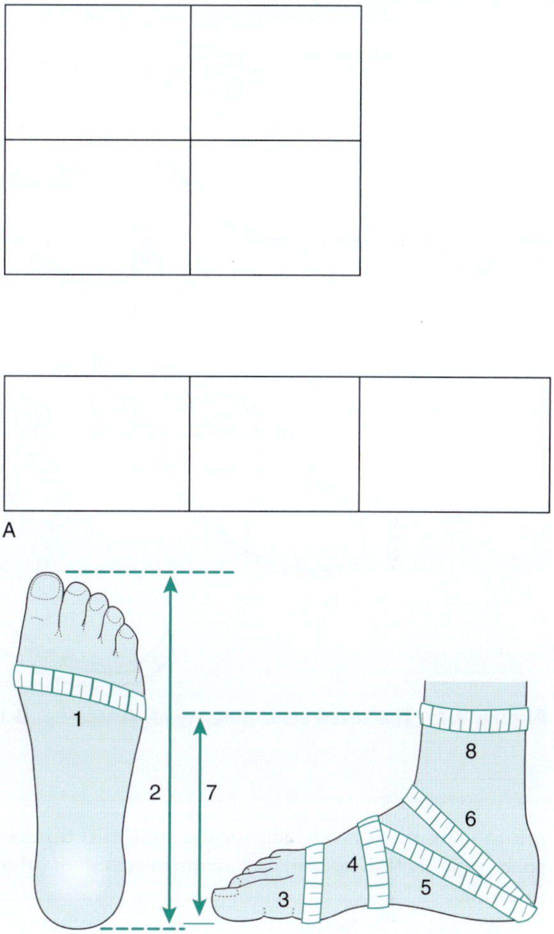

A

B

Figure 9.6 **A** The difference between width and girth: the boxes have the same girth measurement (8 units), but the top one has a width of 2 units and the lower one a width of 3 units. **B** Points at which measurements should be taken to ensure adequate shoe fit: 1 and 3 – joint girth, 2 – foot length, 4 – instep girth, 5 – long heel measurement, 6 – short heel measurement. Measurements 7 and 8 are required for boots: 7 is the boot height and 8 the leg circumference.

Shoe style

There are seven basic shoe styles (Fig. 9.7). The choice of shoe style should be based on the fact that the foot changes in dimension during the various stages of the gait cycle. If the shoe is to be large enough to accommodate the fully loaded foot then it will need to be strapped or laced onto the foot otherwise it will fall off during the swing phase of the gait cycle when the foot is unloaded and of different dimension. Slip-on or court shoes will need to be wedged onto the foot and if they are to stay on the foot during the swing phase they will be too small for the fully loaded foot. They only stay on the foot by a gripping action of the toes. This can lead to the development of corn or callus on prominent toe joints and in some cases can lead to toe deformities through the constant clawing action. Functional straps or laces provide a mechanism for holding the foot back in the shoe and

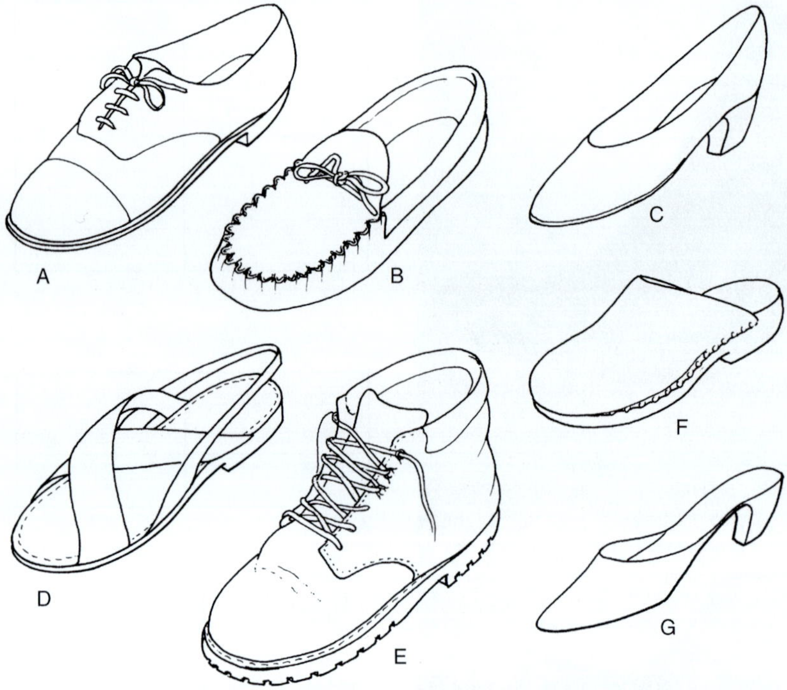

Figure 9.7 The seven basic shoe styles: **A** lace-up, **B** moccasin, **C** court, **D** sandal, **E** boot, **F** clog and **G** mule.

minimising the forward slip of the foot into the toe space of the shoe causing compression of the forefoot.

The heel is the first part of the foot to contact the ground during gait and the heel of the shoe needs to form a firm base for ground contact and for stability in gait. The heel part of the upper (the quarter) needs to be firm to hold and contain the soft tissue surrounding the calcaneus. If this fails the soft tissue will be exposed to excessive tensile stress during heel contact, or splaying over the edge of an open-backed sandal or mule-style shoe, and can result in heel callus or fissures.

The heel height should ideally be about 2.5 cm but no more than 4 cm. The higher the heel the greater the forward displacement of body mass onto the metatarsal heads. An elevated heel also has the effect of changing the body's centre of gravity, and to compensate for this the ankles plantarflex (passively) and there is reduced supination at push off. In addition, the stance knee and hips flex resulting in reduced swing knee flexion (De Lateur et al 1991, Esenyel et al 2003, Gefen et al 2002, Lee et al 1990). There may then be a compensatory action in the lumbar spine. This can lead to discomfort and to arthritic changes in the affected joints. The same basic principles apply to children's footwear with one additional feature, that of growth allowance. The amount of growth allowance will depend on the child's foot length. This will be less in small sizes and up to 14 mm in larger children's sizes.

Footwear should allow free movement of the toes and should be of good fit with adequate length and with quarters of adequate height and shape to grip the heel. It should have good contact with the surface of the foot, and should cradle the foot at this point. The shoe should absorb humidity, limit any increase in foot temperature and be of low weight. In 2002 Brazil became the first country to develop norms for footwear comfort and identified the following factors (World Footwear 2006):

- Mass (weight) of shoe
- Plantar pressure distribution
- Internal temperature control
- Weight carrying capability
- Pronation angle control
- Fitting (individual perception).

See Table 9.2 and **Figure 9.8** for other identified features of a 'good' shoe.

Table 9.2 Assessing shoe fit

Position	*Assessment*	*Possible problems*
First MTPJ (heel to ball length)	The first MTPJ should be located at the widest part of shoe where the shoe flexes	If the joint is situated distal to this point it will result in depressed toe spring and cramping of toes. If it is proximal to this point it will result in additional acquired toe spring and creasing of the vamp
MTPJ width	Adequate width across the joints within the shoe – try to evaluate the fit by running your hand across the upper. Ensure that the foot is not under pressure	Inadequate width will cause compression of tissues, corns, calluses and possible bursitis
Shoe length	The shoe length should allow all toes to lie flat and contain an allowance for extension of foot during walking (10 mm in adults and up to 14 mm in children)	Cramping of toes, foot deformity
Mid-foot	Snug fit, laces parallel when fastened, other fastening correctly placed. Ensure that there is room for adjustment to accommodate any swelling	Too slack a fit will result in the shoe slipping during gait. Too tight a fit may impede circulatory function and irritate dorsum of the foot
Heel	Snug fit with the shape of the shoe reflecting that of the heel. Heel grip can be checked by fastening the shoe on the foot and gently pulling on the back of the shoe so that any slip can be detected	Excessive space at back of the shoe suggests that it is too large and will slip during gait causing the toes to claw in an attempt to grip the shoe
Top-line	Snug fit. Ensure that the shoe sits neatly against the foot but does not encroach on any bony prominences	Gaping – inappropriate shaping, cutting under the malleoli
Tight spots	There should be no localised tight spots	Bunions, toe deformities, corn, callus
Back seam	Height not excessive to cause irritation over Achilles' tendon	Leads to blistering, bursae, bony anomalies
Rearfoot fit	Snug fit of heel counter to prevent slippage. Ensure that it will not rub or cause blisters	Retro-calcaneal lesions

MPTJ, metatarsophalangeal joint.

Shoe sizing and fitting

Shoes that are likely to cause a problem are the ones that do not fit properly. However, just because a shoe corresponds to the size measured does not necessarily means that it fits. Problems with fit are often multifactorial. Feet are asymmetrical and show anatomical variation (Kippen 2004). It has been estimated that 85% of the population walk around in wrong-sized shoes (Prior 2004). However, the determination of shoe size is not as straightforward as most people perceive. Footwear sizing systems developed in different parts of the world, in different time frames, leading to the difference in shoe sizes that we are familiar with today (Janisse et al 1995). In England shoe sizing started during the reign of Edward II

- Functional fastening
-
- Low wide heel – less than 2.5 cm
- Firm heel counter – curved for close fit around the heel
- Top-line curves under malleoli but high enough for adequate fixation, no gaping
- Deep, round or square toe box with at least 1 cm between longest toe and end of shoe when standing
- No localised tight spots, e.g. over hammer toe
- Upper–strong, breathable material
- Cushioned, shock absorbing, slip resistant sole
- Suitable for the activity it is being worn for and for the individual wearing it

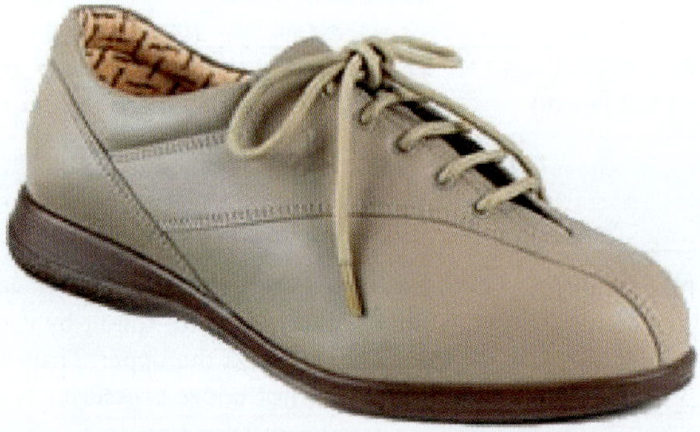

Figure 9.8 Some features of a 'good' shoe (Hughes 1995, Münzenberg 1985, Williams 2005).

where sizes were equated with barleycorns. Over time this evolved to the current measurement of ⅓ inch equating to a shoe size. The English size system starts from a length of 4 inches with the unit of increase between whole sizes being ⅓ of an inch. Children's shoes start at a size 0 of 4 inches and go through to a size 13 (8⅓ inches) Adults sizes then continue from a size 1 (8⅔ inches in length) upwards. The system includes half sizes. The American sizing system has the same unit of increase but starts from size 0 at 3¹¹⁄₁₂ inches. However, in this system sizes are marked up by about 1.5 sizes and become decimalised so a size 4 English becomes 5.5 American.

The Continental or Paris Point system has a unit of increase of ⅔ cm without interruption, starting from 0. The Japanese or Centimetre Size System starts at 0 with a unit of increase of 1 cm with half sizes at 5 mm. **Figure 9.9** compared shoe length measurements and helps explain why there is confusion over shoe sizes.

Even within the same sizing system there is little equity between the various devices which are used to measure length. A particular device from a specific footwear manufacturer may be representative of the size required for that make of shoe but may not be representative for others. It is therefore important that size is taken as a guide and that patients do not rigidly adhere to a given size. This is because the size given will also include a styling allowance which may not be the same even between footwear from the same manufacturer. For example toe shape may dictate that a larger size shoe is needed to accommodate a narrow, pointed toe box profile.

Shoe construction techniques

A variety of footwear construction methods are used by manufacturers. The construction method will be chosen for the function, style and durability required in the finished shoe. In each method of manufacture there are common features. Once the last has been designed patterns are cut for the uppers. The upper parts are prepared from the chosen materials, stitched together, fastening attached, stiffeners inserted and are secured onto the last. The various construction methods discussed below are then used to secure the outer soling unit to the shoe (Fig. 9.10).

Cemented construction

This construction technique is a traditional method which is now commonly used for women's fashion shoes and men's classic shoes:

1. Upper, lining and inner-sole prepared
2. Cement applied to the lasting edge of the upper and inner-sole
3. Stiffener inserted between the upper and lining, in the heel area (heel counter)
4. Last inserted and insole accurately positioned to feather edge

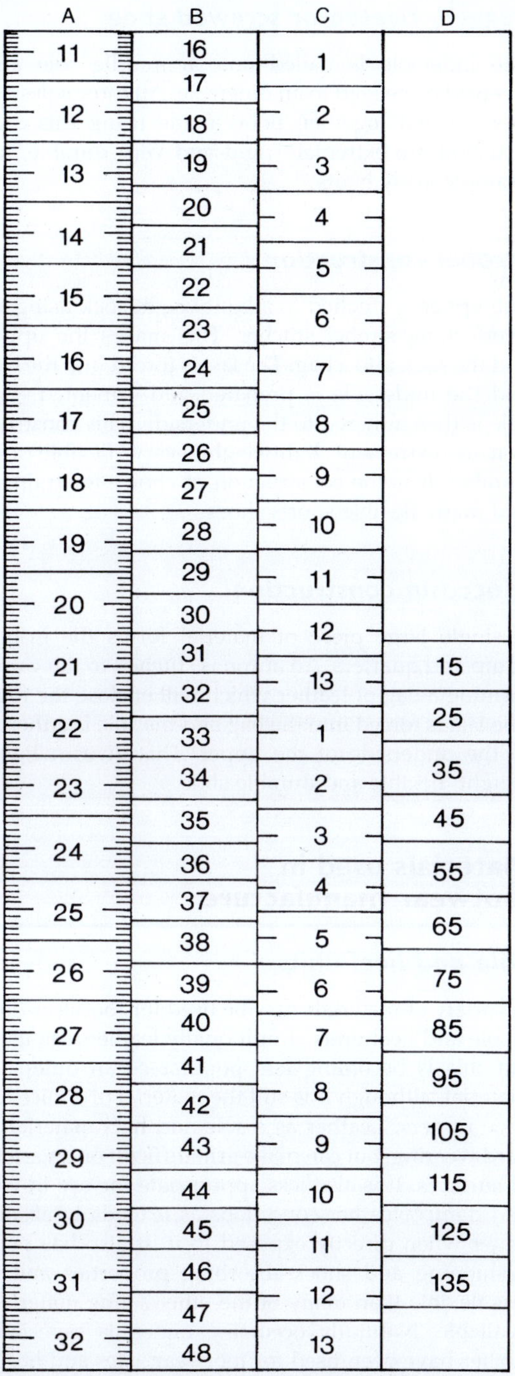

Figure 9.9 Shoe sizing systems: **A** centimetres, **B** Paris Point, **C** English sizes and **D** American women's sizes.

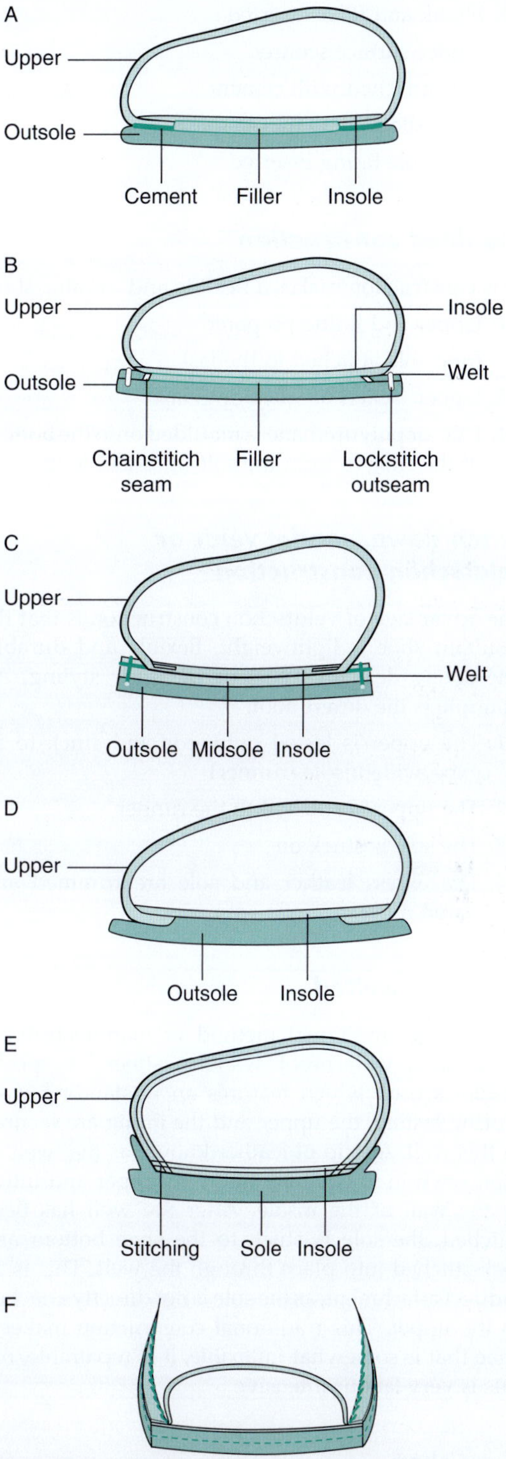

Figure 9.10 Shoe construction: **A** cement, **B** Goodyear, **C** stitchdown, **D** moulded, **E** Strobel-stitched method and **F** stitchdown sandal veldt or veldtschön (field shoe).

5. Shank and filler inserted
6. Under-surface scoured
7. Sole attached with cement
8. Heel attached
9. Innersole lining inserted.

Moulded construction

This construction makes a flexible and durable shoe:

1. Upper and lining prepared
2. Innersole attached to the last
3. Upper tacked or stuck onto last
4. PVC or polyurethane is moulded onto the bottom of the shoe to form the sole and heel unit.

Stitch down, sandal veldt or veldtschön construction

The advantage of veldtschön construction is that the resultant shoe is lightweight, flexible and durable. The soling design is part of the shoe styling. An example is the desert boot:

1. The upper is lasted outwards and stuck to an extra wide insole (runner)
2. The upper is stitched to the runner
3. The sole is stuck on
4. The excess leather and sole are trimmed and pared off.

Machine welted

This is the traditional method of manufacture for well-made, waterproof walking shoes. A special insole is used which features an upstanding wall. During lasting, the upper and the lining are secured to this wall. A strip of leather known as the 'welt' is then sewn in to combine the welt, upper and lining to the wall of the insole. After the welt has been stitched, the sole is stuck to the shoe bottom and lock-stitched into place through the welt. This is an indirect attachment, as the sole is not directly attached to the upper. This traditional construction makes a shoe that is somewhat inflexible; it is repairable, but this is very labour intensive.

Turn shoe

In this construction, the upper is stitched to the sole in a reversed position and then turned inside out to conceal the stitching, for example a ballet shoe.

Pegged, riveted or screwed shoe

The innersole is nailed onto a middle sole and screwed or pegged to an outersole. All three soles are then riveted together. Boots made using this construction are extremely rigid and very durable, for example army boots.

Strobel construction

The upper is stitched to a lightweight sock using an overlocking strobel stitcher. This makes the upper and the sock into a bag. The last is forced into the bag and the underside is prepared and cemented. The sole is then adhered to the underside. This construction is extremely lightweight, very flexible and durable. It is the construction of choice for trainers and many flexible sports shoes.

Moccasin construction

A single large piece of material forms the insole, vamp and quarters. An apron is stitched to the vamp forming a bag of leather which will enclose the foot. The last is forced into the bag and the sole is adhered to the underside of the upper. This gives a lightweight, flexible and durable shoe.

Materials used in footwear manufacture

Sole and heel units

A variety of materials may be used for footwear outersole and heel units. Traditionally leather was used but this is becoming less popular as an outersole material, although it is still the material of choice for shoe uppers. Leather as a sole and heel material is hard wearing, but can make grip difficult on a variety of surfaces. It is also less appropriate for use in wet and damp weather conditions as it tends to absorb water when directly exposed to it. It also has poor cushioning and shock-absorbing properties and is less flexible than many of the other soling materials available. Naturally occurring materials especially rubber have been used for footwear soles and heels, but more commonly synthetics such as ethylene vinyl acetate (EVA), rubber compounds (composition rubber), thermoplastic rubber, and microcellular polyurethane are used. The rubber compounds and polyurethane have the advantage of having good wear properties, flexibility, durability, slip resistance and shock absorption. Microcellular EVA is lightweight and is useful as a mid-sole and for giving improved shock absorption. Table 9.3 lists the common materials used for soling and their properties.

Shoe uppers

Shoe uppers can be made of a variety of materials including cotton, linen, nylon, woven synthetics, plastics and of course leather. Whereas leather may not be the most effective material for soling, it has the advantage over many of the synthetic materials as a shoe upper. It has a unique structure which will allow the passage of moisture vapour from the foot without allowing light rain to penetrate it. This is especially so if treated with appropriate finishes or polishes. Leather has elasticity which means that it has the ability to stretch and recover its original shape, and will so withstand foot flexion without deforming. It also has plasticity which means that it can also be moulded into various shapes and when subjected to heat, moisture and pressure it will retain that shape. As the foot is often warm and damp and the leather is subjected to pressure from the foot it will continue to mould itself to the shape of the foot as it is worn. Leather is durable even though it is a relatively thin material and also has tensile strength which gives it a resistance to permanent creasing. It is also easily cleaned. Few synthetic materials contain all of these properties. When shoes are made of plastic they may be moulded to retain a certain shape but this material lacks the elasticity and permeability

Table 9.3 Properties of soling materials

Soling type	*Recognition*	*Wear merits*	*Use*
Resin rubber	Hard solid rubber, 'heavy' feel, like thick leather soling	Adequate wear performance of thin substances	Men's and women's formal footwear and general
Vulcanised composition rubber	Solid rubber, more resilient than resin rubber	Good to high durability. Good grip and all-round performance	Walking and sports footwear. Industrial applications. School wear
Microcellular EVA	Lightweight, often brightly coloured. Sweet smell	Adequate wear at reasonable thickness, good cushioning	Casual and sports shoes
Microcellular rubber	Medium weight, dull colours. Distinctive smell (sometimes masked by vanilla)	Adequate wear at reasonable thickness, good cushioning	Casuals, lower grades in slipper through soles
PVC	Plastic feel, often has shiny finish. Distinctive smell	Good all round performance	General applications. School wear
Thermoplastic rubber	High friction surface, resilient, often a 'pearly' or crepe appearance. Oily smell	Good wear properties, including slip resistance, especially in cold conditions	General, except for indoor sports (e.g. squash) or oil exposure risks
Microcellular polyurethane	Medium density, resilient. Surface patterns may be 'pin-holed'	Good wear properties, especially durable and grips and cushions well	General purpose, including sports, industrial and school wear
Leather	Usually hard and heavy. Distinctive smell.	Adequate for fashion shoes. Has 'upmarket' appeal	Town shoes
Plantation crepe	Translucent, difficult to distinguish from thermoplastic rubber	Good grip and durability in the highest grades	General purpose, school wear. Degrades on exposure to oil

of leather. Cotton, nylon and woven synthetics can be shaped with the use of folds, gathers and seams but these seams themselves may irritate the foot, and the materials also allow the foot to become wet when worn in rain.

Sports footwear

The production of sports footwear has become a multi-million pound industry. Most people have a pair of trainers even though they may not undertake any sporting activity. Sports shoes have a fashion element, but footwear designed for specific sporting activity does help the feet to function in the most effective way for that activity. All sports footwear has the same basic pattern (Fig. 9.11) but the construction technique used in manufacture will vary according to the type of shoe and the rigidity required within it. The properties of materials used in the various parts of the shoe will vary according to the activity required.

In general when firm footing is required during relatively slow paced walking-type activity the footwear will include fairly rigid soles, stiff heel counters and firm toe puffs. This is the case for golf, rambling, hiking and mountaineering. Where walking over rough terrain is involved such as in rambling and mountaineering, boots are preferred to shoes as they give stability to the ankle joint. The heel counters in such boots will not only be strengthened but will also be extended both proximally from the malleoli and distally through to the mid-foot to give firm control and minimise the likelihood of spraining the ankle. The outer soling of this footwear will contain a ridged pattern to give grip. In the case of golf shoes the outer soling will contain spikes or dimples to hold the feet securely in the turf while the player is taking a shot. Footwear for these activities may also have a selectively permeable lining to allow moisture from the foot to escape while preventing the feet becoming wet from ground conditions and rainfall. The construction methods used in this type of footwear will vary from traditional cemented construction to injection moulding using polyurethane soling materials.

In sports where activity is undertaken at faster speeds the soling will be more flexible to enable the player to move rapidly when necessary. Even footwear for activities such as soccer and rugby will have flexibility in the forefoot. Footwear for rugby still tends to be boot-style, with a higher cut to give ankle support. While this style is good for those who rely on lower body strength for power while scrummaging,

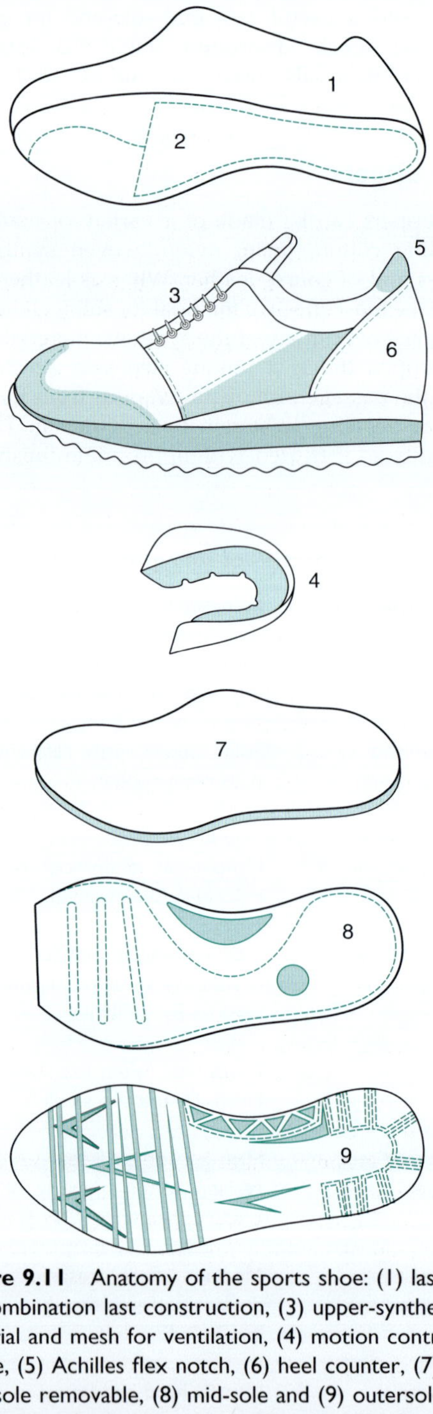

Figure 9.11 Anatomy of the sports shoe: (1) last, (2) combination last construction, (3) upper-synthetic material and mesh for ventilation, (4) motion control device, (5) Achilles flex notch, (6) heel counter, (7) innersole removable, (8) mid-sole and (9) outersole. (Redrawn with permission from Ross JA 2006 Sports medicine and injuries. In: Lorimer D L, French G J, O'Donnell M et al (eds) Neale's disorders of the foot, 7th edn. Churchill Livingstone, Edinburgh.)

some players particularly backs, prefer lower cut soccer-style footwear to give them greater mobility on the pitch. Footwear for soccer is generally low cut with quarter height finishing under the malleoli. All such footwear will have strong heel counters with uppers made either of leather or synthetic material. Leather with its elasticity and plasticity will mould to the foot, but leather uppers can stretch out of shape when worn repeatedly in wet conditions. Synthetic uppers may make the boots lighter and may be cheaper than leather ones. Some manufacturers offer soccer boots with lacing positioned at the side of the boot. This is intended to give a larger top surface area for control of the ball. The outer soling tends to be rigid underneath the heel and midfoot but with flexibility in the forefoot to allow for rapid movement. The soles also contain either screw-in or moulded studs, although boots with soles made up of a series of blades are also available. Blades come in a variety of depths, depending on the model, and some soccer footwear is available with changeable blades. The use of blades is said to make turning easier but concerns have been raised as to whether they increase injuries associated with rapid torsional movements such as knee cruciate ligament injuries.

Shoes for racquet sports again need to be flexible but also need to allow for side-to-side sliding while playing. This side-to-side movement is supported by additional stiffening throughout the medial and lateral borders of the shoe. Shoes for tennis are best with additional reinforcement in the toe box to counter the effect of forefoot drag in the serve follow-though. They also feature a herringbone tread in the outersole to offer greater traction.

The outstanding feature of footwear for faster paced activities is the weight. Shoes for sprinters, hurdlers and those who undertake other track activities are generally extremely lightweight and flexible. The forepart of the outersole contains spikes to maximise performance while running. The spike length may vary according to the activity and the surface on which the athlete is working. Sprint spikes tend to have a slightly stiffer spike plate, distance spikes are more flexible and field spikes are specific to events. For example high jump spikes contain spikes in the heel to ensure traction while planting for the jump. Longer spikes tend to be used when competing on cinder tracks and for cross-country activity and shorter needle spikes are best for rubber-based track surfaces. The uppers of this footwear will tend to be made of mesh and microfibre for lightness and to allow the evaporation of moisture from the foot.

Shoes for running, training and jogging need to have:

- comfortable soft upper
- provide control and stability in the heel
- provide cushioning for the plantar surface of the foot to counter the effects of ground reaction force
- have good traction
- lightweight.

Within these criteria the individual should choose the shoe which is most compatible with their foot shape and foot type. There will be a wide range of choice available for each activity and the clinician should advise their patient on the features of their lower limb biomechanics which should be addressed by the footwear. For example some running shoes will be designed to control pronation and it is helpful for the clinician to be aware of the features of the various styles available so as to advise the patient of the type of shoe to select within the range appropriate for their sport. Needless to say the patients should ensure that the footwear they chose fits them properly following the guidelines for footwear advice in Figure 9.8.

Socks for sporting activity

Sports-specific socks are produced by all major manufacturers. However, this hosiery has certain characteristics which make it appropriate for sports in general rather than specific activity. Socks should be chosen as specific to the shoe rather than the sport itself. The biomechanical movement and stresses of recreational and competitive sporting activities vary greatly but designing socks to mitigate those stresses has resulted in very similar features despite the variety of sporting activity. Double layer socks are useful in reducing blistering as they help to reduce the heat caused by dynamic friction. A variety of materials can be included in the yarn from which the sock is made. Some have a 'wicking' action which draws perspiration away from the skin and allows the foot to remain drier. Socks can also contain material which has shock absorbing capabilities. This varies from a layer of toweling-like fabric to the inclusion of a silicone layer underfoot. Other features include antimicrobial capability which helps reduce foot odour and fungal growth.

The socks to be worn in footwear should be chosen before footwear is fitted to ensure that:

- there is adequate accommodation
- the footwear will not cause damage to the feet because of the additional girth required by the sock.

Therapeutic footwear

Indications for specialist footwear

The need for therapeutic footwear may be dictated by a number of local or systemic conditions or by the fact that a patient's feet are outside the normal size and fitting range of retail footwear. Therapeutic footwear is costly, but is often either the only option available or the most effective way of treating a condition (White 1994). It may be indicated for patients with neurological conditions, connective tissue disorders, endocrine disorders, circulatory impairment, renal pathologies, arthritic conditions, etc.

However, before considering a referral for surgical (orthopaedic) footwear the patient's foot size, shape and biomechanical function should be assessed. It may be that their own footwear can be considered for modification. Once the patient has footwear of a suitable style and material a number of adaptations can be made to it. For example a few millimetres of raise can be added to compensate for a limb length discrepancy, a ball and ring stretcher can be used to stretch leather uppers to accommodate minor problems such as toe deformities or hallux valgus. Tongue pads and heel grips can be included to adjust fitting (Fig. 9.12). Despite these options there will be a few patients whose foot health needs can only be accommodated in specialist footwear.

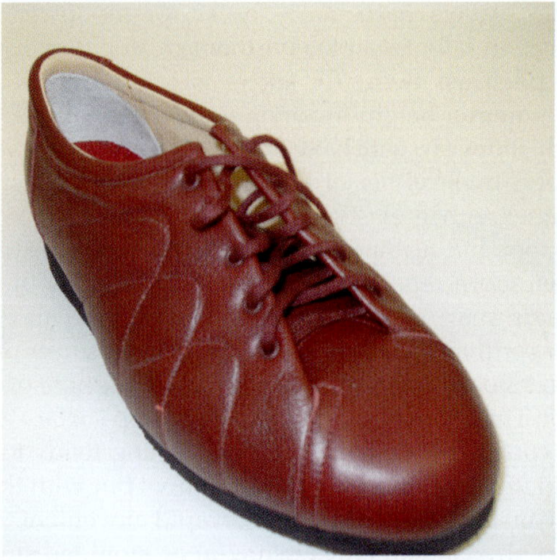

A

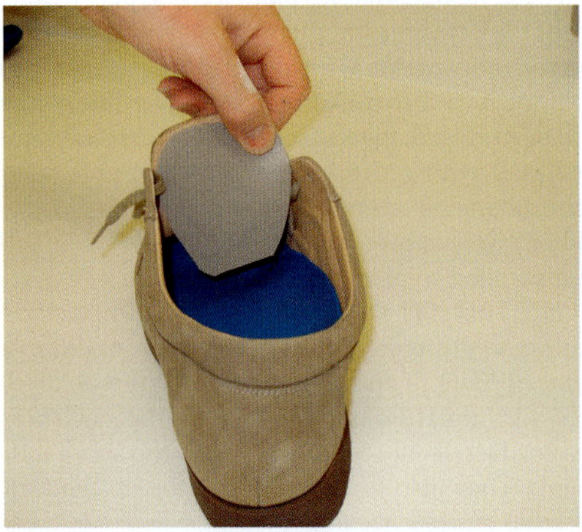

B

Figure 9.12 **A** Adding a heel grip to give a slight length reduction and firmer grip around the heel. **B** Adding a tongue pad.

Several manufacturers provide stock ranges of therapeutic (orthopaedic or surgical) footwear. These shoes are available for immediate delivery. They are in basic colours, usually black or brown, but are made in a wide range of sizes and fittings and at relatively low cost. They are also available on a sale or return basis and so provide an opportunity for the practitioner who is qualified in fitting of stock footwear to fit them on their patient's feet without commitment to purchase. It is possible to fit a high percentage of patients requiring therapeutic footwear from this range. Once a good fitting shoe is identified patients may then move on to footwear made on the same last from the same manufacturer, but in perhaps a different style and colour which would be non-returnable and which would require a financial commitment on ordering the shoes.

For patients whose feet are outside the dimensions of the shoes available from stock, modular or bespoke footwear may be prescribed. For both the modular and bespoke options, complex prescription and precise, detailed instructions need to be given to the shoe manufacturer. Modular footwear involves the modification of a manufacturer's existing last. Additional width, girth, height and length can be added at specific points, for example:

- the inclusion of inserts in the medial quarter to accommodate valgus deformity of the midfoot
- the addition of bunion pockets to accommodate first metatarsal head exostoses
- additional toe box depth to accommodate badly deformed toes
- the inclusion of additional depth in the tarsal region
- an alteration in the height of quarters to prevent irritation on prominent malleoli.

A range of foot deformities can be accommodated within the modular approach but despite the facility to adapt lasts there will be patients with foot shape or deformities which are so severe that modification to existing lasts will not meet their needs. In these cases patients will need fully bespoke footwear and a last will need to be made specifically for each of their feet. This is done by taking plaster of Paris impressions of feet and lower legs and carefully charting a diagram of the foot outline with width and girth measurements identified at specific points on each foot. There is a British Standard for this process (BS5943), which needs to be followed in detail for a successful outcome. Both modular and bespoke footwear is available at a fitting stage so that the patient can try the shoes before they are finished and at a time when modifications can be made to ensure an exact fit.

Footwear success will depend not only on the choice of style and upper material but also upon the choice of sole material and the type of environmental conditions in which the footwear will be worn. Studies on safety footwear (Rowland 1996) show that the wear characteristics of the floor/sole combination must be considered. When prescribing, it is important to consider the patient's occupation and type of activities that the shoe will be used for. For example, certain soling materials may be irreparably damaged by certain chemicals and careful advice needs to be given to patients working in environments where chemicals may spill onto the floor.

In considering the soling material required the lifestyle and activity levels of each patient should be borne in mind. Commando soles with additional grip are helpful for patients who live in rural areas and walk over rough terrain. Certain activities require special soling styles, such as playing bowls where a through wedged sole and heel unit is needed. A lightweight and smooth surfaced outersole and heel could be ideal for a lightweight person with a shuffling gait.

Heels and sole choices can also be invaluable when combating postural instability. A wide heel base leads to more stability than a narrow heel. Narrow heels have been implicated in falls within the elderly community (Rubenstein et al 1988). Certain features can be added to the heel to increase stability. If there are problems with a leg-length discrepancy then a raised sole on the shorter side can be used. Rocker or roller bottom soles are useful to increase the rapidity of the mid stance phase of the gait cycle and to limit the movement at the MTP joints (Wu et al 2004). However, a rocker or roller is only beneficial if the sole of the shoe is not flexible.

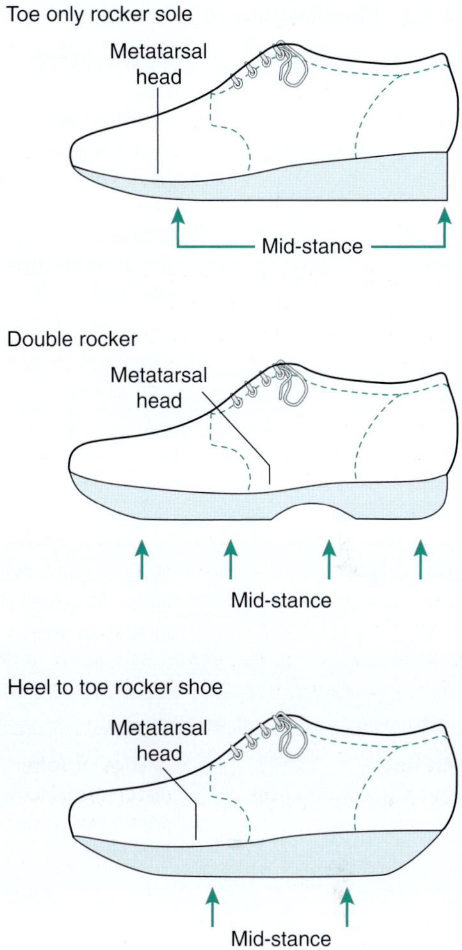

Figure 9.13 Types of rocker sole.

With rocker soles it is important to be aware that there is considerable variation in their effects among individuals, including reduction of forefoot pressures and, therefore, careful consideration must be given when prescribing or assessing rockers for patients (Brown et al 2004, Fuller et al 2001, Hsi et al 2004, Schaff & Cavanagh 1990, Stacpoole-Shea et al 1999, Van Schie et al 2000). Ideally, assessment for rockers should include plantar pressure measurements, but where this is not possible close monitoring of patients following the issue of rocker soled footwear is essential.

A complete discussion of heel and sole modifications available in therapeutic footwear is beyond the scope of this chapter. Some of the common modifications are shown in Figure 9.13 and Table 9.4.

Table 9.4 Modifications to sole and heel

Adaptations	*Where applied*	*Function*	*Use*
Thomas heel Reverse Thomas heel 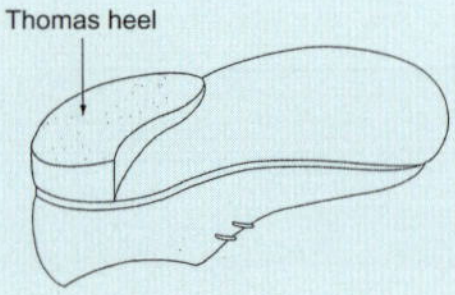	Medial extension to anterior aspect of heel. Or in the case of reverse Thomas heel a lateral extension to the anterior aspect of the heel	Control of excessive subtalar and midfoot motion. Control excessive supinatory forces	Control pronation or supination. Prevent recurrent ankle sprains
Heel flares 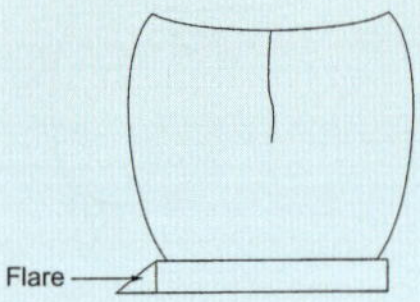	Extension to either side of heel	Correctional moment of force at heel strike. Alter lever arm of ground reaction force	Useful for inversion pathologies (lateral) or eversion pathologies, Charcot neuroarthropathy (medial)
Sole wedges 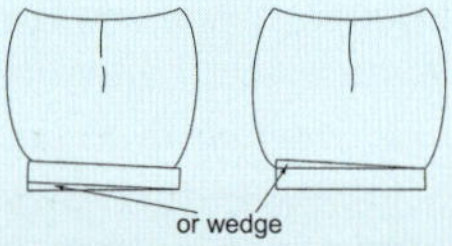	Wedge applied to entire length of shoe or just an area	Achieve tilting of shoe and alter resting foot position	Polio, stroke, Charcot
Sach heel Solid ankle cushion heel 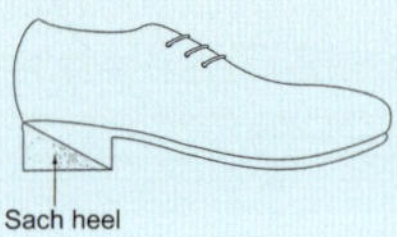	Wedge of softer material replaces portion of posterior heel base	Reduces shock at heel strike and compensates for the absence of ankle motion	Not commonly used today, but occasionally used after ankle fusion
Rocker sole See Figure 9.13	Addition to the sole in curved manner, may be added to forefoot alone, to entire shoe or heel	Alter forward progression of the ground reaction force so loads can be taken off susceptible metatarsal heads. Enables roll off	Hallux rigidus, diabetes, pathologies affecting sagittal plane motion, e.g. arthritis
Shoe raise 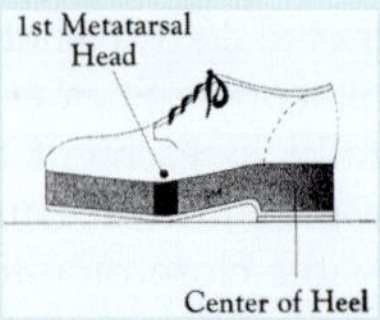	Addition made to entire sole but up to 12 mm may be added to heel before it is necessary to raise the sole	Level hips	Leg length inequality

Heels

Heel height

It has long been understood that there is a relationship between forefoot loading and heel height. The higher the heel, the greater is the forefoot loading and the lighter the heel loading. This should be borne in mind when considering footwear as a therapy for the treatment of foot pathologies (Broche et al 2004). Normal heel height for therapeutic footwear is between 2 cm and 4 cm and averages at 2.5 cm (1 inch). Certain pathological states will require the prescription of a higher than normal heel height.

Consideration also needs to be given to ankle mobility. Limitation of ankle movement due to arthritis, spasticity, or surgery may require the heel height of the prescribed shoe to be altered. Heel height is measured from the point vertically beneath the lateral malleolus. The depth of sole material should be excluded from this measurement as the soling depth runs thoughout the shoe, some common heel modifications are included in Table 9.4.

Using orthoses in shoes

Footwear is a major consideration when prescribing orthoses and the footwear in which the orthoses are intended to be worn should be evaluated before confirming any orthotic prescription. There are several criteria which should be borne in mind.

First careful consideration should be given to the shoe construction itself. Any insert is likely to affect the quality of fit delivered by the shoe. The aim should be to accommodate the orthotic and allow it to perform its prescribed function without impairing the fitting qualities of the host shoe.

If there is a removable innersole or foot bed inside the shoe this might be removed to provide some additional accommodation to house the orthoses. If the footwear is available in half sizes it might be worthwhile evaluating the next half size larger to see if this will give improved fit once an orthotic is placed within it. Consider the shoe construction. Some shoes made by Strobel construction do not use shanks or heel stiffeners of significant strength. Will the inclusion of an orthotic cause stresses within the shoe that may be beyond its design tolerance? To determine this it is necessary to carefully evaluate the orthotic and shoe during gait. Carefully review the functioning and fit of the shoe to ensure that the fitting criteria are met and that the shoe is not distorted by the orthotic.

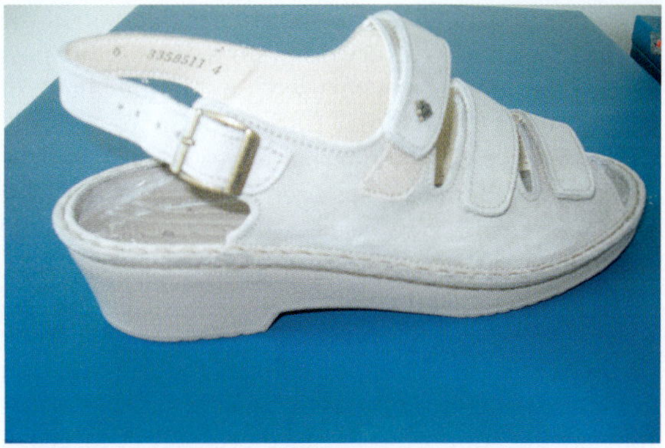

Figure 9.14 Sandal containing a well in which an orthotic may be accommodated.

The shoe heel height must be considered and only in rare circumstances should orthoses be prescribed for a shoe with a heel height of more than 4 cm. The footwear should have an adjustable fastening, deep toe box, and a deep heel counter or well in which the orthoses may sit. Shoes should also have deep sides in the instep area or contain a well where the orthoses may sit. The presence of a heel counter and quarters covering the instep area are important to hold the orthoses in place. Footwear without these features includes sandals and mules. Although orthoses should not be used in mules, sandals with a well can accommodate an orthotic with a low heel cup (Fig. 9.14).

Forensic podiatry

> *Wherever he steps, whatever he touches, whatever he leaves even unconsciously, will serve as silent witness against him. Only human failure to find it, study it and understand it, can diminish its value*
>
> Kirk quoted by Bodziak (2000)

Forensic podiatry involves trying to determine whether a foot impression, foot mark or wear pattern was made by a specific foot. It is a growing area of scientific study and investigation. The first report of a chiropodist being involved in a forensic investigation occurred in 1935. Since that date it has begun to develop into a more exact science (Vernon 1995). The use of podiatric evidence in criminal cases is generally circumstantial. Although it may be possible to identify that an impression at a crime scene was made by a particular shoe and that the shoe belongs to a specific individual, providing conclusive evidence that the shoe was worn by the person at the time of the crime is a very different matter. In the past forensic evidence has focused on identification of marks made by external forces but more recently those marks made by internal forces such as by biomechanical anomalies has been assessed. After all, it is in footwear that we see the result of the dynamic activity of gait.

In compiling a forensic investigation whether it is related to identification of disaster victims or crime scene studies investigation will include impression evidence made by the weightbearing surface of the foot on the supporting surface (Vernon et al 2004). The intensity of this impression on a surface may help determine the body mass of an individual or identify whether an individual may have been carrying a heavy load. Similarly the distance between steps may be of significance in determining cadence. The extent of the impression may give some information about the speed of walking or running.

When a shoe is manufactured it is not designed to wear in a particular manner. The nature and the degree of that wear are dependent on a persons individual characteristics including gait, body mass, occupation, etc. Certain shoe factors also contribute to wear including the shoe style, materials used, construction technique, last shape and the surfaces over which the shoe is worn. There is more and more interest in using footwear as an aid in police investigations and many inferences can be drawn from footwear imprints. Of interest also is the identification of individual footprints. Each is unique. It can provide evidence of biomechanical effects, structural characteristics such as toe deformities, foot size may give a general guide as to individual height, ethnic features in the form of general foot shape.

Wear marks

Wear marks give an indication of shoe–foot interaction during gait and demonstrate the location of pressure areas. They are best seen in well-worn shoes constructed using traditional construction methods and made of leather. The advent of synthetic, durable soling material with heavy tread patterns makes it much more difficult to evaluate the outersole for wear. However the upper, lining, inlay (innersole) as well as the outersole can all give valuable information about the wearer, their dynamic gait, foot pathology and the environment in which they are active. The shoe uppers will crease and deform according to pressure and abnormal frontal, transverse, or sagittal plane motion during gait. If the foot is functioning normally and is in a well-fitting shoe the foot and shoe should work together as a unit.

The wear marks on the upper should comprise of a crease across the vamp where the foot flexes during gait. Other marks may be related to activity, for example kicking a ball or operating machinery, or related to a foot pathology such as toe deformities or exostoses. The heel of the upper should be examined for distortion. The seam at the back of the heel should be straight with no medial or lateral bulging of the counter. In the case of patients with conditions causing a high degree of sub-talar joint pronation the entire upper becomes distorted. The alteration to the topline is caused by adduction and plantarflexion of the talus with the medial shift of the navicular, while the bulge on the medial heel counter is caused by the tilting of the calcaneus (**Fig. 9.15**).

The lining of the shoe will wear in areas where it has been subjected to most friction. Examples of this include: the area overlying the hallux where it is hyper-extended or in cases of onychogryphosis; over the fifth toe with abduction of the forefoot; over the area of the medial eminence of the first metatarsal head in hallux valgus. It is also advisable to examine the heel lining. The most significant wear may be seen on the medial aspect in cases of hyper-pronation where the calcaneus tilts.

Wear marks on the innersole are valuable in assessing shoe fit and excesses of plantar pressure. Where the innersole is removable it may be worthwhile removing it to examine the position of the toes and evaluating the adequacy of the length of the shoe. The width may also be assessed by identifying the positions of the first and fifth metatarsal heads. Areas of excessive pressure will have caused some compression of the innersole or discoloration.

The pressure on the outersole should be fairly evenly distributed so that no one part wears excessively. When looking at the outersole remember that exaggerated wear marks indicate that an area is taking more pressure. A smooth transfer of load from the heel to the forefoot following a centre of pressure line should create normal shoe wear (Hughes 1995). Due to the determinants of gait normal activity will produce wear on the posterior lateral section of the heel, across the tread line, under the ends of the toes and at the tip of the sole of the shoe. Patterns that vary from this can be considered abnormal but before drawing conclusions it is important to remember that some patterns may be indicators of poor shoe fit rather than a true reflection of foot pathology.

The wear occurring under the toes and at the tip should be light in comparison with wear at the heel and under the metatarsophalangeal joints. The extent

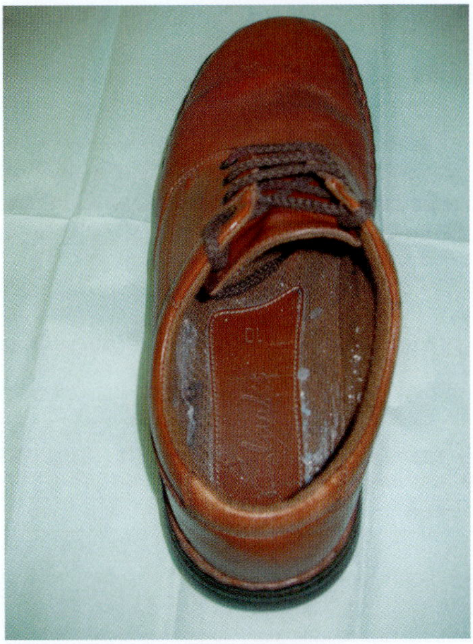

A

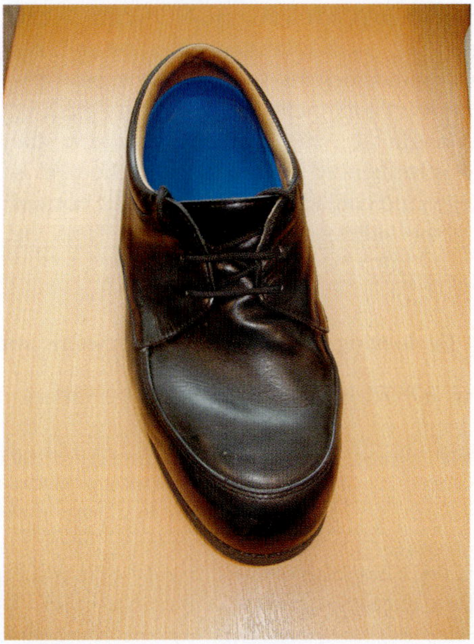

C

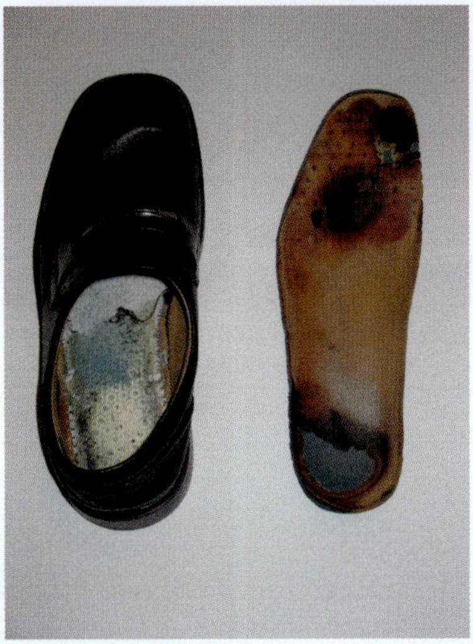

B1

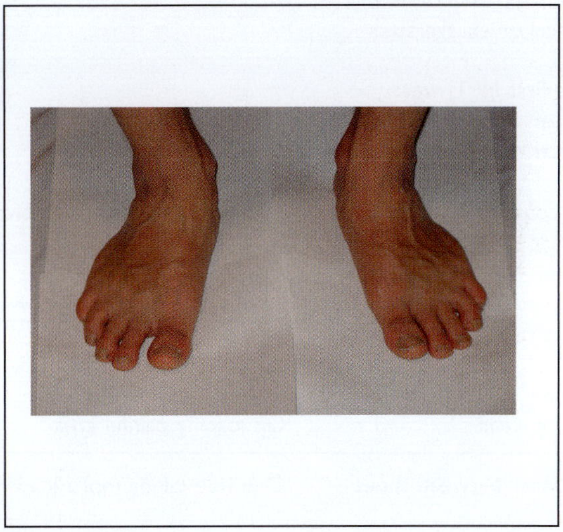

B2

Figure 9.15 **A** Deformation of the shoe topline as a result of pronatory forces. B1 shows the wear marks in footwear worn by the patient photographed at B2. This is a case of tibia varum with mid-tarsal joint pronation and functional hallux limitus. Note that the throat of the shoe is distorted, there is creasing and distortion of the vamp on the medial side with heavy wear at the heel, across the treadline and under the hallux. Also note lateral wear marks on the heel of the insole, under the central plantar metatarsal area and distally under the toes. **C** Abnormal creasing of the vamp in hallux rigidus. Note the flexion on the upper runs from the fifth metatarsophalangeal joint to the interphalangeal joint of the hallux.

to which the toes bear load in normal individuals can vary considerably, but as wear under the toes reduces the tip wear should increase so it is wise to read the two wear marks in conjunction. The wear on the heel reflects the angle at which the heel contacts the ground and is influenced by the fact that the heel is inverted on ground contact as a component of normal late swing phase subtalar joint supination. Thus the wear mark appears on the posterior-lateral part of the heel top piece. In the foot which is pronated throughout the gait cycle the main heel wear mark will be posterior-central. Where the foot strikes the ground in an inverted position and where subtalar supination is constant the wear mark will be lateral (e.g. cavus foot), but where excessive subtalar joint pronation occurs during the mid stance phase of gait

Table 9.5 Evaluating wear marks in footwear: some commonly seen patterns and possible causes

Area of wear – outersole	*Possible cause*	*Seen in*
Excessive tip wear	Insufficient toe spring, shoe flexing in wrong position, shoe too long for foot, loss of toe function	Forefoot instability, cavus foot with retracted toes
Insufficient wear on posterior part of sole + excessive tip wear	Heel–ball length too short, whole shoe too short	
Slight curvature on undersurface of sole not apparent/non-symmetrical or exaggerated	Abnormal toe function	Reduced toe function + short stride length
Excessive first MPTJ wear +ve wear along inner aspect +ve wear outer aspect		Plantarflexed first ray Everted forefoot Inverted forefoot
Circular contact wear marks +ve wear lateral margin heel +ve wear medial heel margin	Metatarsal being used as pivot	Fifth MPTJ with mid-tarsal break Inverted hindfoot/genu varum Everted hindfoot/genu valgum
Outside of heel + inner side of sole		Out-toed gait(external rotation of hip)
Absence of wear	Off loading painful area	
Unequal wear between shoes	One side taking more load	Leg length discrepancy, occupational characteristics
	The upper can also deform in characteristic ways	
Excessive oblique crease		Hallux rigidus
Deformation of upper/medial border		Hallux abductor valgus
Bulges in toe puffs		Hammer/claw toes
Medial border prominence		Over-pronated/flat foot
Scuffed toes		Drop foot deformity

MPTJ, metatarsophalangeal joint.

there will also be a wear mark on the anterior-medial aspect of the heel top-piece. Some of the factors contributing to abnormal wear patterns are given in Table 9.5.

Shoe wear is not always considered in a standard patient assessment and thus a useful diagnostic tool is being missed. If shoes are excessively worn they may actually be causing the patient's foot pathology. So when should a patient discard a pair of shoes?

- If any part of the sole becomes so thin that the cushioning capability is lost.
- If the heel becomes worn so that normal heel contact is jeopardised.
- If the fastening becomes non-functional.
- If the heel counter is so distorted it no longer supports the calcaneus.
- If the lining is damaged causing soft-tissue irritation.

Patient concordance

While we may know what advice to give our patients about footwear this will be of little benefit to their foot health if they do not use it. We may identify footwear as the cause of pathology and be able to advise the patient of the means of resolving their foot problems, but unless the patient is willing to heed the advice and to act on it little will be achieved.

Concordance with footwear advice is generally considered to be low. Research has been undertaken into the use of prescribed footwear but little evidence exists about the success of therapeutic strategies which require the patients to change their footwear and provide themselves with shoes which meet their foot health needs. Both patient and practitioner expectations of what the footwear should achieve require discussion to ensure the footwear is appropriate to that specific patient. What the patient thinks is the most important element of their footwear may differ from the practitioner's view. For example the style and colour may be the most important aspect to the patient but the practitioner would believe that the fit is more important. Irrespective of the style, the fit and size must be appropriate otherwise shoes will cause problems such as rubbing and blistering, which in the neuropathic foot could be the cause of a break in the epithelium, leading to ulceration (Veves et al 1992).

It is important for the practitioner to appreciate that the patient has their own perception of their health. They may not consider their foot condition to be of significance. They may not relate their foot problem to their footwear despite evidence to the contrary. They may not wish to purchase appropriate footwear; or wear prescribed footwear. The clinician will have to consider:

- perceived susceptibility – does the patient believe their condition has risk and do they understand that their foot lesion is related to their footwear?
- perceived severity – does the patient understand/accept the severity of their condition. Do they appreciate that it will not improve unless they modify their footwear choice?
- perceived benefits – is the patient able to recognise the benefits of the treatment/course of action proposed to address their condition?
- perceived barriers – what might be the problems perceived by the patient in adopting the treatment/course of action?
- cues to action – what will prompt the patient to remain true to their health belief and treatment?
- self-efficacy – how will the patient make this happen?

Conclusion

Footwear is not just a fashion item and not solely a protection for the feet. In its various forms footwear can facilitate activity, improve mobility, become an effective therapy, reduce morbidity, and improve and extend quality of life. To ensure that footwear is optimal the clinician needs to understand how the normal foot functions when shod and how the shoe may have contributed to any pathology present. Footwear should be regarded as part of both our diagnostic and our therapeutic strategies.

References

Bodziak W 2000 Footwear impression evidence, detection recovery and examination. CRC Press, Boca Raton, FL

Broche N, Wyller T, Steen H 2004 Effects of heel height and shoe shape on the compressive load between foot and base. Journal of the American Podiatric Medical Association 94:461–469

Brown D, Wertsch J, Harris G et al 2004 Effect of rocker soles on plantar pressures. Archives of Physical Medicine and Rehabilitation 85:81–86

De Lateur B, Giaconi R, Qestad K et al 1991 Footwear and posture. Compensatory strategies for heel height. American Journal of Physical Medicine and Rehabilitation 70:246–54

Esenyel M, Walsh K, Walden J et al 2003 Kinetics of high heeled gait. Journal of the American Podiatric Medical Association 93(1):27–32

Fuller E, Schroeder S, Edwards J 2001 Reduction of peak pressure on the forefoot with a rigid rocker-bottom post-operative shoe. Journal of the American Podiatric Medical Association 91:501–507

Gefen A, Megido M, Itzchak Y et al 2002 Analysis of muscular fatigue and foot stability during high heeled gait. Gait and Posture 15:56–63

Goonetilleke R, Luximon A 2001 Designing for comfort: a footwear application. In: Das B, Karwowski W, Mondelo P (eds) Proceedings of the Computer-Aided Ergonomics and Safety Conference. Available at: www-ieem.ust.hk/dfaculty/ravi/papers/caes.pdf (accessed 20 December 2007)

Hsi W, Chai H, Lai J 2004 Evaluation of rocker sole by pressure-time curves in insensate forefoot during gait. American Journal of Physical Medicine and Rehabilitation 83:500–506

Hughes J R 1995 Footwear assessment. In: Merriman L M, Tollafield D R (eds) Assessment of the lower limb. Churchill Livingstone, Edinburgh

Janisse D, Wertsch J, Del Toro 1995 Foot orthoses and prescription shoes. In: Redford J, Basmajian J, Trautman P (eds) Orthotics: clinical practice and rehabilitation technology. Edinburgh, Churchill Livingstone

Kippen C 2004 The history of shoes: shoe making podiatry. Available at: http://podiatry.curtin.edu.au/shoo.html (accessed 7 December 2007)

Lee K, Shieh J, Matteliano A et al 1990 Electromyographic changes of leg muscles with heel lifts in women. Archives of Physical Medicine and Rehabilitation 71(1):31–33

Menz H, Lord S, McIntosh A 2001 Slip resistance of casual footwear: implications for falls in older adults. Gerontology 47:145–149

Merriman L, Tollafield D 1997 Clinical skills in treating the foot. Edinburgh, Churchill Livingstone

Münzenburg K J 1985 The orthopaedic shoe, indications and prescription. In: Orthopaedic elements: actions and indications. Deutsche Bibliotheck Verlagsgesellschaft mbh, Germany, pp 15–43

Prior T 2004 quoted by Bestick L in Try this for size, The Times, 21 April

Ross J A 2006 Sports medicine and injuries. In: Lorimer D L, French G J, O'Donnell M et al (eds) Neale's disorders of the foot, 7th edn. Churchill Livingstone, Edinburgh

Rowland F, Jones C, Manning D 1996 Surface roughness of footwear soling materials: relevance to slip resistance. Journal of Testing and Evaluation 24(6)

Rubenstein L, Robbins A, Schulman B et al 1988 Falls and instability in the elderly. Journal of the American Geriatrics Society 36:266–278

Schaff P, Cavanagh P 1990 Shoes for the insensitive foot: the effect of a 'rocker bottom' shoe modification on plantar pressure distribution. Foot & Ankle International 11:129–140

Stacpoole-Shea S, Shea A, Armstrong D et al 1999 Do rocker soles reduce plantar pressure in persons at risk for diabetic neuropathic ulceration. Proceedings of the Foot Pressure Interest Group, Leeds

Van Schie C, Albrecht J, Becker M et al 2000 Design criteria for rigid rocker shoes. Foot & Ankle International 21:833–44

Vernon D 1995 The use of chiropody records in forensic and mass disaster identification. Journal of British Podiatric Medicine 50;12:196–200

Vernon W, Parry A, Potter M 2004 Theory of shoe wear pattern influence incorporating a new paradigm for the podiatric medical profession. Journal of the American Podiatric Medical Association 94:261–268

Veves A, Murrey H, Young M et al 1992 The risk of foot ulceration in diabetic patients with high foot pressure: a prospective study. Diabetologia 35(7):660

White J 1994 Custom shoe therapy current concepts, designs and special considerations. Clinics in Podiatric Medicine and Surgery 11:2259–2269

Williams A 2005 Interested in footwear? You should be. Podiatry Now 8,6:32–33

World Footwear, May/June 2006. Norms for Shoe Comfort, pp 46–47

Wu W, Rosenbaum D, Su F 2004. The effects of rocker soles and SACH heels on kinematics in gait. Medical Engineering and Physics 26(8):639–646

CHAPTER

10

Musculoskeletal assessment

Indicates figures on DVD, including colour

Indicates video of assessment on DVD

Chapter contents

Section 10A: Orthopaedic assessment of the lower limb

B Ribbans

Introduction

A thorough musculoskeletal assessment of the whole limb is an essential component of evaluation of a patient's specific and often localised lower limb complaint. Apparent localised foot and ankle problems may have a genesis in proximal regions or, conversely, have secondary untoward effects on other structures. Such an assessment involves both static and dynamic assessment of musculoskeletal function.

Movement of the lower limb involves interaction between the musculoskeletal and nervous systems. The function of both systems can be compromised by vascular pathology. This chapter concentrates on the orthopaedic assessment of the musculoskeletal system. The assessment of the vascular system is covered in Chapter 6 and the neurological basis of movement and assessment of the nervous system are covered in Chapter 7. As the healthcare practitioner becomes competent, experienced and confident, essential components of these three systems will be evaluated seamlessly during the patient evaluation. Although reference is made to the weightbearing examination during this chapter, this subject, including gait analysis, is covered in greater detail in section 10B (functional assessment).

The assessment process begins with a detailed history of the patient's complaint. Subsequent examination of the limbs is based on an approach following the methodology outlined by McRae (2004):

- general observation of the patient
- specific joint observation
- palpation
- examination of movements
- performance of specific tests.

Qualitative, semiquantitative and quantitative measurement techniques are used. The practitioner should be aware of the likely errors that can ensue from such measurements and take these into consideration when interpreting and analysing data from the assessment (see Ch. 4).

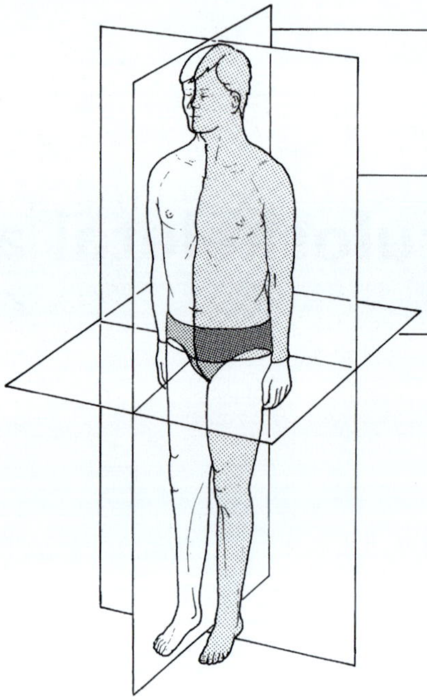

Figure 10A.1 Cardinal planes of the body: sagittal, frontal and transverse. Sagittal divides the body into right and left halves, frontal divides the body into front and back, and transverse divides the body into upper and lower sections. The diagram shows midplanes but the terms refer to any plane parallel to the appropriate midplane.

Terms of reference

The body is divided into three cardinal planes (Fig. 10A.1):

- sagittal
- frontal (coronal)
- transverse.

These planes form the reference points from which are described:

- the position of a part of the body
- joint motion
- the position of a joint
- deformity of a part of the body.

Universal use of these terms of reference is important when communicating with colleagues as one can be safe in the knowledge that they will understand the nature of the pathological process being described.

The position of a part of the body

The cardinal body planes are used as reference points to describe positions within the body:

- **Anterior** (to the front of) and **posterior** (to the rear of) describe positions in the frontal plane, e.g. the patella, or knee cap, lies anterior to the main weightbearing part of the knee joint (tibio-femoral).
- **Distal** (away from the centre) and **proximal** (towards the centre) describe positions in the transverse plane, e.g. the interphalangeal joints of the foot (IPJs) lie distal to the metatarsophalangeal joints (MTPJs) of the foot.
- **Medial** (towards the midline of the body) and **lateral** (away from the midline of the body) describe positions in the sagittal plane, e.g. the navicular lies on the medial side of the foot and the cuboid on the lateral side.
- In the foot, **dorsal** is used to refer to the top of the foot and **plantar** to the sole of the foot. The equivalents in the hand are dorsal and palmar.

Joint motion

Sagittal plane

Motion in the sagittal plane produces **extension** and **flexion**. The terms used to describe sagittal plane

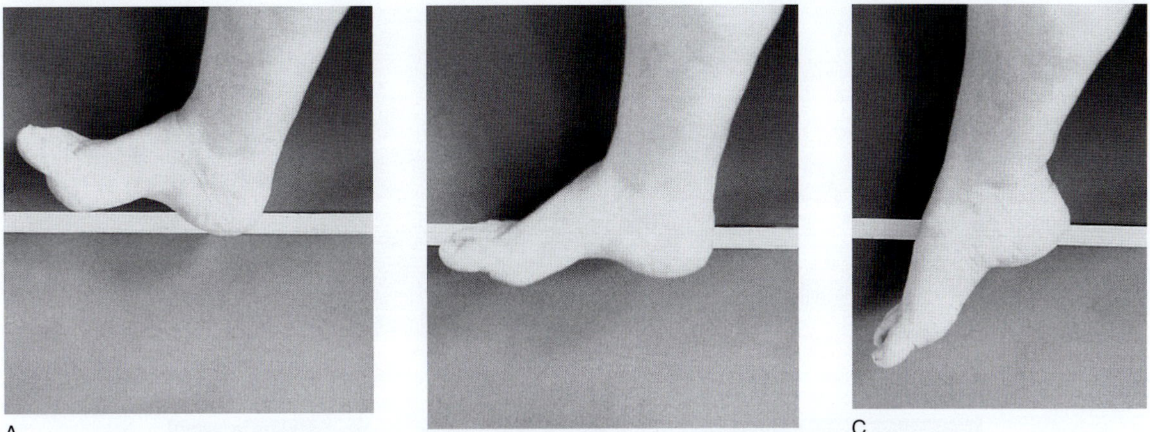

A B C

Figure 10A.2 Sagittal plane motion at the ankle. **A** Dorsiflexion: movement of the foot toward the anterior aspect of the tibia **B** Neutral position. **C** Plantarflexion: movement of the foot away from the tibia.

motion in the foot are slightly different from those used to describe such motion at the hip and knee (extension and flexion).

At the ankle (Fig. 10A.2), the midtarsal joints (MTJs), the MTPJs and the IPJs, sagittal plane motion is termed **dorsiflexion** and **plantarflexion**. Dorsiflexion denotes a raising of the whole or part of the foot towards the leg, whereas plantarflexion denotes the movement of the dorsal aspect of the foot away from the leg.

Frontal (coronal) plane

Motion in the frontal plane produces **abduction** and **adduction** of the thigh and leg and **inversion** and **eversion** of the foot. This is because the foot lies at right angles to the leg, so the terms used to describe movements of the foot differ from those used for the leg and thigh.

Abduction is when the distal segment moves away from the midline of the body and adduction when it moves towards the midline. For example, in order to do the 'splits', gymnasts must abduct their legs. Inversion of the foot is when the plantar aspect of the foot is tilted so as to move towards the midline of the body. Eversion is when the plantar aspect of the foot is tilted so as to face away from the midline of the body (Fig. 10A.3).

Transverse plane

Motion in the transverse plane produces **internal and external rotation** of the thigh and leg and **adduction and abduction of the foot**.

Internal rotation occurs when the anterior surface of the distal segment rotates medially in relation to the proximal segment and external rotation when the opposite occurs – the anterior surface of the distal segment moves laterally in relation to the proximal segment (Fig. 10A.4).

In the foot, the use of the terms adduction and abduction depends upon the site of the reference point: the midline of the body or the midline of the foot. Functionally, the midline of the body is usually used as the reference point:

- Abduction of the foot is when the distal part of the foot moves away from the midline of the body
- Adduction when the distal part of the foot moves towards the midline of the body (Fig. 10A.4).

The mid-axial line of the forefoot is different from that of the hand. For the latter, the middle finger is taken as the mid-axial point. Muscles which abduct (dorsal interossei) and adduct (palmar interossei) the fingers take the middle finger as their reference point. Conversely in the foot the longitudinal axis has shifted pre-axially and the second toe becomes the reference point for the mid-axial line for the actions of the dorsal and plantar interossei. The adductor hallucis is inserted into the lateral side of the proximal phalanx of the hallux and is so termed because it brings about adduction of the hallux – movement of the hallux towards the midline of the foot.

Triplanar motion

The position of the joint axis together with the shape of the articulating surfaces can result in motion in more than one plane for a joint or combination of joints acting together.

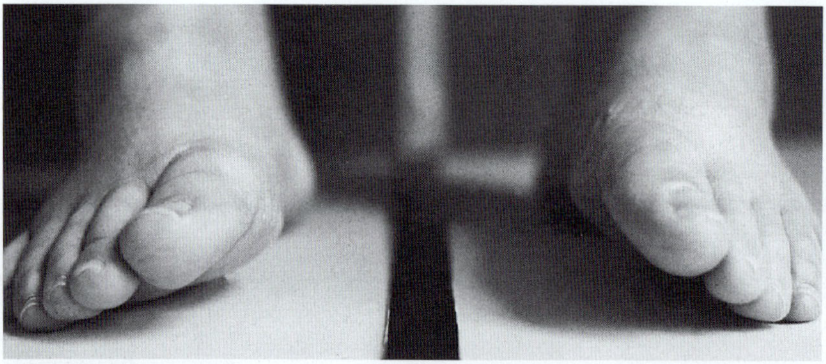

A

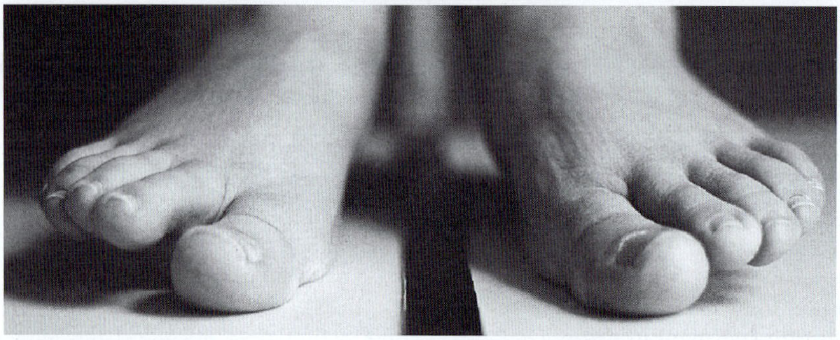

B

Figure 10A.3 Frontal plane motion in relation to the midline of the body (black line). **A** Inversion: the foot is lifted up and away from the line. **B** Eversion: the foot is moved down and towards the line.

If a joint axis is positioned at an angle of less than 90° to all the cardinal body planes triplanar motion can occur, e.g. **pronation** and **supination**:

- Pronation is the collective term for dorsiflexion, eversion and abduction.
- Supination is the collective term for plantarflexion, inversion and adduction.

For example, in the foot triplanar motion occurs at the subtalar and midtarsal joints.

Position of a joint

To describe the position of a joint the suffix '-ed' is used:

- Sagittal plane – **extended** and **flexed** (thigh and leg); **dorsiflexed** and **plantarflexed** (foot)
- Transverse plane – internally and externally **rotated** (thigh and leg); **adducted** and **abducted** (foot)
- Frontal plane – **abducted** and **adducted** (thigh and leg); **inverted** and **everted** (foot)
- Triplanar – **pronated** and **supinated** (foot).

It is important that a distinction is made between joint motion and position; a joint may be moving in the opposite direction to the position it occupies at any one moment. For example, at heel-strike the foot is slightly supinated (position) but as soon as the heel contacts the ground pronation (motion) occurs at the subtalar joint (STJ) in order to absorb shock from ground contact.

Deformity of a part of the body

The term 'deformity' is used to describe an abnormal position adopted by a part of the body.

Terms used to denote deformity often have the suffix **-us**:

- Sagittal plane – **equinus** is when the foot or part of the foot is plantarflexed, e.g. ankle equinus, and **extensus** is when the foot or part of the foot is dorsiflexed, e.g. hallux extensus. **Calcaneus** is used to describe the calcaneus when it is in fixed dorsiflexion, e.g. talipes calcaneovalgus.
- Frontal plane – **varus** and **valgus** (Fig. 10A.5).
- Transverse plane – **adductus** or **abductus**.

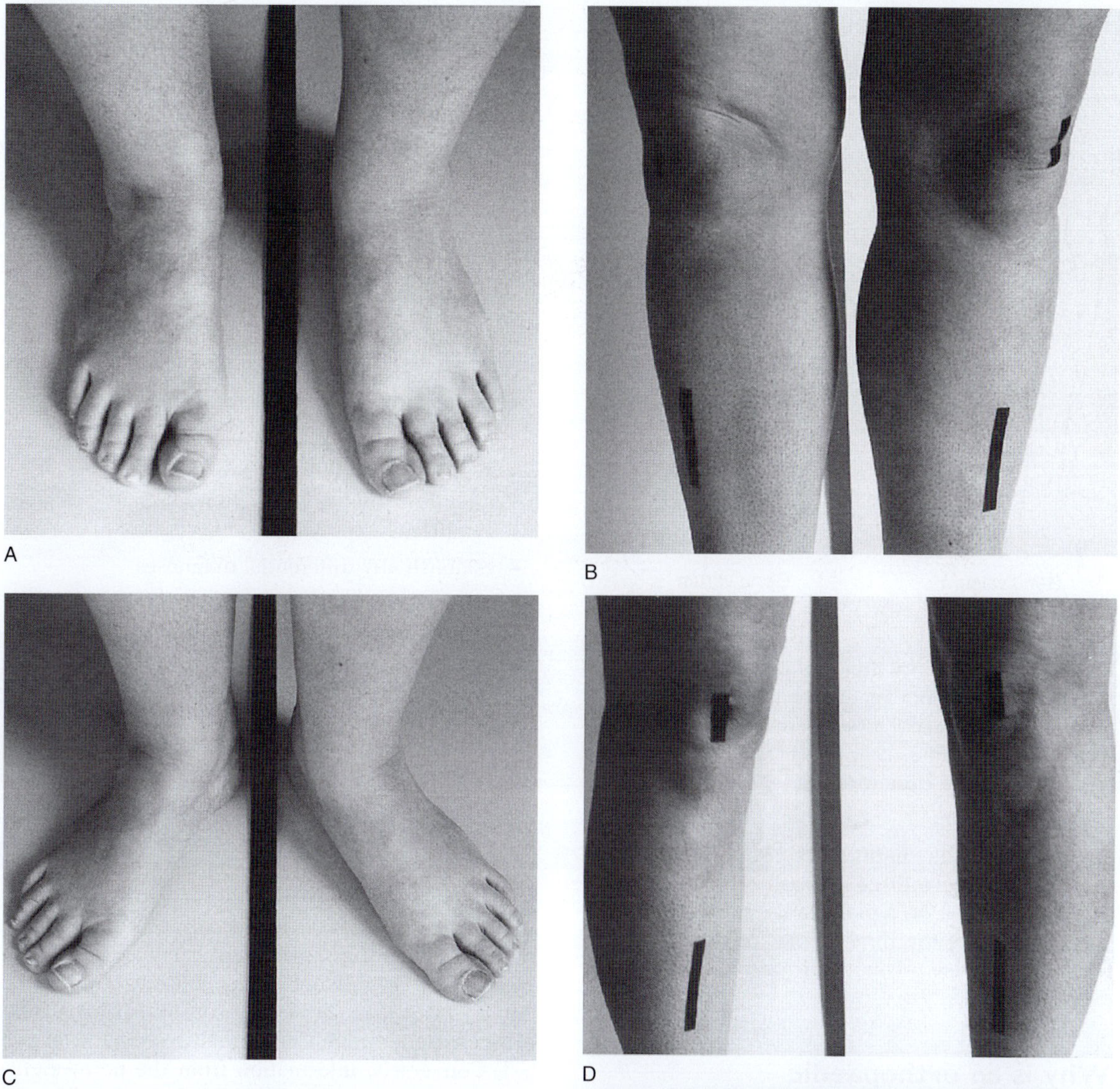

A B C D

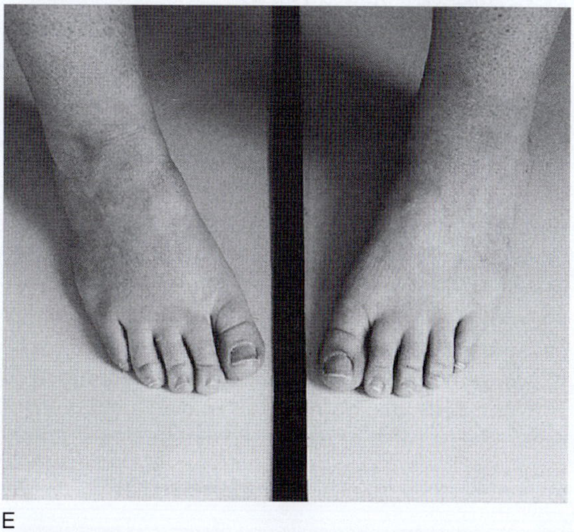

E

Figure 10A.4 Relationship between transverse plane motion in the leg and transverse plane motion in the foot. **A** The feet are mildly abducted; this is the normal standing position **B** The legs are externally (laterally) rotated, which results in abduction of the feet (**C**). **D** The legs are internally rotated (medially), which results in the adduction of the feet (**E**).

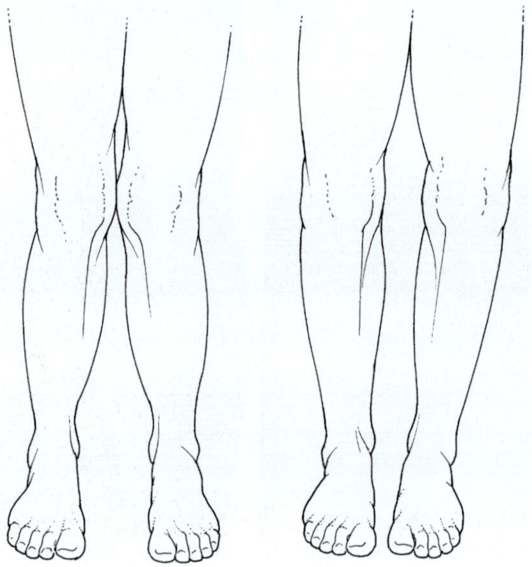

Figure 10A.5 Frontal plane deformity of the legs. **A** Genu valgum (knock knees): the knees are close together and the medial malleoli are far apart. **B** Genu varum (bow legs): the knees are far apart and the medial malleoli are close together.

To reinforce the importance of understanding these terms, **Figure 10A.6** illustrates the three planes of a knee as seen on a plain radiograph and **Figure 10A.7** illustrates the three planes of the ankle and hindfoot as seen on magnetic resonance imaging (MRI).

Why is an orthopaedic assessment indicated?

Normal lower limb function should be free of pain and energy efficient. The main purpose of the orthopaedic assessment is to identify whether the system is functioning within the boundaries of 'normality'. Normal function can be affected by many factors (Box 10A.1). It should be remembered that orthopaedic lower limb problems are not always isolated in origin. They may result from referred pain from a proximal source or can be part of a systemic disorder, e.g. a neuromuscular disease. It is therefore important that the lower limbs are not examined in isolation and that observation and examination of other parts of the body are undertaken where indicated.

In summary the purpose of an orthopaedic lower limb assessment is to:

- establish the main complaint(s), e.g. pain, stiffness, tenderness, numbness, weakness, crepitus
- identify the site of the primary problem, e.g. foot, leg, knee, hip, and try to relate to underlying structures
- identify any secondary problems and relate them to the primary problem, e.g. lesion patterns, pronation due to leg-length discrepancy
- identify the cause of the problem, e.g. abnormal alignment
- establish how the problem evolved
- identify any movement/activity that produces/exacerbates symptoms
- identify movement/activity that relieves symptoms
- establish any differential diagnoses
- utilise the data from the assessment to produce an effective management plan
- utilise the data from the assessment to monitor the progress of the condition.

The assessment process

When undertaking an assessment of the lower limb it is essential that the system is observed weightbearing (dynamic and static) and non-weightbearing. Differences between the two states can help to determine whether compensation has occurred. For example, non-weightbearing assessment may identify the presence of a forefoot varus; observation of the patient's gait may show this problem has been fully compensated through abnormal positioning of the STJ. Conversely, information from the non-weightbearing assessment may explain the cause of a gait abnormality, e.g. a patient may have a bouncy gait due to an early heel lift; non-weightbearing assessment of the ankle joint may reveal that the cause is an ankle equinus secondary to a short gastrocnemius muscle.

To gain a full and detailed picture of the function of the locomotor system, the following factors must be assessed:

- gait
- alignment and position of the lower limb
- joint motion
- muscle action.

The sequence of assessment of the above varies among practitioners. There is no one correct sequence;

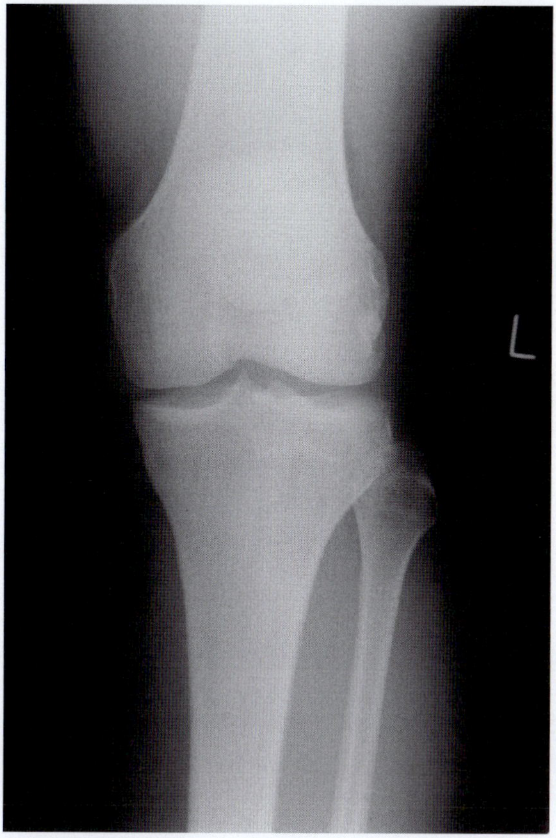

A

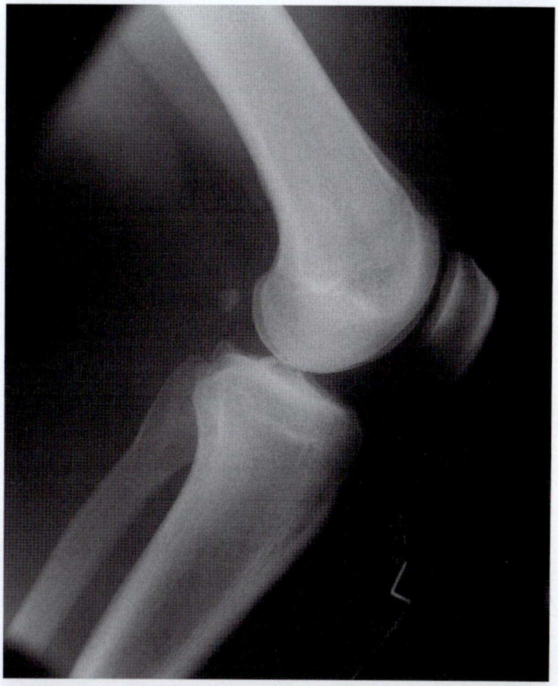

B

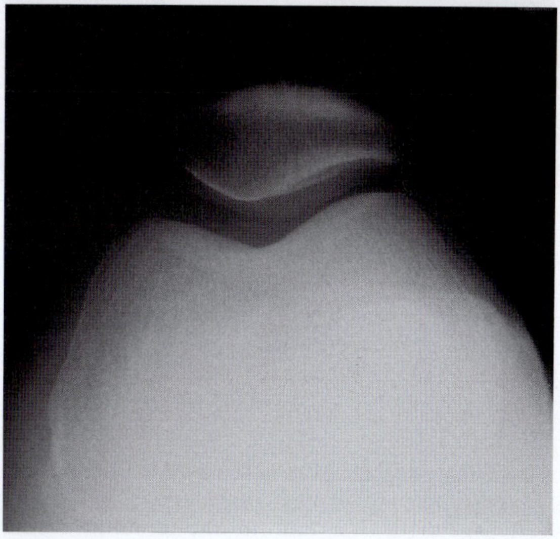

C

Figure 10A.6 Plain X-ray views of a knee joint: **A** anteroposterior or frontal (coronal) view; **B** lateral or sagittal view; **C** and skyline (axial) or transverse view, demonstrating patello-femoral position.

practitioners should adopt the sequence and approach they feel most comfortable with. However, it is essential that a systematic approach is adopted to ensure vital pieces of data are not omitted. For complete assessment, the examination should involve the following three important sections:

1. Non-weightbearing. This will focus on the assessment of joints and muscles.
2. Gait analysis. This will focus on the position and alignment of the body and foot–ground contact during dynamic weightbearing.

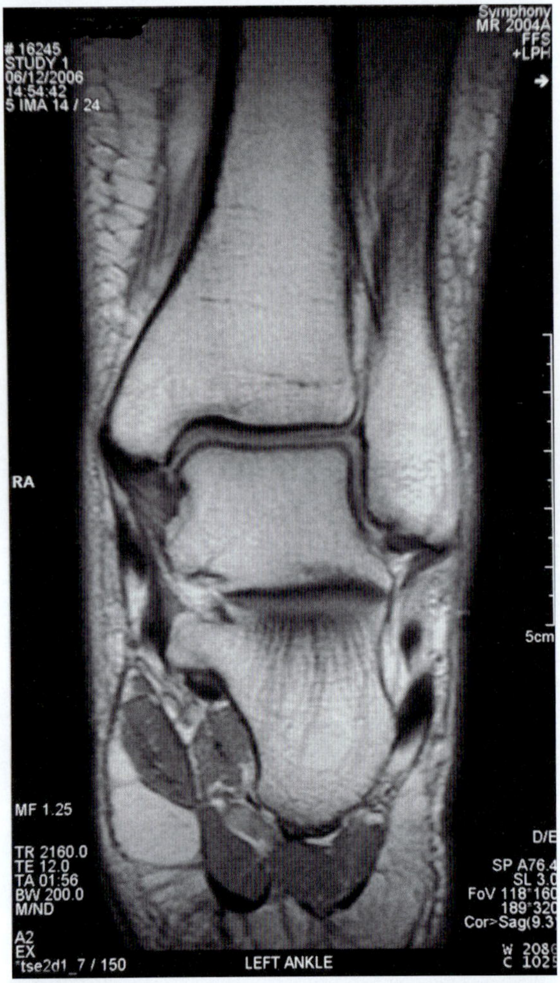

A

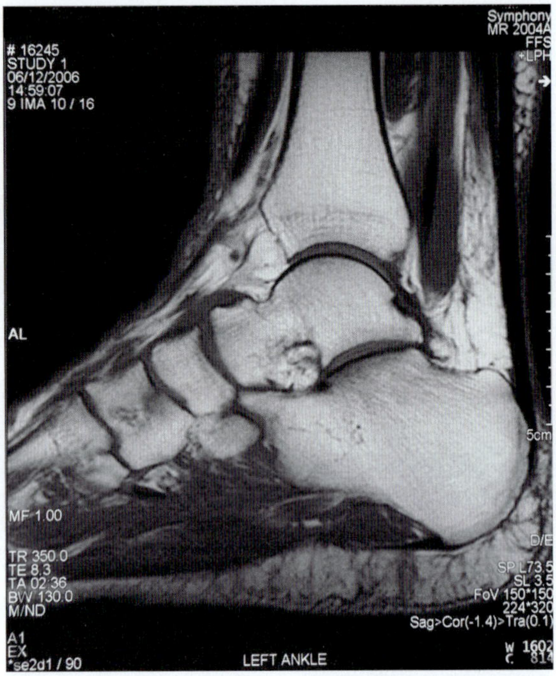

B

Figure 10A.7 MRI of ankle and hindfoot: **A** anteroposterior or frontal (coronal) view; **B** lateral or sagittal view; and **C** axial or transverse view.

3. Static weightbearing. This will focus on the position and alignment of the body and the relationship of the foot to the ground during stance.

Areas 2 and 3 are covered in greater detail in section 10B.

For successful assessment, it is important that the patient is at ease and cooperates with and has confidence in the practitioner. The practitioner should always be sensitive to the patient's needs and explain what they are about to do and why, before undertaking the assessment. Qualitative and quantitative measurement should be undertaken where necessary, but the data must be meaningful and reproducible if they are to be of any use in assessing improvement or deterioration. Various measuring devices may be used; their use will be discussed in the appropriate sections.

General assessment guidelines

- Always observe and functionally assess the joints bilaterally.
- It is valuable to obtain an overview of both limbs, particularly if the onset of the problem is insidious, the pain is diffuse and nonspecific or if during testing a number of joints seem to be implicated.

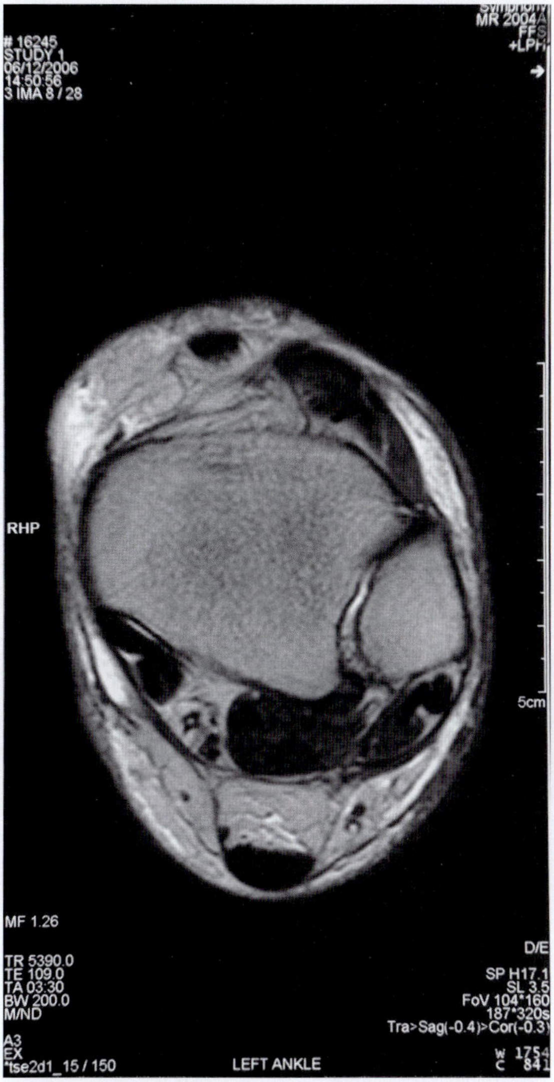

C

Figure 10A.7 *Continued.*

- Where only one limb is affected, it is often helpful to start with the unaffected limb first, then repeat the test on the affected limb. Compare ranges of motion, end feel (the sensation the examiner feels when they push the joint being examined to the end of its range of motion) and muscular strength.
- It is helpful to arrange your testing so that the most painful test is last. This ensures that the condition will not be aggravated by your testing procedure or make the patient apprehensive.

Box 10A.1 Factors that can affect normal function

- Hereditary/congenital problems, e.g. Charcot–Marie–Tooth disease, talipes equinovarus, developmental dysplasia of the hip (DDH)
- Acute/chronic injury causing pain, e.g. slipped capital femoral epiphysis, ankle sprain
- Abnormal alignment secondary to trauma, e.g. femoral/tibial/epiphyseal fracture
- Abnormal alignment (developmental), e.g. internal femoral torsion, genu valgum
- Infections, e.g. tuberculosis
- Neurological disorders, e.g. cerebrovascular accident
- Muscle disorders, e.g. Duchenne's muscular dystrophy
- Neoplasia, e.g. osteosarcoma
- Systemic disease, e.g. autoimmune (rheumatoid arthritis), bone disease (Paget's disease)
- Degenerative processes, e.g. osteoarthritis
- Joint hypermobility, e.g. Marfan's syndrome
- Osteochondroses, e.g. Perthes' disease
- Psychological factors, e.g. attention seeking
- Footwear, e.g. high-heeled shoes

Not all the tests will be required during every lower-limb assessment. The selection of tests used will depend on the findings as the examination proceeds, and should be influenced by the preceding clinical history and observations. However, it is necessary to be thorough enough to rule out alternative pathologies. The exclusion of alternative aetiologies may require the assessment of additional systems, e.g. the cardiovascular system. Referred pain associated with local nerve entrapment or radicular patterns of pain in which spinal nerves or nerve roots are irritated need to be considered.

Remember that a problem that affects one part of the system can lead to problems elsewhere in the system. The lower limb functions as one mechanical unit and as a result a problem in one part may have to be compensated for in another part of the system. Compensation is a change in the structure, position or function of one part in an attempt to adjust to an abnormal structure, position or function in another part. For example, scoliosis of the spine may lead to an apparent leg-length discrepancy, which will affect foot function. Conversely, a problem affecting the foot, e.g. an uncompensated rearfoot varus, may lead to discomfort/pain at the knee.

The process of assessment follows a standard format:

- General observation of the patient
- Specific joint observation
- Palpation
- Examination of joint movement
- Muscle assessment
- Undertaking special tests
- Arranging further investigations.

General observation of the patient

The assessment process starts at the time of introduction. Observation of a patient's demeanour, facial expression, seated posture and how they get up from a chair provides valuable clinical information. In addition, the way in which the patient walks into the clinic, together with use of walking aids, provides more information about mobility and how this might be influencing lower limb/foot function. After history taking, the patient will have to undress appropriately. Observation of the ease with which this is achieved gives an insight into the way a patient copes with certain activities of daily living.

Specific joint observation

Observation of each lower-limb joint before the examination will establish the presence of any clinical features synonymous with pathology, e.g. oedema, contusion, erythema, local muscle wasting, alteration in shape or the presence of scars. Symmetry of contralateral parts, abnormal posture/evidence of limb shortening and abnormal joint movement during gait are additional clinical clues to underlying pathology.

Palpation

Palpation of the limb segment or joint for clinical features such as raised/lowered skin temperature, swelling/effusion, tenderness, pain or abnormal lumps/nodules also provides information to help establish a diagnosis.

Examination of joint movement

Features of an inflamed joint are redness (rubor), heat (calor), pain (dolor), swelling (tumour) and loss of function. Inflammation of a joint may be due to a range of factors, e.g. trauma, arthritis and infection. Examination of the joint, information from the medical and social history and results of radiological and laboratory investigations will enable a diagnosis to be made. If a patient complains of a painful joint, the characteristic features of the pain should be recorded.

Before examining a joint, it is helpful to ask the patient to move the affected limb to assess the likely range of pain-free movement. The process of joint assessment should include the following:

- Range of motion (ROM)
- Direction of motion
- Quality of motion
- Symmetry of motion
- Absence/presence of deformity, including dislocation and subluxation.

ROM is the amount of motion at a joint and is usually measured in degrees. The ROM at a joint can be compared with the expected ROM for that joint, e.g. if only 20° of motion occurs at the first MTPJ when the expected norm is 70° (28% of the normal ROM) it can be concluded that the ability of this joint to carry out normal function is impaired (hallux limitus). Often a guesstimate of the amount of joint motion is made from observation. Protractors, tractographs and goniometers can be used to quantify joint motion (Fig. 10A.8).

A joint may show normal ROM but the direction of the motion may be abnormal. It is, therefore, important to note the direction as well as the range. For example, the total ROM of transverse plane rotation at the hip is 90°; 45° internal rotation and 45°

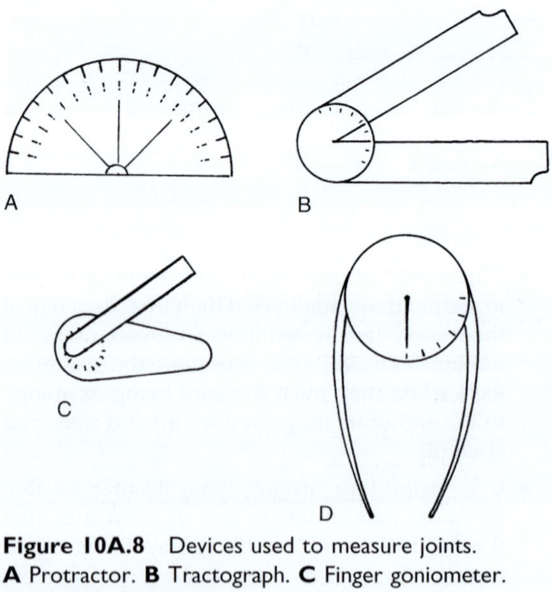

Figure 10A.8 Devices used to measure joints. **A** Protractor. **B** Tractograph. **C** Finger goniometer. **D** Gravity goniometer.

external rotation. If the ROM is 90° but there is 70° of external rotation and 20° of internal rotation then the ROM would be normal but the direction of the motion would be abnormal. Normal joint motion should occur without crepitus, pain or resistance (quality of motion). The ROM and direction of motion of a joint, e.g. hip, should be the same for both limbs (symmetry of motion). The presence of asymmetry of motion should always be noted.

Joint motion can be affected by the ligaments around the joint. It is important as part of joint assessment to identify any dysfunction of the ligaments, e.g. ligament tear or rupture. Finally, joints should be assessed as to whether they are subluxated or dislocated. Dislocation occurs where there is no contact between articulating surfaces of the joint and subluxation where there is only partial contact.

The range of active and passive movement of each respective lower limb joint should be examined, documented, and compared with the contralateral side. It is useful to assess whether passive movement of the joint provokes any pain or guarding (sometimes seen in hallux limitus). In addition, it is valuable to document the response to resisted testing (strong/weak/painless/painful) and stability of the joint. This will determine the integrity of the articulating surfaces and ligaments. Provoking crepitus on joint movement is an indication of joint damage.

Muscle assessment

Muscles allow active motion at joints. They should be tested for:

- strength
- tone
- spasm
- bulk.

Strength

The Medical Research Council (MRC) system is commonly used for grading muscle strength (Crawford Adams & Hamblen 1990):

- 0 = no contraction
- 1 = a flicker from muscle fasciculi
- 2 = slight movement with gravitational effects removed
- 3 = muscle can move part against gravity
- 4 = muscle can move part against gravity + resistance
- 5 = normal power.

Muscle strength can be assessed both by the patient initiating active motion, and by the clinician attempting to prevent active motion – resisted movement.

Tone

All muscles should show tone. Asking the patient to undertake isometric contraction of a muscle is a useful means of identifying tonal quality. Tone can also be assessed by the examiner holding the limb and placing it through a range of movement. Involuntary resistance is indicative of increased tone.

Spasm

Muscles may present in spasm and as a result joint motion is affected. Information from the neurological assessment and medical history aids identification of its causation.

Bulk

Muscle bulk should be observed and comparisons made between the limbs. Atrophy of muscle results in a loss of muscle bulk and may be due to a number of factors, e.g. lack of use, lower motor neurone lesion. Hypertrophy of muscles that show normal tone and symmetrical distribution is considered normal and is usually due to exercise. Unilateral atrophy/hypertrophy can be assessed by observation and recorded by measuring the girth of both limbs with a tape measure.

Undertaking special tests

It may be necessary to carry out specific tests to confirm a diagnosis or to differentiate between similar conditions. Some clinical examination techniques have been developed to test a particular aspect of joint function, e.g. Lachman's test to assess sagittal plane stability of the knee in an anterior direction and thereby the integrity of the anterior cruciate ligament. The section on non-weightbearing examination discusses the specific tests used to assess each of the lower limb joints and their associated structures.

Arranging further investigations

Usually the information obtained from a detailed history and assessment is sufficient to arrive at a diagnosis. Occasionally, specialist investigations may be necessary to confirm the diagnosis or to consider other options. A number of possibilities are available including: specialist imaging techniques and haematological, biochemical and nerve conduction studies and electromyography (EMG). In addition, histological examination of specimens, video/treadmill gait analysis or computerised analysis/forceplate analysis may be indicated.

Non-weightbearing examination

VIDEO

The prime purpose of the non-weightbearing examination is assessment of the joints and muscles of the lower limb and other important soft-tissue structures. A flat couch is required for the patient to lie on. Patients should feel comfortable and relaxed and should not be wearing restrictive clothing. Non-weightbearing examination involves an assessment of the following:

- Hip
- Knee
- Ankle and hindfoot
- Midtarsal
- Metatarsals
- MTPJs
- Digits (proximal and distal IPJs)
- Alignment of the lower limb.

Examination of the hip

The hip joint is regarded as a stable ball and socket synovial joint. It has sufficient mobility to allow economic gait and stance while being more restricted than its counterpart in the upper limb, the shoulder joint (glenohumeral joint), which tolerates greater potential instability in exchange for increased motion. The hip joint's stability is provided by:

- depth of the acetabulum, accentuated by the fibrocartilaginous labrum
- strong capsule, reinforced by capsular ligaments
- surrounding muscles.

History

Hip joint pain (coxodynia) is usually felt as an anterior groin pain sometimes radiating down the front of the thigh as far as the knee. In children, significant hip pathology may present as knee pain due to the shared nerve supply (femoral and obturator nerves).

A frequent diagnostic problem is distinguishing hip from spinal problems, and they often co-exist in elderly people. Low back pain radiating into the buttock, and posterior and lateral aspects of the thigh is more likely to have a spinal origin. Similarly proximal pain which radiates below the knee into the calf and foot is unlikely to emanate from the hip joint. A history of altered sensation or weakness in the limb is more likely to be neurological in origin. With concomitant spine and hip pathology, an intra-articular injection into the hip joint of local anaesthetic (with or without steroid in arthritic conditions) under aseptic conditions and image intensifier control can help distinguish the contribution of the hip from that of the spine.

Examination

Not every patient who presents to a podiatry clinic needs to have their hips examined. However, the hip should be examined if the patient complains of discomfort or pain in the area and/or gait analysis reveals an abnormality which affects normal pelvic and lower limb mobility and mechanics, e.g. weakness or limb discrepancy. The hip should be examined with the patient:

- standing
- lying on the examination couch
- walking.

Preparation for the hip examination

A proper hip examination requires both space and exposure:

- Adequate clinic space is required to allow the patient to stand and be observed standing from all positions and to walk freely.
- The examination couch should ideally not be placed against a wall. The examiner should be free to examine the patient from both sides and be allowed unencumbered assessment of parameters such as hip abduction.
- The patient should be adequately exposed. Ideally, they should be undressed down to shorts or suitable underwear. Both the hip and spinal areas should be exposed to assess linked mobility and posture.

Patient standing

The patient should be observed standing with the spine and lower limbs exposed.

Observe the patient from all positions and look for evidence of the following:

- **Wasting**: Wasting particularly of the thigh and gluteal (buttock) musculature may indicate longstanding hip pathology, such as arthritis, infection and congenital disorders.

- **Scars**: Has the patient had previous surgery or sustained any traumatic injury? A pitted sinus may indicate previous infection, e.g. tuberculosis.
- **Exaggerated lumber lordosis**: This is observed from the side and, if present, may indicate a fixed flexion deformity of the hip joint.
- **Limb attitude**: The position of both limbs will indicate any rotational or frontal plane (abduction/adduction) gross deformities.
- **Evidence of limb-length inequality**: See section on limb-length inequality.

Trendelenburg's test

This test is performed with the patient standing. The patient can be assessed from the front or behind – the latter is usually more reliable. The patient is initially asked to single leg stance on the unaffected limb. Normally the contralateral buttock is elevated and pelvis tilted towards the standing side. This moves the centre of gravity of the body closer to the centre of the standing hip joint. The pelvic tilt is produced by the hip abductors (principally gluteus medius and minimus).

The patient is asked to elevate the contralateral pelvis for 30 seconds, and then they are asked to repeat the test on the affected limb. If the contralateral hemi-pelvis cannot be elevated and held for 30 seconds the patient is said to be Trendelenburg positive. Often the patient will tilt their trunk excessively, bringing the centre of gravity close to or even lateral to the centre of the standing hip joint. A positive Trendelenburg test indicates one or more of the following problems:

- Weak abductors, e.g. in poliomyelitis, muscular dystrophies, post-surgical nerve damage
- Painful arthritic hip joint, which both inhibits gluteal activity and increases friction within the joint opposing abductor activity
- Congenital disorders, e.g. developmental dysplasia of the hip and coxa vara
- Previous injury to the proximal femur, reducing the efficiency of the gluteal system.

Patient lying on the examination couch

Ideally the patient should be able to lie fully flat on the examination couch. The examiner should be able to observe the pelvis and limb position and gain access to the lumbar spine area to assess changes in lumbar position. Usually, the examination is commenced with the patient lying supine. Check that the patient's iliac crests on either side of the pelvis are level and that the lower limbs are placed in identical position. Begin the supine examination with an assessment of limb-length inequality (see end of section 10A).

Palpation

Ask the patient to point and demonstrate the sight of any pain. The centre of the hip joint is deep to the femoral pulse, which can usually be easily palpated. However, the hip is a far deeper joint than the knee and, subsequently, it is more difficult to palpate and has fewer landmarks. However, a systematic examination around the hip joint should include palpation of:

- anterior groin for crepitus, swelling and tenderness – remember the other causes of groin pain including herniae, varicose veins and swollen lymph nodes
- adductor tendon origin
- proximal quadriceps
- lateral structures – including the greater trochanter and gluteal area for evidence of trochanteric bursal pathology
- iliac tuberosity for proximal hamstring pathology
- piriformis tenderness – rarely related to sciatic nerve compression.

Check for evidence of previous scarring from surgery or trauma. Look for healed sinuses which may be evidence of old, deep infection. Look for evidence of wasting of the thigh musculature – indicative of disuse of the joint.

Assessment of hip joint mobility

Hip joint mobility should be assessed in three planes:

- Sagittal: extension and flexion
- Frontal: abduction and adduction
- Transverse: internal and external rotation.

Before commencing formal passive hip movements, it is wise to ask the patient to move each limb actively in turn. This allows a rapid, albeit global, assessment of the amount of pain-free movement that is likely to be available in each limb. Similarly, gently rotating the extended limb internally and externally will indicate the degree of 'irritability' of the joint. Pain from this gentle manoeuvre is unlikely to elicit pain from any pathology except an intra-articular problem.

Sagittal plane movement

To ensure normal forward progression during gait, sagittal plane motion at the hip is essential. There should be approximately 120–140° of flexion and 5–20° of extension, although not all of this is necessary for gait.

Hip extension and Thomas' test

Extension of the hip is assessed by placing one of the examiner's hands under the lumbar spine. At rest the curvature of the lower spine (lumbar lordosis) should be felt. With the hand staying in this position, ask the patient to flex the healthy hip and knee. As the hip progressively flexes, the lumbar curvature should progressively flatten until the lordosis is obliterated.

If during the process of flexing the healthy hip, the damaged hip begins to lift from the couch, the patient is said to exhibit a loss of extension or fixed flexion deformity (FFD), which can be measured in relationship to the horizontal. Many patients when standing and walking attempt to 'mask' moderate degrees of fixed flexion deformities by increasing their lumbar lordosis.

The test can be undertaken 'in reverse' by asking the patient to flex both hips and during this manoeuvre confirm that the lumbar curve has been obliterated. Then, in turn, ask the patient to hold one leg in position with their hands while gradually extending the other hip. In health, a person should be able to place the leg on the couch without increasing the lumbar lordosis as a compensatory mechanism.

If the hip displays no evidence of an FFD, more subtle changes of hip extension may be detected by placing the patient prone. With the pelvis stabilised by the examiner's hand, each limb in turn is lifted from the couch and any difference noted. Normal extension is up to 10–20°.

Hip flexion

The good hip is flexed to allow lumber spine flattening. The comfortable flexion angle is noted and the patient asked to steady the limb with their own hands. The affected hip is then flexed while checking that the pelvis and lumber spine remain static. A comparison is made between the flexion in both hips.

The sagittal ROM is recorded. For example, with an osteoarthritic left hip, the following may be written in the notes:

- Right hip: extension 15°, flexion 120°
- Left hip: extension –30°, flexion 90°

The normal right hip has a total arc of movement of 135° while the diseased hip has only 60° with a significant FFD.

Frontal plane movement

This should be assessed with the patient lying flat and supine, with room to assess both limbs. An exaggerated impression of available hip abduction may be gained if the pelvis is not stabilised by the examiner placing their hand on the contralateral iliac crest as the limb is moved. Then the limb is moved outwards and the arc of movement from the midline noted. If possible, when dealing with unilateral pathology, start with the normal side. Usually, enough abduction is available in the healthy hip to allow the leg to hang dependent over the couch with the knee flexed. This allows further stabilisation of the pelvis and allows comparison with the contralateral side. Normal hip abduction is at least 40°.

Adduction is best assessed after abduction. Less adduction is available than abduction – usually about 25°. It can be assessed in several different ways:

- Each limb in turn can be raised and brought across the midline over the contralateral limb.
- The contralateral limb can be raised by an assistant, allowing the limb being examined to be moved in a more pure frontal plane.
- With the contralateral limb held in an abducted position, e.g. flexed at the knee over the side of the couch, move the limb being examined into the space vacated by the other limb.

Tightness of the adductors on attempted abduction is common in osteoarthritis and other common hip pathologies. In cerebral palsy, it can lead to a scissors-type gait when one or both legs have a tendency to cross over during gait.

Transverse plane movement

Internal and external hip rotation can be assessed in several different ways. The recorded measurement might be slightly different according to the method employed. It is important that the way the assessment was conducted is recorded in the notes. Essentially there are three methods:

- Supine patient with hips and knees extended
- Supine patient with knees and hips flexed
- Prone patient with hips extended and knees flexed.

With the patient supine, rotation can be assessed with the hips and knees extended, i.e. the legs straight. Observe the patient from the foot of the bed and assess rotation in each limb simultaneously. Hold each heel in the palm of your hands and first externally rotate and then internally rotate each limb. In this position, rotation is derived from the hip, unless there is any knee instability. It is useful to observe the movement of the patellae as a gauge of the amount of rotation from the hip. The alternative method with the patient supine is to flex to 90° the hip and knee joints. This may be difficult if hip flexion is painful and restricted. The hip is moved both internally and externally and the angle is measured by comparing the position of the shin with respect to the midline.

With the patient prone, rotation can be assessed by flexing the knees to 90°. The legs can be simultaneously rotated outwards to assess and compare internal rotation. External rotation can be assessed with one limb extended and the other leg moved towards the midline. Alternatively, external rotation can be compared by crossing the legs. For all these manoeuvres it is important that rotation is not exaggerated by the pelvis lifting alternatively off each side.

In health, 45° of comfortable internal and external rotation is possible. In certain conditions, e.g. unilateral excessive femoral anteversion, the total rotational arc may be the same in both hips, but with a skew in one rotational direction in one hip compared to the other. Females tend to show more internal rotation than males (Svenningsen et al 1990). The range of transverse plane motion at the hip decreases with age and most hip pathologies.

Assessment of femoral anteversion

Femoral anteversion is the angle that the femoral neck makes with the shaft of the femur. It varies with age, and there is a difference between the sexes. In males, the neck lies more in line with the femoral shaft than in females – 140° compared with 120° of anteversion. In children, the angle is similar to that in the adult female. It is important for podiatrists to be aware of this because excessive femoral anteversion is one of the most important causes of 'intoeing' – especially in the child (along with tibial internal torsion and persistent metatarsus adductus).

The most accurate clinical evaluation of femoral anteversion is with the patient lying prone and the knee flexed. With the contralateral limb extended, rotate the leg from side to side. Feel the greater trochanter laterally as the hip rotates. When the trochanter is truly facing lateral, the angle between the shin position and the vertical represents the anteversion angle of the femoral neck. On occasions, computed tomography (CT), which can measure this angle more accurately, is required.

Patient walking

Ask the patient to walk up and down the examination area. Make sure that there are no obstructions and the patient can perform at least four to five stride lengths. With regard to hip pathology, the four most common reasons why a patient has a limp are:

- pain – an antalgic gait pattern
- weakness – e.g. abductor weakness causing Trendelenburg's gait pattern
- limb-length inequality
- deformity – e.g. adduction or rotational deformity.

Patients often display one or more of these problems. A thorough examination of the patient on the examination couch will have flagged up likely gait problems, e.g. limb shortening and significant hip pain on motion.

Imaging of the hip joint

X-rays

Conventional radiographic views of the hip joint includes an AP view of the pelvis (Fig. 10.9) and a lateral view of one or both hip joints. The advantage of the pelvic AP view is that the hips can be compared and any other pathology within the bony pelvis can be noted, e.g. Paget's disease. Other views can be requested under specific circumstances but are beyond the scope of this discussion.

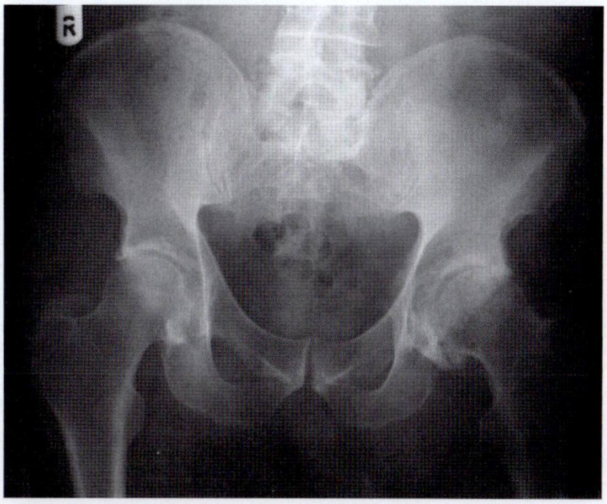

Figure 10A.9 AP pelvis radiograph showing an osteoarthritic hip.

Magnetic resonance imaging

MRI can be used to look for subtle pathology within the hip joint, e.g. labral cartilage tears. Additionally, it allows visualization of the extra-articular soft tissues and may detect conditions that cause hip/groin pain, e.g. bursitis. MRI can also show subtle osseous lesions, for instance early avascular necrosis.

Computed tomography

CT can be useful for looking at bone and joint structure and disease. Modern CT scanners with the ability to collect increasingly smaller, thin slices of information, are capable of detecting ever more subtle lesions. In addition, the ability to reformat the information into a three-dimensional image has helped our understanding of musculoskeletal pathology and planning of corrective procedures.

Isotope scanning

Scanning with isotopes such as technetium-99m is a useful way of determining the presence or absence of pathology in the region of the hip joint. It is helpful in distinguishing the location of discomfort, e.g. hip joint pathology versus spine. It is sensitive for identifying areas of inflammation and abnormal pathology while not being particularly specific about the cause. It is particularly useful in assessing whether an established hip replacement is beginning to loosen and causing symptoms.

Knee examination

The knee joint is a complex synovial joint and should be considered as having three parts:

- Patellofemoral joint
- Medial tibiofemoral joint
- Lateral tibiofemoral joint.

History

A thorough assessment of a knee joint problem requires information about several key issues.

Background information

Knowledge of many background features is important:

- Previous injuries and/or surgery to the knee
- Previous treatment to the joint, e.g. medications, physiotherapy
- Sport(s) and occupation(s) of the patient
- Future activity aspirations of the patient.

History of trauma

The history should include enquiry about the mechanism of injury, direction of injury, experience of tearing, 'popping' or other abnormal sensations, ability to weightbear and the presence or absence of swelling afterwards and its speed of occurrence. In addition, the presence and pattern of any subsequent bruising should be noted.

Swelling within 1–2 hours of an injury is usually due to the presence of blood within the joint (a haemarthrosis). The most common causes of a knee joint haemarthrosis are:

- ruptured anterior cruciate ligament
- fracture – including osteochondral injuries (bone and cartilage fragments) and damage to osteophytes, or bone spurs, in arthritic joints.

Delayed swelling, e.g. the day after, is usually an indication of a synovial swelling (increased volume of normal joint fluid) and is more common after meniscal (cartilage) injuries.

Pain

Ask about location and aggravating factors.

Mobility

Does the patient feel a restriction of movement in any direction? Is the restriction present throughout the day or worse at certain times, e.g. in the morning, or after certain activities, e.g. sitting for long periods? Occasionally, the patient may perceive abnormal movement.

Stability

Does the knee give way? If so when? Does the patient feel the instability is related to the patella or main knee joint?

Locking

Does the knee lock in a position of flexion? True locking never occurs with the knee straight in full extension. Locking may be caused by a number of problems, including:

- meniscal (cartilage) tear
- loose body
- dislocated patella.

Ask the patient in what position and during what activities the knee locks. Often patients unlock the knee themselves and will describe the 'coping manoeuvres' they have developed. 'Pseudo-locking' can occur due to pain and protective muscle spasm following any knee injury.

Swelling

Patients with chronic knee problems often experience swelling. It may be intermittent or permanent, localised or generalised. The popliteal fossa behind the knee is a common site of localised swelling. The swelling is often due to a Baker's cyst, which occurs in patients with arthritis of the knee. Patients of any age, including children, may develop a bursa deep to the semimembranosus muscle and tendon. Anterior swelling may arise from the joint itself or one of the anterior bursae – prepatellar and infrapatellar. Determining which one is the cause requires experience and detailed knowledge of the anatomy.

Change in knee attitude (position)

With long-standing knee problems the resting and/or standing position of the patient may alter:

- The patient may lose extension or stand with the knee flexed for comfort.
- The knee may become bowed (genu varum) or knock-kneed (genu valgum) due to, for instance, medial or lateral tibio-femoral osteoarthritis respectively (see Fig. 10A.5).

Examination

As with the hip, the knee should be examined with the patient:

- standing
- lying on the examination couch
- walking.

Preparation for the knee examination

Similar to the hip, examination of the knee should not be undertaken in cramped surroundings.

- There should be enough space to allow the patient to be observed standing from all positions and to walk freely.
- The couch should not be placed against a wall to allow comparative examination of both joints
- The patient should be adequately exposed.

Patient standing

Initially stand the patient and look at the overall alignment of both limbs. The position of the limb during weightbearing may be quite different from the alignment with the patient supine:

- Does the patient stand with each knee fully extended? If not, is this is a fixed deformity, commonly seen in arthritis, or because the knee is more comfortable for the patient in this position? Some patients have excessive hyperextension (genu recurvatum) – is this bilateral or unilateral? It may be constitutional (normal for the patient, especially in females) or pathological.
- Does the patient have excessive genu valgum (knock-knee) or genu varum (bowed legs) (Fig. 10A.5). An objective recording of genu valgum can be made by measuring the distance between the medial malleoli of the ankle (intermalleolar distance) with a tape. The degree of genu varum can be similarly estimated by measuring the gap between the medial joint lines of the knee using a tape or noting the number of fingers that can fit in the gap. In addition, if a varus or valgus deformity should be noted determine whether it is unilateral or bilateral. In children, the varus/valgus position changes normally as they grow (Ch. 14). However, congenital, traumatic, endocrine and metabolic disorders may cause excessive degrees of angulation. In adults, excessive angulation frequently indicates a degenerative or inflammatory process within the knee with excessive wear on one side of the knee (lateral in genu valgum and medial in genu varum). Trauma to the knee region can alter alignment, e.g. medial collateral ligament injury may cause an increased valgus position at the knee joint.
- Observing the patient standing will also give the examiner an indication of the presence of features such as muscle wasting, scars and swelling.

Patient lying on the examination couch

The patient should be examined both supine and prone for full assessment of the knee. The general principles of look, feel and move apply similarly to the order of examination of the knee joint.

Observation of the knee

Swelling

Is it localised or generalised? Does the swelling outline the extent of the knee joint or extend beyond

Table 10A.1 Local swellings around the knee joint

Type of tissue	*Location*	*Cause*
Solid	Femoral or tibial	Exostoses
	Anterior tibial	Osgood–Schlatter disease
Fluid	Lateral (usually)	Meniscal cyst
	Anterior	Prepatellar bursitis (housemaid's knee)
		Infrapatellar bursitis (clergyman's knee)
	Posterior	Baker's cyst
		Semimembranosus bursa

its boundaries? The knee joint itself can be swollen due the presence of increased amounts of synovial fluid, blood, pus, excessive synovium (synovitis) or a combination of more than one. Swelling that extends beyond the boundaries of the joint may indicate infection, the sequelae of trauma and rarely a neoplastic (tumour) lesion. Local swellings may be solid or fluid (Table 10A.1).

Bruising or discoloration

Bruising usually indicates superficial structure damage, for example medial collateral ligament injury. Redness indicates inflammation, particularly infection. It may be seen in association with an infected prepatellar bursa or septic arthritis.

Abnormal superficial markings

Scarring due to trauma or surgery should be noted. A healed sinus with pitting and tethering of surrounding tissues should raise the possibility of previous infection, especially osteomyelitis. Some patients have prominent varicosities, especially anteriorly and medially with long saphenous incompetence and posteriorly with short saphenous incompetence. Some patients may have skin lesions, for example psoriasis. Psoriasis is more commonly found on the flexion surfaces of a joint and can be associated with an inflammatory arthropathy of the joint.

Muscle bulk

An accurate impression can usually be gauged by observing both limbs from the end of the couch. Ask the patient to contract both quadriceps and observe the degree of muscle development in either limb. A lack of muscle bulk is often seen around vastus medialis with patellofemoral pain syndrome.

Palpation of the knee

Feel the knee with the joint initially extended and then flexed (if comfort allows).

Temperature

Feel the temperature of both joints simultaneously by placing a hand on the front of both joints. Increased local warmth is an indication of inflammation from an arthropathy, infection, trauma or rarely malignancy.

Synovial thickening

One cause of a swollen knee is generalised thickening of the synovial lining secondary to an irritant stimulus such as an inflammatory arthropathy or blood. The thickness of the synovial membrane is best assessed at the margins of the patella. A localised synovial fold is called plica. These folds can occur anywhere in the joint and can cause irritation if they become thickened or inflamed (usually anteromedial).

Knee effusion

A swelling of the knee joint causes bulging principally above the patella (in the suprapatellar pouch) and on either side of the patella. Observation will usually indicate whether a knee has excessive fluid in it, but there are three tests for detecting the presence and amount of excessive fluid:

- **Patella tap test**. Fluid is milked down from the suprapatellar pouch with the first web space of one hand (i.e. between the thumb and index finger). The fingers of the other hand pushes downwards on the central part of the patella. If there is sufficient fluid beneath the patella, the patella will be felt to 'tap' against the femoral condyles. A false-negative result can be obtained if the patella is not stabilised between the thumb and index fingers of the proximal hand or if the effusion is too tense, as it does not allow the patella to be pushed downwards because of resistance.

- **Bulge test**. This is the easiest way of detecting substantial effusions. The thumb and index finger of one hand are placed on either side of the patella while the other hand squeezes fluid down from the suprapatellar pouch as described in the patella tap test. As the fluid is milked distally the fluid bulges and displaces the thumb and index finger either side of the patella.
- **Fluid displacement (or wipe) test**. This test is likely to pick up more subtle effusions within the joint. Empty the suprapatellar pouch as described in the previous two tests. Stroke the lateral side of the joint with the free hand and observe the medial side of the joint. Any excessive fluid will be seen to distend the medial side. The opposite will happen when the fluid is swept back from the medial to the lateral side.

Tenderness

If comfort allows, it is better to start the examination of the knee for tenderness with the joint flexed at 90°. This allows clearer identification of the various anatomical structures. There is no correct order for examining the various structures of the knee. It is important that you adopt an order that is repeatable and complete for yourself. One useful order is to start medially and then move laterally. The following parts should be palpated for tenderness at some stage during the examination with the knee flexed:

- Medial tendons: sartorius, gracilis, semitendinosus
- Medial collateral ligament
- Medial femoral and tibial condyles
- Medial joint line: to assess for medial meniscal pathology
- Tibial tubercle, patella tendon and its posterior relation, the fat pad
- Lateral joint line: to assess for lateral meniscal pathology
- Lateral femoral and tibial condyles and fibula head
- Lateral collateral ligament
- Lateral tendons: biceps femoris and iliotibial band
- Common peroneal nerve as it winds around the fibula neck.

At a later stage, with the knee extended, evidence of tenderness around the patella and distal quadriceps and tendon should be sought. Similarly, with the patient prone, the structures contributing to the boundaries of the popliteal fossa (medial and lateral heads of gastrocnemius, medial hamstrings and biceps femoris) should be palpated along with the structures within (although the popliteal artery pulsation is best palpated with the knee flexed).

Movement of the knee

Preliminary visual inspection and palpation of the knee should provide an indication of the relative comfort of the joint and likely mobility and contained pathology. Now it is necessary to establish the amount of movement that the joint possesses. Establish how much knee flexion and extension is possible with the patient supine.

Extension

Full extension of the knee is recorded as 0°. Any loss of full extension is recorded as a negative reading, e.g. −10° of fixed flexion deformity. Any hyperextension (or genu recurvatum) is, by convention, recorded as a positive reading, e.g. +10° of hyperextension.

Start by asking the patient to push their knees downwards by contracting their quadriceps muscles. The examiner's hands can be placed under the knees to feel if there is an equal amount of extension, i.e. equal pressure on each hand. Both legs can be lifted by the examiner simultaneously from the end of the bed. Any hyperextension becomes more obvious as does any asymmetry. Common causes of an FFD include:

- meniscal injury
- arthritis
- protective spasm of supporting musculature following injury, particularly in the continuing presence of an effusion.

Common causes of hyperextension (genu recurvatum or 'swayback') include:

- constitutional – especially in females
- patello-femoral abnormalities
- cruciate instability problems
- generalised laxity, e.g. Ehlers–Danlos syndrome.

Flexion

Full flexion is limited by apposition of the soft tissues of the calf and thigh. Full flexion is usually no more than 135°. Objective measurements can be obtained by the use of a goniometer or measuring heel to buttock distance with a tape measure. Lack of flexion may be caused by a number of pathologies including arthritis and recent soft-tissue injury.

Tests for instability

The knee displays different patterns of instability, depending on the combination of structures involved (Table 10A.2).

Specific tests for instability

There are a number of tests of instability of various structures around the knee. Knowledge of every stability test is only expected of those working on a daily basis with significant knee problems. However, the reader should be aware of the presence of different patterns and the presence of specific tests to distinguish between each. Specific assessment tests for patella instability are discussed in the section on the assessment of the patellofemoral joint.

Collateral ligament assessment

The collateral ligaments may be damaged in isolation by coronal forces (valgus or varus) or as part of a more complex ligament injury pattern. The medial collateral ligament (MCL) is more commonly injured than the lateral collateral ligament. The medial ligament is a large strap-like structure. It is injured when a valgus force is applied to a knee, for example a rugby tackle from the side. The ligament may be injured anywhere from its origin on the medial femoral condyle to its tibial insertion, four fingerbreadths below the medial joint line. Tenderness and bruising will usually be present in significant injuries. Because it is an extra-articular structure, swelling purely from the ligament injury should be confined to the medial side of the knee.

The stability of the MCL should be assessed with both the knee extended and slightly flexed at about 15–20°. Many patients have slightly lax medial collateral ligaments, particularly from constitutional laxity or from medial joint compartment arthritis which causes the knee to become increasingly varus (bow-legged) and relaxes the tension in the MCL.

Following injury to the MCL, a knee that is stable to valgus stressing in extension will usually repair satisfactorily even if it is slightly lax in 15–20° of flexion. If, however, there is instability in both knee positions, the possibility of long-term significant disability should be considered, especially in the presence of other ligament damage, for example anterior cruciate ligament (ACL) injury. Stress views under fluoroscopy can provide objective evidence of the degree of instability.

An injury to the lateral collateral ligament rarely happens in isolation and is often associated with damage to the biceps tendon and posterolateral corner of the knee. Cruciate ligament injuries are often damaged at the same time. Tenderness and swelling/bruising can often be found after such an injury. Varus stressing should be done in a similar fashion to the MCL with the knee observed in both full extension and slight flexion. Check for damage

Table 10A.2 Patterns of knee instability

Plane	*Direction*	*Likely structures involved*
Coronal	Valgus (lateral)	Medial collateral ligament ± cruciate ligament(s)
	Varus (medial)	Lateral collateral ligament ± cruciate ligament(s) ± biceps femoris tendon
Sagittal	Anterior tibial displacement	ACL ± collateral ligament(s)
	Posterior tibial displacement	PCL ± collateral ligament(s)
Transverse	Usually valgus	Patella instability
Axial (rotatory instabilities)	Anteromedial (medial tibial condyle subluxes anteriorly)	ACL + medial collateral and medial capsule
	Anterolateral (lateral tibial condyle subluxes anteriorly)	ACL ± lateral collateral ligament
	Posterolateral (lateral tibial condyle subluxes posteriorly)	PCL + lateral collateral ligament and associated structures

ACL, anterior cruciate ligament; PCL, posterior cruciate ligament.

to the neighbouring common peroneal nerve, which causes foot drop.

Anterior cruciate ligament assessment

ACL injury is relatively common. The patient often experiences a tearing or popping sensation at the time of injury; the patient also often feels the knee come out of joint and spontaneously relocate. Swelling usually appears within 1–2 hours and indicates haemarthrosis secondary to bleeding from torn vessels on the ligament. Immediate assessment is usually difficult due to swelling, and limitation of movement and pain. In the post-acute stage a more full assessment can be made. The patient can often run in a straight line but experiences instability on changing direction or twisting.

ACL stability is assessed by several tests. The anterior drawer test is performed with the knee flexed to 90° (Fig. 10A.10). Ask the patient to relax their hamstrings, which can mask ACL incompetence. Stabilise the leg by sitting on the foot – warn the patient first! Place your thumbs on the patient's tibial tubercle, index fingers on the medial and lateral hamstring tendons to confirm their relaxation and the other three digits of both hands behind the upper calf. Push the proximal tibia forward and assess the amount of anterior translation. Check the other healthy knee. Some knees exhibit slight laxity but with a definite 'endpoint'. With ACL injuries the anterior translation is excessive and usually associated with a 'soft endpoint', indicating ACL incompetence.

Lachman's test assesses the ACL in a similar fashion but with the knee flexed to only 15–20° (Fig. 10A.11). One hand stabilises the femur while the other grips the upper tibia and assesses the amount of anterior travel of the leg. With large thighs, it is easier to stabilise the femur at the correct degree of flexion by placing the examiner's knee under the patient's thigh and the examiner's hand on the front of the thigh. Lachman's test can often be undertaken at an earlier stage after acute injury when the knee cannot flex fully to 90°. Sometimes the degree of anterior translation will differ for the anterior drawer and Lachman's tests. This is because the two tests assess the ACL in different positions and hence the tautness of the ligament may differ, with different subsections of the ligament having slightly differing roles in various knee positions.

The pivot shift test assesses anterolateral instability associated with ACL incompetence (Fig. 10A.12).

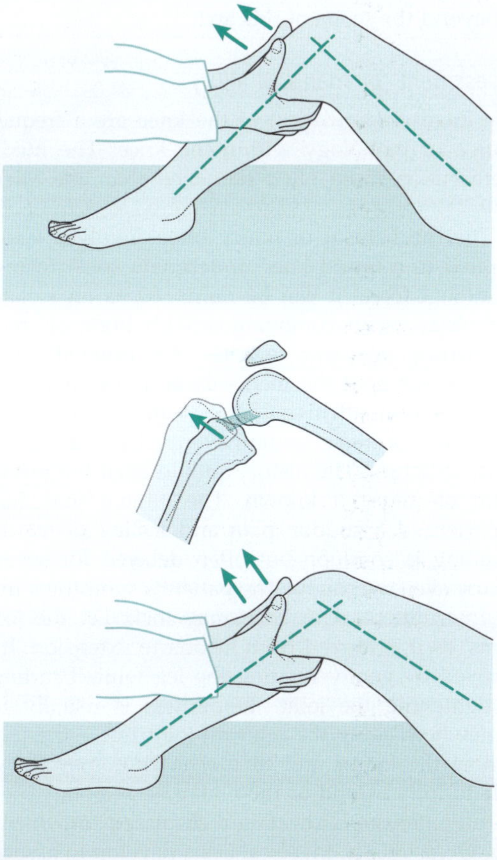

Figure 10A.10 The anterior drawer test of the knee. (Redrawn with permission from McRae R 2004 Clinical Orthopaedic Examination, 5th edn. Churchill Livingstone, Edinburgh.)

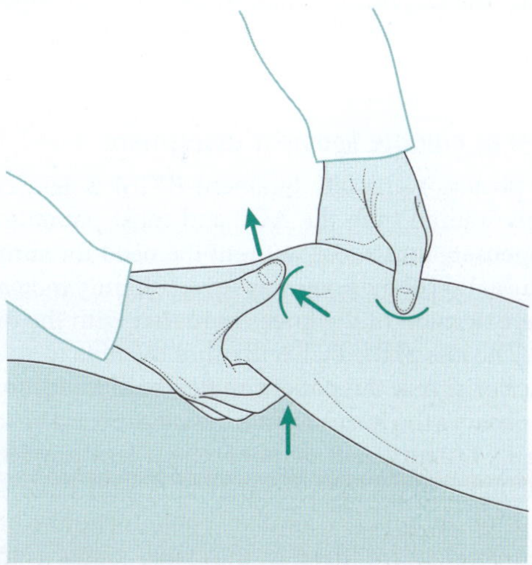

Figure 10A.11 Lachman's test of the knee. (Redrawn with permission from McRae R 2004 Clinical Orthopaedic Examination, 5th edn. Churchill Livingstone, Edinburgh.)

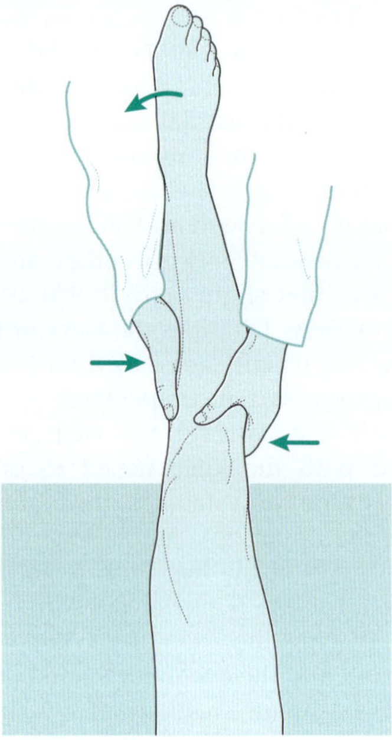

Figure 10A.12 The pivot shift test of the knee. (Redrawn with permission from McRae R 2004 Clinical Orthopaedic Examination, 5th edn. Churchill Livingstone, Edinburgh.)

The test starts by holding the knee extended and the tibia internally rotated. A valgus stress is applied to the knee. In ACL incompetence, the lateral tibial condyle will be in a subluxed position. While maintaining the valgus rotational stress, the knee is gradually flexed. At about 30°, the knee reduces with a clunk.

Posterior cruciate ligament assessment

The posterior cruciate ligament (PCL) is less commonly injured than the ACL and most patients can compensate for its loss without the need for surgery. Examination of the knee may reveal slightly increased hyperextension of the knee compared with the other side. The loss of the PCL will cause the tibia to sublux posteriorly. Ask the patient to flex both knees to 90° and observe the knees from a lateral aspect. The knee with PCL injury will demonstrate a less prominent tibial tubercle as the proximal tibia will have subluxed posteriorly. A similar phenomenon can be demonstrated by flexing the knee over a thigh support to about 20–30°. Gravity will cause the proximal tibia to sag posteriorly (Fig. 10A.13).

A posterior drawer test is performed by flexing the knee to 90° and pushing the proximal tibia posteriorly. Excessive sag is an indication of an incompetent PCL. Other tests for assessing posterior and combined rotatory instabilities involving the PCL include a dynamic posterior shift test and Jacob's reversed pivot shift test. However, a discussion of these tests is beyond the scope of this text.

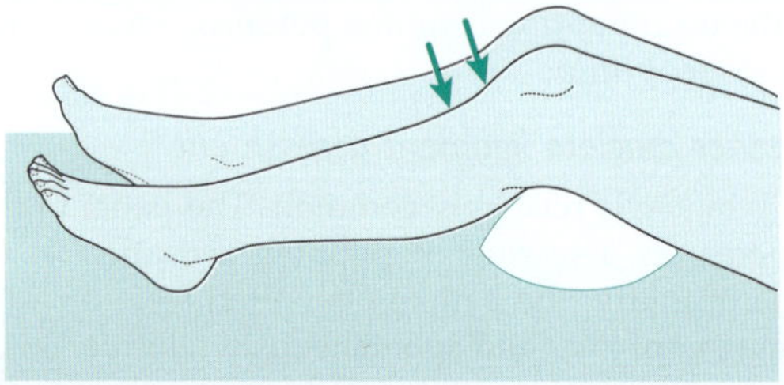

Figure 10A.13 The gravity test of the knee for PCL instability. (Redrawn with permission from McRae R 2004 Clinical Orthopaedic Examination, 5th edn. Churchill Livingstone, Edinburgh.)

Assessment for meniscal injury

The menisci (cartilages) of the knee are a frequent source of pathology within the knee. The medial meniscus is more often damaged than the lateral side.

The mechanism of injury often involves a load applied to a flexed knee undergoing some form of rotational force. It can be damaged as an isolated pathology or in combination with bone or, more frequently, ligament injuries. An isolated single episode can spilt the meniscus or, more frequently, it occurs as an attritional injury with initial weakening of the cartilage leading eventually to a full tear in its structure. The history should elicit the mechanism of injury if known. The patient may have experienced a sudden pain and feeling of tearing. Swelling is common but often delayed for several hours, even overnight. The patient's symptoms may be intermittent. The knee may lock, i.e. the joint 'jams' as it is moved from flexion to extension. It is relieved by gently rotating the leg while bending/straightening the joint. Tenderness is usually felt somewhere along the relevant joint line – the junction of the femur and tibia. The knee may not be able to fully extend or there may be a spongy block to full extension indicating a displaced torn meniscus. Occasionally, meniscal cysts develop in association with meniscal injury. They are far more common on the lateral side. They present as well-circumscribed soft-tissue swellings originating at the level of the joint line.

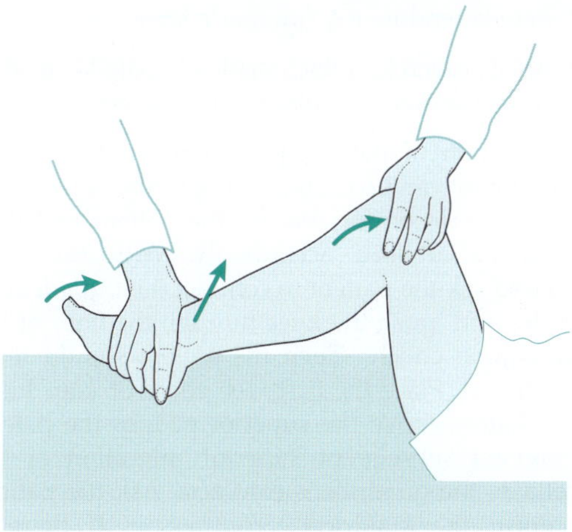

Figure 10A.14 McMurray's manoeuvre for the medial meniscus. (Redrawn with permission from McRae R 2003 Clinical Orthopaedic Examination, 5th edn. Churchill Livingstone, Edinburgh.)

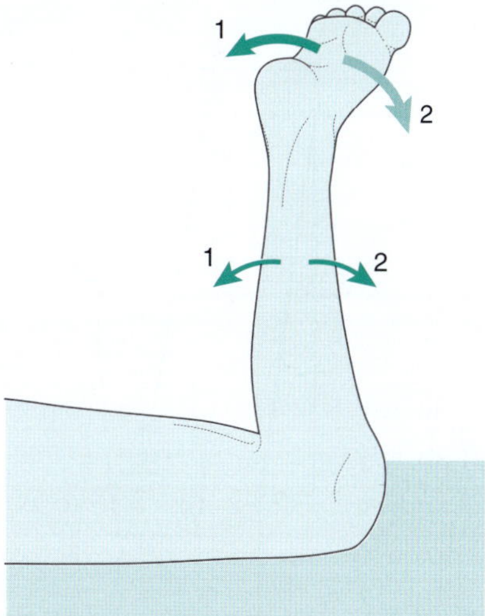

Figure 10A.15 Apley's grinding tests. (Redrawn with permission from McRae R 2003 Clinical Orthopaedic Examination, 5th edn. Churchill Livingstone, Edinburgh.)

With the patient supine, pick up the leg and flex the knee as fully as is comfortable for the patient. Place the thumb and index finger of one hand on both medial and lateral joint lines of the knee. With your other hand hold the ankle and heel. Gradually extend the knee while imparting an external rotational force to the leg. A click and/or pain may be felt over the medial joint line indicating a medial meniscal lesion (Fig. 10A.14). For a lateral meniscal lesion, repeat the test but internally rotate the leg in combination while extending the knee and check for pain and/or a click from the lateral joint line.

Apley's test is used to diagnose meniscal injury and to try to distinguish it from collateral ligament damage (Fig. 10A.15). The patient is laid prone with the knee flexed to 90°. First axial compression is applied to the knee joint. This is done by applying pressure to the joint through the patient's heel. While this is being done the leg is rotated (internally for lateral meniscal and externally for medial meniscus lesions). The knee is gradually extended. Pain is strongly suggestive of a meniscal injury.

For collateral ligament injuries, the same test is applied except for the knee joint being distracted by one of the examiner's hands being placed on the back of the thigh while the heel is distracted at the same time as a rotational force is applied to the leg. Pain on either side of the knee is said to be diagnostic of a collateral ligament injury, since a distracted joint should not experience pain from a damaged meniscus relieved of compression from between the femoral and tibial condylar surfaces.

Assessment of the patello-femoral joint

The patella is shaped like the keel of a boat with two facets – lateral and medial – designed to align with the corresponding surface of the intercondylar groove (trochlea) of the distal femur. Many different variations of patella size and height and facet size angle and relative proportion exist. The patella engages with the groove as the knee begins to flex from full extension and remains in contact with the femur during the rest of the flexion arc. During this process, large forces are generated which, on a flexed knee during single leg stance amounts to several times the patient's body weight. Patients usually complain of anterior knee pain, instability or both in relation to patellofemoral disorders.

The patellae should be assessed with the patient:

- standing
- lying supine
- knees flexed over the end of the examination couch.

The knee should be assessed for the presence of alignment abnormalities known to be associated with patello-femoral abnormalities:

- Genu recurvatum (hyperextension) as described above
- Genu valgum (knock-knee) as described above.

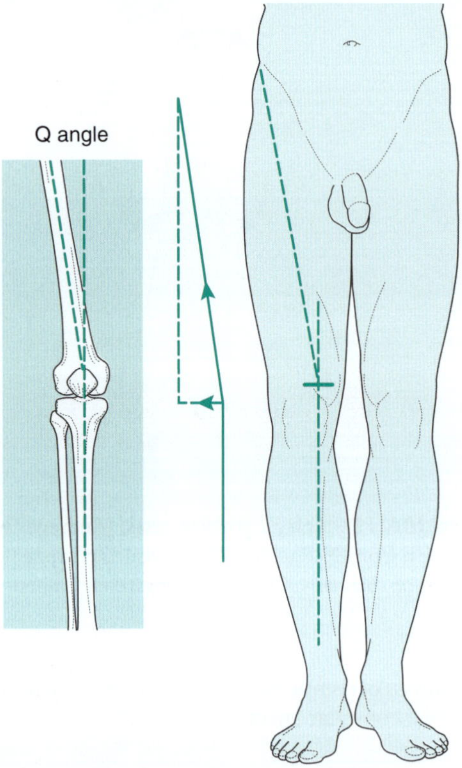

Figure 10A.16 Finding the Q angle. (Redrawn with permission from McRae R 2004 Clinical Orthopaedic Examination, 5th edn. Churchill Livingstone, Edinburgh.)

The Q angle should be assessed and, if thought to be abnormal, formally measured and recorded. The Q angle is the angle between the patella ligament long axis (middle of patella to the tibial tubercle) and a line joining the anterior superior iliac spine (ASIS) and the middle of the patella (**Fig. 10A.16**). The measurement should be taken with patient standing. It is usually about 6–12°, although intra-observer and inter-observer error is common. Angles over 15° are said to be abnormal.

Any painful/tender areas should be elicited by palpating the patella and its associated ligaments. Tenderness may occur at a number of sites, for example:

- quadriceps tendon superior to the patella
- patella itself, e.g. patello-femoral syndrome, patella osteoarthritis, bi-partite patella
- inferior pole of the patella (Sinding–Larsen–Johansson disease)
- Patella tendon, e.g. 'jumper's knee'
- tibial tubercle attachment of patella tendon (Osgood–Schlatter disease in teenagers).

Confirmation of painful pathology in the patello-femoral joint can be elicited using Clarke's test. This test can be uncomfortable for the patient and they should be advised accordingly. With the knee extended ask the patient to contract their quadriceps muscles and 'push the knee through the floor of the examination couch'. Then the patient should relax the muscles. Place the first web space of your hand immediately above the superior pole of the patella to prevent subsequent superior migration of the patella as the quadriceps contracts. Ask the patient to repeat the quadriceps contraction. If there is inflammation and/or cartilage damage from the patello-femoral joint, discomfort and possibly crepitus will be experienced as the patella is prevented from proximal migration and forced against the corresponding surface of the femoral intercondylar groove.

Assess the size of the patella and its position in relation to the femur in extension to establish whether there is a degree of patella alta (high-positioned patella). As the knee is moved through a range of flexion/extension, the examiner's hand should be placed on the patient's patella to assess for crepitus denoting surface irregularity from the patello-femoral joint. If there is concern about the integrity of the extensor patello-femoral mechanism ask the patient to straight leg raise (SLR) from the hip. This will test quadriceps strength. In addition, if there has been damage to the patella, quadriceps or patella tendons, the patient will have difficulty raising the leg or will do so with the knee flexed (extensor lag).

Assess horizontal mobility of the patella. Make sure the patient's quadriceps are relaxed and move the patella laterally and medially. Problems can arise from a patella that is too mobile or too stiff. As the patella is moved to either side, palpate the exposed facet surface for tenderness caused by arthritis or chondromalacia. Excess mobility may produce instability episodes, termed 'patellofemoral instability'. Excessive stiffness may cause pain particularly if it is associated with a tendency for the patella to tilt laterally causing unequal pressures on the facets (lateral pressure syndrome).

The patella is prone to subluxation (partial dislocation) or dislocation. The direction of dislocation is almost always lateral. There are different forms of patella dislocation (Table 10A.3)

Table 10A.3 Forms of patella dislocation

Type of dislocation	*Description*
Congenital	Present at birth. Rare and usually irreducible patella dislocation
Traumatic	Usually direct blow to patella from medial direction. Most commonly seen in adolescent girls
Recurrent	The patella frequently either fully or partially (subluxes) dislocates. Usually follows an initial traumatic episode. The patella dislocates, usually with progressive ease
Habitual	Patella dislocates every time the knee joint flexes. This is rare, but is seen in patients with lax joints or possibly toddlers with fibrosed lateral thigh structures following repeated intramuscular injections into the quadriceps muscles

and many of the common predisposing factors include:

- high positioned patella (patella alta) often in association with hyperextension of the knee (genu recurvatum)
- small patella
- poor tone/strength of quadriceps musculature – especially vastus medialis
- quadriceps contracture/fibrosis – usually secondary to trauma
- congenitally deficient (hypoplastic) lateral femoral condyle
- laterally placed tibial tubercle (where the patella tendon inserts)
- tight lateral structures, e.g. lateral retinaculum
- increased Q angle – causing a resultant force to move the patella laterally.

The apprehension test is performed as part of the assessment of horizontal, or translational, mobility. If, when attempting to displace the patella laterally, the patient experiences the same premonition felt immediately prior to a dislocation episode they will try to stop the test.

Finally, ask the patient to sit on the end of the examination couch with the knees flexed. Ask the patient to extend each knee in turn while observing the 'tracking' of the patella. Compare the pathways described by each patella. Most patients' patellae will follow a straight track. However, some patients will noticeably move their patellae laterally as they perform the last 10–20° of extension. Sometimes, this may be associated with lateral tilting of the patella in terminal extension. Excessive lateralisation of the patella may be associated with pain and instability episodes.

Testing of muscle groups controlling knee function

Quadriceps

The practitioner should inspect the tone of the quadriceps. Wasting of the vastus medialis in particular may occur as a result of knee dysfunction. A tape measure can be used to assess muscle bulk in this area and monitor any change as a result of treatment (Fig. 10A.17). The circumference of both legs should be measured at a standard distance of 10 cm above the superior pole of the patella. The rectus femoris muscle is a weak flexor of the hip but a powerful extensor of the knee. As part of the quadriceps group of muscles, rectus femoris is an important stabiliser of the knee, in conjunction with the vasti, and is needed to swing the leg forward in gait. Pain at its insertion (anterior inferior iliac spine) can arise with a strong kicking action. Examination of the rectus femoris muscle is undertaken with the patient sitting on the edge of the couch with the knees flexed. To assess the strength of this muscle, the patient is asked to extend the knee while the practitioner attempts to resist this active motion.

Hamstrings

The tone of the hamstrings should be inspected. From an extended knee position the strength of the hamstrings is tested by asking the patient to flex their knee (push down) against resistance. The 90:90 test is used to identify tightness and contracture of the hamstring muscle group. Tight hamstrings may cause knee flexion, creating an inefficient antagonist action with the quadriceps and a functional equinus at the ankle joint. The 90:90 test is performed with the patient supine. The knee and hip are flexed to 90°. The practitioner holds the leg and extends the knee until resistance is met. If the knee can be fully straightened or straightened to within 10°, then the

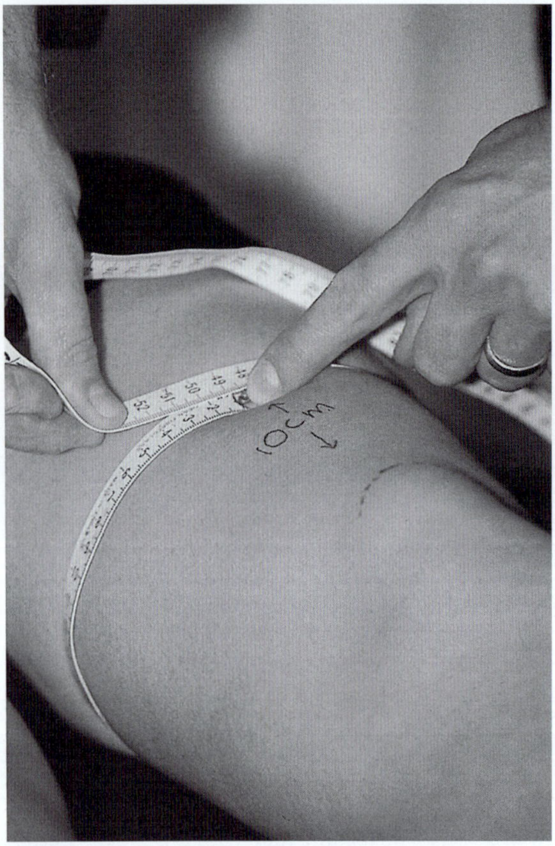

Figure 10A.17 Assessment of muscle bulk (quadriceps) using a tape measure.

hamstrings are within normal limits. If the leg can only be partially extended it indicates tight hamstrings.

Any asymmetry should be noted. To assess whether this is due to a tight biceps femoris (lateral hamstring) or semitendinosus (medial hamstring), the biceps femoris muscle can be stretched by rotating the extended leg medially and the semitendinosus can be stretched by rotating the leg laterally.

Joint aspiration

It may be both necessary and helpful to aspirate a swollen knee. This will relieve discomfort and allow inspection of the fluid. It should be performed under strict aseptic conditions and with local anaesthesia. Examination of synovial fluid is covered in Chapter 13.

Imaging of the knee

X-rays

Imaging of the knee should commence with plain radiographs. The two most commonly requested views are:

- AP – weightbearing wherever possible (Fig. 10A.6(A))
- lateral (Fig. 10A.6(B))

Two other views can also be requested:

- tunnel – for closer inspection of the intercondylar notch area
- skyline view of patello-femoral joint (Fig. 10A.6(C)).

The radiographs should be scanned for abnormal features, including:

- overall alignment, e.g. the development of varus (bow-legged) or valgus (knock-knee) deformities
- skeletal development in immature bones
- recent bone or joint injury
- development of osteoarthritis, e.g. joint narrowing, cysts, osteophytes, and juxta-articular sclerosis (increased bone density close to the joint)
- bone mineralisation
- patella position – seen best on lateral and skyline views
- loose bodies within the joint
- calcification of soft tissues, e.g. origin of the MCL (following injury) and menisci (seen in chondrocalcinosis)
- lesions of the immature joint, e.g. osteochondritis dissecans.

MRI

In the past 20 years, MRI has established itself as the imaging modality of choice for assessing soft tissues in and around the knee, for identifying cartilage lesions, and detecting subtle bone lesions not obvious on plain X-rays (Fig. 10A.18). It has an accuracy for diagnosis of around 98% in experienced hands.

Ultrasound

Ultrasound has a role in imaging of structures around the knee. It is useful for viewing soft-tissue swellings, e.g. cysts behind the knee, patellar tendon pathology. It is particularly helpful when a therapeutic procedure such as drainage of a cyst is required as this can be undertaken under ultrasound guidance.

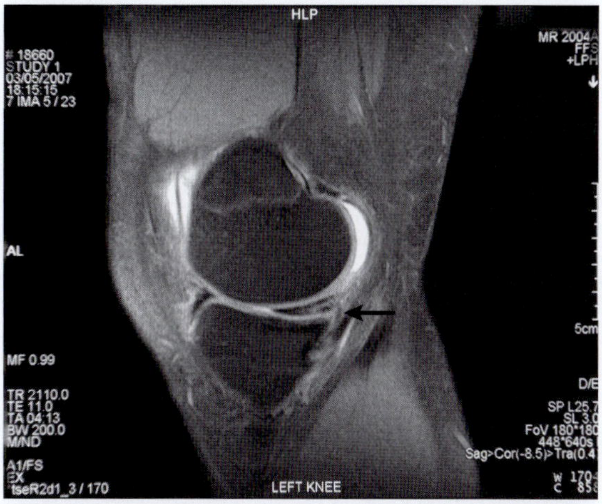

A

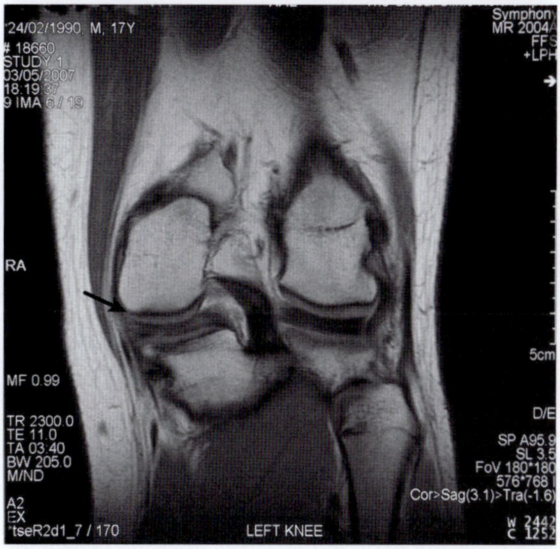

B

Figure 10A.18 MRI of knee demonstrating a medial meniscal tear.

Foot and ankle examination

Ankle and hindfoot examination

When examining the ankle and hindfoot, the following joints should be assessed:

- ankle joint (talocrural joint)
- inferior tibiofibular joint
- STJ (talocalcaneal joint)
- MTJ or Chopart's joint – comprising the talonavicular and calcaneocuboid joints.

Functionally these joints work together in a complex arrangement to allow stable weightbearing and propulsion. All of the major soft tissue structures spanning the ankle and hindfoot should also be examined.

Inman (1976) regarded the ankle as a two-joint system comprising the talocrural joint and the STJ. In addition, Brukner & Kahn (1993) consider the inferior tibiofibular joint to be part of the ankle joint complex. The inferior tibiofibular joint is a syndesmosis supported by the inferior tibiofibular ligament. A small amount of rotation is present at this joint. Elftman (1960) considered the MTJ to be the third member of the ankle complex. The midtarsal and the subtalar joints are often termed the rearfoot complex as the two structures work in tandem with each other. Motion of the foot is primarily controlled through the rearfoot complex, but the whole proximal segment relies on the ankle joint working in concert with this rearfoot complex.

Each of these joints will be considered separately for examination purposes but functionally they should be considered together.

Talocrural (ankle) joint

Assessment of talocrural joint ROM, stability, strength, palpation for tenderness, grading of ligamentous injury and proprioception are important parts of the ankle joint assessment.

Anatomical and biomechanical considerations

The trochlear surface of the talus articulates with the inferior surface of the tibia to form the talocrural joint. The medial and lateral malleoli provide additional articulations and stability to the ankle joint. The talocrural joint is a triplanar joint but, because of the position of its axis and the shape of the joint surfaces, its main motion is in the sagittal plane. The lateral curvature and radius of the trochlear surface of the talus has been found to be variable – the longer its radius, the less dorsiflexion (Barnett & Napier 1952). During midstance there should be at least 10° of dorsiflexion at the ankle to allow the leg to move over the foot. The axis of movement of the ankle is not in a strict sagittal plane but skewed in both transverse and coronal planes. If an imaginary line is drawn from the tip of both malleoli, the axis of the ankle joint will be closely followed passing from medial to lateral both posteriorly and inferiorly. This obliquity varies and is responsible for a small degree of medial-lateral foot deviation during ankle motion. The obliquity of the axis is also important in absorbing the normal rotational motion more proximally in the leg during gait.

Compensatory mechanisms for stiffness of the talocrural joint

If necessary, the body can compensate for a lack of ankle dorsiflexion at the knee and/or rearfoot complex. The STJ has less available sagittal plane motion than the talocrural joint, but if necessary the STJ will increase the amount available through the MTJ. The amount of overall dorsiflexion/plantarflexion available in the subtalar and midtarsal joints is best appreciated following a successful ankle fusion (arthrodesis) that has eliminated ankle motion. In addition, the knee can hyperextend (genu recurvatum) or undergo earlier stance phase flexion as a way of compensating for an ankle equinus.

Talocrural joint motion

The passive range of talocrural joint plantarflexion and dorsiflexion should be assessed and compared for each limb. The total arc of movement is variable. Plantarflexion is usually considerably more than the available dorsiflexion (e.g. 40° compared with 15° respectively). Ankle equinus is traditionally defined as less than 10° of dorsiflexion at the talocrural joint, although some practitioners suggest that less than 5° dorsiflexion leads to abnormal compensation. It may arise from acquired or congenital causes of a soft tissue, osseous, or combination of both types of abnormalities.

Assessing sagittal plane motion at the talocrural joint is difficult. It can be assessed as:

- non-weightbearing – either supine or prone
- weightbearing.

If assessing as non-weightbearing in a supine position, the patient should lie with the knee extended and the foot and ankle free of the end of the couch. The practitioner holds the foot in a neutral position with one hand, places the other hand on the sole of the foot and dorsiflexes the ankle (Fig. **10A.19A**). If STJ pronation is allowed to occur during the examination a falsely elevated dorsiflexion value will result (Tiberio et al 1989, Rome 1996a). The force applied by the practitioner to produce talocrural joint dorsiflexion can vary; this will influence the result. A tractograph can be used to assess the ROM but the practitioner may find it difficult to use, while at the same time keeping the foot in a neutral position (Fig. 10A.19B). In addition the intra-observer and interobserver reliability of non-weightbearing talocrural joint dorsiflexion measurements using a tractograph is questionable (Rome 1996b).

A tight soleus and/or gastrocnemius may prevent talocrural joint dorsiflexion. To differentiate between the two the amount of dorsiflexion with the knee extended and flexed should be measured. With the knee flexed the tendons of gastrocnemius which cross the knee are released from tension and as a result a tight gastrocnemius should not affect talocrural joint dorsiflexion. If the amount of dorsiflexion is still reduced when the knee is flexed the cause is likely to be the soleus. A bony block (osteophytes on distal/anterior tibia or neck of talus) can also limit talocrural joint dorsiflexion with the knee flexed; however, the tendo Achilles in this case will feel slack. Assessment of the talocrural joint end-of-ROM is useful. Soft-tissue limitation, secondary to, for instance, anterior ankle synovitis will result in a springy end-feel, whereas limitation resulting from a bony block will be abrupt.

Examination of the talocrural joint with the patient prone is useful for comparing ankle motion. With the patient placing their knees close together and flexed to 90°, the patient's range of movement can be compared in the ankles. Knee flexion eliminates (or reduces) any contribution to ankle dorsiflexion restriction from gastrocnemius tightness. In addition, this position allows subtalar movement to be assessed and compared, and direct inspection of the sole of the foot for any pathology and the pattern of callus. More consistent results have been achieved when sagittal plane motion is assessed with the patient weightbearing. The patient stands facing a wall with a distance of approximately 0.5 m between the patient and the wall. One leg, with the knee in a flexed position, is placed in front, approximately 30 cm from the wall. The other leg is placed behind the forward foot with the knee extended and the foot held in a neutral position. The patient leans towards and places both hands on the wall and is asked to move their body towards the wall.To do this the patient must dorsiflex the ankle of the limb furthest from the wall. The amount of dorsiflexion can be measured with a tractograph. The lunge test is another method of weightbearing assessment of ankle dorsiflexion and is covered in Chapter 16.

Abnormal talocrural motion

Following significant lateral ligament injury, the patient may experience episodes of instability causing 'recurrent sprains'. The presence of abnormal mobility can be assessed in both the frontal and the sagittal planes.

Varus stressing is undertaken by asking the patient to sit at the end of the examination couch with the leg dependent from the knee. The examiner cradles the relaxed hindfoot in one palm and stabi-

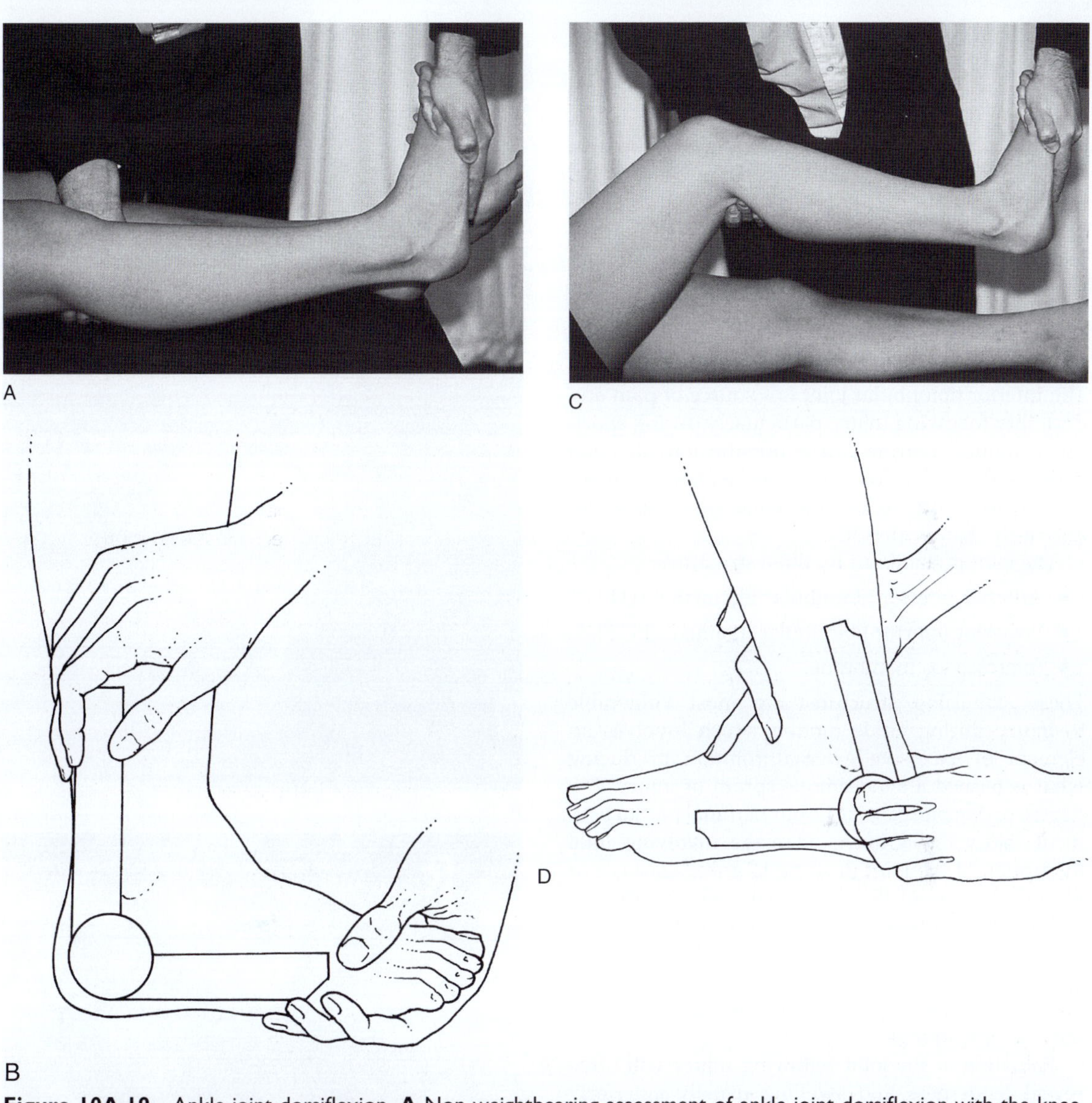

Figure 10A.19 Ankle joint dorsiflexion. **A** Non-weightbearing assessment of ankle joint dorsiflexion with the knee extended and the foot in the neutral position. Restriction of motion may be due to tight gastrocnemius, soleus or bony block. **B** A tractograph is used to measure the amount of dorsiflexion. **C** Non-weightbearing assessment of ankle joint dorsiflexion with the knee flexed and the foot in a neutral position. Restriction with the knee flexed due to a bony block or tight soleus. **D** Assessment of ankle joint dorsiflexion weightbearing.

lises the lower shin with the other hand. Pressure is applied to the hindfoot from the lateral aspect to see if there is excessive talar tilt. It assesses the integrity of the lateral ligament complex overall. A comparison should be made with the other side. More specific testing of the integrity of the anterior talofibular ligament of the lateral ligament complex is undertaken by performing an anterior talar drawer test. The patient should be placed in the same position as for varus stressing. The examiner's hand on the heel pushes the calcaneum forwards while the tibia is stabilised by the examiner's hand placed on the anterior aspect of the tibia. The amount of forward glide of the talus beneath the tibia is noted. Once again a comparison should be made with the other side.

For both tests, it is important that the patient is relaxed and that the hindfoot is isolated from the midfoot and fore-foot. If stressing the ankle is uncomfortable for the patient, local anaesthesia can be applied to the damaged ligament area. Objective evidence can be obtained by repeating the stress testing under fluoroscopy. This allows formal measurement of the angle of talar tilt and amount of forward translation on performing a talar drawer (Fig. 10A.20).

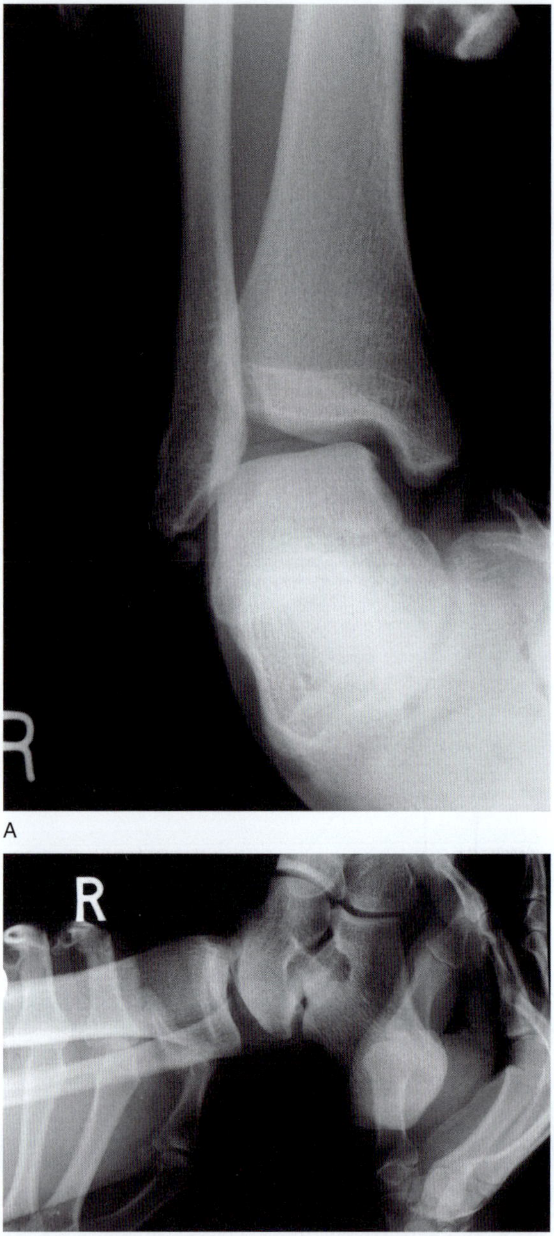

Figure 10A.20 Plain X-rays of abnormal talar tilt and anterior translation secondary to lateral ligament instability of the ankle joint.

Inferior tibiofibular joint

The inferior tibiofibular joint is a source of pain and disability following injury particularly during sporting activities. During ankle dorsiflexion, the gap between the distal tibia and fibula widens by about 1.5 mm to accommodate the talus which is wider anteriorly than posteriorly.

The joint is stabilised by three structures:

- Anterior inferior tibiofibular ligament (AITF)
- Posterior inferior tibiofibular ligament (PITF)
- Interosseous membrane.

These stabilising structures are most vulnerable to injury during ankle motion which involves an element of excessive external rotation producing what is termed a syndesmotic sprain or injury. The degree of damage can vary from minimal partial ligament injury to significant damage involving total disruption of the joint (leading to ankle diastasis or loss of the normal tibiotalar relationship) with disruption of the interosseous membrane in the calf and a high proximal fibula fracture (Maisonneuve's injury). Often there will be a fracture or ligament injury on the medial side of the ankle as well in the more severe injuries.

Palpation of the joint following injury will often reveal tenderness and swelling usually anteriorly and occasionally posteriorly. More widespread lateral swelling and pain usually indicates a combination of injury to the lateral and syndesmotic structures. Three specific tests for syndesmotic pathology have been described:

- Calf squeeze test (tibia-fibula compression test)
- External rotation test
- Cotton (tibiofibular shuck) test.

A positive calf squeeze test is elicited if pain is felt at the syndesmosis when the proximal calf is compressed by manual pressure. This is performed by pushing the fibula and tibia towards each other in the midcalf area which forces the syndesmosis apart reproducing pain at this site if it is torn.

The external rotation test is probably the most reliable test for confirming pathology from the syndesmosis. With the knee flexed over the end of the couch, the examiner holds the heel in the palm of the hand. The calf is stabilised with the other hand. The lower hand external rotates the hindfoot under the tibia. If injured, this manoeuvre will reproduce the pain occurring at the syndesmosis.

The cotton test is designed to detect abnormal increased medial and lateral translation within the ankle mortise. The relaxed, dependent ankle is grasped in one hand while the leg is stabilised with the examiner's hand. The heel is moved medially and laterally. The amount of translation detected is compared with that of the other side.

Subtalar joint (talocalcaneal joint)

The inferior surface of the talus articulates with the superior surface of the calcaneus at three facets. The largest facet forms the posterior joint, which is separated from the others by the interosseous talocalcaneal ligament, which lies in the sinus tarsi. Pain may arise from damage to the sinus tarsi. The STJ produces triplanar motion. Because of the position of its axis, little movement is produced in the sagittal plane but motion does occur in the frontal and transverse planes (ratio of motion 1:3:3). Alteration of the axis can favour motion in one direction at the expense of motion in another. The knee and foot are affected by the axial position of the STJ (Green & Carol 1984).

Joint motion

To measure triplanar motion at the STJ one would have to measure the motion produced in each plane, which is impossible to achieve clinically. The amount of frontal plane motion at the STJ can be measured, and this is used as an indicator of the ROM at this joint. It is important that there is an adequate ROM and appropriate direction of motion at the STJ for normal pronation and supination of the foot. The amount of movement in the STJ varies enormously (Isman & Inman 1969). There is normally twice as much inversion as eversion (ratio 2:1). The range of movement should always be compared with the other side. Sometimes, such as in pes planovalgus deformities, the total range of movement may be normal but with excessive eversion and little inversion, that is the arc of movement has moved towards eversion. Stiffness of the STJ should raise the possibility of conditions such as:

- arthritis of the STJ
- tarsal coalition.

To assess frontal plane STJ motion the patient lies prone with the ankle and foot hanging over the edge of the couch. The distal third of the leg is bisected; this line is used as a reference point for measuring the range and direction of motion. The calcaneus is moved into its maximally inverted position and its posterior surface is bisected. A tractograph is used to measure the angle between the bisection of the leg and the bisection of the posterior surface of the calcaneus. The calcaneus is placed in its maximum everted position and a reading is taken of the angle between the bisection of the leg and the bisection of the posterior surface of the calcaneus. Although this technique is helpful for clinical assessment, it is not considered accurate (Elveru et al 1988). Milgrom et al (1985) examined 272 male infantry recruits and an error in excess of 20% was identified. It is also recognised that for research purposes its reliability and validity are poor (Menz 1995). Some consider it to be so poor as to suggest that this method of examination no longer be used to determine the measurement of STJ movement (see section B and Buckley & Hunt 1997). A weightbearing assessment of STJ ROM would theoretically be a better indicator of the range used during walking.

A more accurate method of assessing subtalar movement is to place the patient prone and ask them to flex their knee to 135° (nearly full flexion for most patients). In this position the axis of the STJ lies close to the horizontal axis. The heel is passively inverted and everted and a goniometer used to assess mobility.

Abnormal pronation

Abnormal pronation, that is excessive STJ pronation during contact phase and/or STJ pronation occurring when the STJ should be supinating during midstance and propulsion, is one of the most common disorders of the lower limb. A large degree of frontal plane motion in the foot (due to uncontrolled STJ pronation) is thought to predispose to forefoot pathology and ankle dysfunction, whereas a greater degree of transverse plane tibial rotation is thought to predispose to leg and knee pathology.

The presence of four or more of the following may indicate abnormal pronation:

- More than 6° between the relaxed calcaneal stance position (RCSP) and the neutral calcaneal stance position (NCSP)
- Medial bulging of the talar head or 'midtarsal break' – quantified using the navicular drift technique (Menz 1998)
- Lowering of medial longitudinal arch – quantified using the navicular drop technique (Mueller et al 1993)
- More than 4° eversion of the calcaneus
- Helbing's sign (medial bowing of the tendo Achilles)

- Abduction of the forefoot at the MTJ (concavity of lateral border of foot)
- Apropulsive gait.

Numerous conditions arising in the lower limb may lead to abnormal pronation, including the following, albeit not exhaustive, list:

- Internal or external torsion of the leg/thigh
- Tibial (genu) valgum/varum
- Coxa vara/valga
- Ankle equinus
- Rearfoot varus
- Inverted forefoot
- Everted forefoot.

For treatment to be effective it is important that the cause and the extent of the abnormal pronation are correctly identified; otherwise, only symptomatic treatment on a trial and error basis can be provided.

Midtarsal joint

The MTJ comprises two synovial joint complexes: talonavicular and calcaneocuboid. This joint is also known as the transtarsal or Chopart's joint, and is an articulation between the rearfoot and forefoot. It has two axes: longitudinal and oblique. The longitudinal axis provides frontal plane motion facilitated by the ball and socket joint of the talonavicular articulation. The oblique axis involves both calcaneocuboid and calcaneo-talonavicular joints and primarily produces transverse and sagittal plane motion. Limitations of motion at the ankle joint are compensated at the oblique axis of the MTJ.

The MTJ assists in reducing impact forces and helps to prepare the foot for propulsion. It can also accommodate walking on uneven terrain without affecting the rearfoot. This means that the forefoot might invert while the heel remains vertical; the converse does not occur. The movement at the MTJ is intimately linked to that at the STJ. This is perhaps best demonstrated following an isolated talonavicular fusion for osteoarthritis. Approximately 70% of hindfoot inversion and eversion is lost.

Joint motion

To assess the motion at the MTJ the practitioner must stabilise the STJ and prevent any motion occurring at this joint by firmly holding the heel with one hand and holding the foot just distal to the MTJ with the other. The MTJ should then be moved in the following planes:

- Sagittal
- Transverse
- Frontal.

There should be most motion in the sagittal and transverse planes and minimal motion in the frontal plane. The position of the axes will affect the amount of motion at the MTJ, for example a high (vertical) oblique axis will result in an increase in transverse plane motion but a reduction in sagittal plane motion. Motion of the MTJ should be assessed in isolation by stabilising the calcaneus in a neutral position in line with the long axis of the leg and the forefoot in parallel to the floor. Abduction and adduction should be assessed. There is usually twice as much adduction as abduction at the joint. The total range should be noted as well as direction. The other side should be compared.

Stiffness of this joint complex occurs in arthritis and gross pes planovalgus deformities. In the latter, it may not be possible to bring the joint into neutral from its fixed abducted position.

Metatarsal and Lisfranc's joint assessment

The articulations between the bases of metatarsals 1–5 and the three cuneiforms medially and the cuboid laterally are known collectively as Lisfranc's joint. It is named after Jacques Lisfranc (1790–1847), a field surgeon in Napoleon's army. Lisfranc described an amputation performed through this joint because of gangrene that developed after an injury incurred when a soldier fell off a horse with his foot caught in the stirrup. Injury to this joint complex is unusual and commonly misdiagnosed. The complex is stabilised by series of ligaments. Significant injury is associated with considerable disability. Osteoarthritis is quite common in this area, particularly in the second and third tarsometatarsal joints often in the presence of gross hallux valgus or flat foot deformity. Instability may occur in one or more of the joints following injury and if left untreated will result in osteoarthrosis. The Lisfranc joint is the commonest site for Charcot's neuroarthropathy (see Ch. 18).

Try to isolate the source of pain and/or instability by isolating each metatarsal in turn and passively mobilising each of the basal joints and asking the patient to identify any symptoms. The first and fifth metatarsals have independent axes of motion and produce triplanar motion. The second metatarsal is firmly anchored to the intermediate cuneiform and has least motion; the third has less motion than the fourth metatarsal. Whereas the first and fifth metatarsals provide triplanar motion, the central three only move in the sagittal plane. The ability of the first metatarsal to plantarflex is important in order that the medial side of the foot makes ground contact during gait and the first MTPJ can dorsiflex during propulsion. Patients commonly present with cutaneous changes associated with dysfunction of the metatarsals, especially the first and fifth. Sometimes one of the metatarsals may be held in a plantarflexed position. The position of the metatarsals can subsequently affect foot mechanics and gait.

Joint motion

Clinical assessment of first and fifth metatarsal motion can only be satisfactorily undertaken in the sagittal plane. Unlike most joints, motion at the first and fifth rays is measured in millimetres, not degrees. To assess sagittal plane motion the patient can be in a supine or prone position. The feet must be allowed to hang free of the couch. The practitioner places one hand, with the thumb to the plantar surface, around the lateral side of the forefoot including the second metatarsal while maintaining the foot in its neutral position. The other hand, again with the thumb to the plantar surface, is placed around the first metatarsal. The first metatarsal is moved into maximum dorsiflexion and plantarflexion. It is usual to find approximately 10 mm in each direction (Fig. 10A.21A,B). Lack of plantarflexion of the first ray is known as metatarsus primus elevatus. The amount of motion can be assessed using the thumb technique (Kelso et al 1982). The Sagittal Raynger is an alternative means of assessing first metatarsal motion (Fig. 10A.21C,D) (Kilmartin et al 1991). Sagittal plane motion of the fifth metatarsal can be undertaken using the same approach. The validity of this technique is questionable, however, as it may not represent the range the first or fifth metatarsal moves through during gait.

Deformity

Deformity of the metatarsals is said to occur when the range or direction of motion of one or more metatarsals is asymmetrical or the metatarsal heads do not lie in the same plane. Table 10A.4 lists the various positions and terms associated with the deformities affecting the rays; these may be congenital or acquired. It is not unusual for a problem affecting the metatarsals to be unilateral.

Metatarsal parabola

The metatarsal parabola should also be assessed and documented using the palpation technique (Spooner et al 1994), as abnormal metatarsal length is known to be associated with pathology. A short first metatarsal can be associated with the development of hallux valgus, whereas a long first metatarsal can cause hallux rigidus. Shortening of a lesser metatarsal (e.g. brachymetatarsia) can result in the development of intractable plantar keratosis, metatarsalgia, hammer or retracted toe deformity.

The metatarsal formula refers to the apparent length of the metatarsals (Box 10A.2). The second metatarsal is usually the longest and the fifth the shortest. A typical metatarsal formula is 2 > 1 > 3 > 4 > 5 or 2 > 3 = 1 > 4 > 5. A weightbearing dorsiplantar radiograph is the most accurate method of establishing the type of metatarsal parabola or cascade. Comparison with the other side reveals how often minor variations occur between the two feet.

It is important that the first metatarsal is shorter than the second to allow normal function during propulsion. When the first MTPJ dorsiflexes the first ray plantarflexes on to the sesamoids; if the first metatarsal is as long as the second this cannot occur and as a result the first MTPJ is not able to dorsiflex, resulting in overloading of the other metatarsal heads, commonly the second. The practitioner should look at the shoe crease to observe the normal oblique angle afforded by the typical 2 > 1 > 3 > 4 > 5 formula. A rare but well-recognised formula is when the fourth metatarsal is congenitally short, known as brachymetatarsia (Tachdjian 1985). In this case the formula is 2 > 1 > 3 > 5 > 4.

The metatarsal formula is important for normal digital function. Abnormalities of the formula may affect forefoot pressure distribution, causing metatarsalgia. Short first metatarsals do not necessarily cause symptoms in the foot (Harris & Beath 1949); a correlation between long first metatarsals and the incidence of hallux valgus has been reported (Duke et al 1982). Minor changes in metatarsal length may not adversely affect forefoot function and weight distribution.

Forefoot to rearfoot alignment

It is important that the practitioner is able to assess the relationship of the forefoot to the hindfoot since it can deliver clues as to underlying pathology, determine management options and assess the outcome of therapy. The plantar plane of the forefoot should lie parallel to the plantar plane of the rearfoot

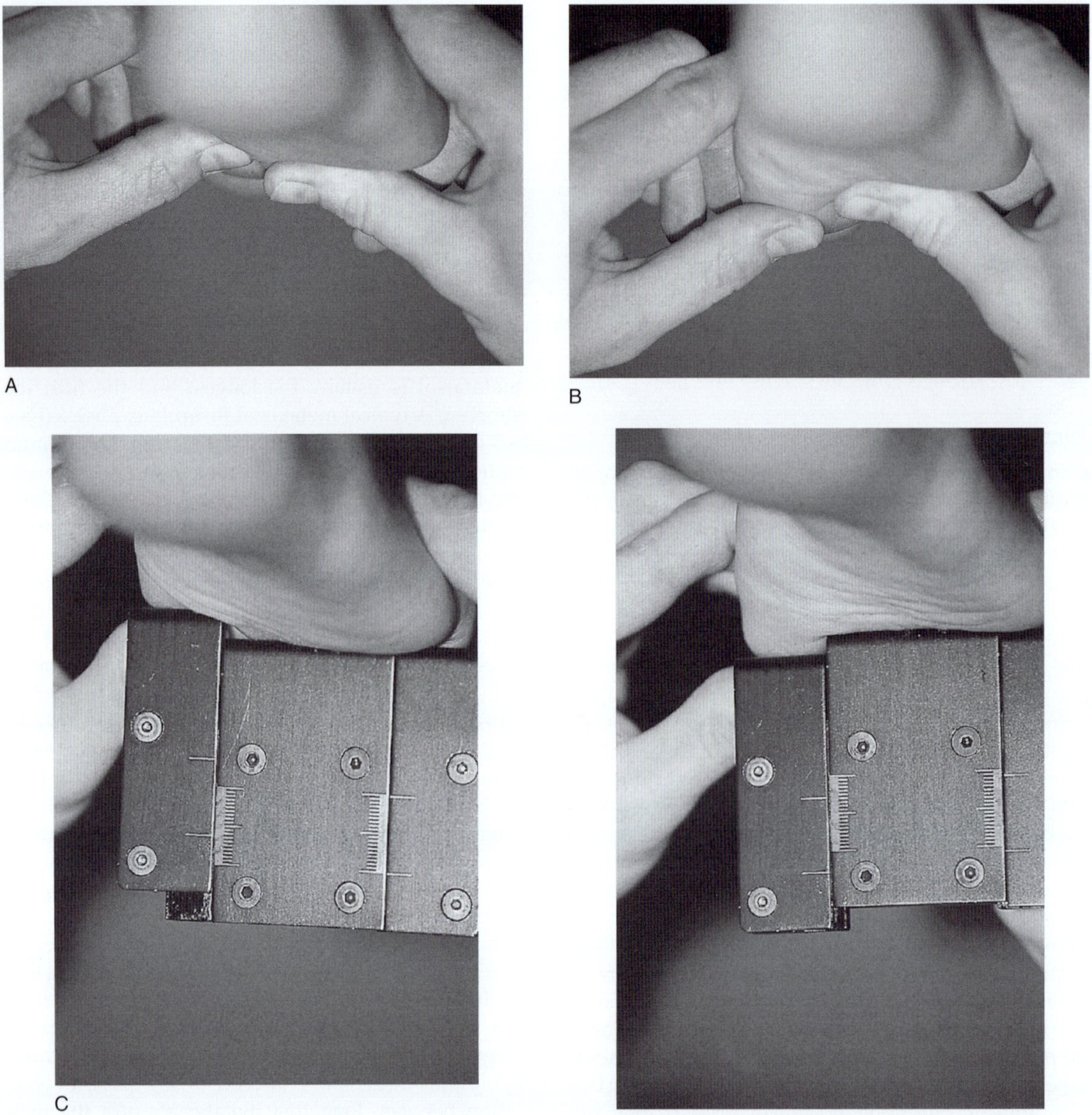

A B C D

Figure 10A.21 Assessment of motion at the first ray. **A** Measurement of dorsiflexion of the first ray using the thumb test. **B** Measurement of plantarflexion of the first ray using the thumb test. **C** Dorsiflexion of the first ray measured with a Sagittal Raynger. (Curtesy of Nova Instruments.) **D** Plantarflexion of the first ray measured with a Sagittal Raynger. (Courtesy of Nova Instruments.)

(Fig. 10A.22B), although minor degrees of variability are unlikely to be of great clinical importance. The relationship of the forefoot to the rearfoot is assessed by the following:

- The foot is placed in its neutral position. This is best assessed by the patient lying prone with contralateral knee flexed at 90° and the foot to be examined hanging over the end of the couch.
- To place the foot into the neutral position the practitioner should feel on the dorsum of the foot for the talar head. The foot should be moved into pronation and supination; while the foot is pro-

Table 10A.4 Abnormal positions of the metatarsals

Position	*Description*
Normal position	The first and fifth metatarsals exhibit equal motion above and below the second/fourth metatarsal of 10–20 mm (5–10 mm in each direction)
Metatarsus primus elevatus	Reduces ability of first metatarsal to bear weight and overloads central (dorsiflexed first metatarsal) metatarsals. Differential diagnosis forefoot varus. Shows limited plantarflexion and cannot be reduced below level of second metatarsal
Flexible plantarflexed first metatarsal	The first metatarsal may appear pronounced on the plantar surface of the foot with a cleft between the first and second metatarsal heads. Most of the movement is in the plantar direction. Loading the metatarsal head produces reduction of the position
Rigid plantarflexed first metatarsal	The first metatarsal cannot be reduced at all from its plantarflexed Position. The forefoot tends to rotate in inversion during weightbearing; this affects rearfoot function

Box 10A.2 Metatarsal formula

Optimal metatarsal length

- 1 < 2 by 1–2 mm
- 3 < 2 by 3.5–4 mm
- 4 < 3 by 6 mm
- 5 < 4 by 12 mm

nating the talar head can be felt protruding on the medial side of the talonavicular joint and while the foot is supinating it can be felt protruding on the lateral side of the talonavicular joint (Fig. 10A.23). Neutral position is achieved when the talar head is felt equally on both sides.

- As the foot is non-weightbearing it is also necessary to 'lock' the MTJ in order to reproduce the position the foot would adopt if it were weightbearing.
- To lock the MTJ the talar head should be held in its neutral position and a slight dorsiflexing force applied to the fourth and fifth metatarsal heads until the foot is at 90° to the leg. The neutral position of the foot therefore acts as a reference point from which joint motion and the position of parts of the foot can be assessed.
- While the foot is held in its neutral position a tractograph or a forefoot measuring device can be used to measure any deviation of the forefoot to the rearfoot in the frontal plane; the forefoot may be everted or inverted to the rearfoot (Fig. 10A.22A,C).
- Minor differences between the forefoot and rearfoot are usually insignificant and are often due to examiner error, but quite high angles of discrepancy can exist in excess of 15°.

The forefoot can assume one of three positions:

- **Neutral**: The metatarsals lie in a plane perpendicular to the axis of the os calcis.
- **Varus**: The forefoot appears supinated with the lateral border of the foot relatively plantarflexed in comparison to the medial border.
- **Valgus**: The forefoot appears pronated with the medial border of the foot relatively plantarflexed in comparison to the lateral border.

The various relationship permutations are shown in Table 10A.5. Once the type of relationship has been established, it is important to determine whether any identified abnormality is rigid or flexible. Clearly, flexible deformities are more suitable for conservative treatments. If hindfoot surgery is undertaken to correct a deformity to render the heel neutral, and compensatory forefoot deformity will only realign itself if the abnormality is flexible. If it is rigid, secondary surgery to realign the forefoot is required as well.

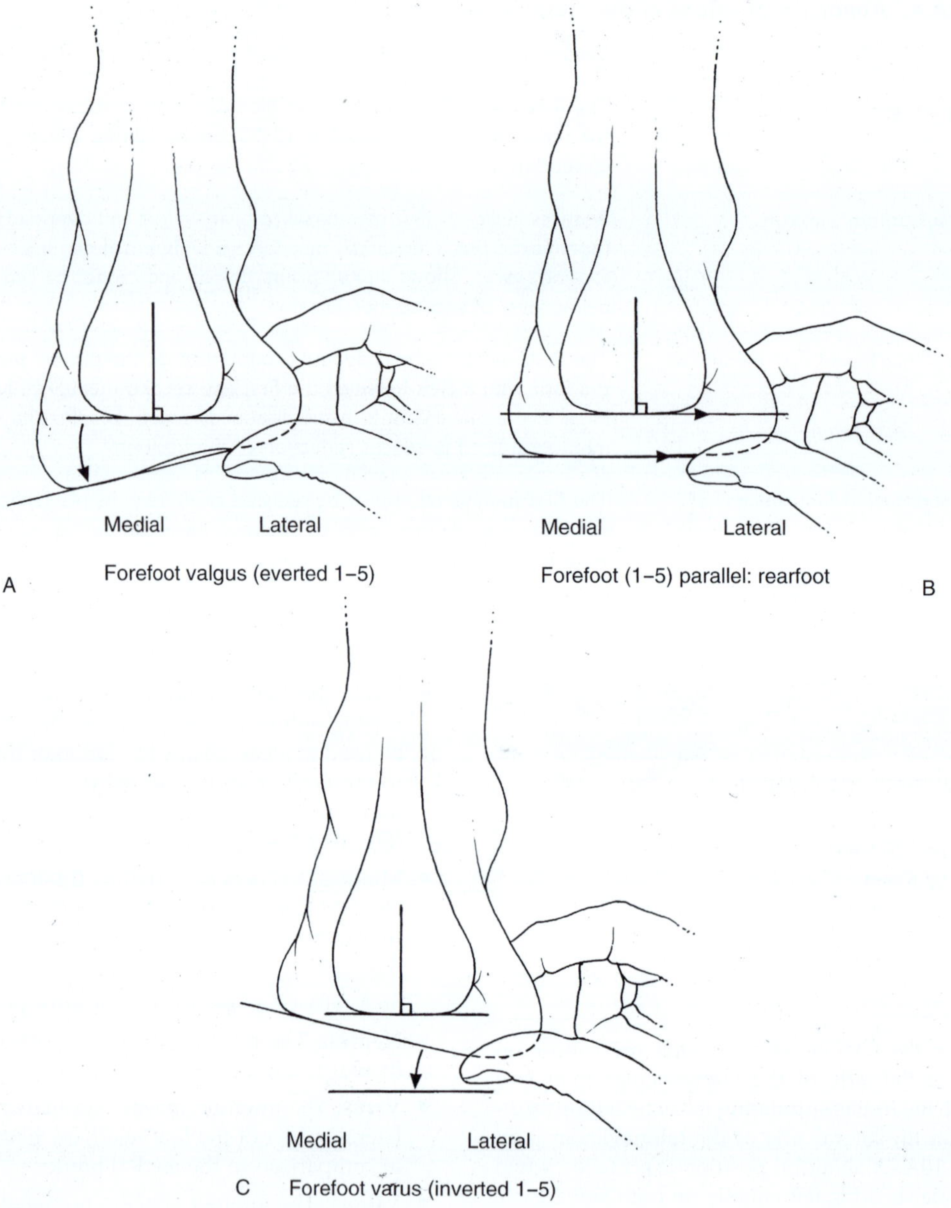

Figure 10A.22 Assessment of forefoot to rearfoot relationship. **A** Everted forefoot: the forefoot is everted to the rearfoot. **B** Ideal forefoot to rearfoot relationship: the forefoot is parallel to the rearfoot. **C** Inverted forefoot: the forefoot is inverted to the rearfoot.

An inverted forefoot may be due to:

- **true forefoot varus**: Bony abnormality, theoretically due to inadequate torsion of the head and neck of the talus during fetal development, but this is not well supported (Kidd 1997). The presence of a true forefoot varus is said to lead to a very flat foot with no longitudinal arch (Grumbine 1987).
- **forefoot supinatus**: Acquired soft-tissue deformity due to abnormal pronation of the rearfoot. The forefoot is held in an inverted position because of soft-tissue contraction. This condition

can be reduced with treatment. It can be difficult to differentiate between a forefoot supinatus and forefoot varus. Various techniques have been suggested. One is to get the patient to stand; the foot is put into its neutral position. With both conditions the medial side of the foot should not be in ground contact. Pressure is applied to the dorsum of the first ray: with a supinatus, there should be some give and the first ray should plantarflex; with forefoot varus, any pressure on the dorsum of the first ray should cause the foot to tilt inwards and the fifth ray to leave ground contact.

- **dorsiflexed first ray (metatarsus primus elevatus)**: May be a fixed or flexible deformity.
- **plantarflexed fifth ray**: As with the first ray this may be a fixed or flexible deformity – depending on the cause, treatment may reduce the deformity.

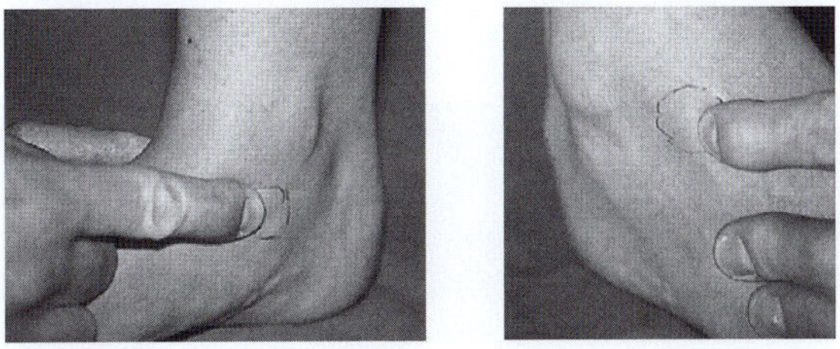

A B

Figure 10A.23 Finding STJ neutral. **A** Locating the talar head on the medial side. **B** Locating the talar head on the lateral side. It is easier to palpate the talar head on the lateral side than it is on the medial side.

An everted forefoot may be due to:

- **forefoot valgus**: Bony abnormality, theoretically due to excessive torsion of the head and neck of the talus during fetal development which holds the forefoot in a fixed everted position that cannot be reduced with treatment.
- **plantarflexed first ray**: A common cause of an everted forefoot position that may be due to a fixed or flexible deformity.
- **dorsiflexed fifth ray**: As with the first ray this may be a fixed or flexible deformity.

The incidence of metatarsus primus elevatus and plantarflexed first ray is thought to be greater than that of forefoot varus and valgus. There may also be malalignment between the forefoot and the rearfoot in the sagittal and transverse planes. The forefoot may appear plantarflexed in relation to the rearfoot or vice versa. This may be a flexible or fixed deformity and may lead to a pes-cavus-type foot. The forefoot may appear adducted on the rearfoot; this may be due to a metatarsus adductus or metatarsus primus adductus; non-weightbearing the lateral border of the foot appears banana-shaped with a metatarsus adductus.

Metatarsophalangeal joints

The MTPJs are the joints between the metatarsals and the proximal phalanges; they produce motion in the sagittal plane. During the propulsive period of gait it is important that dorsiflexion occurs at these joints to facilitate toe-off.

Table 10A.5 Various relationship permutations of forefoot to hindfoot alignment

Forefoot	*Hindfoot*	*Comments*
Neutral	Neutral	
Varus (uncompensated)	Neutral	
Neutral	Valgus (compensated)	A varus forefoot appears flat or parallel to the ground. In the position the heel assumes a compensatory valgus position. This can cause the os calcis and lateral soft tissues to impinge against the lateral malleolus
Valgus (uncompensated)	Neutral	
Neutral	Varus (compensated)	A valgus forefoot is allowed to appear parallel or flat to the floor by compensatory varus hindfoot position

Joint examination

The range and direction of motion in the sagittal plane should be assessed for all MTPJs; they should have a free ROM without pain or restriction (Fig. 10A.24). The first MTPJ has the greatest ROM: approximately 70–90° dorsiflexion and 20° plantarflexion (Bojson-Moller 1979). The range and direction of motion at the first MTPJ can be assessed with a tractograph or finger goniometer. The practitioner should appreciate that the declined angle of the first ray accounts for at least 15° of dorsiflexion at rest.

A lack of dorsiflexion at the first MTPJ is known as hallux limitus, and a complete absence as hallux rigidus. The presence of either of these conditions, but particularly hallux rigidus, will affect toe-off and can lead to an apropulsive gait and overloading of one or more of the other metatarsal heads. Some authors also consider that this interferes with the angular momentum of the body (Miyazaki & Yamamoto 1993) and predisposes to the development of chronic postural complaints (Dananberg 1986, 1993). Hallux flexus is not so common; this is where the proximal phalanx adopts a plantarflexed position. Hallux extensus (trigger toe) is where the proximal phalanx is abnormally dorsiflexed; it is often associated with pes cavus.

Restriction of movement at MTPJs could be due to osteophytes, loose bodies or articular damage, for example osteochondritis dissecans. In Freiberg's disease, there may be an enlargement of the metatarsal head and early osteoarthritic changes; this usually affects the second or third metatarsal. In some patients, particularly younger ones, clinically the joint may appear normal and X-rays may reveal no abnormalities. In these cases spasm of flexor hallucis brevis and/or abductor hallucis can be ruled out with the use of local anaesthetic block.

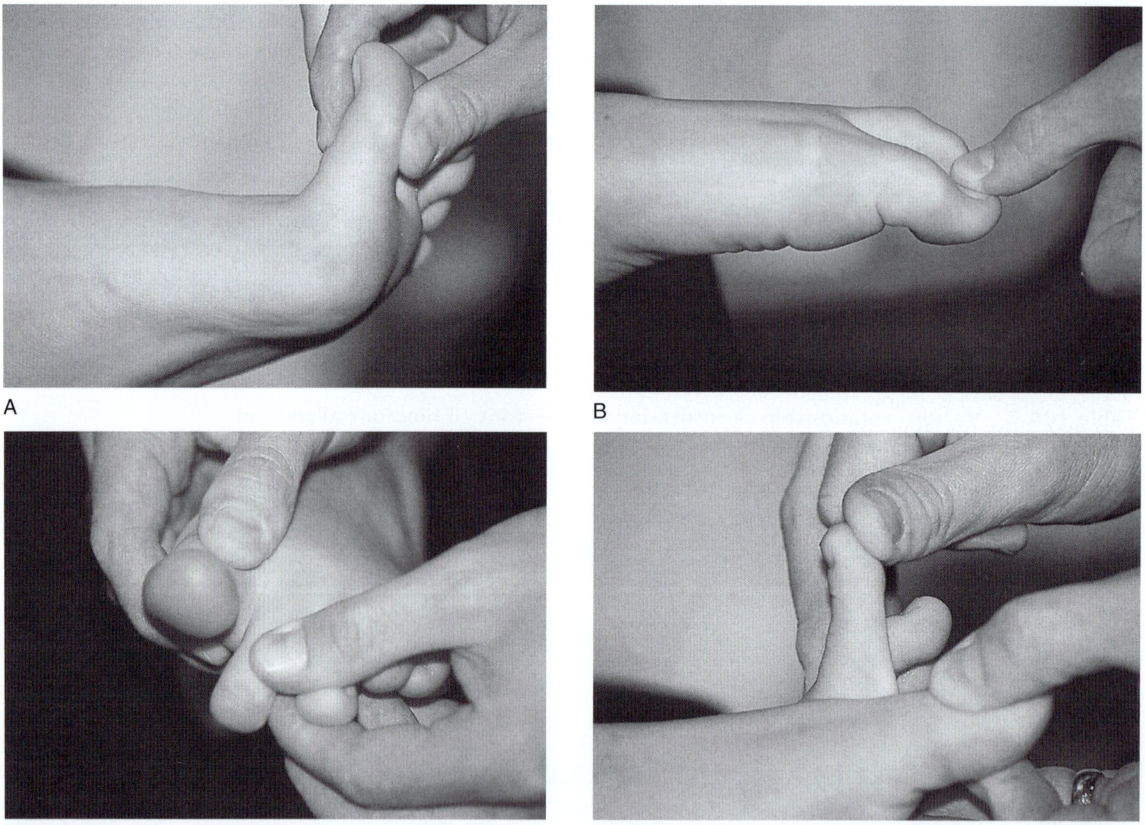

Figure 10A.24 Assessment of motion at the MTPJs. **A** Dorsiflexion of the first MTPJ. **B** Plantarflexion of the first MTPJ. **C** Dorsiflexion of the second MTPJ. **D** Plantarflexion of the second MTPJ. In both cases (first and second MTPJ) dorsiflexion is greater due to the shape of the articular surfaces.

Abnormal movement of the metatarsophalangeal joints

On occasions one of the lesser MTPJs, especially the second and third MTPJs can become unstable. The most common pattern is for dorsal subluxation/dislocation of the proximal phalanx over the metatarsal head. Less commonly, the proximal phalanx may translate/angle laterally or medially. If this occurs with dorsal subluxation it is termed a cross-over toe deformity. The causes include:

- injury
- inflammatory arthropathy
- abnormal metatarsal parabola.

MTPJ stability can be assessed by passively mobilising the joint in a dorsal-plantar direction often in association with longitudinal traction on the digit. The degree of travel of the proximal phalanx can be assessed similar to performing Lachman's test on an ACL deficient knee. A dorsally subluxed MTPJ may be reduced by this manoeuvre and then observed to dislocate again once the examiner's hands release the joint.

Interphalangeal joints

Toes have considerably less functional movement than fingers. The practitioner should note any restriction or fixed deformity affecting either the proximal (PIPJs) or distal (DIPJs) joints.

Joint examination

The PIPJs can plantarflex (approximately 35°) but cannot dorsiflex (Fig. 10A.24A). The DIPJs can dorsiflex to 30° and plantarflex up to 60° (Fig. 10A.24B,C). The patient may be unable to actively move the toes to assess the function of the intrinsic muscles. However, plantarflexion can be assessed by placing the fingers under the apices of the toes and asking the patient to claw the toes around them.

Soft tissue examination of the ankle and hindfoot

It is important to develop a systematic method of assessing the various soft tissues around the ankle and hindfoot. As with other examination areas, it is important to be able to see the patient standing and examine them both prone and supine. The following areas should be examined:

- Anterior
- Posteromedial
- Posterolateral
- Posterior

Anterior examination

The important structures to assess passing anterior to the ankle are:

- anterior ankle joint
- extensor tendons and retinaculum
- deep peroneal nerve and dorsalis pedis artery
- superficial peroneal nerve
- dorsalis pedis artery
- saphenous nerve and long saphenous vein.

Anterior ankle joint

The anterior aspect of the ankle joint is a frequent source of pain and pathology. The problems relating to the adjacent inferior tibiofibular joint and syndesmosis have already been discussed. An effusion of the ankle and/or synovitis is frequently seen best at the front of the ankle and can be confirmed by palpation.

Extensor tendons and retinaculum

There are four tendons that pass across the front of the ankle joint bound down by the extensor retinaculum. From medial to lateral, they are:

- tibialis anterior
- extensor hallucis longus
- extensor digitorum longus
- peroneus tertius.

Tibialis anterior

Tibialis anterior is a powerful invertor and dorsiflexor of the foot and ankle. It attaches principally to the medial cuneiform. It is easily palpated when the patient is asked to dorsiflex their ankle against resistance.

Extensor hallucis longus

Lateral to the tibialis anterior tendon is the extensor hallucis longus (EHL) tendon. This powerful tendon attaches to the distal phalanx of the great toe and dorsiflexes the digit and helps tibialis anterior dorsiflex the ankle. Resisted great toe extension demonstrates the activity and route of this structure.

Extensor digitorum longus

Extensor digitorum longus lies lateral to EHL. It supplies tendons to each of the lesser four toes and extends the MTPJs and IPJs of these digits. Each tendon is joined from its lateral side by smaller slips from extensor digitorum brevis (EDB) and together they form the extensor hood over the dorsum of the proximal digit to which the intrinsic muscles contribute. The tendon and its branches can be visualised by resisted dorsiflexion of the lesser toes.

Peroneus tertius

Peroneus tertius is the most lateral and least important of the four tendons of the anterior compartment of the leg. Its tendon passes anterolaterally across the ankle to insert into the dorsum of the base of the fifth metatarsal. It is responsible for dorsiflexion of the ankle and eversion of the hindfoot.

Deep peroneal nerve and dorsalis pedis artery

This nerve is the continuation of the tibial nerve that supplies the anterior compartment of the leg. It passes anterior to the ankle joint deep the extensor retinaculum between the EHL and extensor digitorum longus tendons. It supplies sensation to the dorsum of the first web space between the great and second toe. It may be injured during trauma (including surgical) and can be compressed by dorsal osteophytes (spurs) in the midfoot secondary to degenerative changes in the area. Rarely, the web space may be rendered numb following an anterior compartment syndrome of the leg (either trauma or exercise induced) causing damage to the nerve.

The dorsalis pedis artery is the continuation of the anterior tibial artery. It accompanies the deep peroneal nerve across the front of the ankle deep to the extensor retinaculum. Its pulse can be felt as it passes across the dorsum of the midfoot. It terminates by passing deep between the bases of the first and second metatarsals.

Superficial peroneal nerve

This nerve emerges from the peroneal compartment above the ankle joint and passes superficially across the anterolateral aspect of the ankle. In thin individuals, its main trunk and some branches can be seen under the skin – especially if the skin is placed under tension by plantarflexing the ankle and supinating the foot.

The nerve divides into a number of branches, which are responsible for supplying sensation to the dorsum of the foot with the exception of the first web space (deep peroneal nerve territory). The nerve(s) are at risk from traction damage following injury, for example inversion sprains of the ankle, and from injudiciously placed surgical incisions. Look for areas of tenderness and sensitivity along the course of the nerve, and for altered sensation of the dorsum of the foot.

Saphenous nerve and long saphenous vein

The saphenous nerve is a branch of the femoral nerve. It is the only sensory nerve that is not derived from the sciatic nerve below the knee. It passes immediately anterior to the medial malleolus accompanied by the long saphenous vein. It supplies sensation to the medial border of the foot as far as the hallux. It can be damaged by trauma. It may be injured during vein surgery or possibly during an ankle arthroscopy.

The long saphenous vein is the largest of the superficial veins. It drains blood from the medial side of the foot. It passes medial to the knee into the thigh before piercing the cribriform fascia in the groin to enter the femoral vein. Incompetence of the system and its communications with the deep veins of the calf can produce swelling, varicose eczema and varicosities along its course.

Posteromedial examination

The order of structures lying behind the medial malleolus of the ankle can be remembered by the mnemonic: Tom, Dick And Harry. Tom is the tibialis posterior tendon, Dick is the flexor digitorum longus tendon, And represents the posterior tibial artery, nerve and veins, and Harry is the flexor hallucis longus tendon.

Tibialis posterior

The tibialis posterior tendon passes into the foot to the posterior aspect of the medial malleolus in its own sheath. It is a strong musculotendinous unit with little excursion on contraction. It attaches to a number of structures in the foot but principally to the navicular. Failure of this tendon will cause a progressive planovalgus deformity of the foot. It inverts and plantarflexes the foot. Swelling secondary to synovitis along its course may be seen in the early stages of pathology. While the patient is being viewed from the posterior aspect look for evidence of swelling 'filling in' the sulcus between the medial malleolus and Achilles tendon.

To test its function ask the patient to invert the foot against the resistance of the examiner's hand while the ankle is in slight plantarflexion. Another useful dynamic test to assess tibialis posterior function is to ask the patient to undertake tip-toeing. The test should be performed with both feet and legs exposed. Ask the patient to stand in front of a wall and place their hands on the wall for balance. On tip-toeing, the hindfoot should swing into varus as well as plantarflexing since the tibialis posterior tendon is stronger than the peroneal tendons. Ask the patient to double-stance tip-toe:

- Can they perform this without pain?
- Do both hindfeet swing into varus?

Then, in turn, ask the patient to undertake single-stance tip-toe:

- Is the patient able to lift the heel?
- Is there a difference between the two feet?
- Does the hindfoot swing into varus?

Flexor digitorum longus

Flexor digitorum longus (FDL) lies immediately behind the tibialis posterior tendon in its own sheath. It divides into four tendons to serve digits 2–5. It crosses the FHL tendon at the knot of Henry (see below). It plantarflexes these toes by its insertion into the distal phalanx. Functionally, its loss has little functional effect on the foot and it is used to reconstruct a ruptured tibialis posterior tendon.

Posterior tibial nerve and artery

The posterior tibial nerve and accompanying artery and veins run between the FDL and the flexor hallucis longus (FHL). The nerve divides into its terminal branches the medial and lateral plantar nerves to supply sensation to the sole of the foot, medial side of the heel, and supply the intrinsic muscles of the sole.

Compression of the nerve on the medial side of the foot produces a tarsal tunnel syndrome similar to a carpal tunnel syndrome in the wrist, although it is much rarer than its upper limb counterpart. Irritation of the nerve may be found by direct palpation. Light tapping (percussion) along the line of the nerve may produce tingling (positive Tinel's test). The nerve gives off medial calcaneal branches to the medial side of the hindfoot that are at risk of localised compression and often misdiagnosed as plantar fasciitis.

Flexor hallucis longus

The FHL is the most posterior of these structures. At the ankle it is almost in the midline. It passes medially enclosed in a fibro-osseous tunnel beneath the sustentaculum tali of the os calcis. On the medial border of the foot, it crosses the FDL at the knot of Henry – often fibres between the two tendons interconnect. It inserts into the distal phalanx of the great toe and flexes the hallux. The function of the FHL is tested by asking the patient to flex the IPJ of the great toe against resistance.

The FHL is a source of posteromedial pain behind the ankle. It can become inflamed and swollen. Occasionally, the entrance into its fibro-osseous tunnel can become stenosed (narrowed) causing restriction of FHL movement and a functional limitation of great toe flexion (hallux saltans).

Medial (deltoid) collateral ligament of the ankle joint

This ligament is less commonly injured than the lateral complex. However, when injured it can occur in association with significant fractures around the ankle. With a diastasis of the joint, the talus moves abnormally laterally tearing the deltoid ligament. The two ends can become folded into the joint preventing anatomical reduction of the joint.

As the ligament lies deep to the tibialis posterior and FDL, it can be difficult to palpate separately. However, pain and swelling on the medial side of the ankle following injury, which involves an element of eversion should raise the suspicion of a deltoid ligament injury.

Posterolateral examination

The important structures to assess behind and below the lateral malleolus are:

- peroneal tendons and sheath
- sural nerve and short saphenous vein
- lateral ligament complex of the ankle joint.

The presence of posterolateral swelling secondary to significant pathology is often best appreciated, as for posteromedial pathology, by observation of both ankles viewed in the standing position from behind. Be aware that in post-menopausal women there may be swelling in this area from localised adipose deposition, which is a normal finding.

Peroneal tendons and sheath

The peroneal (lateral) compartment of the leg contains the peroneus brevis and longus tendons. The third peroneal tendon (peroneus tertius) is the most lateral of the tendons in the extensor (anterior) compartment as it crosses the ankle joint. The two tendons are named according to tendon length. As the tendons curve posteroinferiorly around the lateral malleolus, the longus tendon lies more posteriorly and superficial. The two tendons are contained within the peroneal retinaculum. On the lateral aspect of the foot, beyond the lateral malleolus, the two tendons occupy separate sheaths and are sometimes divided by a prominent bony tubercle, the peroneal tubercle.

The sheath may be swollen secondary to synovitis. This may be caused by injury or a systemic inflammatory condition, for example rheumatoid arthritis. Palpate the tendons along their courses for areas of swelling and tenderness. The brevis tendon is attached to the base of the fifth metatarsal. The longus tendon winds around the lateral border of the foot before disappearing under the cuboid bone until it attaches itself to the base of the first metatarsal. These tendons may sustain splits and tears. The peroneal tubercle is variable in size and may cause discomfort.

Ask the patient to dorsiflex and plantarflex the ankle while observing the tendons in their groove behind and below the lateral malleolus. Deficiencies of the retinaculum, usually due to trauma, can cause the tendons to sublux, or frankly dislocate, over the lateral malleolus. This causes pain and increases the risk of tendon splitting. Test the function of the tendons by asking the patient to actively evert the foot with and without resistance.

Sural nerve and short saphenous vein

The sural nerve accompanies the short saphenous vein down the back of the calf until they both move laterally to pass behind the lateral malleolus. The nerve innervates the lateral border of the foot. It is a surprisingly large nerve and can be damaged by trauma – including during surgery.

Test sensation over the innervated area. Trace the course of the nerve for signs of tenderness indicative of a neuroma. Percussion of the nerve with the index finger (Tinel's test) may localise the site of a neuroma and cause tingling in the distal distribution of the nerve.

The short saphenous vein drains the lateral structures of the foot. It passes posteriorly in the calf before piercing the fascia of the popliteal fossa to join the popliteal veins. Incompetence of the system and its communications with the deep veins of the calf can produce swelling, varicose eczema and varicosities along its course.

Lateral ligament complex of the ankle joint

The lateral ligament complex of the ankle joint comprises three significant structures:

- Anterior talofibular ligament (ATFL)
- Calcaneo-fibular ligament (CFL)
- Posterior talofibular ligament (PTFL).

Following inversion injury, the ankle can sustain a ligament sprain to one or more of these three elements. Usually the ligaments are injured in order from anterior to posterior. Thus, the mildest injury would be a grade I (partial) injury to the ATFL. The worse would be a grade III (complete rupture) of all three ligaments.

The CFL can be palpated in slim individuals deep to the peroneal tendons. The ATFL is a short structure leading anteriorly from the fibula tip lying close to the sinus tarsi. Following injury lateral swelling with or without bruising is common. More severe injuries lead to bleeding within the ankle joint (a haemarthrosis). This may cause bruising to become evident on the medial side – an important sign of significant damage following an inversion injury. Methods of determining abnormal mobility following lateral ligament injury are detailed in the section on the Talocrural joint.

Posterior examination

The posterior aspect of the ankle and hindfoot is a frequent source of pathology. It is important to consider the following:

- Achilles tendon
- Posterior aspect of the calcaneum and related structures
- Structures deep to the Achilles.

Achilles tendon and posterior aspect of the calcaneum

The Achilles tendon is a common source of pain and disability. The patient may present with one or more of the following:

- Equinus deformity lack of ankle dorsiflexion secondary to contracture
- Stiffness – especially in the morning and after exercise
- Swelling of the tendon itself
- Pain
- Acute rupture.

With Achilles tendon problems, the first issue to resolve is whether the problem is related to the tendon itself (non-insertional) or to its attachment to the calcaneum (insertional). The causes of non-insertional Achilles tendinopathy include:

- tendinosis – degeneration of the tendon itself
- peritendinitis – inflammation of the paratenon around the tendon
- combination of the above two pathologies
- rupture – full or partial.

The causes of insertional Achilles tendinopathy include:

- bursitis
- Haglund's deformity

- inflammatory arthropathies, e.g. gout
- insertional Achilles tendinopathy
- 'pump bump' – prominent lateral calcaneal ridge
- systemic enthesopathies, e.g. Reiter's disease, ankylosing spondylitis.

An equinus deformity of the ankle joint may be caused by a contracture of the gastrocnemius–soleus complex. It is possible to distinguish between a contracture of the gastrocnemius and the Achilles itself by applying the Silfverskiöld test. The patient is examined supine on an examination couch. The knee is initially extended and the degree of loss of ankle dorsiflexion assessed. The knee is then flexed to relax the gastrocnemius, which takes origin from above the knee joint on the posterior femoral condyles. If this allows the ankle to fully dorsiflex, it can be deduced that the contracture involves the gastrocnemius muscle itself (gastrocnemius equinus). If the restriction of dorsiflexion remains then the problem is determined a gastrocsoleus deformity – almost certainly from the tendo Achilles itself.

Structures deep to the Achilles tendon

Patients may present with deep pain in the posterior aspect of the ankle. It is often attributed to Achilles tendon pathology. Frequently other structures are involved. Posterior impingement of the ankle joint can cause both deep posterior ankle pain and restriction of full ankle plantarflexion.

The potential causes of this presentation include:

- inflamed FHL tendon
- large posterior tubercle of the talus (Stieda process)
- os trigonum
- shepherd's fracture of the posterior talar tubercle.

Clinical features include:

- swelling behind the ankle – usually medial
- tenderness to deep palpation
- restriction of ankle plantarflexion
- pain reproduced by passive ankle plantarflexion combined with axial compression on the calcaneum – for osseous lesions.

Examination of the forefoot

Assessment of the painful forefoot is covered in Chapter 17. In terms of orthopaedic examination, when inspecting the forefoot, the following features should always assessed:

- Observe the colour of the digits – do they appear well-perfused?
- Is sensation in the forefoot normal? If not is it local, e.g. from a Morton's neuroma, or more diffuse? Does it follow the distribution of a peripheral nerve or dermatome?
- What is the appearance and alignment of the great toe – is there evidence of bunion and hallux valgus deformity, dorsal osteophytes or clawing.
- On weightbearing do each of the digits reach the ground and contribute to load bearing?
- What is the relative length of the toes:
  - Egyptian foot type: great toe longer than the second toe
  - Greek foot type: second toe longer than the great toe
  - square foot type: great toe length equal to that of the second toe?
- On weightbearing do the lesser toes splay indication a space-occupying lesion in the web spaces, e.g. Morton's neuroma, or instability of the joints?
- Are there any swellings of the lesser toes? Either at the MTPJs or within the digits?
- Are they any deformities of the lesser toes?
- Always inspect the sole of the foot. Look for the presence of callus formation as an indicator of the pattern of wear and relative forces passing through different parts of the foot.

Imaging of the foot and ankle

The indications for different types of imaging modality of the foot and ankle are covered in Chapter 12.

Limb-length inequality

Assessment of limb-length inequality (LLI) should be an essential part of any complete assessment of the lower limb. It is usually assessed once gait analysis, non-weightbearing and static weightbearing examinations have been completed, although there is no strict convention to the order.

VIDEO

A significant LLI can have profound effects on the functioning of the musculoskeletal system, affecting any section of the lower limb, the spine, and sacroiliac joints. However, what constitutes a significant LLI remains controversial. The consequences are undoubtedly variable with some people being able to compensate for discrepancies of greater than 1 cm without any obvious disability and attaining high levels of sporting achievement. Overall, however, the more sedentary a person's lifestyle is, the lesser the importance of a relatively small LLI.

Patients may be aware of the presence of an LLI either as a result of previous consultations with other healthcare professionals or from personal observation, for example an increased tendency to limp. Indeed, some patients may already have modifications to their footwear.

Assessment of limb-length inequality

Formal measurement of lower limb lengths, even by an experienced practitioner, can be inaccurate when using either visual assessment or the tape measure. One should be aware of the potential shortcomings of the findings. If greater accuracy is required, it is possible to use scanograms with plain radiographs or computed tomography (CT).

The presence of an LLI may become apparent at several points during the orthopaedic assessment:

- The patient may volunteer during the history taking section that they are aware of a LLI
- Observation of the patient during standing and gait may reveal an obvious LLI
- Observation of the patient lying supine on the examination couch may indicate a clear relative difference in the distal extent of the lower limbs
- A LLI may only become clear on formal assessment of limb lengths.

A leg-length discrepancy may be:

- real (true)
- apparent.

A real limb-length discrepancy is due to a true difference in the segment length of the femora, tibiae or both. An apparent limb length discrepancy is present when one limb appears shorter than the other when formal assessment reveals equal limb lengths. This is caused by an abnormal positioning of one of the limbs. For instance, adduction of the hip causes the affected limb to appear shorter. It has been calculated that every 10° of adduction adds a further 3 cm of apparent shortening to any real shortening present (Ireland & Kessel 1980). In addition, an environmental limb-length discrepancy may exist due to uneven footwear or camber of roads.

Observation during patient standing and walking for limb-length inequality

The presence of a limb-length discrepancy can be observed during standing and gait.

Standing

- Hip and knee flexed on the long side
- Ankle plantarflexed in equinus on the short side
- Asymmetric lower gluteal (buttock) crease
- Pelvic tilt/obliquity*
- Shoulder tilt to one side
- Foot supinated on the short side and pronated on the long side

*Pelvic obliquity (or tilting) as observed from the front or back can be due to:

- limb shortening
- hip abduction or adduction
- spinal deformity.

Walking

- Unequal arm swing
- Marked limp during gait.

If there is evidence of limb-length inequality, wooden blocks of increasing height can be placed under the shortened limb until the iliac crest lies horizontal. This is particularly helpful when assessing a prescription to equalise limb length by providing a shoe raise. The patient's perception of a comfortable equalised limb length does not always match the observed difference as the patient is often more comfortable and confident with a long standing limb discrepancy not fully corrected.

Observation with the patient supine

Patient positioning

The patient should be examined, if possible, fully supine on an examination couch. The patient's lower limbs should be fully exposed and access is required to identify:

- a midline structure in the trunk (either the umbilicus or xiphisternum)
- the ASIS.

Reliable results cannot be obtained by attempting a limb-length assessment through layers of clothing. Similarly, care should be taken when assessing overweight patients, as identification of the ASIS can be difficult.

The patient's position should be observed and, if necessary, adjusted. Ideally this should allow the legs to be parallel to each other and the sides of the examination couch and perpendicular to an imaginary line joining the anterior superior iliac spines. If this position is possible, it is extremely unlikely that there is a significant apparent leg-length discrepancy.

If the patient has a fixed deformity of one limb, e.g. fixed hip adduction, causing an apparent LLI, then an accurate comparison of true differences can only be obtained by simulating the abnormal position in the normal limb, i.e. by placing it in a similar position of adduction.

Measurement of apparent shortening (Fig. 10A.25)

With the patient supine, the legs should be parallel and the pelvis perpendicular to the limbs. If the pelvis is tilted, it may be caused by, and masking, an apparent leg-length inequality. Apparent shortening is assessed using a midline reference point above the pelvis, either the umbilicus or xiphisternum. The limbs are measured in the position comfortable to the patient with no attempt to correct any pelvic tilt or abnormal limb position. A flexible, non-stretch tape is placed on the selected midline point and measures the distance to each medial malleolus of the ankle. Any difference between the limbs is noted.

Measurement of true (real) shortening (Fig. 10A.26)

A true measure of leg length should calculate the distance between the top of the femoral head and the middle of the ankle joint. This can be done with imaging scanograms. However, both landmarks are difficult to identify accurately in the patient and, by convention, the ASIS proximally and the medial malleolus distally are used instead.

Is there true shortening?

In the absence of any apparent shortening, the pelvis should be perpendicular to the couch with an imaginary line between the ASISs at right angles to the couch edges and the alignment of the limbs. In this position, observation of the distal extent of both heels will reveal if there is a significant difference in the length of each limb. Confirm your visual assessment by taking a flexible non-stretch tape measure and placing on the ASIS. The ASIS can be difficult to reliably identify in obese patients and hence repeat the same position accurately on the other side. The other end of the tape is then placed on the medial malleolus and the distance noted. The procedure is repeated on the other side and any differences noted. If there is apparent shortening of the limb due to for example, a hip adduction deformity, the good leg should be adducted to the same extent as the affected leg when measuring from the ASIS to the medial malleolus (Fig. 10A.27).

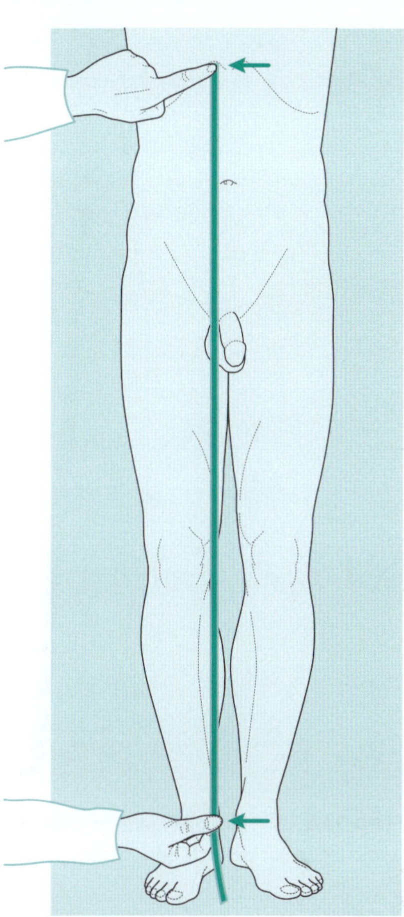

Figure 10A.25 Measurement of apparent shortening. (Redrawn with permission from McRae R 2004 Clinical Orthopaedic Examination, 5th edn. Churchill Livingstone, Edinburgh.)

Is the true shortening coming from above or below the knee or both? (Fig. 10A.28)

To assess the relative contribution of the segments above and below the knee to limb inequality, the next stage is to flex the knees equally (to about 90°). The soles of the feet should remain in contact with the

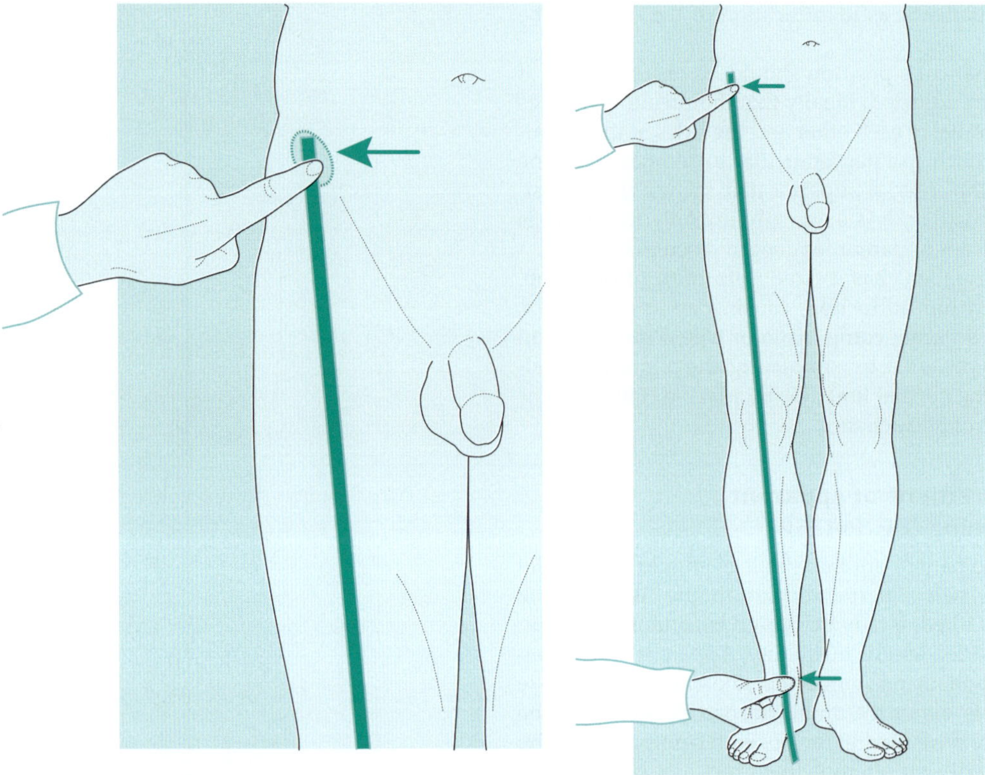

Figure 10A.26A, B Measurement of true shortening. (Redrawn with permission from McRae R 2004 Clinical Orthopaedic Examination, 5th edn. Churchill Livingstone, Edinburgh.)

couch and the examiner checks that the posterior aspects of the heels are in the same position. From this position, observe the patient from the side at the level of the knees:

- Femoral inequality: If the femora are of unequal lengths, the knee on the shorter side will not extend distally as far as the other side.
- Tibial inequality: If the tibiae are of unequal lengths, the distal thigh on the shorter side will be at a lower level than the other side.
- Combined inequality: If both the femora and tibiae are of unequal lengths combinations of the above will exist.

Confirmation of differences can be made by using a tape measure. Feel and mark with a felt tip pen the following landmarks:

1. Greater trochanter
2. Lateral joint line of the knee – felt with knee flexed as the soft area between the end of the femur and top of the tibia laterally
3. Medial joint line of the knee – felt with knee flexed as the soft area between the end of the femur and top of the tibia medially
4. Medial malleolus.

Measurement 1–2 will measure femoral length below the greater trochanter. Measurement 3–4 will measure tibial segment length. Accurate identification of the greater trochanter is prone to inaccuracy, and also to inter-observer and intra-observer error in obese patients.

Is any femoral shortening coming from above or below the greater trochanter?

If the assessment above indicated that the limb shortening was coming from above the knee, a decision has to be made as to whether it comes from above or below the greater trochanter, that is if the problem is associated with the hip or not.

In a thin patient, tape measurement from the greater trochanter to the lateral knee joint line will

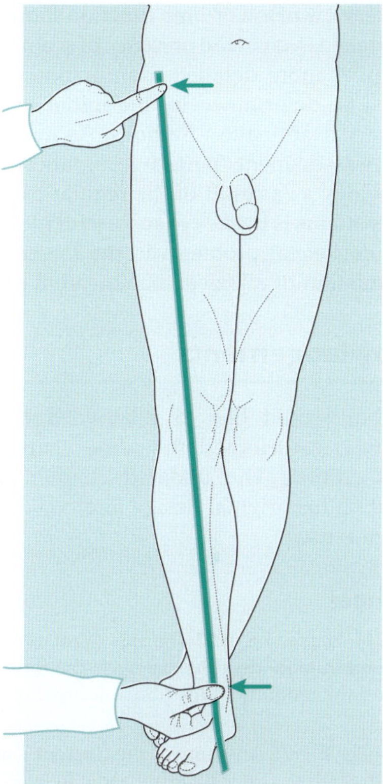

Figure 10A.27 Measurement of true shortening in the presence of an adduction deformity. (Redrawn with permission from McRae R 2004 Clinical Orthopaedic Examination, 5th edn. Churchill Livingstone, Edinburgh.)

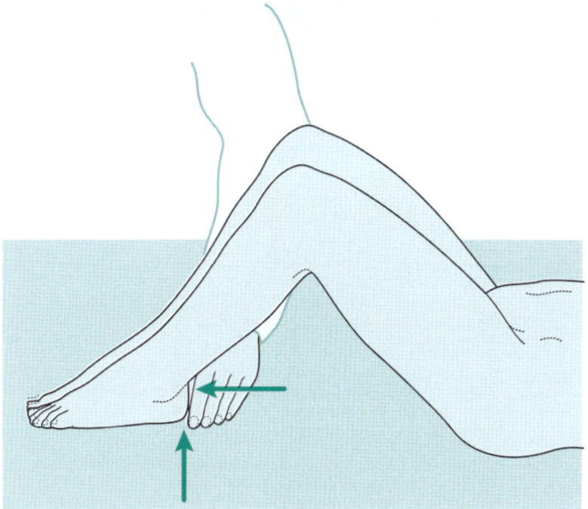

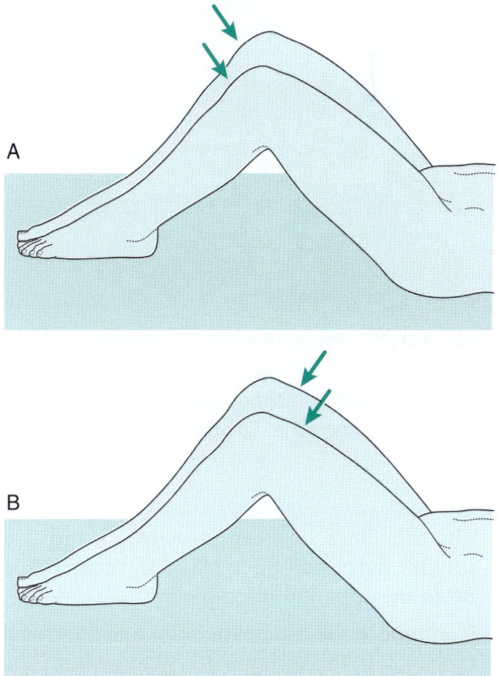

Figure 10A.28A, B Measurement of true shortening – distinguishing between **A** femoral and **B** tibial shortening. (Redrawn with permission from McRae R 2004 Clinical Orthopaedic Examination, 5th edn. Churchill Livingstone, Edinburgh.)

give an indication of the relative lengths of the femoral shafts. Alternatively, by lying the patient supine with the hips and knees extended, place your thumbs simultaneously on both ASISs. Place your middle fingers simultaneously on the greater trochanters. Assess whether the gap between your digits is shorter on one side than the other. If it is, the indication is that there is shortening above the greater trochanter (Fig. 10A.29).

Combined apparent and true shortening

Occasionally, the patient will display a combination of apparent and true shortening, for instance in advanced osteoarthritis of the hip:

- True shortening: Articular cartilage wear with or without deformity of the femoral head.
- Apparent shortening: Secondary shortening of the thigh adductors.

To assess the relative contribution of each carry out the following:

1. Measure the apparent shortening (Fig. 10A.25).
2. Compare true leg lengths by placing the normal limb in the same position as the affected limb when measuring from ASIS to medial malleolus.

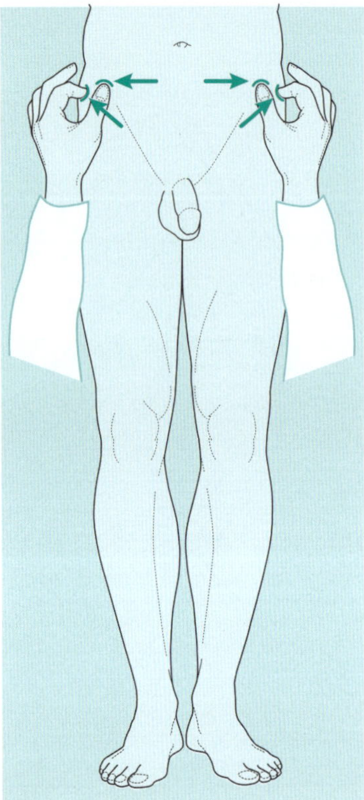

Figure 10A.29 Measurement of true shortening – above the trochanter. (Redrawn with permission from McRae R 2003 Clinical Orthopaedic Examination, 5th edn. Churchill Livingstone, Edinburgh.)

3. The difference between measures 1 and 2 will provide the contribution of the adductor deformity to the apparent discrepancy.
4. Continue to determine the source of the true discrepancy, in this example likely to be from above the greater trochanter.

Summary

Assessment of problems involving the lower limb requires a methodical and open-minded approach from the examining practitioner. Pathology will often be located to one discrete structure, but the possibility of referral of symptoms from other areas of the limb and more proximally should never be discounted. In addition, one should always consider the possibility of secondary problems developing in adjacent structures as a result of pain, disability or deformity in the primary area.

An overview of lower-limb function should always be undertaken even in the presence of seemingly local pathology. A more detailed examination of specific areas will be determined by the initial history and preliminary examination findings. As in all areas of healthcare assessment, 'pattern recognition' of potential pathology as a result of the regular examination of many patients is the key to successful identification of musculoskeletal problems in the lower limb and the formulation of a logical management plan.

Acknowledgements

The author would like to acknowledge Mr Paul Beeson who contributed the same chapter in the previous edition. The updated chapter has been modelled on his original design and certain sections have been reused.

References

Barnett C H, Napier J R 1952 The axis of rotation at the ankle joint in man. Its influence upon the form of the talus and the mobility of the fibula. Journal of Anatomy 86:1–9

Bojson-Moller F 1979 Anatomy of the forefoot – normal and pathological. Clinical Orthopaedic Related Research 142:10–18

Brukner P, Khan K 1993 Clinical sports medicine. McGraw Hill, Sydney, p 438

Buckley R E, Hunt D V 1997 Reliability of clinical measurement of subtalar joint movement. Foot and Ankle International 18(4):229–232

Crawford Adams J, Hamblen D L 1990 Outline of orthopaedics, 11th edn. Churchill Livingstone, Edinburgh, pp 280–283, 353

Dananberg H L 1986 Functional hallux limitus and its relationship to gait efficiency. Journal of the American Podiatric Medical Association 76(11):648–652

Dananberg H L 1993 Gait style as an etiology to chronic postural pain. Part 1: functional hallux limitus. Journal of the American Podiatric Medical Association 83(8):433–441

Duke H, Newman L M, Bruskoff B L et al 1982 Relative metatarsal length patterns in hallux abductovalgus. Journal of the American Podiatric Association 72:1–5

Elftman H 1960 The transverse tarsal joint and its control. Clinical Orthopaedics 16:41–46

Elveru R A, Rothstein J M, Lamb R L 1988 Goniometric reliability in a clinical setting. Physical Therapy 68(5): 672–677

Green D R, Carol A 1984 Planal dominance. Journal of the American Podiatry Association 74:98–103

Grumbine N A 1987 The varus components of the forefoot in flatfoot deformities. Journal of the American Podiatric Medical Association 77:14–20

Harris R I, Beath T 1949 The short first metatarsal: its incidence and clinical significance. Journal of Bone and Joint Surgery (Am) 31A(4):553–565

Inman V T 1976 The joints of the ankle. Williams & Wilkins, Baltimore, p 65

Isman R E, Inman V T 1969 Anthropometric studies of the human foot and ankle. Bulletin of Prosthetic Research 10–11:97–129

Ireland J, Kessel L 1980 Hip abduction/adduction deformity and apparent leg-length inequality. Clinical Orthopaedics 153:156–157

Kelso S F, Ritchie D H, Cohen I R et al 1982 Direction and range of motion of the first ray. Journal of the American Podiatry Association 72(12):600–605

Kidd R 1997 Forefoot varus – real or false, fact or fantasy. Australian Journal of Podiatric Medicine 31(3): 81–86

Kilmartin T E, Wallace A, Hill T W 1991 First metatarsal position in juvenile hallux abductovalgus – a significant clinical measurement? Journal of British Podiatric Medicine 46:43–45

McRae R 2004 Clinical Orthopedic Examination, 5th edn. Churchill Livingstone, Edinburgh, pp 1–9

Menz H B 1995 Clinical hindfoot measurement: a critical review of the literature. The Foot 5(2):57–64

Menz H B 1998 Alternative techniques for the clinical assessment of foot pronation. Journal of the American Podiatric Medical Association 88(3):119–129

Milgrom C, Giladi M, Simkin A et al 1985 The normal range of subtalar inversion and eversion in young males as measured by three different techniques. Foot and Ankle International 5:143–145

Miyazaki S, Yamamoto S 1993 Moment acting at the metatarsophalangeal joints during barefoot level walking. Gait Posture 1:133–140

Mueller M J, Host J V, Norton B J 1993 Navicular drop as a composite measure of excessive pronation. Journal of the American Podiatric Medical Association 83(4):198–202

Rome K 1996a ankle joint dorsiflexion measurement studies – a review of the literature. Journal of the American Podiatric Medical Association 86(5):205–211

Rome K 1996b A reliability study of the universal goniometer, fluid goniometer, and electrogoniometer for the measurement of ankle dorsiflexion. Foot and Ankle International 17(1):28–32

Spooner S K, Kilmartin T E, Merriman L M 1994 The palpation technique for determination of metatarsal formula: a study of validity. The Foot 4(4):198–200

Svenningsen S, Trejesen T, Auflem M et al 1990 Hip rotation and in-toeing gait. A study of normal subjects from four years until adult age. Clinical Orthopaedics and Related Research (251):177–182

Tachdjian M O 1985 The child's foot. W B Saunders, Philadelphia

Tiberio D, Burdett R G, Chadran A M 1989 Effect of subtalar joint position on the measurement of ankle dorsiflexion. Clinical Biomechanics 4:189–191

Section B: Functional assessment

A Redmond

Introduction

This section aims to introduce the principles of functional assessment of the lower limb and the locomotor system and to provide a practical model to follow. Along with scalpel and other instrument-based skills, and neurological and vascular assessment, a thorough investigation of the musculoskeletal system forms the cornerstone of podiatric and other healthcare practitioners', practice.

The purpose of the functional assessment, in podiatric practice often called the 'biomechanical examination', is to gain an understanding of how the lower limb might function during real-world activities. There is a slight problem though, in that this understanding must be based, not on the quantification of the actual functions that might cause the presenting symptoms, but on assumptions drawn on a limited and structured set of measures undertaken in a clinical setting. For the correct therapies to be implemented the clinical tests should represent actual function, and the assessment must provide a sensitive enough quantification to allow a therapy to be prescribed. It must also be practical enough to have clinical application in a world where appointments last 20–30 minutes, space is limited and high-tech resources are often unavailable.

With the development of microcomputer-based motion analysis technologies it is now perfectly possible, given enough time, money and expertise, to quantify accurately and in detail all of the exact movements or functions that might be contributing to musculoskeletal pathology. A detailed, and one might argue, 'proper' laboratory biomechanical examination yields a vast amount of data and is very information-rich. However, it does take hours to collect and sometimes days to analyse these data. In practice of course, apart from in research laboratories, the resources and facilities required to conduct such assessments are not available and so the day-to-day biomechanical evaluation is a series of compromises, each of which is slightly less than ideal. The key to a good functional assessment therefore is to maximise the practical utility, while minimising the degree of compromise resulting from missing information, that is achieving the ideal compromise between the time and resources required and the loss of information richness of the resulting data. Laboratory analysis is dealt with in detail in Chapter 11.

The rest of this section will focus on the practical observations and measures that make up a workable clinical functional assessment, a compromise solution for getting a broad idea of a patient's function within the constraints of typical clinical practice. It will take a critical look at the range of techniques available; such critique is necessary because *all* of the techniques covered outside the laboratory setting are compromises and should be used with due consideration of their shortcomings. However, each critical review is followed by a section on application in which the best compromises are outlined and the implementation described.

Definitions

Biomechanics

The most commonly used definition of (human) biomechanics is that of Hay (1973):

> ***Biomechanics is the science concerned with the internal and external forces acting on the human body and the effects produced by these forces.***

The field of biomechanics thus encompasses a range of disciplines including fluid dynamics and detailed study of joint forces such as finite element analysis, which are not of direct relevance to day-to-day clinical practice. Although the practitioner in clinical practice might attempt to form a mental model of the forces affecting joints (joint kinetics), in most cases the clinical assessment is based on the evaluation of no more than joint angles. Proper scientific measurement of the angular relationships and movements between bony segments is termed 'kinematics', although in clinical practice any measurement is rather more arbitrary. The use of the term biomechanics in association with the simple functional assessment conducted in clinical practice infers a level of scientific investigation not actually present in the assessment process and many would argue should be avoided.

Function

The *Oxford English Dictionary* defines function as:

> ***The action of performing. Discharge or performance of something. Activity, action in general.***

From a clinical perspective, we are usually concerned with the activities of daily living that may contribute to, or be affected by musculoskeletal pathology. Often for the purposes of the clinical assessment, the term function is taken to mean simple walking in a straight line. Although it is difficult to assess variations from straight-line walking, the practitioner should pay some attention to the mix of functions performed by the patient in the course of daily life and attempt to factor these into the clinical decision making. Variants of straight-line walking can be assessed, for example observation of sit to stand performance, stair climbing and running. These aspects are covered later.

Functional assessment

As outlined above, a proper 'biomechanical examination' would be expected to yield, as a minimum, a quantification of directly measured joint motions (kinematics measured in degrees to an acceptable degree of accuracy) acquired during the performance of a specific function or range of functions of choice. For this reason the term 'functional assessment' is used to describe the broad evaluation of static and subjective dynamic parameters that make up the typical non-laboratory evaluation of musculoskeletal function. The term biomechanical examination has a common usage in podiatry so will receive acknowledgement from time to time in this chapter but as a rule the term functional assessment will be used in its place.

Theoretical concepts

Weightbearing versus non-weightbearing movement

Most of the function that concerns us as a risk factor for musculoskeletal injury occurs with the limb in a load bearing or 'weightbearing' state. The unloaded or non-weightbearing state is in contrast usually relatively harmless, and unloaded movements rarely contribute significantly to injury. Importantly, the function of a joint in the non-weightbearing state may be very different from its function when fully loaded. Differences between loaded and unloaded measures have been reported to be up to 9.4° at the talonavicular joint and 4.4° at the subtalar joint (STJ) (Kitaoka et al 1995), equivalent to 20–30% of the joint's total range of motion. This has ramifications for the clinical assessment process and great care must be taken so as not to draw inappropriate conclusions about weightbearing function from a non-weightbearing assessment. The mechanical explanation for these differences is based on the concepts of open kinetic chain and closed kinetic chain movements.

An **open kinetic chain** is said to exist where a part moves relative to one fixed point but where the remainder of part is free to move in space. Movement of the arm and hand about the shoulder joint is a typical example of open kinetic chain motion where the distal part of the arm is unconstrained and can move freely in space. The foot and leg, however, more usually function in a closed kinetic chain. In a **closed kinetic chain** the part will be constrained at both ends. In the case of the leg, the constraint at the proximal end of the weightbearing limb derives from the hip articulation and the inertia of the body, and at the distal end the motion is constrained by the interface with the ground. In the case of the many interdependent relationships occurring in the joints of the feet this becomes particularly important. Our knowledge of the anatomy of the leg and foot has derived historically from anatomical principles drawn from the study of cadaveric specimens, all naturally non-weightbearing (i.e. open kinetic chain). In the twentieth century the study of anatomy has focused more on the functional anatomy (acknowledging the closed kinetic chain) and on attempting to understand the relationship between form and function. There remain, however, legacies of the early morbid work, and the nomenclature of the soft tissues and motions often describes the original open chain findings from the morbid specimens rather than the function of the part in closed chain 'natural' function.

Assessment of the closed chain functional anatomy of the lower limb is problematic, as it has proved difficult to re-create real-life (*in vivo*) situations in the laboratory (*in vitro*) in anything but the simplest forms – such as loading of a single tendon or small groups of tendons (Kitaoka et al 1997). In vivo studies themselves are necessarily limited by the degree of invasion that can be tolerated before the experiment itself interferes with the function of the limb. Thus the understanding of the precise function of the lower limb remains limited especially in the case of the multiple small functional units of the foot. Evaluation of the foot and leg complex has therefore been subject to two conflicting demands. It is possible to reasonably accurately quantify motion and function in the open chain but this is not particularly reflective of the true function and so the measures have little validity (Lattanza et al 1988, McPoil & Hunt 1995, Weiner-Ogilvie & Rome 1998). In contrast, while it is increasingly possible to objectively assess the limb *in vivo* in closed kinetic chain, the resources and time required are great and the accuracy is still limited. Clinical measures are quite poor at quantifying real-life dynamic function and so static and quasi-functional tests predominate. Most agree now that closed kinetic chain assessment is the method of choice as far as possible, with supplementary measures from open kinetic chain assessment performed where appropriate (Astrom & Arvidson 1995, Kitaoka et al 1995, Lattanza et al 1988, McPoil & Hunt 1995, Sell et al 1994).

Pathology – position versus symptom

The definition and quantification of foot pathology is not as straightforward as might immediately appear (Keenan 1997, Menz 1995, Saltzman et al 1995). In medicine generally there are different conventions for defining the presence of a pathological state and this is especially the case for the type of functionally mediated problems we see affecting the foot. Certain disease states, such as congenital clubfoot, are clearly abnormal and can be confirmed clinically in individuals, for instance through histology. The variation in the physical postures from 'normal' can be described statistically relative to the population at large but in the absence of clear 'physical' characteristics to define a pathological state, definitions can become confused. The most common method is to define a normal population using centiles (commonly the 5th to 95th centile) or the value encompassing two standard deviations from the mean to describe a 'normal' range. The pathological state is then defined as any state associated with values outside this range. This method is easily understood but it has limitations. First, some unwanted states carry risk of other pathology at values far less than two standard deviations from the mean, and second, it assumes that all diseases have the same prevalence in every population (100 – 95 = 5%).

Until the advent of the Root-informed philosophies of the 1980s the most universally accepted classifications of foot type had historically been based on readily recognised and relatively extreme co-existing orthopaedic pathology, such as the talipes deformities resulting in the clubfoot/cavo-varus deformity, or pes plano-valgus secondary to cerebral palsy. In these cases the pathology is usually accompanied by identifiable neurological and profound histological change (Staheli 1987). In the presence of such a characteristic clinical picture, even subjective classifications have strong face validity. Such discrete classifications (e.g. 'clubfoot' versus 'normal' or 'pes planus') require no statistical definition of normal ranges and remain in widespread use. Greater difficulty arises when there exists in clinical practice, a need for foot posture/function evaluation that relates to more subtle variations from the 'normal' or 'ideal' foot type (McPoil & Hunt 1995, Staheli 1987). Also identification of potential associations between foot type and secondary pathology or symptoms using such simple, subjective, dichotomous classifications is often inadequate.

The problem is highlighted with the definition of a class of potential deformities sometimes called 'postural' deformities. These are relatively minor variations from normal occurring in otherwise healthy people. They have no overtly pathological characteristics such as neurological involvement or histological change and often lie well within the mathematically accepted bounds of 'normality'. The postural deformities cover undesirable ranges of movement at hips, knees, ankles and feet as well as subtle positional variations in rigid segments such as femora and tibiae.

Early pioneers in the field of podiatric biomechanical theory described a number of subtle variations from normal and made sometimes ambitious claims for their importance. In disciplines used to dealing with major deformity this concern with variations from normal regarded as trivial, caused disagreement among practitioners and often between entire disciplines. Dispute has existed over the need for any intervention, the types of interventions available, and the evaluation and efficacy of any such intervention for postural problems. These difficulties with definition and 'diagnosis' have also impacted on our scientific understanding of the epidemiology and natural history, and subsequently the management of these conditions.

In the absence of any definitive cut-off points for normal and in the presence of some theoretical overenthusiasm from both extremes of the debate a strong case can be made for adopting a flexible approach to interpreting the outcomes of a functional assessment. This is especially true in defining postural states as normal or frankly abnormal and keeping an open mind is often helpful in interdisciplinary practice.

Primary 'deformity' and compensation

Another layer of complexity arises in the definition of pathology where the undesirable consequences (usually symptoms) occur as a result of compensations rather than as a result of the underlying 'deformity'. To illustrate this we can consider the example of a tibial varum, a pathological state in which the tibia is angled towards the midline more acutely than 'normal'. No scientifically derived population studies of tibial varum have defined an adequate normal range for this measure but we might usually expect to see a varus angulation of between 5° and 12° in the frontal plane. If a larger angle exists, say, for example 25°, then the primary deformity would tend to orientate the foot so that it was inverted in line with the varus tibia. On weightbearing this angulation would tend to overload the lateral side of the foot. Function on this type of foot might be expected to result in problems associated with lateral loading, such as the formation of a callus over the fifth metatarsophalangeal joint (MTPJ) or even a stress fracture to the fifth metatarsal. In practice, what happens in most people is that in the presence of a tibia aligned excessively in varus, the ankle and subtalar joints combine to allow the heel to rotate in the frontal plane, compensating for the underlying abnormality. The foot is thus able to bear weight in a plantigrade position with an even distribution of load. Unfortunately this compensation mechanism can itself cause problems. With the heel moving into a valgus position relative to the leg, the foot is likely to become excessively pronated and functionally hypermobile. If this happens then other symptoms such as central MTPJ callus or first MTPJ functional limitation might occur.

The example above uses a rigid bony segment and so is conceptually relatively simple but the dilemma extends further when normal or abnormal postures have to be considered relative to joints. In the case of joints there can be variations in normal relating to the end of the range in either (or many) directions, to the total range available, or to the joint's functionally ideal or reference position. When postures are considered relative to joints, the definition of deformity or normality becomes little more than a faith position. As a consequence there is much debate in the literature about conceptual deformities such as forefoot varus and valgus. Do they exist? How would you define them? How do they present clinically and can the link be validated scientifically? The ability of theorists to invent new and complex mechanisms or 'paradigms' to explain these linkages and patterns of compensation far exceeds the capacity of scientists to test the hypotheses properly. The result is a large gap between what is *thought* and what is *known*. This gap further contributes to difficulties of defining what is mechanically normal and, indeed, in understanding the results of our functional assessments.

Experience in both clinical and scientific fields suggests strongly that there is a case to be made for a pragmatic approach. For many of the conditions or proposed mechanisms there is little or no scientific justification, but there is often a clinical need, some coherently thought-out theory and some empirical evidence for success using a biomechanical approach. In these circumstances the author would have no hesitation in advocating intervention along functional lines – despite the absence of good science. Conversely, in the absence of a strong experimental base the discerning practitioner should remember that the biomechanical paradigms are still largely theory and not science. The wise practitioner will temper their practice, avoiding the most dogmatic definitions of deformity and outlandish claims for efficacy, respecting the healthy scepticism sometimes afforded by others in their own and other disciplines.

Principles of assessment

The principles of assessment outlined in this chapter involve nothing more complex than an ordered passage through a number of discrete systems. Using four simple systems (Box 10B.1) the practitioner can ensure that the information acquired covers all of the necessary detail without gathering unnecessary information or conducting irrelevant and time-consuming tests.

The last point in Box 10B.1 is important. There is no need to collect all the information potentially available on every patient. One is perfectly entitled to of course, but it is time consuming and an inefficient use of clinical resources. Instead we try to steer the assessment process so that we filter out areas of little or no relevance and focus our attention on more productive lines of enquiry. Achieving this 'higher state' is arguably what constitutes clinical expertise. It is certainly a skill that develops with experience.

There is at present no formally validated assessment protocol for assessing the foot and little consensus across disciplines regarding the 'ideal' assessment. Medical students are now taught a simple GALS (gait, arms, legs and spine) screen (Doherty & Doherty 1992) which includes at least some observation of walking and a brief examination of the lower limb (see Box 10B.2).

Box 10B.1 Systematic approaches to assessment

- History → Observation → Examination
- Large to little
- Proximal to distal
- Bone → Joint → Soft tissue → Skin

Musculoskeletal specialists in the medical disciplines (mainly rheumatology and rehabilitation medicine) are being introduced to a new, validated assessment protocol, REMS (Regional Examination of the Musculoskeletal System) (Coady et al 2004), which includes more detail on the foot (see Box 10B.3) but again is meant for use as part of a whole-body assessment and is too limited for a podiatric evaluation.

In the absence of a standardised foot assessment we have developed a preferred protocol for foot assessment at the Leeds unit of musculoskeletal disease, which is based on a history–observation–examination (or history + look–feel–move) model (Fig. 10B.1).

History, observation, examination

The history–observation–examination model allows the assessment process to start with a broad range of possible avenues to follow and for these to be refined sequentially as the assessment progresses. The history will usually start with the most general information, which is then supplemented by directed enquiries specific to the musculoskeletal complaints under suspicion.

History

After recording the requisite clerking information, the history-taking process starts to focus on those factors that might be indicative of the pathology being investigated. It is essential to investigate any systemic disease that might be manifesting as a local musculoskeletal problem so it is important to look for the red flags of systemic disease (see Box 10B.4). If the patient is known to have systemic disease, this should be explored further. If a definitive diagnosis has been made, it should be recorded although at times patients might have difficulty accurately recalling specific diagnoses, for example differentiating between osteoarthritis and rheumatoid arthritis and this should be cross-checked if there are concerns. If there is a confirmed diagnosis of systemic disease

Box 10B.2 Gait-arms-legs-spine screen

GALS

First three simple questions:

1. Do you have any pain or stiffness in your muscles, joints or back?
2. Can you dress yourself completely without any help?
3. Can you walk up and down the stairs without any help?

Followed by a brief structured examination of the gait, arms, legs and spine.

Gait

- Symmetry and smoothness
- Stride length
- Ability to turn normally

Arms

- Wrist/finger swelling deformity
- Squeeze test across metacarpals
- Inspect hands for muscle wasting
- Pronation/supination of forearm
- Grip
- Elbow extension (arms out straight)
- Can patient place their hands behind their head

Legs

- Knee swelling and deformity
- Quadriceps muscle bulk
- Knee effusion
- Crepitus during knee flexion
- Internal and external rotation
- Squeeze test across metatarsals
- Check for foot callosities

Spine

- Scoliosis
- Symmetrical muscle bulk
- Level iliac crests
- Tenderness over mid-supraspinatus
- Kyphosis
- Flexion (ability to touch toes)
- Neck lateral flexion (shoulder to ear)

then current treatments and related disease control should also be documented.

In the absence of systemic disease the history of any presenting musculoskeletal pain can be documented, paying particular attention to any previous history of similar problems, the onset of the current problems, the date/duration of onset and any precipitating, exacerbating or relieving factors (see Ch. 3). The history of the presenting complaint should dictate the rest of the functional assessment allowing for exploration of causal links which may help with potential management.

Box 10B.3 The Regional Examination of the Musculoskeletal system assessment protocol

- Examine sole of patient's feet
- Recognise hallux valgus, claw and hammer toes
- Assess the patient's feet in standing
- Assess for flat feet (including patient standing on tip toe)
- Recognise hind foot/heel pathologies
- Assess plantarflexion and dorsiflexion of the ankle
- Assess movements of inversion and eversion of the foot
- Assess the subtalar joint
- Perform a lateral squeeze across the metatarsophalangeal joints
- Assess flexion/extension of the big toe
- Examine the patient's footwear

Observation

The observation phase can be broken down into two parts, the *non-weightbearing observations* and the *weightbearing observations*. The patient is usually seated for the history taking and review of location of pain, and so the natural progression for this part of the functional assessment is to review the non-weightbearing observations first.

Box 10B.4 Red flags for systemic disease

- History of trauma, infection or fever immediately prior to onset
- Generalised morning stiffness
- Involvement of several joints (especially if symmetrical)
- Progressive deformity
- Unremitting pain
- Numbness/paraesthesia
- Flaccid muscle paralysis
- Pain away from typical structures (e.g. bone pain)

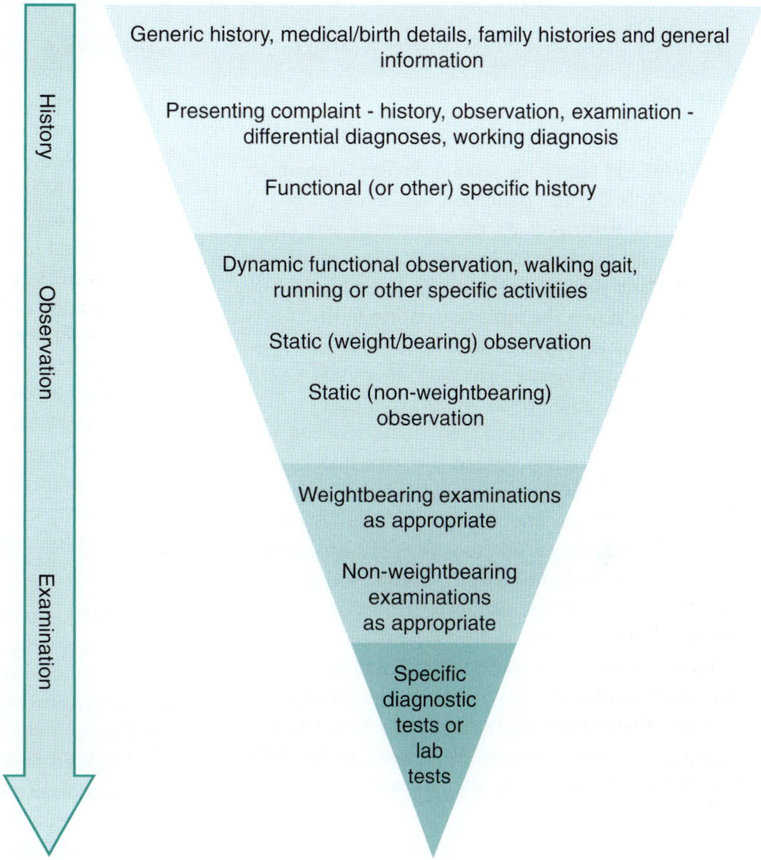

Figure 10B.1 The history–observation–examination model.

At this point the history–observation–examination model can be further refined using an appropriate anatomical model. There are several ways in which this can be followed, although all are complementary. The 'large to little' anatomical approach simply advocates starting with the large joints (such as the hip and knee) or large problems (significant deformity) before progressing to the smaller joints (the ankles and feet) or smaller, that is potentially less significant problems. For example, there is little merit in pursuing a 4° valgus forefoot deformity if the patient has a 25° valgus knee deformity.

The large to little approach also coincides well with the proximal to distal model. Finally, the entire system can be refined further by considering the structures involved, thus prioritising the observations according to importance of the anatomical structures as well as by region (Box 10B.5). The bone, joint, soft tissue, skin model ensures that significant deformities of bony segments are prioritised over deformities of joints, visible abnormalities of soft-tissue structures and visible signs in the skin (Box 10B.6). This reflects the fact that bony deformity is largely irreducible except by surgical means, that joint deformity is usually acquired and may be reducible, that soft-tissue deformity (e.g. displaced tendons, bursae or scars) are the consequence of bone/joint problems, and that skin lesions by and large are useful pointers to underlying function but are the consequence, and not usually the cause, of functional pathology. All of these assessment models will enhance a systematic approach and the clinician can adapt and match which ever is most convenient and relevant to their own purposes.

Observation (weightbearing)

At this stage in the assessment, we are concerned with making broad observations only and this part of the process mainly focuses our later, more involved hands-on assessment. As such we are looking for and documenting general clinical features. The next step is to have the patient make the transition from the **non-weightbearing** to the **weightbearing**

Box 10B.5 Observation (non-weightbearing)

Limb alignment

Observe the position/orientation of the hip/femur (if relevant and upper leg visible). Progress down to the knee checking for significant varus, valgus or fixed flexion deformity. At the same time you can consider soft tissue (muscle mass, bursae, joint swellings) and skin lesions down to knee level.

Continue down the limb, estimating tibial alignment (varus/valgus) as well as rotation and observing for soft tissue signs such as muscle atrophy. At the ankle observe for significant deformity (e.g. fixed valgus), soft-tissue swelling and the passage of tendons around the joint if visible.

In the foot, first document more major deformity such as hallux valgus and digital deformity. Try to classify the foot into a simple type (e.g. high-arched, normal or low-arched) before assessing for soft-tissue change (swelling, bursae) and skin lesions (scars, callus patterns).

At this stage, the observations should be a quick overview, a more thorough investigation can be conducted later once likely candidates have been prioritised. It may, however, be helpful to document the site and dimensions of skin lesions at this point.

Box 10B.6 Callus patterns

It has long been recognised that callosities – physiological skin thickening, as well as painful, pathological calluses – can give an insight into foot function. Note: All of the most useful callus patterns occur in the forefoot, and heel callus is not considered further here.

It should be remembered though, that interpreting callus patterns is a black art, that the relationships are incomplete, that there are many examples of inconsistencies and that no formal process of associating specific callus patterns with functional features has yet been validated. Nevertheless, some patterns may act as useful clinical pointers, and they are listed here in order of diminishing confidence in the relationship between observation and underlying pathology:

- Lateral callosities fifth metatarsophalangeal joints (MTPJ), lateral side of the fourth MTPJ. Suggest an uncompensated varus deformity (the level of the varus deformity may lie between hip and forefoot and needs separate investigation).
- Lateral callosities (fifth MTPJ), combined with localised first MTPJ callus. Indicates a tripod type function usually associated with a rigid, supinated/ cavus type foot.
- Callosity over the first interphalangeal joint. Indicates defective function of the first ray. The underlying cause may be difficult to establish but this lesion pattern indicates that *something* is wrong.
- Diffuse callosities over the second /third MTPJs. Often associated with a pronated/hypermobile foot.
- Localised callosity under the second MTPJ. May be associated with limited ankle dorsiflexion.

Combinations of these patterns can co-exist where compensation mechanisms occur but are inadequate to completely compensate an underlying deformity. In this case the compensations produce their own pattern of callus and the patterns associated with the underlying (e.g. varus) deformity manifest also.

state, observing any changes that occur. This provides some insight into the mechanisms by which any obvious deformities might be affecting function and how the musculoskeletal system is behaving to compensate for any minor shortcomings in its make-up.

Obvious signs to document are significant aberrations in the angle of gait (pointers to rotational problems in proximal segments) and base of gait (pointers to problems with balance or of frontal plane alignment). As the patient rises from the couch and takes their weight, observe whether varus/valgus problems in hips and knees are improved or worsened. Pay particular attention to the feet. Feet that appear high arched or rigid while non-weightbearing can look normal on weightbearing, while perfectly normal-looking non-weightbearing feet can become significantly pronated when required to compensate under load. Simple documentation of the change in state can provide valuable information as to the cause and the nature of any functional abnormalities.

Once the patient is weightbearing this is usually a sensible time to take a look at their walking, a part of the assessment process often referred to as **observational gait analysis (OGA)**. The first part of the OGA is usually confined entirely to observation and so fits neatly into the history–observation–examination schema. At the end of the walking observations we will start a transition into a more directed, examination-oriented protocol.

Many functional assessment protocols that were developed in the 1980s and 1990s placed the *non*-weightbearing examination nearer the front of the assessment process. The goniometer or 'tractograph' was the main weapon in the war on musculoskeletal pain and OGA was mainly used to confirm (although rarely to refute!) the findings of the detailed goniometric examination.

Following the principle laid out at the beginning of the chapter that the assessment process is a filtering mechanism, our preferred assessment model places more importance on OGA as a method for refining the requirement for later hands-on examination. There are other advantages to this. The whole functional assessment process is a surrogate for being able to quantify in detail, actual dynamic function. It makes sense therefore to get at least an empirical picture of that function early on in the assessment process. It must be remembered that OGA is highly dependent on the viewer's interpretation of events and so unless deformities are significant, OGA is relatively unreliable, especially in terms of consistency between different observers (Novacheck & Walker 2000, Saleh and Murdoch 1985). Nevertheless, despite its shortcomings OGA remains, especially for the experienced practitioner, arguably the most informative part of the functional assessment.

The kinematics of the human gait cycle have been well documented (Wright et al 1964). There is some minor dispute over the precise angulations observed, particularly in the small segments of the foot but in the main, these disputes arise due to controversy over the definition of starting reference positions and clinical protocols (Cornwall & McPoil 1999 , McPoil & Hunt 1995, Pierrynowski & Smith 1996) and while the precise values are debated, the underlying patterns of motion seem fairly clear (McPoil & Cornwall 1996, Pierrynowski & Smith 1996) and are described in detail in the chapter on gait analysis.

Observational gait assessment is the simplest approach to evaluating these patterns as they occur during walking and is inherently limited by the ability of the human eye to capture what can be subtle variations and the ability of the brain to process events occurring over very short time periods. The Leeds model uses a top-down approach, ignoring the foot at first. This reflects the fact that while podiatrists may be primarily interested in abnormalities of foot function it is important not to neglect abnormality elsewhere in the musculoskeletal system. A top-down approach ensures that the foot is always contextualised in the bigger picture.

Position yourself so that the patient can walk away from and towards you over a distance of approximately 7–10 m. If possible, the assessment setting should be arranged so that you can also get a side-on view during the assessment process; this demands more space though and may be difficult. Ask the patient to walk at normal speed and allow them time to relax before the assessment of walking starts in earnest. A thorough OGA may take several passes up and down the walkway and the patient should be warned to expect this:

- First, get a feel for the **overall gait type** – is the patient rigid, fluid, relaxed, upright, hunched, hypermobile? Specific gait patterns are associated with a range of systemic disease presentations (Box 10B.7).
- Determine whether the **walking speed** is normal and consistent and whether segments accelerate and decelerate noticeably.
- Observe the **head carriage** and the levels of the shoulders – is one side higher or lower than the

Box 10B.7 Specific gait patterns

- Festinating gait – characterised by tiny, shuffling steps and difficulty with starting and stopping.
- Trendelenburg's gait – where hip abductor weakness allows the non-weightbearing side to drop with each step.
- Rombergism – a wide, unsteady base of gait.
- Scissor gait – caused by adductor tightness (spasticity or contracture) resulting in consecutive footsteps crossing the midline.
- Hemiparetic gait – where a unilateral paralysis causes significant asymmetry. Often the paralysed leg is 'hitched' through swing phase with the hip circumducting to raise and swing the whole leg up, outwards and forwards.
- Antalgic gait – occurs in an attempt to avoid painful stimuli. There are no specific patterns per se, but the viewer will see evidence of efforts to avoid loading painful joints or structures.
- Marionette/drop foot gait – a high stepping gait style occurring in the presence of distal weakness or paralysis. The leg is lifted high to provide extra ground clearance if the foot cannot be dorsiflexed adequately during swing phase.
- Ataxia – a usually profound variation from normal, reflecting an inability to coordinate subtle interactions between muscle groups. Characterised by jerky and uncoordinated movements.

other? Different authors give different importance to small differences in shoulder height. The scientific understanding of the subtleties of 'functional scoliosis' and limb-length differences is generally weak and so common sense is advised when interpreting these signs.

- Look for **scoliosis** of the spine – either primary to spinal deformity or secondary to external factors such as malalignments elsewhere, muscle imbalance or habitual factors such as load carrying.
- Observe **upper limb carriage**. Is there evidence of flexion at elbows or of asymmetry in arm carriage?
- Observe **pelvic tilt** both in the frontal plane, i.e. left to right side tilt, and also in the sagittal plane (anteroposterior). Make a point of checking for Trendelenburg's gait (see Box 10B.7).
- Observe the **knees** from the front – are they internally rotated, externally rotated, pointing directly ahead? Check for signs of knee valgus/varus (Q angle) but beware that internal rotation and knee valgus can be difficult to distinguish during OGA.
- It is helpful at this stage to try to get a side-on view. Re-check the head carriage for anteroposterior carriage, and observe the spine for kyphosis and/or lordosis.
- Observe the knees from the side – are they fully extended, hyper-extending or permanently flexed?
- Qualitatively estimate **tibial varum**.
- Qualitatively estimate the **foot placement angle**.
- Qualitatively estimate **base of gait**.

Only once we know what is happening above the ankle do we observe the foot in function:

- Observe to get a feel for the **general function of the patient's feet**. Are they a matching pair, is the function symmetrical? Does one or both function generally about a neutral, pronated, or supinated position? Does the foot posture exhibit the normal pronation/re-supination cycle as expected through the stance phase (see Box 10B.8)?
- At first contact (often termed loading response) observe the effect of weight acceptance. Does the foot make **ground contact** at the heel, midfoot or forefoot? While even 'normal' runners will sometimes make first contact at the midfoot or forefoot at higher speeds, normal *walking* should always start with heel loading. Failure to load the heel in walking indicates significant ankle equinus, drop foot or excessive knee flexion. The knee should be close to full extension at first contact.
- **Calcaneal position.** Are the heels perpendicular to the ground in midstance or are they everted or inverted. Does this position change?
- **Medial arch height.** Is adequate arch contour maintained in midstance? Is the foot rigid and the arch profile abnormally high throughout the stance phase? Is the pronation/re-supination cycle evident?
- Does the **ankle dorsiflex** to maximum late in midstance?
- **Forefoot position.** Is the forefoot aligned with the hindfoot or is it adducted or abducted?
- It is also prudent to listen carefully while the patient is undertaking this walking assessment. Some patients exhibit an obviously heavy heel-strike which may be a relevant clinical feature.

With practice, just from watching the patient walk you should be able to get close to a functional diagnosis. Certainly you should aim to understand broadly what the lower limb is doing during gait from its outward appearance. The above protocol describes an essentially qualitative approach in which the patient's gait is observed and broad inferences

Box 10B.8 Clinical note

The normal foot goes through a pronation/re-supination cycle in stance phase.

Early pronation is counteracted by external rotation of the leg on the fixed foot, inverting the heel re-supinating the foot prior to heel-off. This mechanism can become defective if external demands on the foot are great or if the coupling mechanisms that control re-supination are inadequate.

Causes of excessive demand include:

- in-toed/out-toed gait patterns, valgus or varus knee/tibial positions, intrinsic foot malalignments. Limited ankle joint dorsiflexion (ankle equinus) creates a demand for pronation late in midstance resulting in an increase in pronation in late stance sometimes associated with an abductory twist of the whole foot at heel-off.

Coupling mechanisms can be affected by:

- antalgic gait patterns, frank arthritis, local or systemic joint hypermobility.

made. A variety of techniques are also available that document in more detail the functional or standing observations and allow a semi-quantitative approach to be applied. Using these techniques requires at least some learning – akin to learning a simple language and so these are not detailed in this chapter. Some techniques that interested reader might think worthy of further investigation include Benesh's movement notation and Valmassy's gait homunculus representation.

Observations of function other than walking

While walking is the most commonly performed assessment of locomotor function it is worth bearing in mind that some disorders will have unique presentations in specific activities. In addition to the observation of straight-line walking it is sometimes helpful, therefore, to have patients perform specific activities, such as stair climbing, or to have them perform actions that represent simple clinical tests. Foot-specific tests are detailed later but many simple variations on walking can be informative:

- **Stair climb** – stair climbing (and descending) requires proximal extensor muscle power as well as coordination.
- **Heel/toe and medial and lateral border walking** – ask the patient to walk on tip toe, then on their heels alone, and finally to walk on the medial and then the lateral border of the foot. This is evaluating a number of systems including neuromuscular coordination, distal muscle power, tendon integrity and antalgia.
- **Gower's sign** – most commonly associated with muscular dystrophy, this is a feature rather than a test per se. In the presence of profound proximal weakness the patient cannot raise themselves from a sitting position on the floor without assisting their weakened quadriceps activity with their arms, either placing the hands on the front of the knees to lever themselves up or using nearby features (e.g. a door frame or couch) to assist them.
- **Morgan's test** – a simple squat and raise test. The patient squats down so that the buttocks are close to the heels and then raises him or herself. This is difficult in the presence of distal muscle weakness.

Temporal and spatial parameters of gait

The temporal and spatial parameters of gait are the simplest of the dynamic parameters of walking and while they are best measured in the laboratory, some are simple enough that they can be measured in the clinical setting. **Temporal parameters** are those that reflect timing of gait (e.g. stance phase duration, double support vs single support periods) and are probably best left to the laboratory analysis. **Spatial parameters** reflect the position of the limb (e.g. step/stride length, base of gait, foot placement angle) and can be quantified fairly simply using readily available materials such as chalk on paper. Temporal and spatial parameters are useful indicators of functional capacity with healthier function known to be generally associated with faster walking, shorter periods of double support, longer step/stride length. These parameters can be estimated by observation but a quantitative record can be obtained clinically if so desired.

Evaluation of running

In sports practice it is not uncommon to want to see the patient engaged in activities more demanding than normal walking. Evaluating the patient running introduces more problems than the evaluation of walking because the patient is moving toward or away from you more quickly and the events of interest are shorter in duration. Some sporty practitioners are happy to take to the streets and run with patients but for most a treadmill assessment is the only option.

Treadmill running provides a reasonable approximation of gait but there are known systematic differences from over ground walking and these should be considered in the interpretation of either running or, indeed, walking patterns when the patient is moving on a treadmill. The two main complicating factors are a tendency to shorten the stride length and to lean forward. The first factor is of relatively minor importance but the transfer of load anteriorly can impact on evaluation of events such as heel loading, heel-off, ankle dorsiflexion and line of progression.

Footwear assessment

The observational component of the functional assessment should close with at least some consideration of the best available indicator of long-term function – the patient's footwear (see Ch. 9). In evaluating the contribution of mechanical factors to a clinical presentation, it is important not to miss the environmental factors as well as the intrinsic factors. The **wrong type of footwear** for an activity can precipitate symptoms (lack of lateral support or adequate cushioning for example), as can footwear characteristics, such as a runner seen by the author who developed anterior shin soreness after buying new shoes with a relatively long posterior extension to the sole in the heel region. These had increased the plantarflexion moment at heel-strike causing an overuse problem in the tibialis anterior muscle.

Old shoes also tell a tale, with **sole wear patterns** and upper distortion adding valuable information to the clinical picture.

Weightbearing static evaluation: the border between observation and examination

This phase of the assessment lies on the cusp between simple observation of presenting features and the start of the formal examination process. Simple estimation of a position or posture constitutes no more than observation but for some observations the addition of a simple line or measure helps to quantify the posture and add detail. Here we cross the border into examination. In this section all of the observations of natural standing are covered – even if a quantification technique is also added. Once manipulation of the part is required such as positioning into a neutral or reference position, or movement through an artificial range, these assessments are considered under the hands-on examination phase.

Relationship between static and dynamic measures

There is a widely held assumption among clinicians that the static posture gives the clinician a useful indicator of the likely function of that foot (Menz 1998). Bevans in 1992 reported a link between static standing measures and the site of ulceration in patients with diabetes, supporting this view. Formal investigation of this link has proved difficult, however, and the results of studies exploring the closeness of any link are equivocal, with some authors suggesting that foot morphology can be useful in predicting function and others questioning the strength of the relationship. This equivocation appears to be a product of the measures employed (both the static and dynamic measures) and to an extent the interpretation of the researchers.

Early work by Nigg and co-workers (1993) had reported a co-efficient of determination of 0.27, for the explanation of variability in transverse plane shank motion by single plane measurement of arch height. The limitation imposed by single plane measures is supported by the findings of Song et al (1996) in their evaluation of two new, experimental methods for assessing foot function. In a discriminant analysis performed by these investigators, inclusion of three measures in the model enhanced the ability of the analysis to classify correctly, planus and rectus foot types in a small sample.

The relationship between foot morphology and the resulting pressures underneath the weightbearing foot have also been investigated by Cavanagh et al (1997). Cavanagh's study of the relationship between static radiographic measures and dynamic plantar pressures under the heel and first MTPJ found that some 35% of the variation in pressures was explained by changes in foot morphology, although to attain this relatively high degree of prediction a combination of four radiographic angles were required, with individual measures explaining no more than 13% of the variance in actual dynamic function. Other data exploring the relationships at other sites in the foot have demonstrated a medial shift in load associated with pronation of the foot and a lateral shift in load occurring with supination (Arangio et al 2000). In a novel variation, Freychat et al (1996) derived foot prints from both static and dynamic passes over a specially designed apparatus. The relationship between the static and dynamically derived foot print angles was very weak with the static measures explaining only 14% of the variance in the dynamic data. Cashmere et al (1999) found even weaker relationships between standing medial arch height, and the arch compression during gait, findings supported by Hunt et al (2000) for measures of medial arch height and heel eversion with their dynamic equivalents.

It is possible however, that the relationship between static and dynamic measures varies according to site. Nawoczenski et al (1999) reported a high correlation between the static and dynamic measures of hallux dorsiflexion using an electromagnetic motion tracking system. It is likely that this finding reflects the larger ranges of motion seen at the first MTPJ, and the simplicity of attaching markers to the segments proximal and distal to the joint under investigation. Using a compound measure such as the foot posture index (FPI) improves the capacity of a static measure to predict variance in subsequent dynamic walking data to 40% (Redmond et al 2006) but this is only marginally more than the amount reported by Cavanagh.

Given the ready availability of static measures and the limited application of dynamic measures in routine clinical practice, static measures will continue to play a part in the assessment of the human foot. It

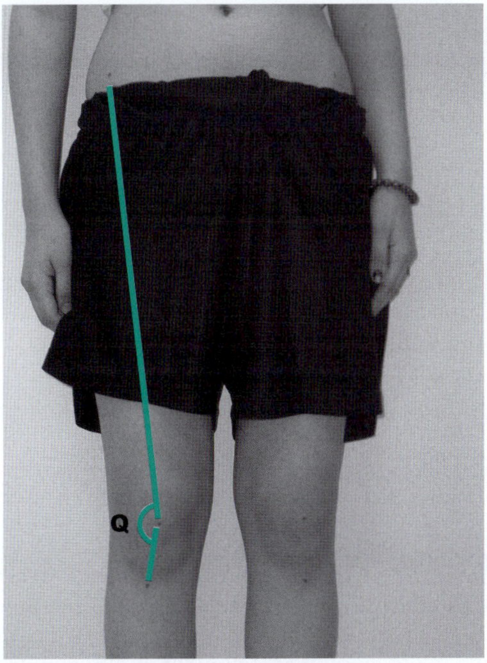

IMAGES

Figure 10B.2 The 'Q' angle.

is important though, that the practitioner recognises that the limitation of employing a static clinical measure instead of a high-tech dynamic measure introduces a significant degree of compromise to the information obtained from the assessment process. This may therefore compromise treatment especially in complex cases.

Q angle

The quadriceps angle (Q angle) is the frontal plane angle of the knee to the lower leg (Fig. 10B.2). It is the angle formed between lines drawn from the anterior superior iliac spine (ASIS) of the pelvis to the centre of the patella, and the centre of the patellar to the tibial tuberosity. The normal angle is 14° for males and 17° for females (Aglietti et al 1983) although the reference range for normal should allow for quite a few degrees variation from this. The Q angle is **best measured standing** as this reflects better the functional position, although it must be borne in mind that when measuring the angle standing, with the knee in full extension, the Q angle may be artificially altered by medial or lateral displacement of the patella. For this reason, some authors advocate measuring the Q angle non-weightbearing, although in the author's experience this simply substitutes one set of shortcomings for another.

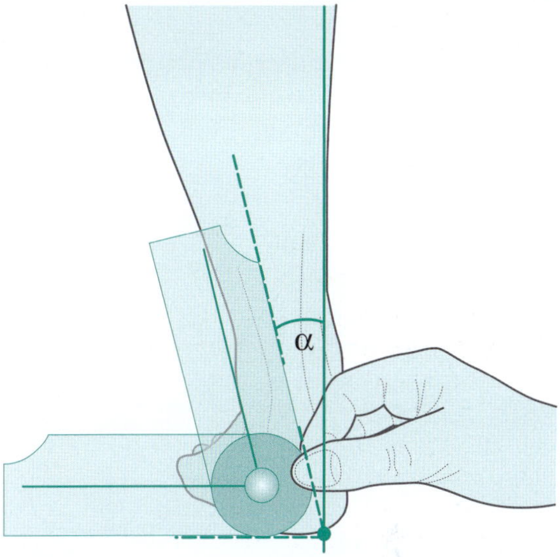

Figure 10B.3 Measurement of the tibial varum.

Tibial varum

Tibial varum is the angle formed between a bisection of the lower third of the tibia and the supporting surface. It can be measured at the same time as the relaxed calcaneal stance position (RCSP). There is some controversy over whether tibial varum should be measured in the resting or neutral calcaneal stance position. In the neutral position, all external factors are (in theory) excluded, but this is not the position from which the foot is functioning during gait. In the resting position tibial varum may appear worse because of medial displacement of the ankle–STJ complex in the pronated foot. Nevertheless, this is representative of the position about which this subject's limb is functioning. The author's preference is for RCSP measurement of tibial varum.

The angle is measured by placing the outside edge of one arm of the tractograph along the bisection of the tibia (either visualised or inked-in) and referencing the other arm of the goniometer to the weightbearing surface. The angle of the bisection of the lower leg is noted and checked by eye (Fig. 10B.3). Note that the convention is to reference the deviation of the tibia relative to a perpendicular to the floor (dotted line). Any varus deviation of the tibia relative to the perpendicular (angle α) is noted as 'α° varus' or as '–α°' as in the figure, while a valgus deviation would be described as 'α° valgus' or as '+α°.'

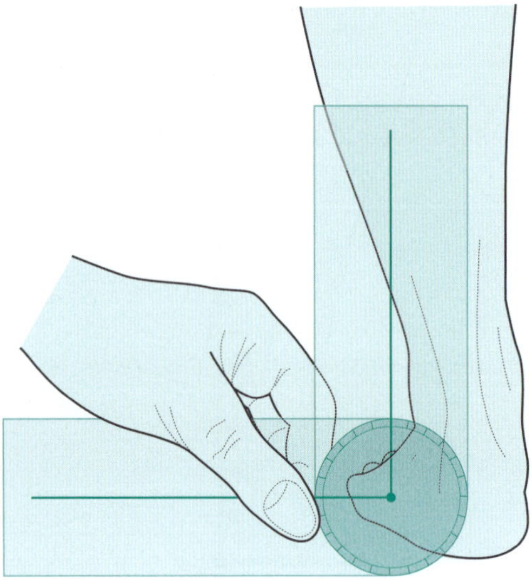

Figure 10B.4 The relaxed calcaneal stance position.

Relaxed calcaneal stance position

Techniques involving measurement of the angles and positions of anatomical landmarks directly on the foot are probably the most common approaches. Of these techniques, the most common are measurements of the angle relationships of the calcaneus, either relative to the leg or the floor.

Measurement of the calcaneal angle has been reported widely in the literature. Estimates of the reliability of the techniques vary greatly (Jonson & Gross 1997), but the majority of accounts suggest generally poor reliability (LaPointe et al 2001, McDowell et al 2000, Pierrynowski & Smith 1996, Weiner-Ogilvie & Rome 1998, Williams et al 1999). Typical figures were provided by Pierrynowski et al (1996) in their report that showed experienced practitioners can place the rearfoot within ±3° of the true position on 90% of occasions. While this precision may sound commendable, a range of 6° would encompass error of the order of 50–100% of the total variation encountered in clinical practice.

Practically, RCSP is measured in a manner similar to tibial varum described above by placing the outside edge of one arm of the tractograph along the bisection of the posterior aspect of the calcaneus (again either visualised or inked in) and referencing the other arm of the goniometer to the weightbearing surface (Fig. 10B.4). The angle of the bisection of the calcaneus is again noted and checked by eye. As with tibial varum the convention is to define varus or valgus explicitly or to denote varus angles with a negative sign and valgus positions as positive.

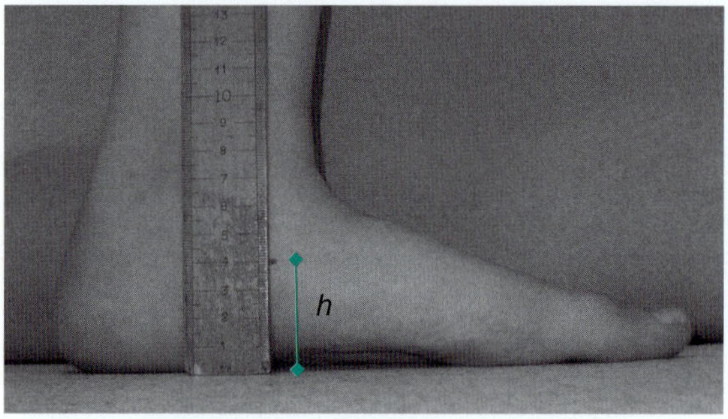

Figure 10B.5 Navicular height.

IMAGES

Navicular height

The direct measurement of the height of the medial arch of the standing foot, has been reported several times, again employing a number of different protocols. In its simplest form this involves direct measurement of either arch height, the height of the navicular tuberosity, or the height of the dorsum of the foot at a specific point. More complex techniques normalise these measures against various interpretations of foot length.

To measure the navicular height the patient is allowed to stand in their natural angle and base of gait. The tuberosity of the navicular is palpated carefully and if required, marked with a pen. A ruler is then placed alongside the tuberosity of the navicular and the distance from the floor (h) measured in millimetres (Fig. 10B.5).

In theory, measurement of arch height should be simple in concept and execution, and it is supposed that the height of the arch should also be a reasonably close indicator of foot function (Atkinson-Smith & Betts 1992). If the raw height of an anatomical landmark is used, however, the value of the measure tends to be limited to repeat measures within individual patients, as inter-subject variation makes between-subject comparisons inappropriate. More recent modifications have advocated a normalised version of this measure in which the height of the navicular from the floor is divided by the foot length (either whole foot length or length to the MTPJs), although this has the disadvantage of providing a measure that has no units and that makes comparisons between individuals inconsistent. Intra-rater reliability of raw measures of arch height and navicular height has been found to be acceptably high

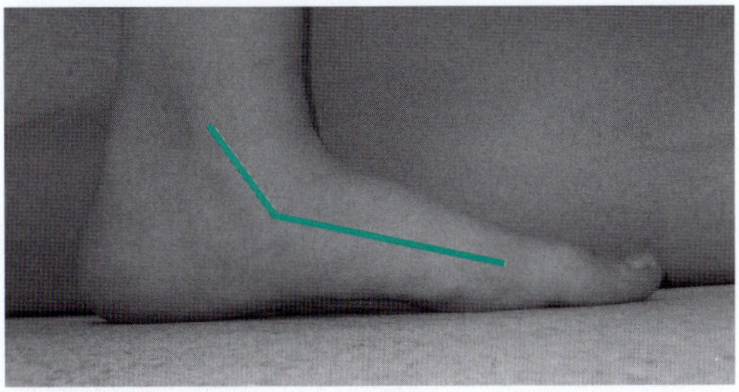

Figure 10B.6 The arch angle.

(Weiner-Ogilvie & Rome 1998), although again the inter-rater reliability is criticised.

The arch angle or the 'Feiss' line is an angle formed by lines drawn from the medial malleolus to the tuberosity of the navicular to the head of the first metatarsal (Coplan 1989, Franco 1987, Giallonardo 1988, Jonson & Gross 1997). The arch angle (**Fig. 10B.6**) is simply a variation of the other measures of navicular height, with the navicular tuberosity acting in this case as the origin of the angle between proximal and distal landmarks. The angle thus changes as the navicular tuberosity moves either dorsally or plantarward with changes in foot posture. The measurement of the arch angle has been reported to be adequately reliable (Jonson & Gross 1997), although is not in widespread use.

Complex approaches to static assessment – the foot posture index

A multifactorial approach to static standing foot type assessment was proposed by Cook et al in 1988, who examined the correlation between three standing measures. Dahle et al (1991) also explored a criterion-based, multifactorial rating scheme and found that practitioners could reliably classify foot type against clinical signs. A wide-ranging, criterion-based system for the classification of foot types was proposed by Scherer & Morris (1996) but by presenting a system with no evaluation of reliability or validity, they undermine its adoption.

To rectify this omission the author has recently developed and published a fully validated system for evaluating foot postures in all three body planes and in multiple foot segments (Keenan et al 2007, Redmond et al 2006). The so-called foot posture index is a simple classification system for quantifying standing foot posture without the need for expensive equipment or time-consuming protocols. The FPI scores six observations against set criteria and applies a common rating system to the observations (positive scores for signs associated with pronated/planus postures and negative scores for signs associated with supinated/cavus postures). The application of a common scoring system across the component measures is novel and is potentially the most important aspect of the new instrument. The five-point system is observational, but adherence to clearly defined criteria introduces objective boundaries and minimises the subjectivity.

The FPI predicts about 60% of the true variance in standing posture relative to expensive laboratory testing and about 40% of the variance observed by laboratory analysis of walking. While these coefficients of prediction do not sound especially high, they are approximately twice as good as those achieved by traditional measures such as calcaneal stance position and navicular height. The six criteria which make up the FPI rating scale are the following:

1. Talar head palpation
2. Supra and infra lateral malleolar curvature
3. Calcaneal frontal plane position
4. Prominence in the region of the talonavicular joint
5. Congruence of the medial longitudinal arch
6. Abduction/adduction of the forefoot on the rearfoot.

Further information, manuals and extra datasheets can be downloaded free from the FASTER website (www.leeds.ac.uk/medicine/FASTER/FPI/).

Foot print and other indirect static measures

One group of potentially useful objective measures are those derived from indirect footprints. Most of these estimate function according to angular relationships of anatomical landmarks or the calculation of relative area of different parts of the print. These have proved to be relatively reliable (Cavanagh & Rodgers 1987, Freychat et al 1996) and can yield useful clinical information. The relationship between the foot print and complex dynamic function is incomplete however, and measures such as the **arch index** (Cavanagh & Rodgers 1987) (Fig. 10B.7), are often criticised for failing to take into consideration the many other factors affecting dynamic gait. One critical study (Hawes et al 1992) reported that apart from a very general association at the extremes, footprint parameters were not related to directly measured arch height.

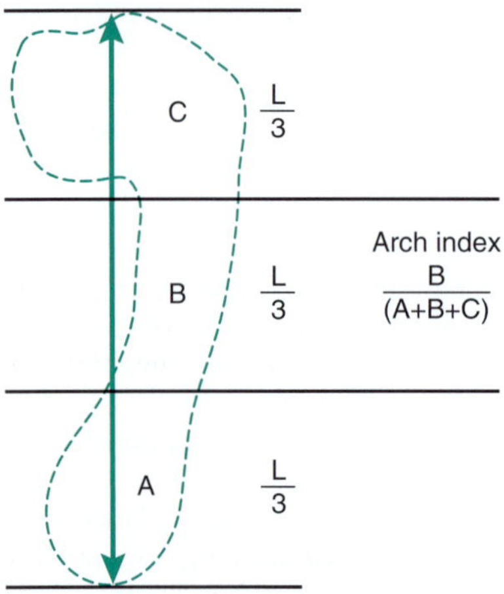

Figure 10B.7 Arch index. (Redrawn with permission from Cavanagh P R, Rodgers M M 1987 The arch index: a useful measure from footprints. Journal of Biomechanics 20(5):547–551.)

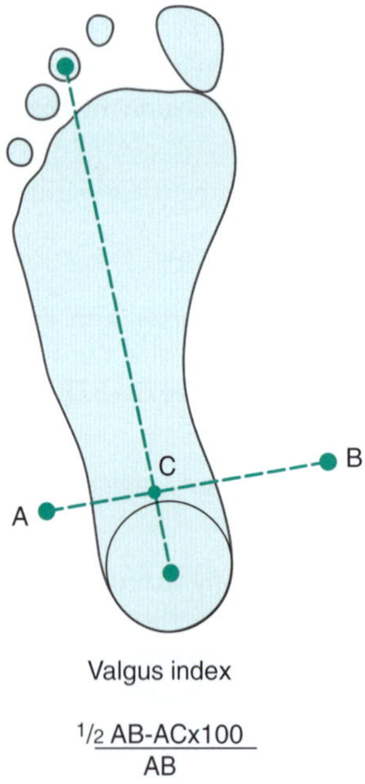

Figure 10B.8 Valgus index.

Foot print measures e.g. arch index and valgus index (Figs 10B.7, 10B.8) have appeal because they are objective and simple, although it may be naive to hope to use observations from only one plane to attempt to give a reliable indication of the overall foot morphology and all must be considered to have significant limitations (Kitaoka et al 1994, Smith & Ocampo 1997, Menz 1998). As with radiographic measures, it is also important to note the significant between-subject variability in these measures. For one set of angular measures derived from footprints from a normal population of 17-year-olds' mean angles of 42.9–46.3° were associated with 95% confidence intervals of 23.5° to 65.3°. Area-based measures were even worse, and the arch index yields a 95% confidence interval for the normal range equal to –0.1 to 0.99 for males and 0.13 to 0.93 for females, almost the entire possible range (Forriol et al 1990). While changes in footprint-derived measures can provide some indication of group effects in large group studies, individual comparisons must be made with care.

Radiographic measures

Radiographic measures have been widely used in the evaluation of foot type as they are reported to provide an accurate basis for the quantification of the relationship between bony segments. In a review for this chapter we found more than 100 papers that reported the use of radiographic measures. It is probably the case that despite some concerns over the effects of magnification associated with radiographic measures (Camasta et al 1991, Perry et al 1992) they are the most reliable of the measures available to the clinician. However, routine exposure of humans to X-ray radiation in the pursuit of clinical measurements is not desirable and their use remains limited. In the past most conventional radiographic techniques involved imaging the foot non-weightbearing and the resulting information is of limited help in understanding function. Conventional X-ray machines can be used in conjunction with raised platforms to make weightbearing images and modern machines are capable of imaging directly to floor level. As a result weightbearing images are becoming increasingly available and should be sought as far as possible for any applications in which foot structure or function is the purpose of the investigation.

One recent study has added another factor into the equation, as the effects of the Wolfe–Davis law may become relevant in the case of bony measurement following long-standing deformity. In a study of the morphology of the bones of the rearfoot undertaken by Anderson et al (1997) significant morphological differences were demonstrated between the shape of the bones of individuals with flat feet and normal controls. It is not clear whether such changes are the cause or the consequence of long-term flat-footed function but the findings call into question the validity of applying values derived from normal samples in the assessment of flat feet.

Examination: moving on from observation only

All of the techniques described previously have involved no more than either simply observing relationships that exist in the patient or, at their most sophisticated, quantifying those observations through simple measurement. In the next phase of the assessment process we now come to techniques that require manipulation of the parts – the true hands-on examination phase.

It is in this phase of the assessment process that the compromises of the clinical versus laboratory assessment become most relevant. Ideally we would like to quantify the actual function of the parts being studied in their day-to-day activities. In practice of course we cannot do that with simple instrumentation so we constrain the examination to fit the available instrumentation and techniques. All of the clinical hands-on techniques are either static (e.g. measures of position), quasi-functional (e.g. measures of a range derived from a fixed measure) or estimations of function (e.g. eyeballing a range or estimating quality of joint motion).

The implications of this compromise *must* be considered when performing and interpreting these tests.

Quasi-functional tests

A variety of tests have been proposed that blur the boundary between static and dynamic evaluation. Among these is Jack's test (or Hubscher's manoeuvre), in which the first toe is dorsiflexed during standing (Jack 1953), standing to tip-toe (Gould 1983), and the lateral 'block test' for rigidity of cavo varus deformity (Coleman & Chesnut 1977). Each of these tests provides further information to the observer of the standing posture, and in particular of the likely behaviour of the foot in dynamic function.

Limb-length evaluation

Measurement of limb length is a useful component of the lower-limb functional assessment as it can highlight both underlying pathologies and compensations. Techniques for measuring limb length include **direct measures** of the length of individual or multiple bony segments, or **indirect methods** whereby functional disparities are addressed progressively and the change quantified. Non-weightbearing measurement has been covered in Section 10A and the two techniques described here are conducted with the patient standing.

Direct weightbearing assessment of limb length can be based on many similar but subtly different protocols and care should be taken in recording and comparing results. The simplest approach is to use a metre rule to measure the height of either the ASIS or the greater trochanter of the femur from the floor. The distance can also be quantified with a tape measure. Variations on the direct approach involve measuring from the chosen proximal point (ASIS, greater trochanter or navel) to the lateral or medial malleolus. The measurement error for any of these protocols is in the region of 1–2 cm so **'diagnoses' of less than 2 cm difference between limbs should be viewed with caution**.

Limb length can also be measured indirectly. With this method the ASIS is either marked or the patient places their index finger tip on the ASIS to act as a reference. The clinician then checks to establish whether the finger tips/ASIS are level, perhaps using a horizontal line of sight. (Charts are available but often a window ledge, door frame or similar provides a reasonable horizontal reference). If one side is deemed to be lower this side is raised using solid blocks (of wood or plastic) of known thickness, usually 2–3 mm. When sufficient blocks have been added to restore the pelvis to level, the thickness of the stack indicates the degree of compensation that may be required. This is a relatively handy approach if heel-raise-type treatment is being considered.

Neutral calcaneal stance position

One of the most profound changes to affect the study of foot function was the theory proposed by Root et al (Root 1964, Root et al 1971), which outlined the concept of a measurable neutral position about which the foot was supposed to function. The Root theoretical model and its later adaptations have become widely adopted among practitioners treating disorders of the foot as it promises a supposedly more sophisticated and scientific basis for the quantification of foot posture and function. Originally, the Root model defined the neutral position for the foot based on the total range available in the STJ during a non-weightbearing examination, a practice which has been largely discredited (Ball & Johnson 1993, Sell et al 1994). Later refinements have attempted to define the subtalar neutral according to weightbearing criteria but problems remain with applying theoretical definitions to real-life anatomy because of several confounding factors such as the shape of segments and joints (Sell et al 1994, Sobel & Levitz 1997) and dubious reliability because of operator dependency, among other things (Dahle et al

1991, Elveru et al 1988, Weiner-Ogilvie & Rome 1998).

Astrom & Arvidson (1995) proposed that the 'ideal' foot functioning around 'neutral' is based on an invalid theoretical concept and a proper reference should be based on clinical observations rather than on theoretical considerations. They also proposed that the theoretically 'normal' foot is a rarity and suggested that it is likely that the range of theoretical definitions of pathology that actually encompass variations of normal is quite large. Despite these reservations the concept of the neutral calcaneal stance position (NCSP) as a reference point from which to quantify amounts of foot pronation or supination remains attractive.

It is possible to identify empirical characteristics associated with various types of foot morphology and these can be helpful to the practitioner. Among these are the concepts of talar head palpation and arch congruence as used in the FPI. It is then theoretically possible to manipulate the weightbearing foot into a posture that can be considered functionally neutral and to quantify the frontal plane position of the calcaneus with the foot in this position using a goniometer/tractograph, much as one would when measuring the RCSP. It is important, however, that the practitioner is aware of the amount of error that is associated with this approach, both in the establishment of the 'neutral' foot posture and in the measurement of the calcaneal position. There is some appeal in undertaking a supposedly scientific and accurate quantification of NCSP but the real scientist and diligent practitioner will recognise that the data derived are so flawed so as to be scientifically almost worthless. For this reason the author does not recommend using NCSP as anything other than an empirical guide to foot structure.

Navicular drop

A quasi-functional component is introduced to the navicular height measures described previously by the use of composite measures such as navicular drop, in which the foot is measured in its resting state and again in an artificially induced 'neutral' position, with the difference between the two measures providing an estimate of the behaviour of the foot under different conditions.

Composite measures such as navicular drop involve two measures on each individual, one to determine the starting height and a second in a predetermined reference position such as STJ neutral. This approach improves the comparability of the results between subjects, but at the expense of decreased reliability, as the repeated measures introduce more potential for error and, as has been discussed in detail above, because the establishment of the neutral reference position is itself of questionable validity and reliability. The reliability of double measure techniques such as navicular drop is low for inexperienced practitioners (Picciano et al 1993), although has been reported to be acceptable in intra-rater evaluations of more experienced practitioners, yielding an intra-class coefficient of approximately 0.7–0.8 and a standard error of the measure of approximately 2 mm (Mueller et al 1993, Sell et al 1994).

The conduct of the navicular drop measure is presented in **Figure 10B.9**. The tuberosity of the navicular is marked and the patient stands in their relaxed stance position (Fig. 10B.9A). The distance from the navicular to the ground is then recorded in millimetres (Fig. 10B.9B). With the foot manipulated into a neutral position (Fig. 10B.9C) the distance to the ground is again recorded (Fig. 10B.9D). The difference between the height with the foot in neutral and in the resting position is the navicular drop.

Navicular drop is considered by a number of authors to be a more valid indicator of foot function than the traditional rearfoot measurements employed in the Root approach (Sell et al 1994, Menz 1998, Weiner-Ogilvie & Rome 1998), although it is a single-plane measure only and provides an incomplete clinical picture. Navicular drop predicts 24–30% of composite forefoot/rearfoot position (Mueller et al 1993) values that are similar to those found by Cavanagh et al (1997) discussed above. This suggests that the fundamental limitation associated with measuring motion in only one plane persists over a range of selected paired measures.

Weightbearing tests of first metatarsophalangeal joint function (Jack's test/Hubscher's manoeuvre)

This common test, first described by Jack (Jack 1953), and later by Hubscher, involves the examiner manually dorsiflexing the hallux while the patient stands in their relaxed double-limb stance position. If the test is successful the hallux is able to dorsiflex freely and the hallux dorsiflexion is associated with a tightening and raising of the medial longitudinal arch, a mechanism sometimes called the '**windlass effect**' (Hicks 1953). A failed test is recorded where the examiner is unable to dorsiflex the hallux from the weightbearing surface without the application of

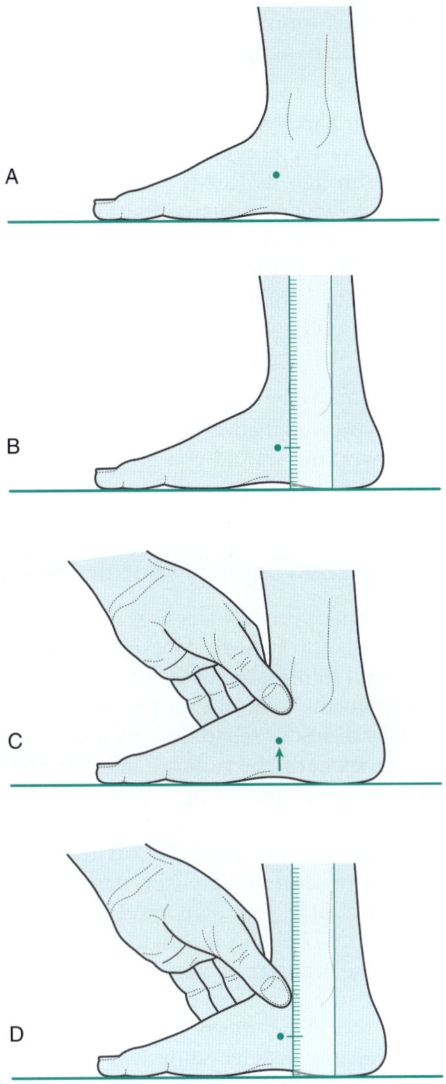

Figure 10B.9 Measurement of navicular drop.

excessive force. In a person with a good range of motion at the first MTPJ when non-weightbearing, a failed Jack's test is supposed to indicate functional hallux limitus (impaired first MTPJ function during gait). In a series of studies conducted by the author's research team, however, Jack's test has proved to be no better than chance at differentiating between patients with normal motion at the first MTPJ and those with actual deficit during walking (Halstead & Redmond 2006). Again, the discerning practitioner needs to make sure that the appeal of a simple test does not cloud their judgement over the actual clinical merit of the results.

Axis orientation

One other factor that has been widely proposed to affect the degree of coupling between the foot and the leg is the orientation of the axis of rotation of the STJ (Lundberg & Svensson 1993, Nawoczenski et al 1998, Nester 1997, Nester et al 2000). The behaviour of this axis has been demonstrated to be extremely complex in dynamic studies, and a number of in-vitro studies have shown substantial variation in axial orientation between specimens (Engsberg 1987, Engsberg & Andrews 1987, Isman & Inman 1969, Manter 1941). Only one study has demonstrated the axes of rotation in vivo, using permanently implanted tantalum markers in each of the tarsal bones in healthy volunteers (Lundberg & Svensson 1993). Such invasive methods are clearly not applicable to clinical practice. A method for ascertaining the STJ axis of rotation was proposed by Morris & Jones (1994). The method is highly subjective and, unfortunately, the authors report no reliability analysis on the 18 subjects they used to illustrate the application of the technique.

The inclusion of an estimate of rearfoot joint axis is clinically appealing and has been advocated for clinical studies (Aquino & Payne 2001), however the reliability of such techniques is questionable. Kirby describes a method whereby the functional axis of the STJ can be determined clinically by a non-weightbearing loading of the joint by thumb pressure in a linear sequence along the plantar surface of the calcaneus. The validity of the technique has not really been established though and the reliability of such complex and technically difficult measures has historically been low. There may be merit in including some estimation of subtalar axis into the clinical decision-making process but the results of such a potentially limited test should be treated with due caution. A modification of this concept, the '**supination resistance test**', was described by Noakes & Payne in 2003 using a protocol performed either manually or using a test device. In the manual test, participants stand in their natural angle and base of gait while the practitioner places two fingers under the talonavicular joint and attempts to supinate the rearfoot. The estimated amount of force needed is recorded by the clinician. The test has been reported to be adequately reliable and the authors suggest that it may have clinical merit, informing choice and prescription of orthoses. At the time of writing the link between theory and application is not well developed but this approach may prove to be of some use as the concept matures.

Non-weightbearing static examination

Before considering the non-weightbearing examination of the foot one important concept must be grasped. The non-weightbearing examination is heavily dependent on extrapolation of clinical findings through theoretical models of foot function (i.e. making an interpretation of the findings), and combining the two to provide an estimate of what functions we would expect to find if we were to actually measure the function directly. **Non-weightbearing assessments mostly do not measure function**, they simply represent parameters that we can enter into a conceptual model. The interpretation of non-weightbearing measures are subject, therefore, to both the vagaries of the testing process and flaws in the models used to interpret the information. Given the limited extent to which most of the complex theories of foot function ('Root' theory, sagittal plane facilitation, rotational equilibrium to name but three) have been tested formally and scientifically, it is obvious that the assessor must be mindful of the leap of faith that is required to interpret many of the non-weightbearing tests.

Foot function is known to be a product of the combined motions occurring at the subtalar and midtarsal joints and at distal joint complexes. The science underpinning the inter-relationships of the joints of the foot have been discussed at a theoretical level in a number of papers (Benink 1985, Bojsen-Moller 1979, Elftman 1960, Kitaoka et al 1995, Lundberg et al 1989, Nester 1997) and some of the theory has been substantiated by in-vivo studies (Cornwall & McPoil 1999, Lundberg et al 1989, Ouzounian & Shereff 1989, Winson et al 1994), and by the intervention studies of Astion et al (1997). The scientific substantiation of the theoretical understanding remains fairly simplistic relative to the complex theories that have evolved, however, and this should be factored into clinical decision-making.

The non-weightbearing static examination process

Remember: Look, Feel, Move.

When carrying out your non-weightbearing examination the temptation is great to pitch straight in with the range of motion (ROM) checks, so remember to take time to assess the joints first. For each joint to be assessed:

- **Look** for signs of deformity, swelling – either soft tissue or bony and discoloration.
- **Feel** for deformity and swelling, note the presence of pain on palpation, note temperature differences.
- **Move** the part – first observe active movement initiated by the patient and then move the part slowly through its ROM. Assess the **quality of motion**, feel for **crepitus**, or **resistance to motion**, note the presence of **pain on movement** and finally **estimate the ROM**. Does it appear to be normal? The joint ROM should be assessed both passively with observer moving the part, and actively, the patient moving the part for themselves.

Only when you are satisfied that you understand *how* the joint is working should you go on to *measure* the ROM.

Measuring the range of motion of joints

The measurement process is less accurate than most of us would like to believe. Measured data provide us with useful information, but for most joint measurement protocols is it wise not to place too much faith in the validity or reliability of the data. Quantified measurement can be valuable in informing treatment decisions and providing a broad indication of response to therapy, but with few exceptions should not be interpreted too rigidly. Be wary of joint ROM assessment procedures that rely on standardised protocols and be clear in your own mind how differences between the protocol and real-world function might impact on the transfer of results into the clinical setting. As a rule of thumb the larger the joint and the greater the ROM, the better chance there is of obtaining reliable results with less error. This is certainly something to bear in mind when measuring small foot joints with small ROMs. Furthermore, most joint ROM measures are operator dependent, with variation introduced by differences in the magnitude of force applied to move the joint, interpretation of the end-of-range point, and variability in measurement/goniometric technique. The error between observers is almost always higher than for repeat measures made by the same individual.

Passive and active movement

Comparing passive and active motions is important for many reasons. The most important is that allowing the patient to move the joint actively allows the examiner to get an idea of the available range and the impact of pain, stiffness and deformity. This can help prevent nasty surprises later during the passive examination.

Range of motion

ROM examination entails the estimation or quantification of the total range through which a joint can be moved. The range can be described in several planes or directions of motion (see subsequent section). The ROM in a joint can sometimes be described empirically in terms of the total movement available (e.g. jaw opening) but because most joints function either side of a central (or 'neutral') position it is more common to describe motions in two (or more) directions from a **central reference position**. Examples of the latter are hip medial and lateral rotation, ankle joint dorsiflexion and plantarflexion, and inversion and eversion of the heel. Individual joint examinations are detailed in the next section, but in all joints the range is evaluated by stabilising one part, usually the proximal part and moving the other part until movement is resisted by the joint's intrinsic elastic limits. The feel of reaching this limit – the '**end feel**' – is often used subjectively to provide clinical information with certain characteristics indicative of underlying clinical findings. Hence a sudden 'bony' end feel, indicates a blockade possibly related to joint surface shape or loose-body impingement while a soft end feel might indicate swelling or interposition of soft tissues, such as in synovitis.

How far a joint can be moved will vary with pain, the applied force, the speed of movement, guarding and a host of minor factors and so again, the practitioner should be mindful of the limits of validity and reliability when assessing ROM. It is without question useful to estimate joint ranges, but care should be taken not to place too much emphasis on the precision with which the various techniques can provide detailed quantitative information.

Direction and quality of motion

Arguably, the most important information in the assessment of joints non-weightbearing comes from the assessment of total range. The path taken by the segments can also be highly informative, however, and in moving the joint through its range the practitioner should also consider the direction of movement and the quality of the motion.

Depending on joint structure, normal motion may be quite flexible such as in the ball and socket construction of the hip, or it may be quite constrained such as the hinge-type mechanism seen in the ankle. The practitioner should pay attention to the direction in which motion occurs and be aware of the consequences that may arise from disordered alignment. Problems can arise from compensations required in neighbouring joints where constrained joints are malaligned, from instability where joints are relatively unconstrained, or directly from the penalties imposed by inappropriate directions of movement.

Quality of motion may also be informative with the presence of crepitus (grinding), squeaking, stiffness or uneven resistance indicative of disorders as wide ranging as osteoarthritis, spasticity or **parkinsonian** syndromes.

Hip

Look and feel for joints such as the hip must be approached with caution because of the potentially personal nature of the examination. Careful judgement should be exercised in selecting those cases where this is appropriate and the presence of a chaperone is encouraged. The hip ROM can be assessed by several possible methods, depending on the facilities available and the nature of the problem.

Hip position – frontal plane

Frontal plane deviations at the hip (coxa vara and coax valga) are extremely difficult to identify clinically and there are no definitive prevalence data. Coxa vara and valga are usually subclinical in impact. There may be signs of an awkward gait, and **apparent genu varum/valgum**, although the hip position is the primary deformity (McCarthy & Gessner 1993, Thomson 1993). Clinical measures are so unreliable as to be worthless so if coxa vara/valga is suspected and is of sufficient severity to warrant intervention then X-ray confirmation is required.

Rotational (transverse plane) motions at the hip

The terminology used in this area is highly inconsistent. In this overview, semantics such as differentiating between torsion, position, rotation and the various connotations are acknowledged but not developed in detail. Intoed or adducted presentations will be used in conjunction with the terms medial (or internal) position/rotation, while out-toed or abducted presentations will be used in conjunction with the terms lateral (or external) position/rotation.

Intoeing is a rotation deformity of the lower limb where the foot is medially rotated, that is rotated toward the midline of the body (Aston 1979, Katz et al 1990, Lanier 1971, Weseley et al 1981). The range within two standard deviations of the normal

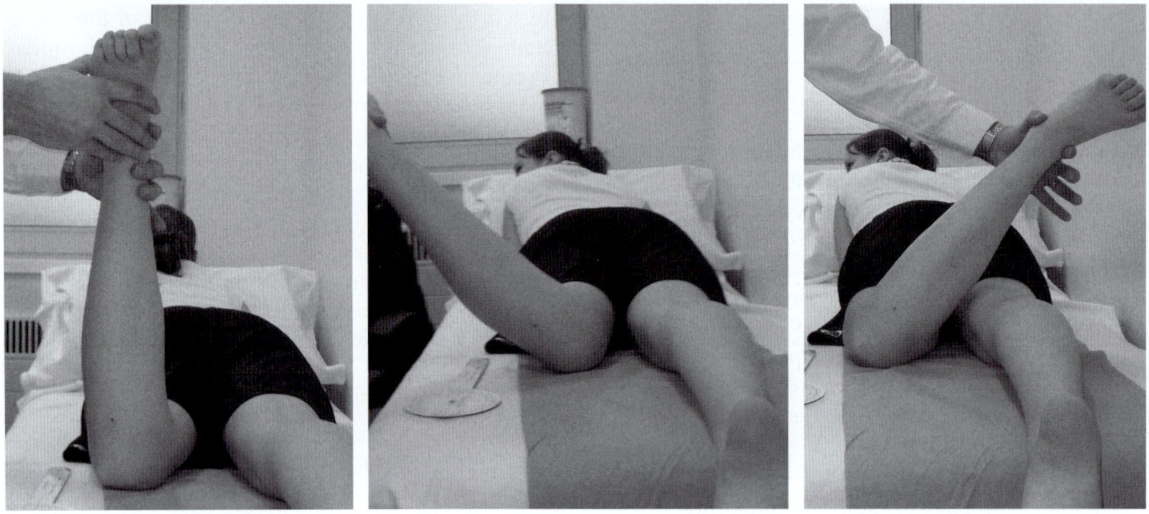

A B C

Figure 10B.10A–C Hip ROM prone by 'eye balling'.

population mean covers –2.5° (adduction) to +20° (abduction) at birth; to –2° to +15° at 15 years (Staheli et al 1985). Intoeing is thus often defined as more than 3° of adduction during walking (Staheli 1986). Pathological **out-toeing**, is more difficult to define precisely, as the wide range of 'normal' external rotation – up to 20° of external rotation – encompasses all but the most extreme cases. Intoed and out-toed gaits can arise from postural variations at the hip, femur, knee, tibia and fibula, or in the foot. At the hip, excessive capacity for medial rotation will result in intoed gait, while excessive lateral rotations cause out-toeing.

The US Orthopaedic Society recommends that **hip ROM is assessed with the patient prone**, with the hip extended and the knee flexed to 90°. The hip joint is put through its ROM allowing gravity alone to establish the range. This method is repeatable in adults, although in children there may be a problem with getting the subject to relax sufficiently. The angle is estimated by eye using the vertical alignment as the reference position (Fig 10B.10A) with the angle of motion being reported as either internal (Fig 10B.10B) or external rotation (Fig 10B.10C) around this baseline.

Quantification can be undertaken using the same basic protocol and a goniometer (Fig. 10B.11). Note, however, that in recording the angle in this manner the horizontal surface is used as the reference position. As the reference line is perpendicular to the vertical reference position for the joint some agile mental arithmetic is required to record position correctly. For example, a reading on the goniometer 60° (relative to the horizontal reference surface) represents 30° of external rotation relative to the (vertical) reference position for the joint.

Perhaps less intimidating for the patient as a first-line assessment is a **sitting technique** where the hip is put through it ROM with the patient seated, hip and knee flexed to 90°. The degree of internal external rotation is estimated using either an angle or a clockface approximation (Fig. 10B.12). Or it can be quantified using a goniometer (Fig. 10B.13).

Non-weightbearing assessment of limb length

The non-weightbearing assessment of limb length is a straightforward technique. It is similar to the tape-measure protocols described previously under weightbearing assessment but with the patient lying supine. The simplest approach is to use a tape to measure the distance from either the ASIS, greater trochanter or navel to the lateral or medial malleolus. This technique can be confounded somewhat by the

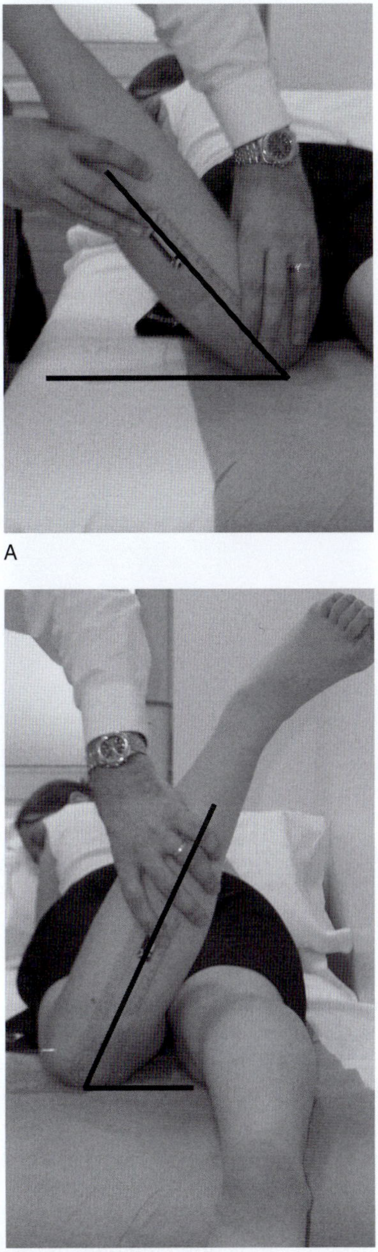

A

B

Figure 10B.11A, B Hip range of motion prone using goniometer.

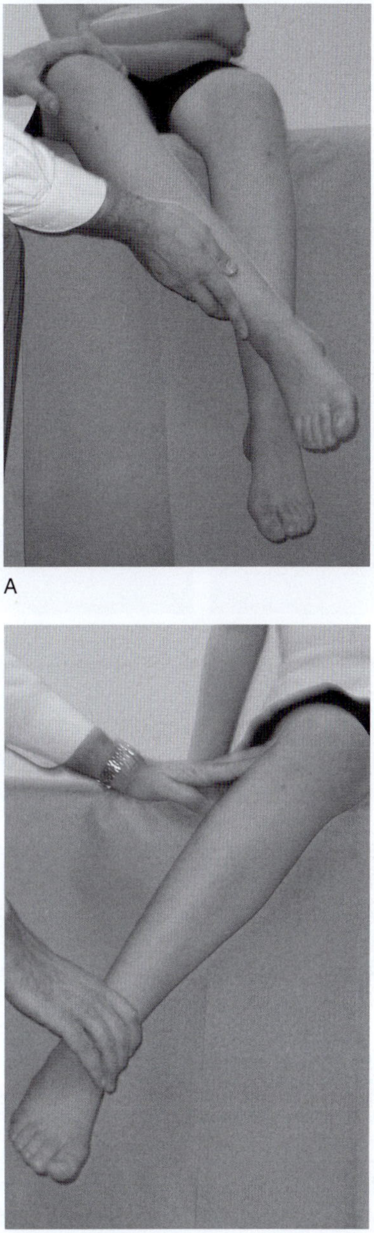

A

B

Figure 10B.12A, B Hip range of motion sitting by 'eye balling'.

passage of tape over large thighs. The measurement error for this type of approach is in the region of 1–2 cm so again 'diagnoses' of less than 2 cm difference between limbs should be viewed with caution.

Alternative techniques are sometimes advocated in which individual segments are evaluated using the back rest or platform base as a reference, with estimation (or direct measurement) of tibial and femoral segments superimposed. With such a variety of essentially flawed techniques available the choice is a personal rather than a scientific one.

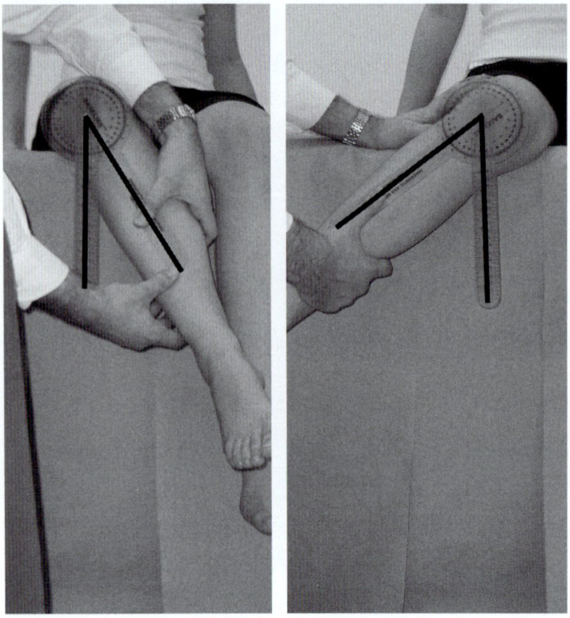

A B

Figure 10B.13A, B Hip range of motion sitting using goniometer.

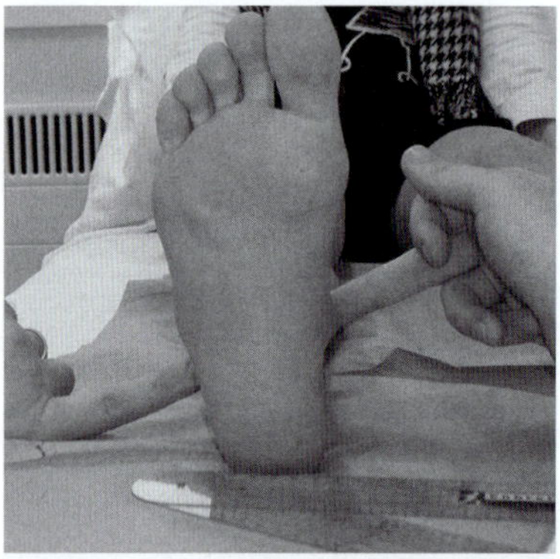

A

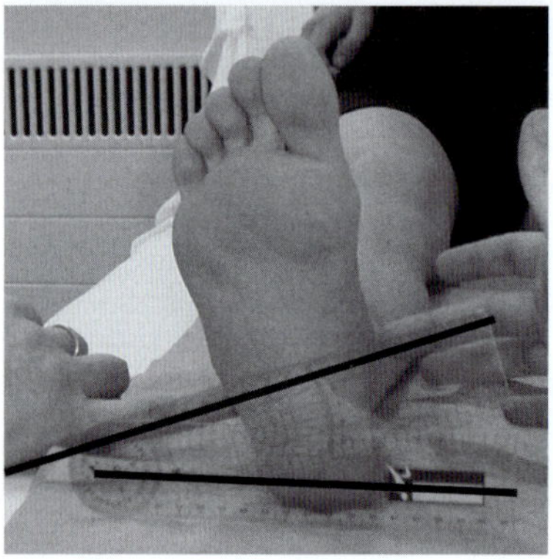

B

Figure 10B.14A, B Malleolar torsion.

Knee

Approximately 15–20° of **genu varum** (**bow leg**) is a normal finding at birth straightening out by approximately 2 years and moving towards 5–15° of valgus before returning to a straight position by 6–12 years. **Genu valgum** is often seen in later years, especially in obese individuals. Genu valgum can be measured directly by aligning a long arm goniometer along the long axes of the femur and tibia but the clinical surrogate of the Q angle (see weightbearing section) is arguably more informative.

Malleolar torsion

Malleolar torsion is a surrogate measure for the amount of positional rotation arising along the long axis shaft of the tibia. It is best measured with a gravity goniometer, although it may be measured with a regular goniometer (**Fig. 10B.14B**). With the patient supine and the knee extended and the leg resting on the bench, the leg is manipulated so that the patella is perpendicular to the supporting surface and the rotation of the malleoli is gauged relative to the supporting surface. The angle of the malleolus can be evaluated by eye using the fingers for assistance (Fig. 10B.14A), or can be quantified using a goniometer (Fig. 10B.14B).

Tibial varum angle

The term tibial varum describes a clinically entity in which the tibia lies in a varus position relative to the supporting surface. It is therefore preferable to take this measure with the patient weightbearing as described earlier.

Ankle dorsiflexion

Following observation and palpation of the joint, the ankle should be moved through its range of motion to assess quality and characteristics of the motion as well as empirically assessing the range. Limitation of ankle joint dorsiflexion can present in both **uncompensated and compensated forms**. In uncompensated forms, the heel will either fail to make ground contact or will be lifted early in the stance phase. The knee and hip will be flexed, significantly compromising the ergonomics of gait. Milder degrees of **equinus** will be compensated in the rearfoot and midfoot through STJ hyper-pronation, and subluxation of the midfoot. **Bony or soft-tissue restrictions** can be differentiated, based on the relative ankle joint ROM measured alternately with the knee flexed and extended (Fig. 10B.15) and the end feel when the limit of movement is reached.

The ROM is measured formally with the STJ in the neutral position (Fig. 10A.16A). The foot is grasped at the fourth and fifth MTPJ and dorsiflexed to resistance, the patient is then asked to assist in the dorsiflexion (Fig. 10B.16B). From the lateral side the angle between the lateral side of the leg and the plantar surface of the foot is visualised and measured with a goniometer (Fig. 10B.16C). Remember to check your measurement with what you can actually see.

A

B

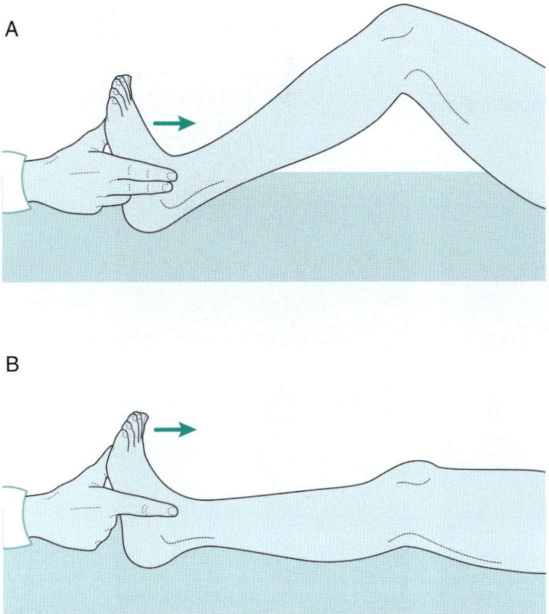

Figure 10B.15 Estimation of ankle joint range of motion.

Subtalar joint motion

Following observation and palpation of the subtalar area, the joint should be moved through its ROM to assess quality and characteristics of the motion as well as empirically assessing the range. It is common for the STJ to have a roughly **similar range in inversion or eversion**, although a predominance towards inversion is the norm. The author no longer measures the subtalar range formally except in unusual circumstances because of serious limitations in the reliability and validity of the formal measurement techniques. However, eyeball evaluation is essential and often informative.

A

B

C

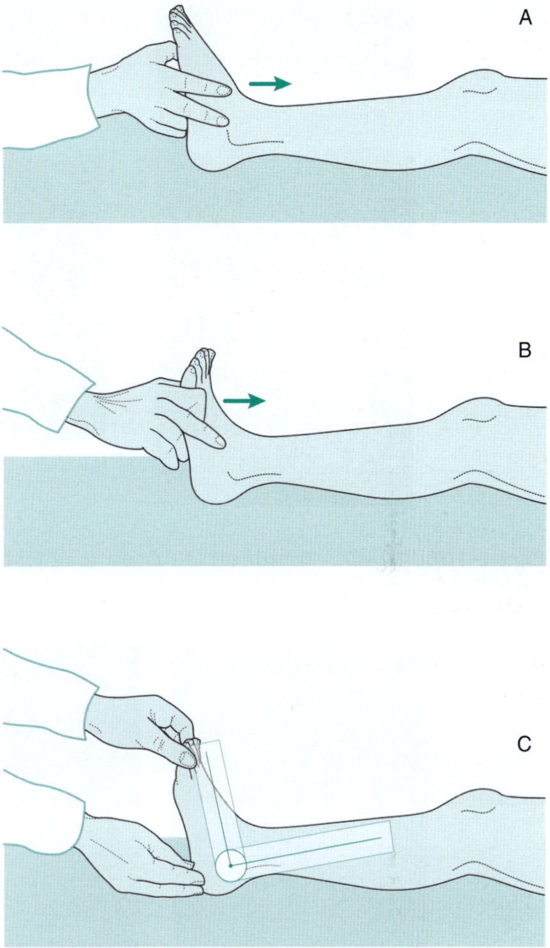

Figure 10B.16 Measurement of ankle joint dorsiflexion. **A** subtalar joint neutral and passive dorsiflexion. **B** Patient assists with dorsiflexion **C** Measure and check.

For a quick screen, assessment of the STJ can be undertaken with the patient sitting (Fig. 10B.17). The ROM is assessed by stabilising the tibia, grasping the heel and inverting and everting the calcaneus. For a clearer view it is necessary to have the patient lying prone and this enables the practitioner to measure the STJ ROM if required (Fig. 10B.18).

Midtarsal joint motion (Box 10B.9)

Following observation and palpation of the midtarsal area the **talonavicular** and **calcaneocuboid** joints should be moved through their ROM to assess quality and characteristics of the motion, as well as empirically assessing the range. It must be emphasised that the scientific understanding of the function of these

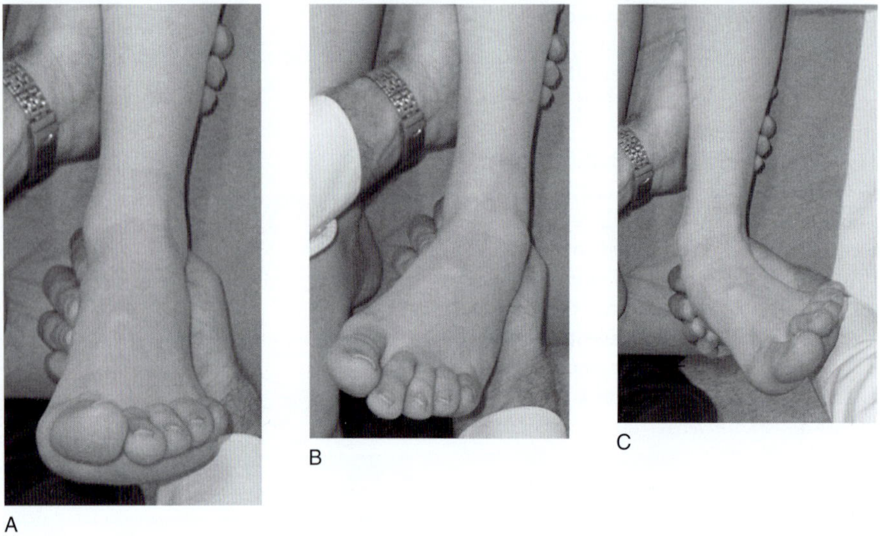

Figure 10B.17A–C Assessment of subtalar joint range of motion supine.

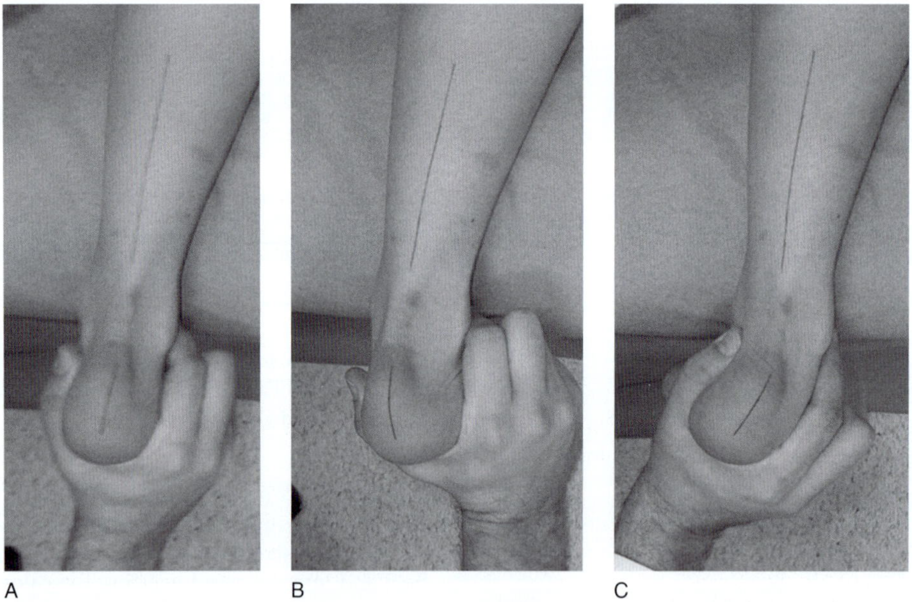

Figure 10B.18A–C Assessment of subtalar joint range of motion prone.

subtle joint complexes is limited and there is great potential for theoretical debate to overwhelm the capacity of the current technologies to confirm or refute these hypotheses. In the midtarsal region two popular theories compete, proposing either a ball and socket-type articulation encompassing a multiple joint complex or a more constrained two-axis model. The clinical assessment process will be similar in both cases with only the observer's interpretation differing significantly.

The single axis/ball and socket model supports a more forgiving evaluation of range, direction and quality of motions at the midtarsal joint. The two-axis model differs mainly in the theoretical separation of the motions observed into discrete axes of rotation. There is no room in this chapter for a wide-ranging

Box 10B.9 Clinical note: Forefoot varus/supinatus and forefoot valgus

There is great dispute in the literature about the existence, definition, clinical evaluation and differentiation of these subtle deformities of limited scientific provenance (Kidd 1997, Kidd 2000, McPoil et al 1987). Technical definitions describe forefoot varus and supinatus as inversion problems of the forefoot. The term forefoot varus is usually used to describe a primary pathology while forefoot supinatus commonly refers to secondary adaptations. Some authors have suggested that the entire concept of forefoot varus/supinatus is flawed and that the deformities do not exist (Kidd 1997, Kidd 2000). Conversely others have claimed that inversion of the forefoot can be detected in as many as 87% of all people (Garbalosa et al 1994).

The reported prevalence of forefoot valgus is also variable, probably a reflection of the paucity of solid epidemiological data but perhaps, more tellingly, reflective of the problems associated with defining 'pathologies' in the face of competing theory and weak scientific justification of the underpinning concepts (Garbalosa et al 1994, McPoil et al 1988). In primary forefoot varus/supinatus, the inverted forefoot position is assumed to primarily cause an eversion moment on forefoot loading. If sufficient compensatory motion is available in the subtalar complex the foot should evert into full ground contact and any secondary symptoms will usually be characteristic of the over-pronation type syndromes. If there is not enough compensatory motion available in the midtarsal joint complex to provide adequate compensation, inversion of the forefoot is proposed to result in increased loads on the lateral border of the foot, causing callosities and occasionally more severe overuse injuries such as fifth metatarsal stress reactions. In the case of forefoot valgus theoretical models propose that impaired locking and instability in the midfoot region during midstance cause most problems. In some patients with particularly demanding foot biomechanics the rearfoot will invert to stabilise the midfoot.

philosophical debate and so from this point we will describe only a clinical assessment protocol and leave its interpretation open to debate.

The author's preference is to assess the midtarsal complex holistically, evaluating empirically the overall ROM in the region and its coupling with the proximal structures. The STJ is placed in as neutral position as can be achieved clinically, to ensure some consistency in the constraint of the distal joints and then the motions of the midtarsal joint complexes are estimated. If a more axial approach is preferred then with the STJ in neutral, the long axis is assessed by grasping the foot between forefinger and thumb from the lateral side and inverting and everting the forefoot on the rearfoot. The oblique axis is assessed by flicking the forefoot in the directions of plantarflexion/adduction/inversion and dorsiflexion/abduction/eversion.

The position of the forefoot on the rearfoot, particularly in the frontal plane (varus/valgus) can, in theory, be quantified through the use of either a forefoot goniometer or a tractograph, although almost all objective evaluations of this approach have suggested it to be invalid. The midtarsal joint can be assessed with the operator interpreting the findings as either a two-axis response (**Fig. 10B.19A–C**) and independently (Fig. 10B.19D,E) or as a ball and socket model (Fig. 10B.19A–E).

First and fifth rays

The first and fifth rays are more mobile than the central rays (second to fourth) and are thought to have a more profound effect on foot function, although, again, the subtleties are not well understood. It is thought that both the first and fifth rays function most effectively from a neutral position, that is a point somewhere midway between maximum dorsiflexion and maximum plantarflexion. To assess the first and fifth rays we first observe and palpate the individual components of the rays; navicular–medial cuneiform–first metatarsal–hallux and cuboid–fifth metatarsal–fifth phalanx. Following the initial assessment, the STJ is placed in an approximation of neutral and with the midtarsal joint close-packed in maximum eversion, the appropriate MTPJ (either first or fifth) is grasped and alternately plantarflexed and dorsiflexed about the axis at the base of the metatarsal. Roughly equal amounts of dorsiflexion and plantarflexion are normal.

Eyeball evaluation of the available motions is usually adequate for clinical purposes, although quantification using specific equipment such as Kilmartin's 'Sagittal Raynger' may be useful in certain applications (see Section 10A). To estimate plantarflexion and dorsiflexion of the first ray by eye the foot is placed in subtalar neutral and the midtarsal joint locked by the application of load to the fourth and fifth MTPJs. The first MTPJ is then dorsiflexed and plantarflexed to resistance. The examiner can get an

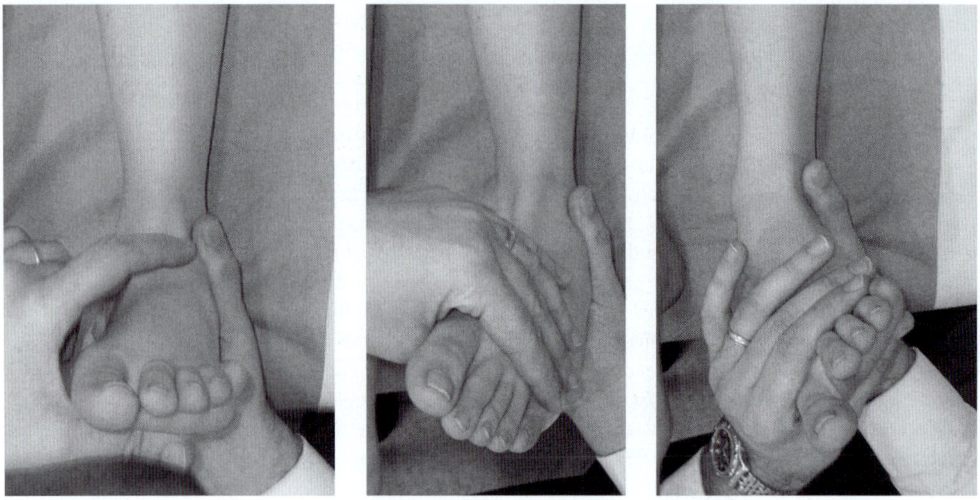

A B C

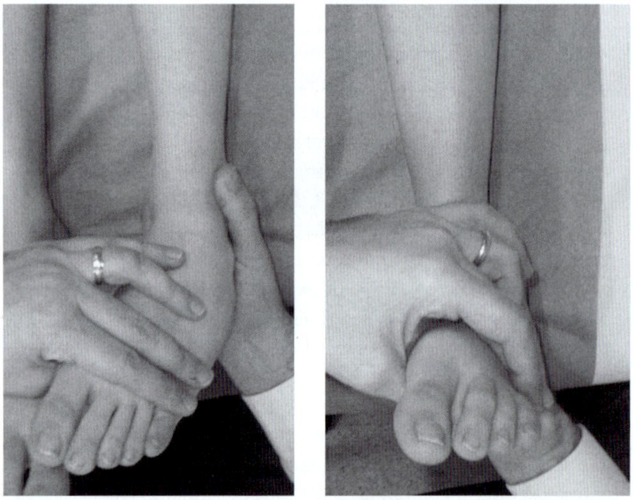

D E

Figure 10B.19A–E Measurement of the midtarsal joint range of motion.

impression of the displacement of the first MTPJ by estimating the relative positions of their own thumbs as they grasp the two segments (Fig. 10B.20). The procedure for evaluating the fifth ray is essentially the same, but transferred to the lateral side of the foot (Fig. 10B.21).

Metatarsophalangeal joints

In the distal joints, subjective assessment of function, joint integrity and quality of motion are arguably more important than ROM measurement and the subjective, empirical findings should be emphasised. Observation of the metatarsal area for soft tissue and bony swellings, and for dermal/epidermal lesions is of paramount importance. Palpation should be undertaken in an ordered fashion and all aspects of the joints should be inspected and palpated. Quality of motion must be carefully assessed as this is often compromised in syndromes such as hallux valgus and in systemic disorders such as rheumatoid arthritis. Note must be made of pain on motion and the overall range.

The first MTPJ is an important functional element and is subject to restriction in the ROM in a number of conditions with both functional and systemic aetiologies. It is thought that for normal functioning of the foot to occur, approximately 60° of hallux dorsiflexion must be available. This is readily estimated by eye or measured using a small goniometer. To measure hallux ROM, the foot is placed in the neutral position and from the medial side the hallux is dor-

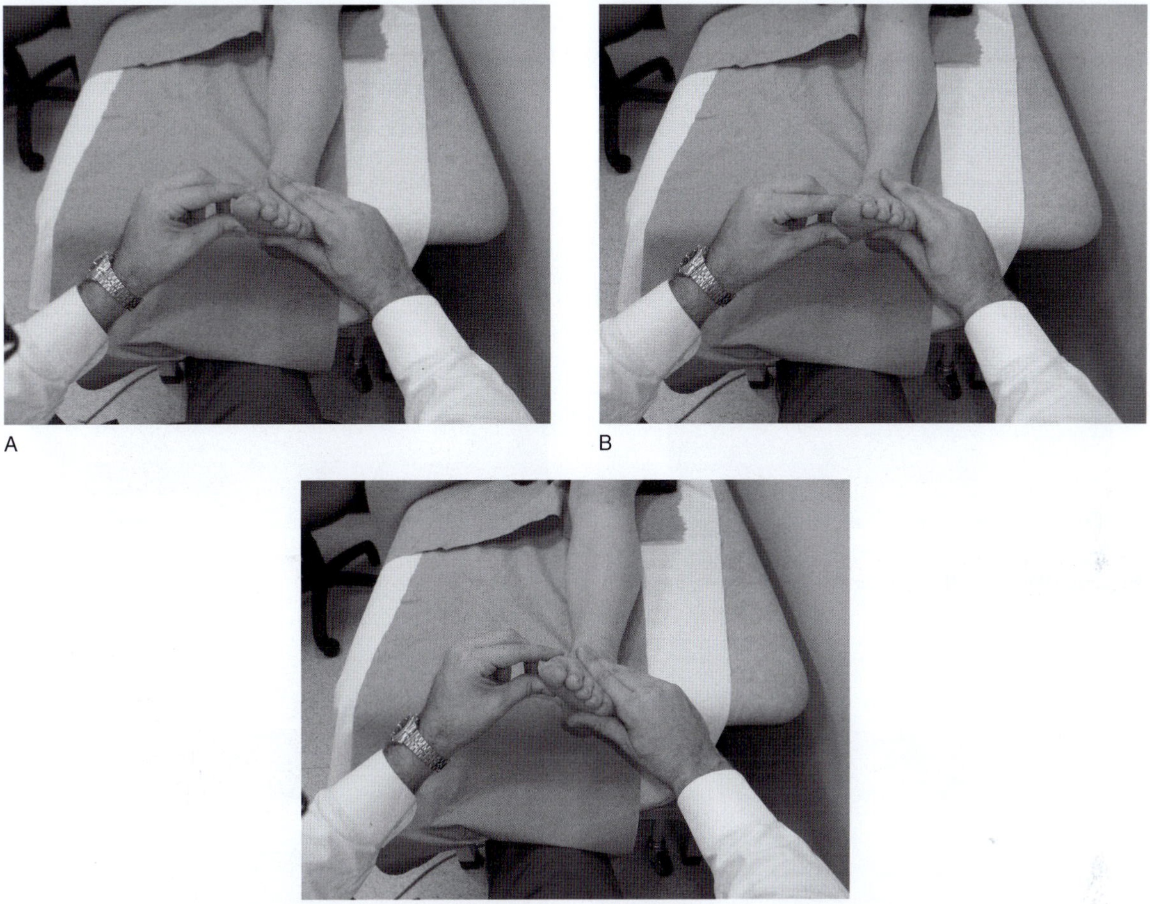

A B C

Figure 10B.20A–C Measurement of first ray range of motion.

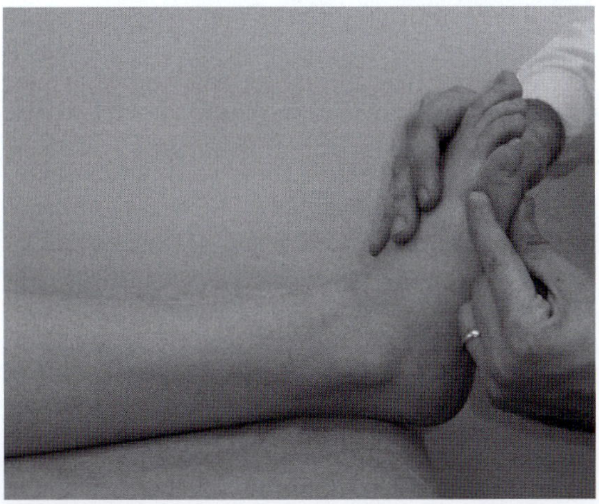

Figure 10B.21 Measurement of fifth ray range of motion.

siflexed passively. The patient can also be asked to assist. The angle formed between the phalanx and the metatarsal is measured on the medial side (Fig. 10B.22A). The same process may be repeated for plantarflexion (Fig. 10B.22B). It is good practice to undertake a similar examination of the lesser MTPJs (Fig. 10B.23).

Interphalangeal joints

As for the MPTJs above the most important aspect of the interphalangeal joint assessment is subjective. **Inspection, palpation and movement** are far more important than measurement of the ROMs.

Secondary features

This final subsection will cover some of the secondary features that arise as a consequence of disordered function and are therefore useful pointers towards

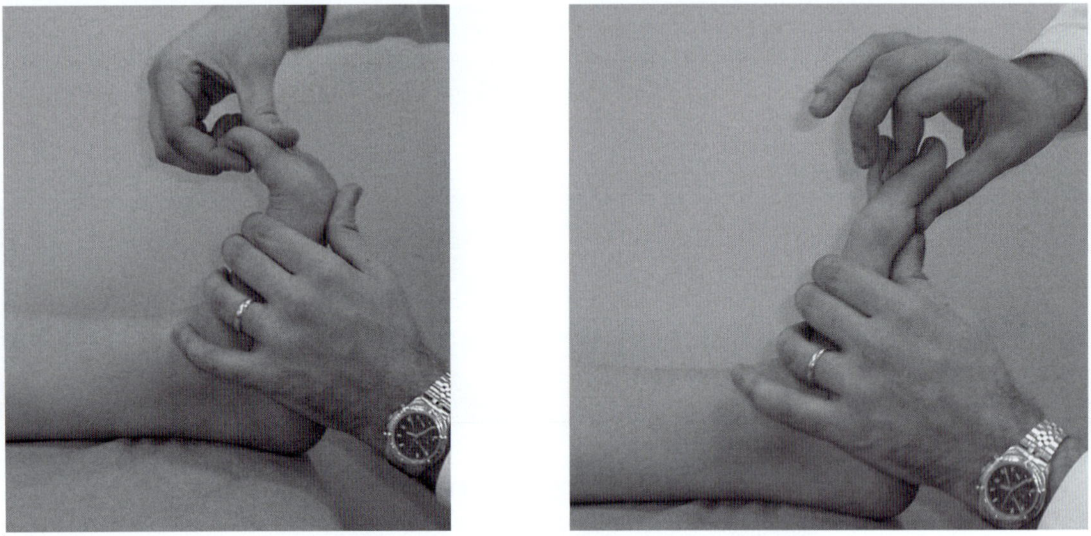

A B

Figure 10B.22A, B Measurement of first metatarsophalangeal range of motion.

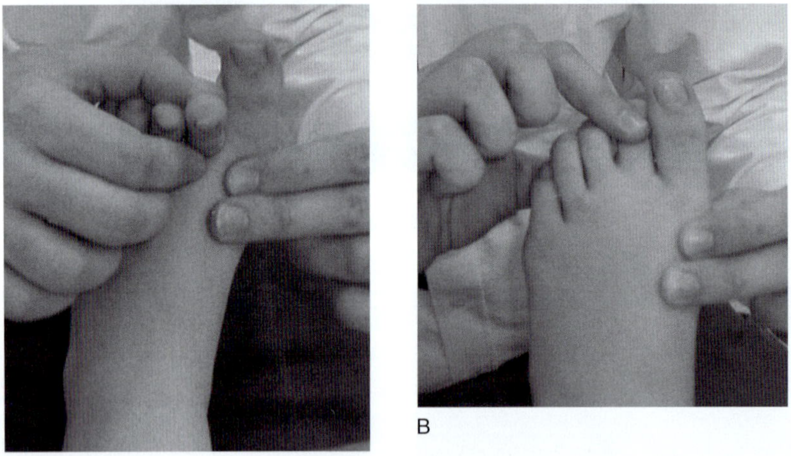

A B

Figure 10B.23A, B Measurement of lesser metatarsophalangeal range of motion.

underlying biomechanical impairment or other musculoskeletal disorder. Secondary features can include bony alterations such as posterior heel (retrocalcaneal exostosis), osteophyte formation at joint margins, soft tissue changes such as bursa formation, or telltale changes in the skin, perhaps in response to altered pressures.

Bony change (osteophytes, retrocalcaneal exostosis)

New bone is often laid down at the margins of joints in response to joint damage or degeneration. Osteophyte formation is often associated with osteoarthritis change but can occur independently. Common sites for osteophyte formation in the foot are the first and fifth MTPJs and first metatarsal–medial cuneiform joint. A **retrocalcaneal exostosis** or 'pump bump' is a bony overgrowth occurring on the posterolateral aspect of the calcaneus. These can be asymptomatic or can cause significant discomfort, especially if irritated by footwear. They are sometimes referred to as a **Haglund's deformity**, although this is often incorrect as a true Haglund's deformity is a bony prominence that occurs on the posterior/superior projection of the calcaneus and can only be properly visualised on X-ray.

Many theories have evolved linking these secondary presentations with underlying mechanical variances but in the absence of compelling scientific evidence for any of these theoretical links, specific mechanisms will not be discussed here. It is accepted, however, that such osteophytes and bony overgrowths are indicative of impaired function and their presence would suggest a need for a thorough functional assessment using whatever paradigms the individual practitioner prefers.

Hallux valgus/limitus/rigidus

Again there are many, sometimes competing theories linking hallux valgus/limitus/rigidus with a range of mechanical variants and it is not possible in this chapter to provide any great detail. In the context of a functional assessment it is appropriate to say, however, that the mere presence of deformity or limitation to movement of the first MTPJ is indicative of impaired function somewhere in the foot. The presence of first MTPJ dysfunction should, therefore, precipitate a thorough functional assessment using the practitioner's preferred methods.

Soft tissue

Soft-tissue structures are relatively responsive to altered function and the presentations can vary. Common signs of impaired foot function include:

- joint swelling in response to disease or physical demands
- contracture or clawing of the digits possibly due to faulty function of intrinsic musculature
- tendon subluxation or bowing, as seen in hallux valgus
- bursa formation in response to external irritation to a joint or other synovial structure
- muscle atrophy and hypertrophy in response to disease or altered demands.

Skin

The most common presentation of altered musculoskeletal function manifesting through changes in the skin is the development or **corns and callus** over regions that are exposed to increased loads or unusual application of loads such as sheer. This was covered earlier in the chapter in more detail but even in the absence of a clear understanding of the precise relationship between function and the patterns of corns or callus, their mere presence indicates a need for a functional evaluation.

Summary

The functional assessment protocol should swing into action once you have reason to believe from your routine history taking or initial observation that a presenting complaint has a functional aetiology. Experience will help the practitioner learn to recognise functional traits and to develop a working understanding of the process of human locomotion.

The most thorough assessment involves a systematic protocol, working from general to specific. In this way the practitioner can, with experience, learn to be selective as to which tests are performed and will develop a familiar framework for the functional assessment.

We recommend a protocol that uses a **Look → Feel → Move** approach and emphasise that the 'Look' component should start with observing gait so as to get an immediate feel for overall function. Individual, non-weightbearing assessments of *all* joints is not usually required and can be prioritised according to observational findings.

It is important not to overestimate the importance of measured, supposedly 'objective' results. The errors associated with most of these techniques are enormous and in many cases your eye is as good a clinical and diagnostic tool as a goniometer. Quantification is sometimes helpful in expressing the magnitude of a variation from normal but in few cases are precise measures required, or of adequate validity, to make a diagnosis. Conversely, the importance of the subjective assessment of the joints must not be underestimated. In functional assessment, observation and palpation have made more diagnoses than measurements.

References

Aglietti P, Insall J N, Tria A J Jr 1983 Patellar pain and incongruence. I: measurements of incongruence. Clinical Orthopaedics & Related Research (176):217–224

Anderson J G, Harrington R, Ching R P et al 1997 Alterations in talar morphology associated with adult flatfoot. Foot & Ankle International 18(11):705–709

Aquino A, Payne C B 2001 Function of the windlass mechanism in excessively pronated feet. Journal of the American Podiatric Medical Association 91(5):245–250

Arangio G A, Phillippy D C, Xiao D et al 2000 Subtalar pronation – relationship to the medial longitudinal arch loading in the normal foot. Foot & Ankle International 21(3):216–220

Astion D J, Deland J T, Otis J C et al 1997 Motion of the hindfoot after simulated arthrodesis. Journal of Bone and Joint Surgery (Am) 79(2):241–246

Aston J W Jr 1979 In-toeing gait in children. American Family Physician 19(5):111–117

Astrom M, Arvidson T 1995 Alignment and joint motion in the normal foot. Journal of Orthopaedic and Sports Physical Therapy 22(5):216–222

Atkinson-Smith C, Betts R P 1992 The relationship between footprints, foot pressure distributions, rearfoot motion and foot function in runners. The Foot 2:148–154

Ball P, Johnson G R 1993 Reliability of hindfoot goniometry when using a flexible electrogoniometer. Clinical Biomechanics 8(1):13–19

Benink R J 1985 The constraint-mechanism of the human tarsus: a roentgenological experimental study. Acta Orthopaedica Scandinavica Supplement 215:1–135

Bojsen-Moller F 1979 Calcaneocuboid joint and stability of the longitudinal arch of the foot at high and low gear push off. Journal of Anatomy 129(1):165–176

Camasta C A, Pontious J, Boyd R B 1991 Quantifying magnification in pedal radiographs. Journal of the American Podiatric Medical Association 81(10):545–548

Cashmere T, Smith R, Hunt A et al 1999 Medial longitudinal arch of the foot: stationary versus walking measures. Foot & Ankle International 20(2):112–118

Cavanagh P R, Morag E, Boulton A J et al 1997 The relationship of static foot structure to dynamic foot function. Journal of Biomechanics 30(3):243–250

Cavanagh P R, Rodgers M M 1987 The arch index: a useful measure from footprints. Journal of Biomechanics 20(5):547–551

Coady D, Walker D, Kay L et al 2004 Regional examination of the musculoskeletal system (REMS): a core set of clinical skills for medical students. Rheumatology 43(5):633–639

Coleman S S, Chesnut W J 1977 A simple test for hindfoot flexibility in the cavovarus foot. Clinical Orthopaedics & Related Research (123):60–62

Cook A, Gorman I, Morris J 1988 Evaluation of the neutral position of the subtalar joint. Journal of the American Podiatric Medical Association 78(9):449–451

Coplan J A 1989 Rotational motion of the knee: a comparison of normal and pronating subjects. Journal of Orthopaedic & Sports Physical Therapy 10(9):366–369

Cornwall M W, McPoil T G 1999 Three dimensional movement of the foot during the stance phase of gait. Journal of the American Podiatric Medical Association 89(2):56–66

Dahle L K, Mueller M, Delitto A et al 1991 Visual assessment of foot type and relationship of foot type to lower extremity injury. Journal of Orthopaedic & Sports Physical Therapy 14(2):70–74

Doherty M, Doherty J 1992 Clinical examination in rheumatology. Wolfe Publishing, Aylesbury

Elftman H 1960 The transverse tarsal joint and its control. Clinical Orthopedics 16:41–45

Elveru R A, Rothstein J M, Lamb R L et al 1988 Goniometric reliability in a clinical setting :subtalar and ankle joint measurements. Physical Therapy 68(5):672–677

Engsberg J R 1987 A biomechanical analysis of the talocalcaneal joint – in vitro. Journal of Biomechanics 20(4):429–442

Engsberg J R, Andrews J G 1987 Kinematic analysis of the talocalcaneal/talocrural joint during running support. Medicine and Science in Sports and Exercise 19(3):275–284

Forriol Campos F, Maiques J P, Dankloff C et al 1990 Foot morphology development with age. Gegenbaurs Morphologisches Jahrbuch 136(6):669–676

Franco A H 1987 Pes cavus and pes planus: analyses and treatment. Physical Therapy 67(5):688–694

Freychat P, Belli A, Carret J P et al 1996 Relationship between rearfoot and forefoot orientation and ground reaction forces during running. Medicine and Science in Sports and Exercise 28(2):225–232

Garbalosa J C, McClure M H, Catlin P A et al 1994 The frontal plane relationship of the forefoot to the rearfoot in an asymptomatic population. Journal of Orthopaedic and Sports Physical Therapy 20(4):200–206

Giallonardo L M 1988 Clinical evaluation of foot and ankle dysfunction. Physical Therapy 68(12):1850–1856

Gould N 1983 Evaluation of hyperpronation and pes planus in adults. Clinical Orthopaedics & Related Research (181):37–45

Halstead J, Redmond A C 2006 Weight-bearing passive dorsiflexion of the hallux in standing is not related to hallux dorsiflexion during walking. Journal of Orthopaedic and Sports Physical Therapy 36(8):550–556

Hawes M R, Nachbauer W, Sovak D et al 1992 Footprint parameters as a measure of arch height. Foot and Ankle 13(1):22–26

Hay J C 1973 The biomechanics of sports techniques, Prentice-Hall, Englewood Cliffs, New Jersey

Hicks J 1953 The mechanics of the foot I: the joints. Journal of Anatomy 87(4):345–357

Hunt A E, Fahey A J, Smith R M et al 2000 Static measures of calcaneal deviation and arch angle as predictors of rearfoot motion during walking. Australian Journal of Physiotherapy 46(1):9–16

Isman R E, Inman V T 1969 Anthropometric studies of the human foot and ankle. Bulletin of Prosthetics Research Spring: 97–104

Jack E A 1953 Naviculo-cuneiform fusion in the treatment of flat foot. Journal of Bone and Joint Surgery 35B:75–82

Jonson S R, Gross M T 1997 Intraexaminer reliability, interexaminer reliability, and mean values for nine lower extremity skeletal measures in healthy naval midshipmen. Journal of Orthopaedic and Sports Physical Therapy 25(4):253–263

Katz K, Naor N, Merlob P et al 1990 Rotational deformities of the tibia and foot in preterm infants. Journal of Pediatric Orthopedics 10(4):483–485

Keenan A M 1997 A clinician's guide to the practical implications of the recent controversy of foot function. Australasian Journal of Podiatric Medicine 31(3): 87–93

Keenan A M, Redmond A C, Horton M et al 2007 The Foot Posture Index: Rasch analysis of a novel, foot-specific outcome measure. Archives of Physical Medicine and Rehabilitation 88(1):88–93

Kidd R 1997 Forefoot valgus: real or false, fact or fantasy? Australasian Journal of Podiatric Medicine 31:81–86

Kidd R 2000 Forefoot supinatus: another fictitious pathology, or have we missed the point? Australasian Journal of Podiatric Medicine 34:81–85

Kitaoka H B, Alexander I J, Adelaar R S et al 1994 Clinical rating systems for the ankle-hindfoot, midfoot, hallux, and lesser toes. Foot and Ankle International 15(7):349–353

Kitaoka H B, Lundberg A, Luo Z P et al 1995 Kinematics of the normal arch of the foot and ankle under physiologic loading. Foot and Ankle International 16(8):492–499

Kitaoka H B, Luo Z P, An K N et al 1997 Effect of the posterior tibial tendon on the arch of the foot during simulated weightbearing: biomechanical analysis. Foot and Ankle International 18(1):43–46

Lanier J C 1971 The intoeing child: treatment with a simple orthopedic appliance. Journal of the Florida Medical Association 58(12):19–23

LaPointe S J, Peebles C et al 2001 The reliability of clinical and caliper-based calcaneal bisection measurements. Journal of the American Podiatric Medical Association 91(3):121–126

Lattanza L, Gray G W, Kantner R M et al 1988 Closed versus open kinematic chain measurements of subtalar joint eversion: implications for clinical practice . . . nonweightbearing (NWB) and weightbearing (WB) positions. Journal of Orthopaedic & Sports Physical Therapy 9(9):310–314

Lundberg A, Svensson O K, Bylund C et al 1989 Kinematics of the ankle/foot complex. Part 2: pronation and supination. Foot and Ankle 9(5):248–253

Lundberg A, Svensson S 1993 The axes of rotation of the talocalcaneal and talonavicular joints. The Foot 3:65–70

Manter J T 1941 Movements of the subtalar and transverse tarsal joints. Anatomical Record 80(4):397–410

McCarthy D J, Gessner R 1993 Anatomical basis for congenital deformities of the lower extremities. Part I: the hip and thigh. Journal of the American Podiatric Medical Association 83(1):18–28

McDowell B C, Hewitt V, Nurse A et al 2000 The variability of goniometric measurements in ambulatory children with spastic cerebral palsy. Gait & Posture 12(2):114–121

McPoil T, Cameron J A, Adrian M J 1987 Anatomical characteristics of the talus in relation to forefoot deformities. Journal of the American Podiatric Medical Association 77(2):77–81

McPoil T G, Cornwall M W 1996 Relationship between three static angles of the rearfoot and the pattern of rearfoot motion during walking. Journal of Orthopaedic and Sports Physical Therapy 23(6):370–375

McPoil T G, Hunt G C 1995 Evaluation and management of foot and ankle disorders: present problems and future directions. Journal of Orthopaedic and Sports Physical Therapy 21(6):381–388

McPoil T G, Knecht H G, Schuit D et al 1988 A survey of foot types in normal females between the ages of 18 and 30 years. Journal of Orthopaedic and Sports Physical Therapy 9(12):406–409

Menz H B 1995 Clinical hindfoot measurement: a review of the literature. The Foot 5:57–64

Menz H B 1998 Alternative techniques for the clinical assessment of foot pronation. Journal of the American Podiatric Medical Association 88(3):119–129

Morris J L, Jones L J 1994 New techniques to establish the subtalar joint's functional axis. Clinics in Podiatric Medicine and Surgery 11(2):301–309

Mueller M J, Host J V, Norton B J 1993 Navicular drop as a composite measure of excessive pronation. Journal of the American Podiatric Medical Association 83(4):198–202

Nawoczenski D A, Baumhauer J F, Umberger B R 1999 Relationship between clinical measurements and motion of the first metatarsophalangeal joint during gait. Patient Care Management 81(3):370–376

Nawoczenski D A, Saltzman C L, Cook T M 1998 The effect of foot structure on the three-dimensional kinematic coupling behavior of the leg and rear foot. Physical Therapy 78(4):404–416

Nester C J 1997 Rearfoot complex: A review of its interdependent components, axis orientation and functional model. Foot 7(2):86–96

Nester C J, van der Linden M L et al 2000 Some effects of foot orthoses on joint motion and moments, and ground reaction forces. 24th Annual Meeting, American Society of Biomechanics, Chicago, IL

Nigg B M, Cole G K, Nachbauer W 1993 Effects of arch height of the foot on angular motion of the lower extremities in running. Journal of Biomechanics 26(8):909–916

Noakes H, Payne C 2003 The reliability of the manual supination resistance test. Journal of the American Podiatric Medical Association. 93(3):185–189

Novacheck T F, Walker K R 2000 Progress in neuromuscular disorders. Current Opinion in Orthopedics December 11(6):454–460

Ouzounian T J, Shereff M J 1989 In vitro determination of midfoot motion. Foot and Ankle 10(3):140–146

Perry M D, Mont M A, Einhorn T A et al 1992 The validity of measurements made on standard foot orthoroentgenograms. Foot & Ankle 13(9):502–507

Picciano A M, Rowlands M S, Worrell T 1993 Reliability of open and closed kinetic chain subtalar joint neutral positions and navicular drop test. Journal of Orthopaedic & Sports Physical Therapy 18(4):553–558

Pierrynowski M R, Smith S B 1996 Rear foot inversion/eversion during gait relative to the subtalar joint neutral position. Foot & Ankle International 17(7):406–412

Pierrynowski M R, Smith S B, Mlynarczyk J H 1996 Proficiency of foot care specialists to place the rearfoot at subtalar neutral. Journal of the American Podiatric Medical Association 86(5):217–223

Redmond A C, Crosbie J, Ouvrier R A 2006 Development and validation of a novel rating system for scoring standing foot posture: the Foot Posture Index. Clinical Biomechanics 21(1):89–98

Root M L 1964 An approach to foot orthopedics. Journal of the American Podiatry Association 54(2):115–118

Root M L, Orien W P, Weed J et al 1971 Biomechanical Examination of the Foot. Los Angeles, Clinical Biomechanics Corporation

Saleh M, Murdoch G 1985 In defence of gait analysis: observation and measurement in gait assessment. Journal of Bone & Joint Surgery (Br) 67(2):237–241

Saltzman C L, Nawoczenski D A, Talbot K D 1995 Measurement of the medial longitudinal arch. Archives of Physical Medicine and Rehabilitation 76(1):45–49

Scherer P R, Morris J L 1996 The classification of human foot types, abnormal foot function, and pathology. In: Valmassy R L (ed) Clinical biomechanics of the lower extremities. Mosby, St Louis, pp 86–93

Sell K E, Verity T M, Worrell T W et al 1994 Two measurement techniques for assessing subtalar joint position: a reliability study. Journal of Orthopaedic & Sports Physical Therapy 19(3):162–167

Smith S D, Ocampo R F 1997 Subtalar arthrorisis and associated procedures. Clinics in Podiatric Medicine and Surgery 14(1):87–98

Sobel E, Levitz S J 1997 Reappraisal of the negative impression cast and the subtalar joint neutral position. Journal of the American Podiatric Medical Association 87(1):32–33

Song J, Hillstrom H J, Secord D et al 1996 Foot type biomechanics. comparison of planus and rectus foot types. Journal of the American Podiatric Medical Association 86(1):16–23

Staheli L T 1986 Torsional deformity. Pediatric Clinics of North America 33(6):1373–1383

Staheli L T 1987 Evaluation of planovalgus foot deformities with special reference to the natural history. Journal of the American Podiatric Medical Association 77(1):2–6

Staheli L T, Corbett M, Wyss C et al 1985 Lower-extremity rotational problems in children. Normal values to guide management. Journal of Bone & Joint Surgery – American Volume 67(1):39–47

Thomson P (ed) 1993 Introduction to podopaediatrics. W B Saunders, London

Weiner-Ogilvie S, Rome K 1998 The reliability of three techniques for measuring foot position. Journal of the American Podiatric Medical Association 88(8):381–386

Weseley M S, Barenfeld P A, Eisenstein A L 1981 Thoughts on in-toeing and out-toeing: twenty years experience with over 5000 cases and a review of the literature. Foot and Ankle 2(1):49–57

Williams D, McClay I et al 1999 A comparison of between day reliability of different types of lower extremity kinematic variables in runners. 23rd Annual Meeting of the American Society of Biomechanics, University of Pittsburgh

Winson I G, Lundberg A, Bylund C et al 1994 The pattern of motion of the longitudinal arch of the foot. Foot 4(3):151–154

Wright D G, Desai F M, Henderson W H et al 1964 Action of the subtalar and ankle-joint complex during the stance phase of walking. Journal of Bone and Joint Surgery (Am) 46:361

Part 3

Laboratory and hospital investigations

CHAPTER

11

Methods of analysing gait

C B Payne, A R Bird

Indicates figures on DVD, including colour

Chapter contents

Introduction

Gait analysis is the systemic assessment and analysis of human locomotion. Gait is a complex activity that has many inter-related components and, as such, there are many different ways of analysing gait. Gait analysis and a thorough musculoskeletal assessment are powerful tools for identifying pathomechanical mechanisms, making treatment decisions, guiding therapeutic interventions and monitoring the outcome of interventions. However, the differentiation of cause from effect is often difficult because of variable individual compensations that operate during the gait cycle and the occurrence of more than one pathology at the same time.

Gross abnormalities, such as a patient with a marked limp or a child who is a toe walker, are relatively easy to visually identify. Minor variations from the 'normal' are harder to spot and describe in a meaningful way. This is not surprising given that it only takes 650 ms to complete one full gait cycle and the human eye cannot perceive events that occur in less than 83 ms (Gage & Ounpuu 1989). Practitioners are, therefore, increasingly looking towards methods of investigating gait in a systematic way that provides accurate, reproducible and quantitative data.

There is no one single satisfactory method of analysing and quantifying gait. In addition, technological advances in this field are rapid, especially the development of software to assist in the collection, analysis and interpretation of data that can be collected by several different methods. As new systems are continually being developed, it is therefore recommended to regularly review the relevant literature.

How can gait by analysed?

Gait can be analysed by observation or by a variety of methodologies which produce quantitative data:

- Temporal and spatial parameters
- Kinematics
- Kinetics
- Accelerometers
- Electromyography
- Energy expenditure.

Clinically based gait analysis methods include observation and simple quantitative methods that can provide useful data. Observation of a patient's gait can be assisted by the use of video and treadmills. Simple quantitative measures can be made with techniques using paper, pen, tape measure and stop watch. Clinically based methods are simple to use, provide repeatable data, and are relatively easy and quick to interpret. They are also relatively low tech.

Gait laboratory methods rely on sophisticated and expensive equipment. Often, specialist knowledge is required to use and interpret the data. Purpose-designed gait facilities can provide an adjunct to the clinical examination but are used mostly for research purposes.

Observation of gait

Observational or visual gait analysis is the analysis of a subject's gait without the use of any equipment, and is one of the more useful and widely used clinical tools available to practitioners. The analysis of gait in this way is subjective and needs a substantial understanding of normal gait (Kirtley 2006, Perry 1992, Whittle 2001).

Observational gait analysis involves watching a person walk up and down an area that allows sufficient space for up to 10 steps, usually a corridor in the clinical setting. Any relevant deviations from the assumed normal are noted. Observational gait analysis is best done by systematically concentrating on one body part at a time, then another, and usually one limb at a time. However, this skill takes time to develop, with novices more erratic in their observation of body regions (Ford 2001) (Fig. 11.1).

With experience many gait deviations can be observed. The difficulty of observing one body part at a time is that multiple movements in multiple segments are occurring concurrently. Checklists, such as the one provided in Box 11.1, are usually helpful to work through, especially when learning. Traditionally, the approach is to observe the limb as it moves through the different periods of the stance phase – heel contact, mid-stance and propulsion. Another approach (Pathokinesiology Service 1993) is to divide gait into weight acceptance (initial contact and loading response), single limb support (period when body progresses over single limb), and swing limb advancement (time when one limb is unloaded and the other limb is loaded) and note variations from normal during these phases.

In clinical practice, observational analysis of gait is usually done after taking the history and carrying out a physical examination of the patient in order to evaluate the presence of any abnormal function that may be responsible for the patient's presenting complaint. The subsequent more detailed static and non-weightbearing biomechanical evaluation can be guided to particular areas of interest by the gait analysis. Of importance at this stage of the clinical evaluation is a consistency between the observed gait and the findings of the biomechanical evaluation. For example, if a lot of transverse plane motion of the midfoot is observed in stance during the gait analysis, a similar increase in the transverse plane direction of motions at the subtalar and midtarsal joints should generally be observed.

There is a tendency in clinical practice to focus on frontal plane motion during the gait analysis, but motion in the transverse and sagittal planes is just as important to appreciate gait. This primarily occurs for several reasons. Most clinics only have long corridors available which facilitate the observation in the frontal plane but hinder sagittal plane observation. The traditional teaching of clinical biomechanics places great importance on frontal plane compensation for different pathomechanical entities, which encourages the use of observation of gait to assess frontal plane motion of the posterior aspect of the calcaneus. The observation of the calcaneus in the frontal plane is easy, but is not necessarily indicative of any abnormal or compensatory gait patterns. For example, any abnormal compensatory movement of the calcaneus in the frontal plane is entirely dependent on the range of motion of the joints of the rearfoot complex and the orientation of the assumed position of the subtalar joint axis. If the axis is more vertical than the assumed normal, there will be very little motion of the calcaneus in the frontal plane, with more in the transverse plane. If the axis is more horizontal, there will be more motion in the frontal plane, which may not be pathological. Observational gait analysis is also limited by the ability to observe transverse plane motions and the difficulty to observe and interpret motion in all three planes simultaneously, as well as the motion occurring simultaneously at several joints. In a clinical setting in patients with pathology, the observation of gait requires walking for some time, which can be tiring for the patients. The endurance of the patient needs to be considered.

There is no permanent record from observational gait analysis – no opportunity to review the data at a later date. The analysis is very dependent on the skill and experience of the observer. All the data are

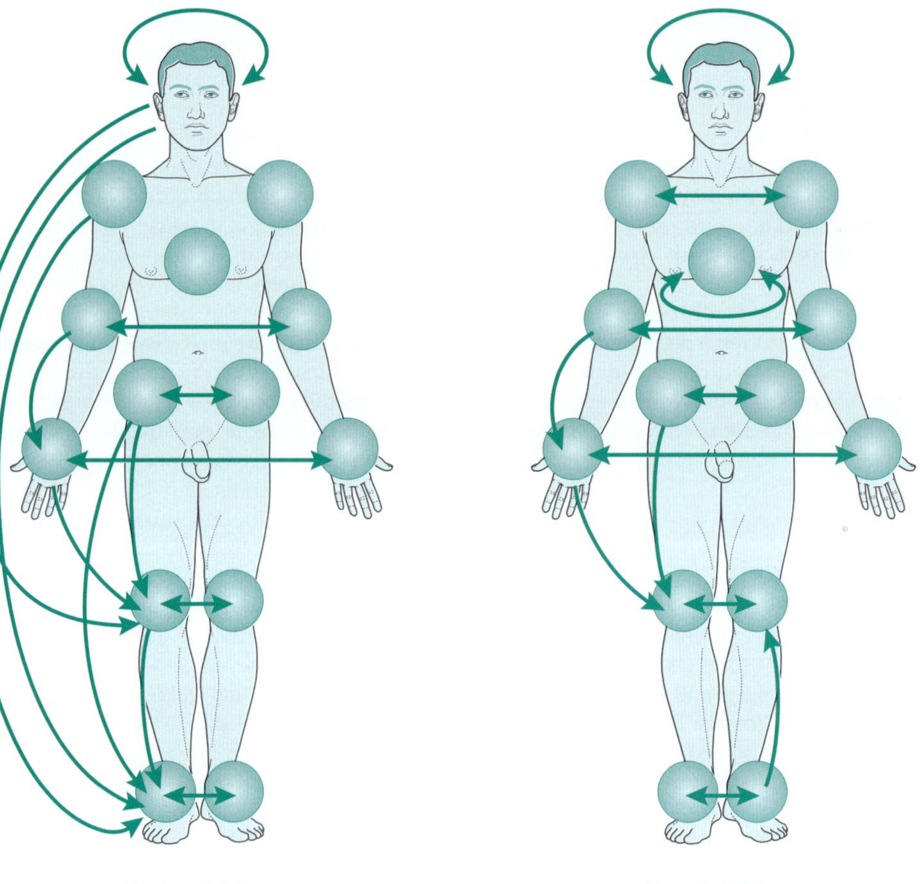

Figure 11.1 State transition diagrams demonstrating visual transitions and fixations with a probability higher than 0.2 in novice and expert clinicians. Expert clinicians made a greater number of transitions to adjacent body regions (e.g. feet to knees). Novice clinicians made a large number of transitions between body regions that were anatomically distant (Ford 2001).

subjective and qualitative. When one observes an individual standing on both feet, it is impossible to predict whether the load (distribution of force) under both feet is equal. This highlights the fundamental drawback of observation of gait: you cannot observe forces and the eye can be easily deceived. Reliability studies on observational gait analysis show that it is somewhat unreliable (Brunnekreef et al 2005, Krebs et al 1985, Saleh & Murdoch 1985). Despite these limitations, observational gait analysis provides a good overall impression of gait and requires no equipment. Experienced observers use observational gait analysis to make critical judgements, assist in diagnosis and determine the outcomes of interventions such as foot orthoses.

Treadmill

One of the most debated areas of gait analysis is the length of walkway required to achieve 'normal' walking patterns: 4–6 m is considered the minimum, but 8–10 m is more appropriate. Some practitioners use treadmills rather than an overground walkway. This is for several reasons: to view running, allow use of video systems or due to a lack of clinical space. If a treadmill is used, one must ensure that the participant has every opportunity to adapt to treadmill walking before the analysis. This usually requires at least 15 minutes of walking on the treadmill. The more exposure to treadmills, the shorter the time recorded to acclimatise and perform consistently

Box 11.1 Practical observational gait analysis

- Observe for amounts and timing of events
- Look for asymmetry
- Concentrate on one aspect at a time
- Bisection of calcaneus and posterior aspect of leg is often helpful
- A mark on the medial side of the navicular is also helpful
- Be aware that many individuals may consciously or subconsciously alter gait while being observed
- At least an 8–10 m walkway is desirable and provision for watching clients from behind/in front (frontal plane) as well as from the side (sagittal plane)
- Patient should be wearing shorts (have different sizes available in your clinic)
- Observe with and without shoes, and with and without orthoses

Frontal plane observations

Upper body

- Head/eyes level or tilted
- Shoulders level
- Height of finger tips
- Symmetrical arm swing
- Pelvis level or tilted

Lower limb

- Position of knee
- Q angle/patellar position
- Timing of knee motion
- Position of tibia
- Timing of tibial rotation

Foot

- Timing/amount of rearfoot motion
- Timing/amount of heel contact/off
- Timing/amount of midfoot motion
- Transfer from low gear to high gear during propulsion
- Angle and base of gait
- Abductory twist?
- Prominent extensor tendons (extensor substitution)
- Clawing of digits (flexor stabilisation)

Sagittal plane observations

Upper body

- Forwards or backwards tilt
- Symmetrical arm swing

Lower limb

- Position/timing of hip joint motion
- Position/timing of knee joint motion
- Position/timing of ankle joint motion

Foot

- Timing/amount of heel lift
- Timing/amount of midtarsal joint motion
- Timing/amount of first metatarsophalangeal joint motion

(Tollafield 1990). Clearly, older clients, children and clients with medical conditions are likely to tire more quickly. No matter how sophisticated the system is, participants must feel relaxed and comfortable when being observed. Most authorities now accept that in order to achieve this objective, clients should be allowed to walk at their own cadence rather than being artificially constrained by walking in time to a metronome or some other timing device.

For visual observation, treadmills facilitate closer inspection of the gait as well as easy observation of gait in the sagittal plane. In addition, treadmills are relatively inexpensive. There are subtle kinematic and kinetic differences between overground and treadmill gait (Riley et al 2006), however the principal consideration is that people should feel comfortable when using the treadmill.

Video

Video recording of gait for subsequent analysis (overground or on a treadmill) offers a different perspective than visual gait analysis. Observational gait analysis is limited by the high speed at which motions occur. It has been observed that events that happen faster than 83 ms (1/12 second) cannot be perceived by the human eye (Gage & Ounpuu 1989), so the use of slow-motion video and freeze-frame can enhance observational gait analysis. For example, some of the motions at the first metatarsophalangeal joint can be

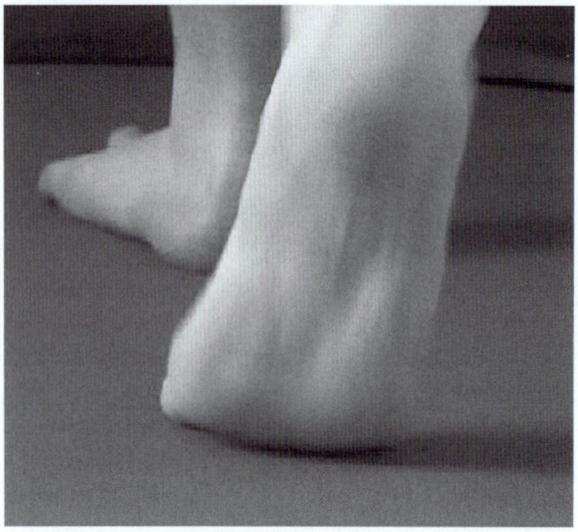

Figure 11.2 This freeze-frame digital video recording allows the observation of a foot that is propelling off the lateral metatarsal heads – which would not have been observed during a visual gait analysis.

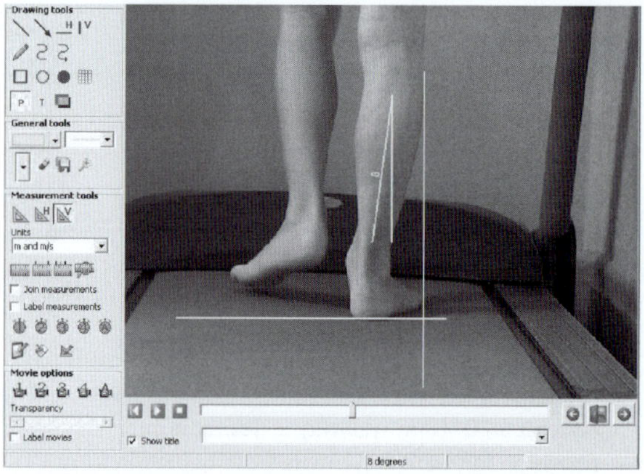

Figure 11.3 Screen shot of a typical analysis software for two-dimensional digital video recording of gait.

observed (Fig. 11.2). With good pause and slow-motion facilities the more subtle features of gait that would otherwise be missed can be observed. This will depend on the frequency of sampling: below 30 Hz may be insufficient, 50 Hz is an ideal for slow walking and 100 Hz will generally be required for running. If these sampling rates are not used, too much movement happens between each sampling frame to be useful for interpretation. Unfortunately, the standard frame rate for consumer-level video cameras is 25 Hz (PAL) and 30 Hz (NTSC). This means that the frame rate for such cameras makes it difficult to see fast-moving parts of the gait cycle: particularly around heel contact and heel and toe off. Some video software systems interpolate video (mathematically create a new video frame between two existing frames) to get around the low frame rate problem, with varying levels of success.

If two cameras and a video mixer are used, it is possible to view gait in two body planes simultaneously on the same split screen eliminating the problem of cross-plane interpretation. Most new digital video cameras allow for video to be downloaded, viewed and archived on a computer. Videos of persons walking with and without footwear and interventions (e.g. taping or foot orthoses) can be easily compared. Some systems (e.g. Dartfish, Contemplas, Silicon Coach) allow the drawing and calculation of angles between segments, the generation of gait analysis reports and the linking of the recorded gait into the patient's computerised records. Such systems also make it easy to show clients their own gait after it has been recorded, which can be a powerful tool to explain abnormalities in their gait for educational purposes (Fig. 11.3).

Disadvantages of the use of video gait systems are:

- the rotational deviations in the transverse plane cannot be seen
- movements out of the plane of the camera can also distort joint angles and influence interpretations, e.g. if sagittal plane knee motion is being observed, the angle may seem less than it really is due to internal rotation of the limb
- analysis of the video is still qualitative and has been shown to be only moderately reliable (Eastlock et al 1991, Keenan & Bach 1996). However, techniques to improve reliability and gather quantitative information from the two-dimensional digital video have been developed (Zammitt & Payne 2007).

Methods of quantitative gait analysis

Temporal and spatial parameters

As gait is repetitive, the measurement of the temporal (time) and spatial (distance) parameters are an aid to evaluating critical events that occur during gait. These parameters include stride length, stride time, step length, step time, double support time, mean walking velocity, cadence and the ratios of left to right of these parameters. It also includes toe-out/

toe-in angles and width of the walking base (base of gait). These parameters are useful as a measure of an individual's functional ability of ambulate: for example, less time will be spent in single limb support if that limb is painful.

Step length

This parameter is the distance from initial heel strike of one foot to the heel strike of the opposite foot.

Cadence

This parameter is the number of steps taken per unit time, usually per minute. For practical purposes, practitioners tend to count the number of steps taken during a period of 10–15 seconds. When measuring cadence it is important that participants are told to walk at their normal walking speed and as naturally as possible. The observation count starts once the subject is walking at normal speed. To estimate average cadence per minute the following formula should be applied:

$$\text{Cadence (steps per minute)} = \text{steps counted} \times 60/\text{time (s)}$$

Stride length

Stride length is the distance between two successive placements of the same foot and therefore consists of two step lengths; this parameter is usually measured in metres.

Base of gait

Also known as stride width, the walking base is the distance between the feet, usually measured at the midpoint of the heel; it is recorded in millimetres.

Toe-out and toe-in

Toe-out and toe-in are a measure of foot position in relation to the line of forward progression. It has been shown that foot position in relation to the line of forward progression constantly changes during gait. To produce an 'average' the position the foot adopts for 10 steps is recorded and the mean is calculated.

Velocity of walking

This parameter, measured in metres per second, is the distance covered by the body in a given time in a particular direction. The mean velocity can be calculated as the product of cadence and stride length. The cadence is measured in half strides per 60 seconds or full strides per 120 seconds. The velocity can be calculated by the following formula:

$$\text{Velocity (m/s)} = \text{stride length (m)} \times \text{cadence (steps/min)}/120$$

The above parameters can be recorded with basic equipment and can provide valuable clinical information (Kippen 1993). Poster paints, talcum powder, chalk, plaster of Paris, carbon paper and various coloured inks have been used to obtain footprint impressions (Wilkinson & Menz 1997). These footprint impressions provide a permanent record of the foot placements during gait and can be used to calculate a variety of parameters (Fig. 11.4).

Foot switches can be used to determine temporal measures; these are inexpensive and simple to use. The switches are either of a compression closing type or force sensitive type. They are typically used under the heel, first metatarsal and fifth metatarsal incorporated into an insole or strapped to the area of the foot. They are activated when a certain threshold of pressure is applied. Foot switches can be used in combination with other systems, such as electromyography, so that the timing of critical events such as heel contact, forefoot contact, heel off and toe off can be determined in relation to other variables or parameters being measured.

Gait mats (e.g. GaitRite, GaitMat) consist of a long strip of walking surface that has embedded in it an array of switches running along the length and width of the mat. As an individual walks on the mat, the switches close and open, allowing the computer to calculate the timing of each switch. As the geometry of the mat is known, many of the temporal and spatial parameters of gait, such as cadence, timing of single and double support duration and stride length, can be determined. These systems have the advantages of being relatively low cost and portable, and the temporal and spatial parameters are calculated automatically.

The measurement of temporal and spatial parameters can highlight pathology and changes associated with disease or rehabilitation. Patients such as those with rheumatoid arthritis, Parkinson's disease or paralysis will all show significant deviations from 'normal' parameters, e.g. short stride length, or slow or fast cadence. However, it must be recognised that assessment of these parameters on their own is not sufficient for a comprehensive overview of gait. Spatial and temporal parameters vary during walking and from one period of walking to another. Consequently, it is important to view the data with caution and to obtain a mean average for any parameter.

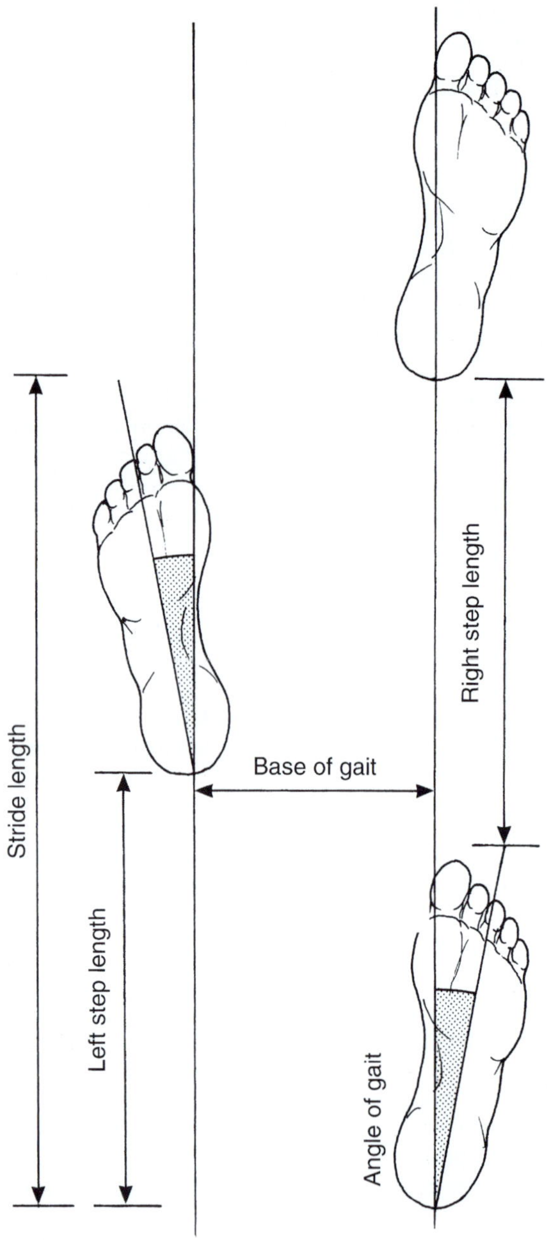

Figure 11.4 Spatial parameters that can be measured using a simple walkway.

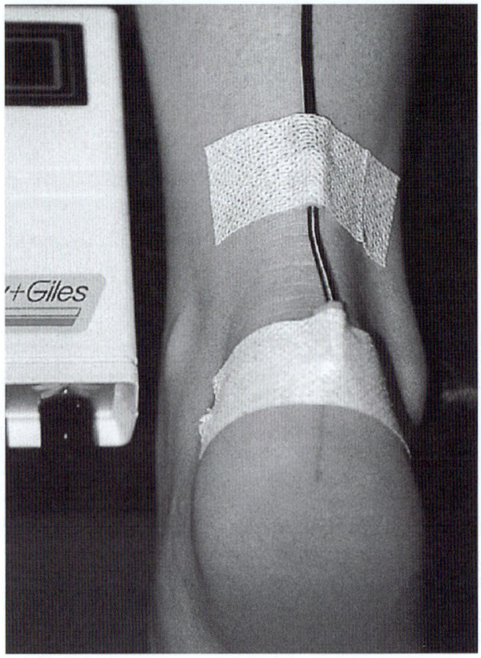

Figure 11.5 Electrogoniometer with transducer capable of reading 0.1° of motion (Penny & Giles, Gwent, UK). The goniometer has been attached to the foot to record frontal plane subtalar motion.

Kinematics

Kinematics is mostly concerned with the measurement of motion, describing angular movement and displacement of joints and the body throughout space. These data can be measured directly and indirectly using a variety of ways.

Direct methods

Direct measurement can be made by using goniometers (Chao 1980). These measure joint angle changes. The use of goniometers is becoming increasingly common, especially electrogoniometers and flexible goniometers (Fig. 11.5). Electrogoniometers (e.g. Biometric) are electromechanical devices that span a joint, being attached proximal and distal to the joint in the plane of motion that the joint generally moves in. They consist of two rigid links connected by a potentiometer that gives a voltage output proportional to the change in angle between the two rigid links. The angle the joint moves through is recorded in a data collection unit. Foot switches can be used to record events such as heel contact and toe off, so the timing of the motion can be determined.

Electrogoniometers can be used to measure two or three-dimensional joint motion. They are of low cost and are relatively easy to use. However, the equipment requires careful calibration and setting up in order to achieve valid and reproducible results. Some patients complain of being impeded by the measurement systems. This will affect the results obtained. Measurement of the small joints within the foot during gait has been more of a challenge and has led to the development and production of small flexible goniometers.

Indirect methods

Cine photography was the principal technique for gathering kinematic data before the introduction of video systems. Muybridge (1955) pioneered the use of cine photography in a classic study of human and animal locomotion. In the book *Human walking*, Inman et al (1981) demonstrated how the use of cine photography and still pictures can provide valuable information about joint angles and limb placement during locomotion. Data analysis of limb movement became much easier and quicker, although it was still too slow and time-consuming for routine clinical applications, following digitisation of the images (Sutherland & Hagy 1972).

Modern cine and video recording devices can be directly interfaced with a computer for reconstruction and analysis. Video motion-based systems (e.g. Optotrak, Vicon, Peak Performance, MacReflex) use one or more cameras to track markers that are attached to subjects at various locations. The markers are either active or passive. Active markers are infrared light-emitting diodes and the passive markers are reflective solid shapes. The video cameras keep track of the coordinates of the markers: in three-dimensional systems, the computer software keeps track of the three-dimensional coordinates of each marker based on the two-dimensional data from two or more cameras.

Two-dimensional analysis is cheaper than three-dimensional analysis because fewer cameras are needed and also less sophisticated software is needed for the analysis. Inaccuracy can occur if the segment being investigated rotates away from being perpendicular to camera. It can be useful, for example, to record the motion of a marker on the navicular to monitor motion in the sagittal plane or to monitor frontal plane motion of the calcaneus. However, the analysis of frontal plane motion of the calcaneus from a two-dimensional system may be problematic, due to range of motion of the rearfoot complex, the position of the assumed subtalar joint axis and being out of plane, which can distort the true angle of motion.

In three-dimensional analysis, the computer tracks several sectors at once, allowing the observation of multiple joints and multiple segments in all three body planes simultaneously. Cardan angles are used to measure kinematics, by comparing orientation of a distal segment relative to a proximal segment. Linked segment models that are based on a joint being composed of two segments are used to describe the kinematics of gait. The foot can be modelled as many linked segments. Three measurable points on a segment are needed by the analysis software to determine the position and orientation of the body segments in all three body planes. The three markers are used to define directions within segments and build segmental coordinate systems in three dimensions. The joint centres are calculated using these segmental coordinate systems. From the joint centres, anatomically aligned coordinate systems are constructed and used to calculate joint angles during walking trials.

To minimise errors, systems need to be calibrated before use. The placement of markers on the skin relative to osseous landmarks is crucial if models that have been developed for various systems are to be used with any reproducibility and if subjects are to be evaluated on different days or if different participants are to be compared with each other. Movement of the skin marker over osseous landmarks also needs to be taken into account during the modelling of gait or the evaluation of an intervention.

As well as calculating and providing graphs of kinematics, software can compute the kinetic variables of the net joint moments, forces and powers based on the kinematics and ground reaction force from the force platform.

Electromagnetic tracking systems

These systems (e.g. Polhemus, Skill Technologies, Flock of Birds) are beginning to be used more frequently. The information they provide is similar to the information provided by the video-based gait analysis systems. However, these tracking systems use electromagnetic sensors to track the motion of a 'marker' attached to the skin in three dimensions, therefore removing the need for cameras and the use of multiple markers on each segment.

Kinetics

Kinetics is the study and measurement of forces and moments exerted on the body that influence movement. Of direct relevance to the practitioner is the recording of forces at the foot/floor interface, measured, for example, via force platforms. Lesion patterns give an indication of the site of excess stresses but quantitative information cannot be gained by observation (Duckworth et al 1985). Consequently, some method of examining the plantar load distribution must be used.

Many clinicians and authors unfortunately use the terms 'force', 'load' and 'pressure' interchangeably. The terms have different meanings;

Force

As defined by Newton's second law of motion, force is mass multiplied by acceleration. This law means that any time a force is applied to an object, the object accelerates. Since acceleration is the change in velocity divided by the change in time, a force applied to an object will produce a change in the object's velocity. Force can therefore be considered as change in momentum divided by change in time. Force is a vector quantity, having both magnitude and direction.

Load

A weight or mass that is supported.

Pressure

Pressure is force divided by area: the larger the area the lower the pressure. This unit has important implications when comparing different measurement systems for measuring pressure under the foot. For example, systems which have large, discrete element sizes may not be able to measure the true pressure under a small area of the foot.

Researchers and practitioners are interested in the interaction between the foot, the shoe and the ground. Some of the fundamental questions being asked are the following:

- Is there a correlation between the loading characteristics of the shod and unshod foot?
- What happens at the foot–shoe interface?
- Is there a correlation between the loading characteristics measured at the shoe–floor interface and those at the foot–floor interface?
- Are the effects of foot orthoses influenced by the type of footwear?
- As forces can damage body tissues, what is the size of these forces and how can they be altered?

History has seen the development of a variety of systems designed to study the way in which load is distributed over the plantar surface of the foot. In addition, reviews of clinical findings from the use of particular equipment are continually being published. Many systems described in the literature are designed as part of research projects. These systems have not appeared on the market because of cost, lack of repeatability and technical difficulties that make them impractical to use clinically.

The systems currently available to practitioners are:

- force plates
- pressure platforms
- in-shoe force measurement.

Force plates

Force plates allow the measurement of vertical and shear forces and centre of force application under the foot. Force plates (e.g. Kistler, AMTI, Bertec) are fixed to the ground and are used to measure the ground reaction forces exerted as the patient walks on the plate during gait. The plates usually need to be set in epoxy concrete to prevent interference from vibration, although these vibrations can usually be identified and ignored on gait data. Force plates consist of a top plate that is mounted level with the surrounding floor. The top surface of the plate can be glass, aluminium or steel. The top plate is separated from the bottom frame by force transducers mounted at each corner. The forces transducers are either piezoelectric – which use quartz transducers to generate an electric charge when stressed – or strain gauges.

In the Kistler force plate, the plates incorporate four quartz rings that exhibit a piezoelectric effect, thus ensuring the system is sensitive to force in three planes: x, y, z. The control unit outputs continuous analogue data via 13 channels, of which eight are normally used. The only limitation of the system is the speed at which data can be received and stored and the analogue-to-digital converter interface, which can limit the resolution in time. Each channel can be sampled up to 3000 times per second. The collected data can be displayed on a computer screen as raw data or as a series of graphs showing force against time before obtaining a hard copy print. The system provides detailed numerical and graphical data on the forces applied to the foot (**Fig. 11.6**). The system has poor spatial resolution and does not analyse discrete pressures on the plantar surface of the foot. However, it should be noted that it can be calibrated and has been used to calibrate other force measurement systems.

Pressure platforms

A number of platforms are available to measure plantar forces and pressures, and a number of parameters are calculated from these. They measure the interaction between the foot and the walking surface (i.e. floor). Different systems use different technologies to measure these. They can be optical (e.g. pedobarograph); capacitative (e.g. EMED™); or piezoresistance (e.g. Tekscan™). There are technical issues

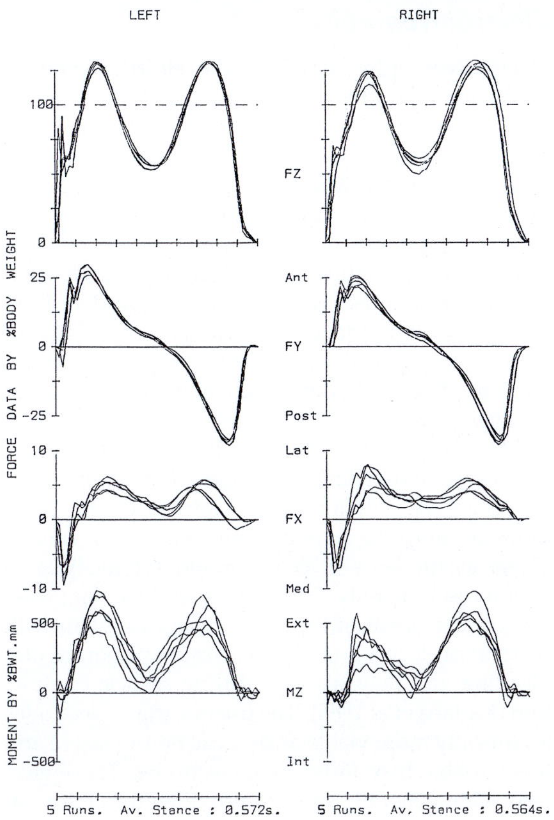

Figure 11.6 Data display from Kistler force plate.

associated with each of the sensor technologies, such as accuracy, linearity, hysteresis, creep and the effects of temperature on the sensors, which necessitate the need to accurately know the dynamic range for the sensors used and the need to calibrate the sensors prior to use.

Many collection protocols are used for the collection of data, but generally involve the subject walking barefoot for several steps before and after the platform. The two-step method involves collecting data from the subject's second step and has been shown to be reliable (Bryant et al 1999). For data to be analysed, the foot can be divided into discrete areas, often called masks, and several parameters are calculated for each mask (e.g. peak pressure, peak force, pressure time integral, force time integral, contact time). The masks are usually created under the heel, midfoot, first metatarsal head, lateral metatarsals, hallux, and lateral toes, but there are many variations in areas measured. Parameters such as the timing and direction of the centre of pressure can also be analysed.

Pressure platforms can be used clinically to determine areas of high pressure (especially in those with pressure lesions) and the timing and direction of the centre of pressure (especially in those with biomechanical problems).

In-shoe pressure and force measurement

Historically, many methods have been developed for recording foot loading while the foot is shod. Piezoelectric discs have been attached to the plantar surface of the foot to record the different effect of heel height on forefoot loading (Schwartz & Heath 1947). Capacitive pressure transducers have been adhered to the sole of the foot to record peak pressures in predetermined areas during gait in patients affected with Hansen's disease (Bauman & Brand 1963).

The current in-shoe pressure measurement systems use similar technology and types of analysis as the platform systems (e.g. Pedar, F-scan). The Pedar system uses individual sensors which are formed electronically at the intersection of rows and columns of conductive material (Nicol & Henning 1978). The F-Scan insole system consists of a printed insole approximately 300 mm long, 105 mm wide across the forefoot, 70 mm wide across the heel and 0.02 mm thick. The insole is a multilayer, piezoresistive, screen-printed sensor, sandwiched in a moisture-resistant coating. The layers are held together by small glue spots at a repeat distance of 1 cm square (**Fig. 11.7**). This allows the sensor insole to be cut to fit any size of shoe down to an adult size 4, providing care is taken not to cut through any required silver connecting tracts.

Often insole sensors used do not show a linear relationship between resistance and pressure; algorithms in the software are used to assign levels to pressure. Since this is not linear, different ranges can be achieved for high or low pressures. The insoles have a range from 0.57 kg/cm^2 (56 kPa) to 8.85 kg/cm^2 (868 kPa). The insole unit may be sensitive to temperature and moisture changes. However, well-controlled protocols may be able to reduce these characteristics. Repeatable data-collection runs are achievable provided that the sensors are undamaged and the system is calibrated prior to data collection.

The advantage of the in-shoe systems is that they provide a method for measuring plantar loading of successive steps of each foot while the foot is shod. This can be analysed with and without foot orthoses or another intervention. The types of parameter that can be analysed are similar to those of the platform systems.

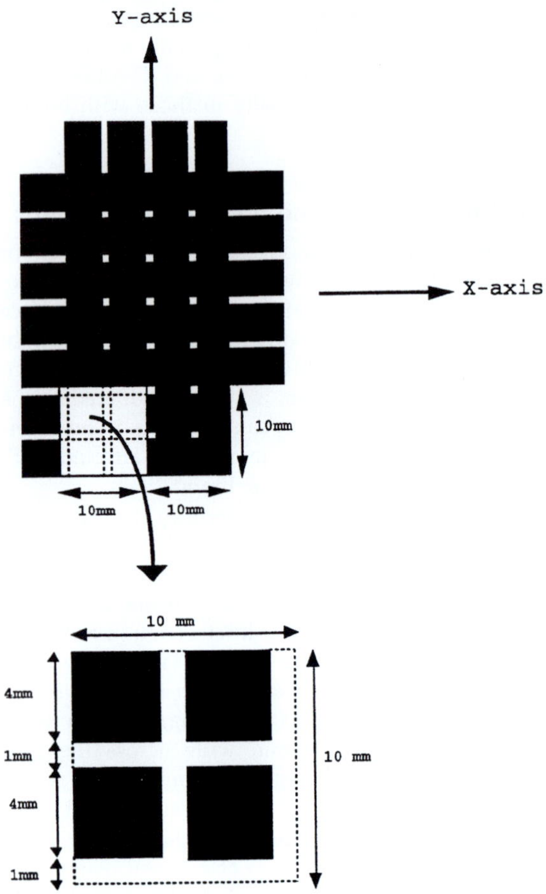

Figure 11.7 Diagrammatic representation of F-Scan.

Accelerometers

The use of accelerometers in gait analysis has generally been confined to the measurement of impact forces (such as those seen at heel strike) and acceleration of body parts in motion (Morris 1973). Much work has been undertaken by sports footwear manufacturers in the quest for the ideal shock-attenuating insole unit. The 'shock meter' system has been used to investigate shock waves transmitted during gait (Johnson 1990). A few experiments have been undertaken using accelerometers mounted on pins and then screwed directly into the bones of volunteers, although this method is clinically unacceptable. Accelerometers have been used in research but in clinical practice they may not be of much value (Collins & Whittle 1989).

Electromyography

Electromyography (EMG) is the electrical voltage associated with muscular contraction. EMG analysis can provide information about timing and intensity of muscle contraction. Such information provides data that indicate whether muscles are contracting in the correct order (phasic), at the right time and in an appropriate way. From this phasic muscle activity, tone, continuous and clonic muscle contraction or no muscle activity can be recorded. Data can assist with the assessment and aetiology of movement abnormality or in the review and assessment of physical therapies, rehabilitation or surgical interventions.

Electromyographic data can be collected by using surface or indwelling electrodes. Indwelling electrodes are more definitive than surface electrodes in terms of sampling activity from a particular muscle. These electrodes are also required for analysis of deep muscle activity, for example in the deep posterior compartment of the calf. A major problem with this sort of electrode is that it can cause intramuscular bleeding and may displace during muscle contraction (Kadaba et al 1985). The use of surface electrodes is clinically more viable as they are non-invasive and less variable than indwelling electrodes. These electrodes are generally used to provide gross information about the activity of muscle groups (Winter 1990) and are therefore less selective. There is also an increased risk of 'cross-talk' – picking up activity from other muscles that are not directly under investigation. Electromyography is therefore commonly used to identify gross phasic muscle activity prior to the fitting of orthoses designed to affect muscle activity, or for preoperative planning prior to tendon transfer or lengthening. For routine clinical practice the system is of little value.

Energy expenditure

Patients who exhibit gross abnormalities in their gait are likely to use more energy than patients with a more efficient gait pattern. This is not surprising since the structure and function of the locomotor system is designed to be energy-efficient in terms of its ability both to store and use energy. The determination of energy expenditure in gait has been undertaken since the 1950s. Many investigations have looked at normal and abnormal gaits in terms of energy cost. Estimation of the energy cost of walking usually involves the measurement of oxygen consumption (Inman et al 1981) or calculation of potential and kinetic energy levels of body segments from their motions and masses (Quanbury et al 1975).

A commercially available device called Caltrac measures the total number of calories used by subjects during walking. An alternative approach is to monitor heart rates as an indication of energy expenditure during activity (Rose et al 1989). In this method the 'physiological cost index' (PCI) is calculated as an estimate of energy used. The following formula is used:

PCI = (heart rate walking – heart rate resting)/velocity

Where heart rate is in beats/min and velocity is in m/min, or beats and velocity are per second. This is probably more useful in clinical practice than the measurement of oxygen consumption and carbon dioxide production during activity.

The measurement of oxygen consumption requires an analysis of the subject's exhaled air. Usually this requires the use of a Douglas bag, which allows the respiratory quotient to be calculated. Exercise is generally undertaken on a treadmill. Since the equipment required is bulky, this type of assessment is not routinely undertaken in the clinic.

Summary

Gait analysis is a complex task. The collection and analysis of quantitative data can aid observation of gait. One of the main problems with these methods is the difficulty in establishing what is normal. Gait may alter with every step a person takes; as a result, repeatability is a major problem. The practitioner must also be wary of highly technical equipment which will provide complex data that can be difficult to process and interpret.

In the research field, quantitative analysis of gait is making a contribution to our understanding of the complexities of this activity. In particular, research into gait is being used to design and evaluate therapeutic interventions, working in conjunction with clinical trials.

References

Bauman J H, Brand P W 1963 Measurement of pressure between foot and shoes. Lancet 3:629–632

Brunnekreef J J, van Uden C J, van Moorsel S et al 2005 Reliability of videotaped observational gait analysis in patients with orthopedic impairments. BMC Musculoskeletal Disorders 6:17

Bryant A R, Singer K, Tinley P 1999 Comparison of the reliability of plantar pressure measurements using the two-step and midgait methods of data collection. Foot & Ankle International 20(10):646–650

Chao E Y S 1980 Justification of triaxial goniometer for the measurement of joint rotation. Journal of Biomechanics 13:989–1006

Collins J J, Whittle M W 1989 Impulsive forces during walking and their clinical implications. Clinical Biomechanics 4:179–187

Duckworth T, Boulton A J M, Betts R P et al 1985 Plantar pressure measurements and the prevention of ulceration in the diabetic foot. Anatomical Record 59:481–490

Eastlock M E, Arvidson J, Snyder-Mackler L et al 1991 Inter-rater reliability of videotaped observational gait analysis assessments. Physical Therapy 71:465–472

Ford N E 2001 Visual cues and decision making in observational gait. PhD thesis. La Trobe University.

Gage J R, Ounpuu S 1989 Gait analysis in clinical practice. Seminar in Orthopaedics 4(2):72–87

Inman V T, Ralston H J, Todd F 1981 Human walking. Williams & Wilkins, Baltimore, MD

Johnson G R 1990 Measurement of shock acceleration during walking and running using the shock meter. Clinical Biomechanics 5:47–50

Kadaba M P, Wootten M E, Gainey J et al 1985 Repeatability of phasic muscle activity: performance of surface intramuscular wire electrodes in gait analysis. Journal of Orthopaedic Research 3(3):350–359

Keenan A M, Bach T M 1996 Video assessment of rearfoot movements during walking – a reliability study. Archives of Physical Medicine and Rehabilitation 77:651–655

Kippen S C 1993 A preliminary assessment of recording the physical dimensions of an inked footprint. Journal of British Podiatric Medicine 48(5):74–80

Kirtley, C 2006 Clinical gait analysis: theory and practice. Churchill Livingstone, London.

Krebs D E, Edlestein J E, Fishman S 1985 Reliability of observational kinematic gait analysis. Physical Therapy 65:1027–1033

Morris J R W 1973 Accelerometry: a technique for the measurement of human body movements. Journal of Biomechanics 6:729–736

Muybridge E 1955 The human figure in motion. Dover Publications, New York

Nicol K, Henning E M 1978 Measurement of pressure distribution by means of a flexible large surface mat. In: Asmussen E, Jorgenson K (eds) Biomechanics VI-A. University Park Press, Baltimore, pp 374–380

Pathokinesiology Service and Physical Therapy Department 1993 Observational gait analysis handbook. Rancho Los Amigos Medical Centre, Downy, CA

Perry J 1992 Gait analysis: normal and pathologic function. Slack, Thorofare, NJ

Quanbury A D, Winter D A, Reimer G D 1975 Instantaneous power and power flow in body segments during walking. Journal of Medical Engineering and Technology 7:273–279

Riley P, Paolini G, Della Croce U et al 2006 A kinematic and kinetic comparison of overground and treadmill walking in healthy subjects. Gait and Posture 26:17–24

Rose J R, Gamble J G, Medeiros J et al 1989 Energy cost of walking in normal children and those with cerebral palsy: comparison of heart rate and oxygen uptake. Journal of Pediatric Orthopedics 9:276–279

Saleh M, Murdoch G 1985 In defence of gait analysis. Journal of Bone and Joint Surgery 67B:237–241

Schwartz R P, Heath A L 1947 The definition of human locomotion on the basis of measurement. Journal of Bone and Joint Surgery 29(1):203–214

Sutherland D H, Hagy J L 1972 Measurement of gait movements from motion picture film. Journal of Bone and Joint Surgery 54:787–797

Tollafield D R 1990 A reusable transducer system for measuring foot pressures: a study of reliability in a commercial pressure pad. BSc thesis, Department of Health Sciences, Coventry Polytechnic

Wilkinson M, Menz H 1997 Measurement of gait parameters from footprints: a reliability study. The Foot 7:19–23

Winter D A 1990 Biomechanics and motor control of normal human movement, 2nd edn. John Wiley & Sons, New York

Whittle MW 2001 Gait analysis: an introduction, 3rd edn. Butterworth-Heinemann, Oxford

Zammitt G, Payne C B 2007 Kinematic changes with foot orthoses and clinical outcomes. Journal of the American Podiatric Medical Association 97(3):207–212

CHAPTER

12

Diagnostic imaging

C McCarthy

Indicates figures on DVD, including colour

Indicates video of assessment on DVD

Chapter contents

Introduction

As the number and complexity of cases referred to the foot specialist continues to increase, diagnostic imaging will develop a more important role in the practitioner's assessment of foot and ankle pathology. Imaging is usually required to confirm a clinical diagnosis and thus guide subsequent management.

The plain radiograph remains the most important and widely available initial imaging modality. This chapter provides practical information on ordering and interpretation of plain radiographs, together with relevant pathological detail. The principles, indications and limitations of other current imaging techniques including magnetic resonance imaging (MRI), computed tomography (CT), ultrasound and nuclear isotope scanning are highlighted to help the practitioner select the most appropriate imaging modality for suspected pathology of the foot and ankle. The radiological features of important bone disorders, such as infection, trauma and tumours, the arthropathies and soft-tissues pathology, including soft-tissue masses, tendon and ligament disease are described and illustrated in more detail.

The interpretation of X-rays and, in particular, the other imaging modalities is complex and these examinations are usually reported by a radiologist. In the light of the radiologist's report, practitioners may add their own knowledge, skills and clinical findings to complete the diagnosis and direct appropriate treatment. A number of excellent references are given in the further reading section at the end of this chapter which should be seen as a starting point for further reading around diagnostic imaging of the foot and ankle.

Plain radiographs

Generation of radiographs

Conventional radiographs

Conventional X-rays are generated by the passage of a high voltage through a heated coiled tungsten wire (the cathode) in a toughened glass tube containing a vacuum, producing free electrons in a process known as thermionic emission. At the other end of the tube is the anode, consisting of a heavy metal disc, usually tungsten, embedded in a copper bar, which rotates to absorb heat. When a high potential difference is applied between the electrodes, the electrons from the cathode stream at high velocity towards the anode and bombard the tungsten target. If a positive nucleus of a target atom is bombarded by fast-moving free, negatively charged electrons from another source, a repulsion and braking effect (the bremsstrahlung process) takes place. The electrons decelerate and emit energy in the form of radiation and if the energy levels are high enough, the radiation is in the form of X-rays.

When an X-ray beam passes through tissues, such as the foot, and strikes a sensitive film emulsion, it produces a chemical change and forms a negative image of the tissues, which may be viewed once the film has been processed. Tissues that lie in the path of the X-ray beam absorb or attenuate X-rays to differing degrees. Dense tissues that result in most X-ray absorption such as bone or calcium produce a white shadow on the X-ray and this area of increased density is known as *increased radiopacity*. Tissues that result in least X-ray absorption such as air produce a black shadow on the X-ray and this area of decreased density is called *increased radiolucency*. These differences account for the radiographic image (Table 12.1).

In practice it takes quite a large amount of radiation to alter the film. To reduce the patient dose, the film is usually placed in a cassette containing a rare earth intensifying screen. These screens fluoresce when struck by relatively small amounts of radiation and it is the fluorescence that changes the film. This reduces the radiation dosage required by up to 90%, depending on the type of screen, and it is therefore safer for the patient and the operator.

Table 12.1 Attenuation of the X-ray beam

X-ray attenuation	*Tissue*	*Effect on radiograph*
Least	Air or gas	Black image
⇩	Fat	Dark grey image
⇩	Soft tissue	Grey image
Most	Bone or calcium	White image

Digital radiographs

Many radiology departments have become filmless, that is they are using digital radiographs. There are two methods of obtaining digital X-rays:

- *Digital radiography.* Digital radiographs are obtained using new digital X-ray machines usually with large flat panel detectors that allow efficient conversion of X-rays directly into a digital signal with rapid production of images. This usually requires that the entire existing X-ray room is replaced with expensive digital acquisition devices.
- *Computed radiography.* Computed radiography uses standard X-ray machines so there is no need to change existing machines as is required with digital radiology. Only the recording device requires a change. In computed radiography, the image is exposed on a phosphor plate rather than a film. The phosphor plates, like film, are stored in cassette format. As X-rays pass through the patient, the phosphors absorb and store X-ray energy. This trapped energy comprises a latent image. The exposed cassette is transferred to a computed radiography unit which extracts and digitises the information stored in the plate to produce a digital image. The image is then transferred to a reader where it is displayed on a monitor. The digital image can be modified to adjust the exposure, which reduces the number of image retakes. Once the quality is approved, the image is usually stored in a digital format and viewed on a work station, although the image may be printed on film in a laser camera if required.

All imaging modalities including digitised radiographs are sent to and managed with a picture archiving and communication systems (PACS). PACS is essentially an information management system with the capability of acquiring, displaying, transmitting and archiving radiological images.

Digital images have many advantages over conventional radiographs. Digital images are of better quality and may be manipulated using a variety of image processing capabilities while being viewed at a workstation. This includes image contrast and brightness optimisation by manipulation of window width and level settings, magnifying, measuring and labelling certain structures. PACS allows multiple copies of the same image to be viewed simultaneously at different locations by a range of practitioners allowing discussion over diagnoses. The clinical history associated with the imaging examination and final report may be viewed in conjunction with the images. PACS systems may be integrated into the electronic patient record (EPR) which allows access to all patient details including clinical information and laboratory results. Image storage and retrieval is more efficient as all patients' previous radiographs are immediately available whenever their record is accessed thus preventing lost radiographs and the need to search for old films. Transmission of radiographic images is greatly facilitated allowing images to be sent electronically to other institutions for advice or patient referral. Although PACS inevitably results in increased IT support costs, expensive film and costs associated with film storage and handling are significantly reduced.

Ordering radiographs

The plain radiograph remains the most readily available imaging modality and should always be available for comparison when other radiological techniques are used. For an investigation to be of maximum use, any relevant clinical history, potential diagnoses and the information sought together with the views required, and it must be clearly specified on the X-ray request form whether they should be taken weightbearing. Relevant clinical information is essential as it justifies the investigation (ionising radiation regulations), results in views that best demonstrate the suspected abnormality, and allows the correct prediction and interpretation of pathology.

It is important that at least two views of the ankle and/or foot are obtained. As an X-ray is a two-dimensional rendition of a three-dimensional object, pathological changes cannot be properly assessed without more than one perspective. Also remember that an X-ray image will inevitably be subject to some enlargement and distortion of the actual structures.

In general weightbearing views are of most use allowing certain biomechanical features to be deduced as well as pathological features. Ordering X-rays for routine biomechanical assessment, however, is not good practice as it involves unnecessary radiation exposure.

The effects of radiation on tissue

Ionising radiation is harmful to living tissue and all radiological examinations must be justified. It is an established principle that the advantage to the patient of having a radiographic examination should outweigh the associated radiation hazard. Effects of radiation may be somatic or genetic. The sensitivity to radiation is related to oxygen saturation of the cells. Neural tissue is the least sensitive, and blood cells and bone marrow are the most easily damaged, leading to anaemia and leukaemia in severe cases of overexposure. The thyroid gland and the lens of the eye are also vulnerable. The gonads are radiosensitive and sterility, or even genetic mutations, can be caused by excessive irradiation of the gonads of a person of reproductive age. It is particularly important that a careful history is obtained from female patients of childbearing age to protect a developing fetus from potential radiation exposure.

Radiographs of the foot, if taken correctly, usually present minimal risk as the dosage is low, the beam is not angled towards the abdomen and gonad protection can be used.

Radiographic views

Some of the more commonly requested views of the foot and ankle are discussed below. Bear in mind that there are variations in radiographic technique between different radiology departments.

Dorsiplantar view

Radiographic technique

This view is taken either weightbearing or non-weightbearing with the X-ray beam angled 10° towards the heel (so that it is perpendicular to the metatarsals) and directed to the base of the third metatarsal.

Anatomical review areas

See Box 12.1.

This general purpose view shows the majority of the foot from the midtarsal area distally (Fig. 12.1). The neck of the talus, the distal edge of the calcaneum, the tarsus, metatarsals and phalanges are clearly seen. The calcaneocuboid and talonavicular joints which make up the midtarsal (Chopart) joint are

Box 12.1 Dorsiplantar view: review areas

- Neck and head of talus
- Distal calcaneus
- Midtarsal (Chopart) joint
- Navicular, cuneiforms and cuboid bones
- Tarsometatarsal (Lisfranc) joint
- Metatarsals
- Metatarsophalangeal joints
- Phalanges

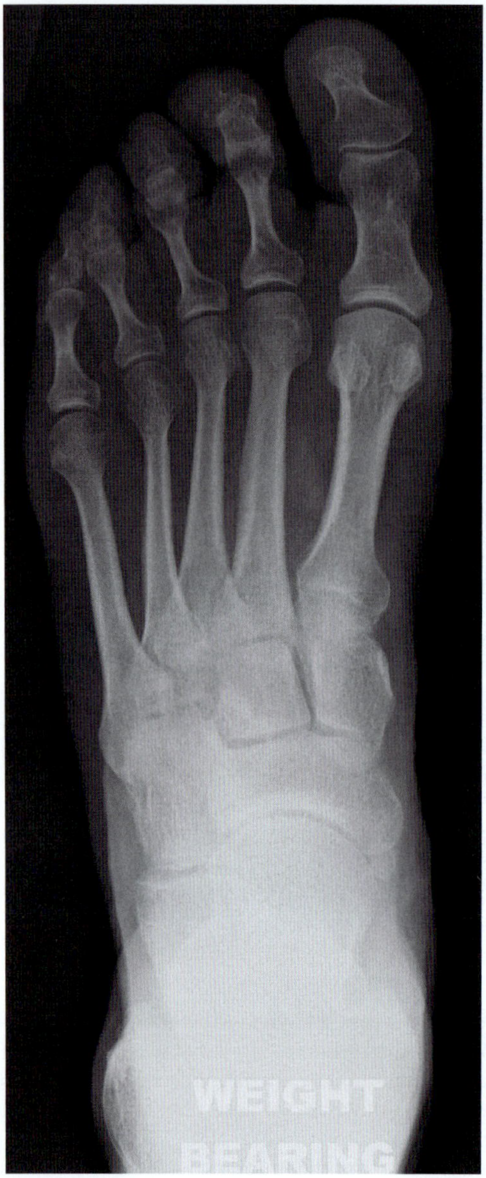

Figure 12.1 Dorsiplantar view.

visualised as are the tarsometatarsal (Lisfranc) joints. The sesamoid bones are seen through the head of the first metatarsal. Usually the bodies of the talus and the calcaneum are occluded by superimposition of the lower ends of the tibia and fibula.

Dorsiplantar oblique view

Radiographic technique

The oblique view is a non-weightbearing view which may be taken in several ways. In the most common method, the patient sits and inclines the plantar surface of the foot 45° to the cassette, with the X-ray beam directed to the base of the third metatarsal perpendicular to the dorsum of the foot.

Box 12.2 Dorsiplantar oblique view: review areas

- Anterior subtalar joint
- Midtarsal (Chopart) joint
- Navicular-cuneiform joint
- Navicular, cuneiform and cuboid bones
- Tarsometatarsal (Lisfranc) joint
- Metatarsals
- Metatarsophalangeal joints
- Phalanges

Anatomical review areas

See Box 12.2.

This view gives a distorted image of the midtarsal area, but is particularly useful for the open view given of the articular facets in the area, particularly the talonavicular, navicular-cuneiform and calcaneocuboid joints (Fig. 12.2). It should be possible to see the outlines of the cuneiforms, but it can be difficult to see the facets of all the intercuneiform joints due to superimposition. The anterior aspect of the subtalar joint and the tarsometatarsal joints are also well seen. Good views of the distal calcaneus, metatarsals and phalanges are obtained.

Lateral view (weightbearing)

Radiographic technique

This is taken with the X-ray beam perpendicular to the foot, centred on the base of the fifth metatarsal with the medial side of the foot against the cassette in the neutral position.

Anatomical review areas

See Box 12.3.

This view shows the tibial and fibular malleoli superimposed over the trochlear surface of the talus which should be domed and smooth in outline. The posterior lip of the tibia, also known as the posterior or third malleolus, is best seen on this projection. The facets of the subtalar joint and the calcaneus are well seen as are the calcaneocuboid and talonavicular joints. The sustentaculum tali and sinus tarsi are usually apparent.

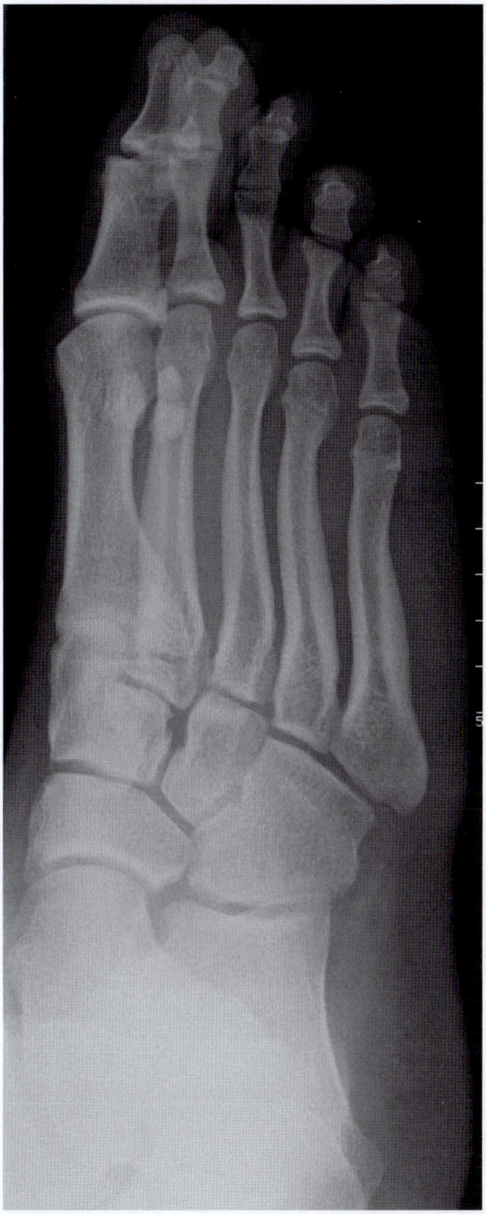

Figure 12.2 Dorsiplantar oblique view.

The midtarsal complex is partially obscured by the multiple superimpositions of the cuneiforms and metatarso-cuneiform articulations, although the first metatarso-cuneiform joint is usually well seen. Just proximal to this joint is the second and third metatarso-cuneiform joints which can be visualised with some superimpositions. The lesser metatarsals are partially superimposed over each other, although the first metatarsal, hallux, and first metatarsophalangeal joint should be easily distinguishable (Fig. 12.3).

Box 12.3 Lateral radiograph: review areas

- Posterior malleolus
- Distal fibula
- Tibiotalar joint
- Talus
- Subtalar joint
- Calcaneus
- Midtarsal (Chopart) joint
- First metatarso-cuneiform joint
- ⅔ metatarso-cuneiform joints

Anteroposterior ankle

Radiographic technique

This view is taken with the X-ray beam directed along the longitudinal axis of the foot towards the ankle, centred on a point midway between the malleoli.

Anatomical review areas

See Box 12.4.

The ankle mortise including the trochlear surface of the talus and the articulations with the tibial plafond and malleoli are well seen with this view (Fig. 12.4). It is useful if ankle injury is suspected and avulsion fractures, which occur with inversion and eversion injuries, can usually be seen on this view. Virtually no detail of the forefoot is seen due to marked superimposition.

This view is sometimes taken as a non-weight-bearing *stress radiograph* in which the foot is held in inversion or eversion and the amount of ligamentous damage is checked by assessing the degree of tilt of the talus within the joint (Fig. 12.5). This may be a painful procedure and the patient may require local anaesthesia.

Axial sesamoid view

Radiographic technique

The X-ray beam is angled towards the sesamoids with the foot flexed at the metatarsophalangeal joints. A special positioning platform may be used in some departments, but more commonly the patient lies in a prone position with the all of the toes dorsiflexed and resting on the cassette or in a supine position using a loop of bandage to retract the toes.

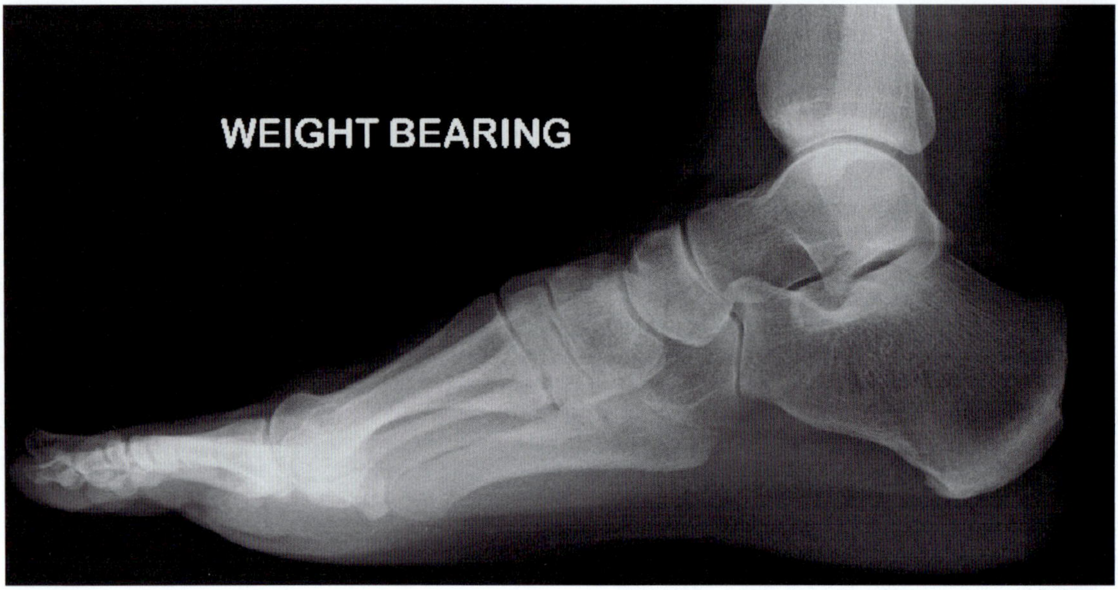

Figure 12.3 Lateral weightbearing view.

Box 12.4 Anteroposterior ankle radiograph: review areas

- Tibial plafond
- Medial malleolus
- Lateral malleolus
- Ankle mortise
- Body of talus (trochlear and malleolar facets)

Anatomical review areas

Although not commonly standard, this view clearly demarcates the sesamoids which should be smooth in outline and positioned under the head of the first metatarsal on either side of the intersesamoidal ridge. The ends of the lesser metatarsals are also seen and may determine whether a long or plantarflexed metatarsal disturbs foot dynamics (Fig. 12.6).

Basic radiographic assessment

A vast amount of information can be gleaned from a plain radiograph. The ABCS system of radiological

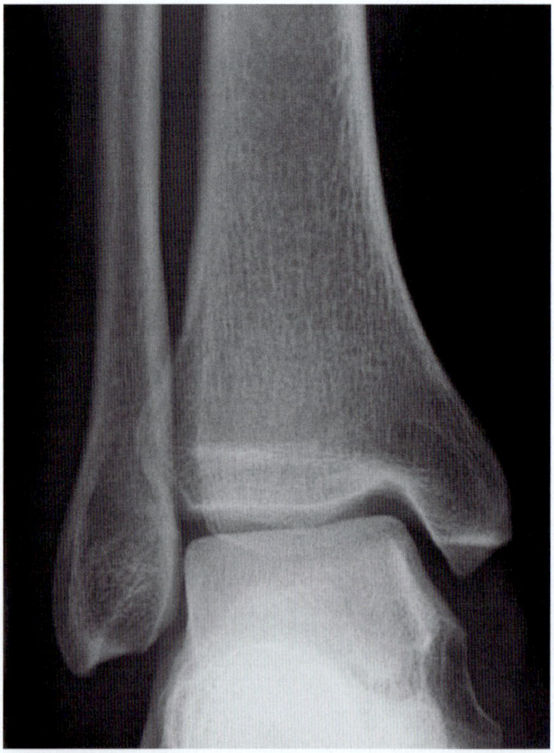

Figure 12.4 Anteroposterior ankle view.

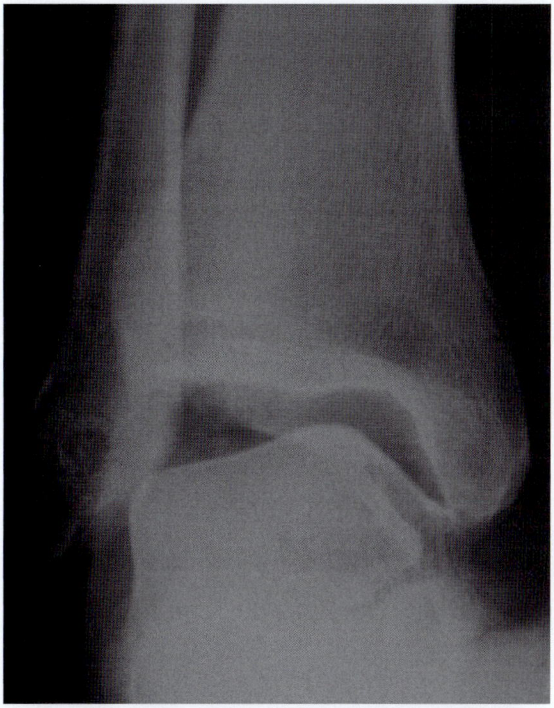

Figure 12.5 Stress radiograph. Anteroposterior ankle view with inversion stress of the talus shows varus tilt of the talus and widening of the lateral ankle joint space secondary to lateral ligament injury.

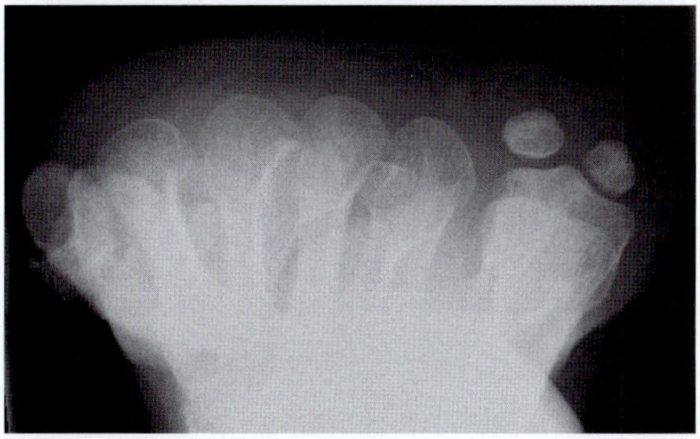

Figure 12.6 Axial sesamoid view.

assessment may be useful, where:

- A = Alignment and Anatomical variations
- B = Bone density
- C = Cartilage
- S = Soft tissue

Alignment

In order to make judgements about the biomechanical features of a foot on an X-ray, dorsiplantar and lateral weightbearing radiographs are obtained in normal angle and base of gait to provide an accurate representation of the foot in its functional position. The angles quoted below should be considered as guidelines only.

Dorsiplantar view

Commencing at the hindfoot, the *longitudinal axis of the hindfoot* is a line parallel to the distal portion of the lateral border of the calcaneus. In the normal foot, it is parallel to the long axis of the fourth metatarsal (Fig. 12.7). The *talocalcaneal angle* is measured between the longitudinal axis of the hindfoot and a line along the midline axis of the talus (Fig. 12.7). There is usually a 15–35° more lateral axis of the calcaneus compared with the talus. A smaller angle means that the calcaneus is directed closer to the midline and there is *hindfoot varus* or *supination* with increased superimposition of the talus on the calcaneus. A larger angle means that the calcaneus is directed further from the midline and there is *hindfoot valgus* or *pronation*.

Forefoot varus and valgus is often discussed as a relationship between the talus and the first metatarsal, even though these bones are not truly adjacent. Simply put, the midline axis of the talus normally goes through the base of the first metatarsal (Fig. 12.7). If the axis of the talus lies lateral to the first metatarsal, the metatarsal is directed closer to the midline and there is *forefoot varus* or *supination* (also referred to as inversion). The bases of the metatarsals tend to converge more than normal and the proximal metatarsals are superimposed. If the axis of the talus lies medial to the first metatarsal, the metatarsal is directed further from the midline and there is *forefoot valgus* or *pronation* (also referred to as eversion). The metatarsals are less convergent than normal, more parallel with less overlap.

The *longitudinal axis of the lesser tarsus* is perpendicular to a line that transects the lesser tarsus which extends across the tarsus from halfway between the medial aspect of the talonavicular joint and the medial aspect of the first tarsometatarsal joint to halfway between the lateral aspect of the calcaneocuboid joint and the lateral aspect of the fifth tarsometatarsal joint (Fig. 12.8).

Normally, 75% of the head of the talus articulates with the navicular. In a pronated foot the head of the talus moves out of alignment with the cupped surface of the navicular and there is progressive abduction of the lesser tarsus. The *lesser tarsus abduction angle* is the angle between the longitudinal axis of the lesser tarsus and the longitudinal axis of the hindfoot

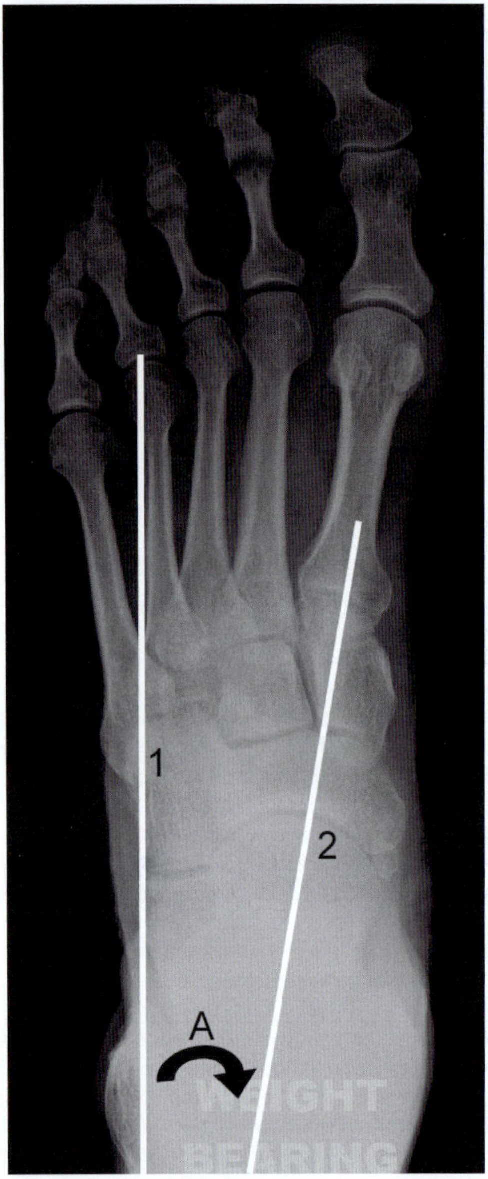

Figure 12.7 Alignment dorsiplantar view. Line 1 – longitudinal axis of hindfoot. Line 2 – midline axis of talus. Angle A, talocalcaneal angle.

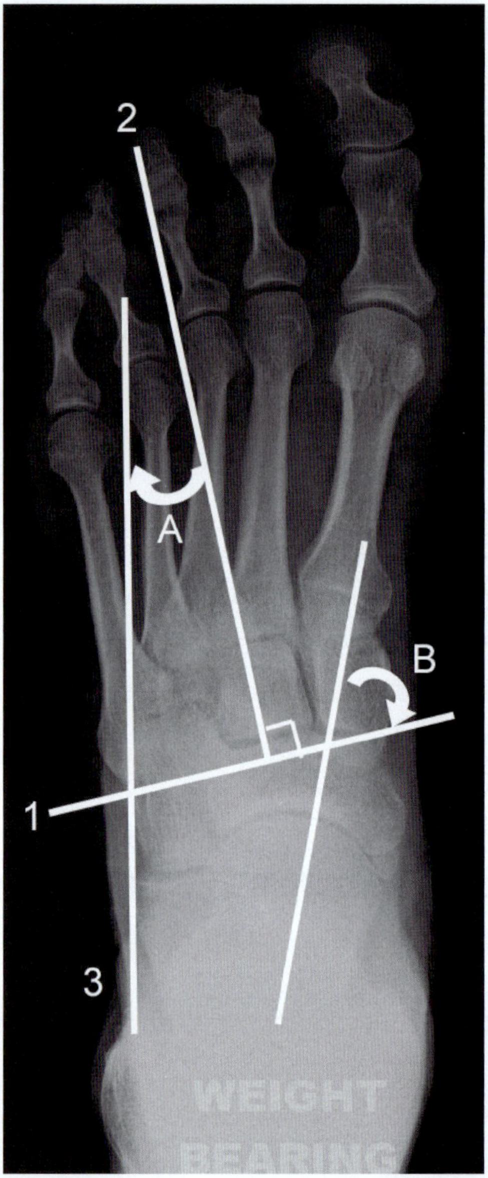

Figure 12.8 Alignment dorsiplantar view. Line 1 – bisection of lesser tarsus. Line 2 – longitudinal axis of lesser tarsus. Line 3 – longitudinal axis of hindfoot. Angle A – lesser tarsus abduction angle. Angle B – talonavicular angle.

(Fig. 12.8). This angle increases with pronation and decreases with supination. The *talonavicular angle* is between the midline axis of the talus and the bisection of the lesser tarsus (normal 60–80°) (Fig. 12.8). This angle is greater than 80° in the supinated foot and less than 60° in the pronated foot.

The *longitudinal axis of the metatarsus* is a longitudinal bisection of the second metatarsal (Fig. 12.9). The *metatarsus adduction angle* is the angle between the longitudinal axis of the metatarsus and the longitudinal axis of the lesser tarsus (normal <15°) (Fig. 12.9). A higher figure indicates that metatarsus adductus or deviation of the forefoot to the midline is present. Severe metatarsus adductus is associated with hindfoot valgus. The *metatarsus primus adductus*

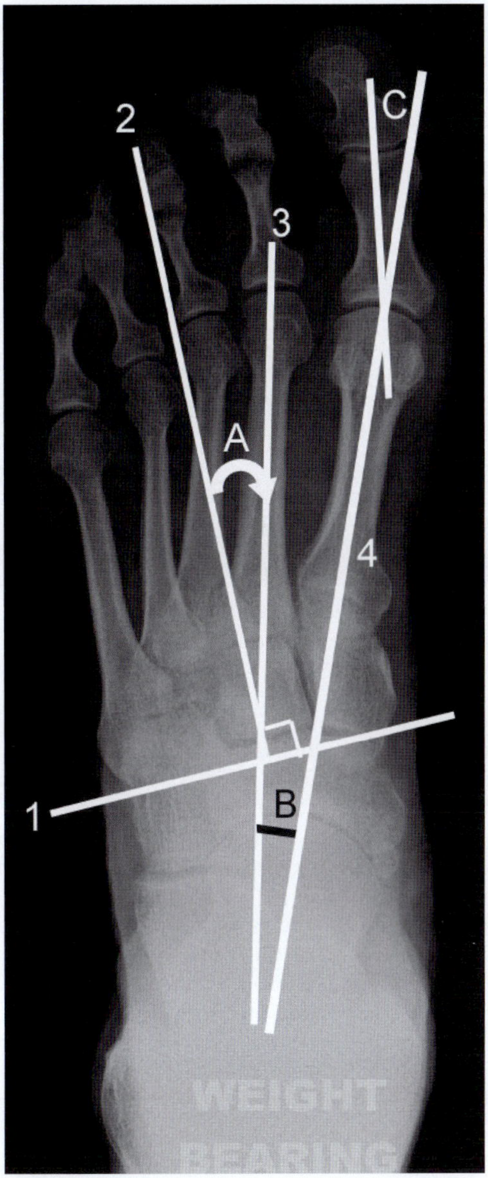

Figure 12.9 Alignment dorsiplantar view. Line 1 – bisection of lesser tarsus. Line 2 – longitudinal axis of lesser tarsus. Line 3 – longitudinal axis of metatarsus. Line 4 – midline axis of first metatarsal. Angle A – metatarsus adduction angle. Angle B – metatarsus primus adductus angle. Angle C – hallux valgus angle.

angle, also known as the *metatarsus primus varus* or *first intermetatarsal angle*, by strict definition refers to a varus relationship of the first metatarsal with respect to the medial cuneiform. In everyday practice, metatarsus primus adductus is measured by considering the angle between longitudinal bisections of the first and second metatarsals (it is assumed that the second metatarsal axis gives a reasonable approximation of the medial cuneiform axis) (Fig. 12.9). An angle of more than 10° is considered abnormal and is associated with hallux valgus.

In hallux valgus, the proximal phalanx of the great toe (hallux) is directed further from the midline with respect to the first metatarsal. If a longitudinal bisection of the first proximal phalanx is compared with a longitudinal bisection of the first metatarsal, the *hallux valgus angle* can be measured (Fig. 12.9). The hallux may normally deviate laterally by a small amount and an angle of less than 15° is generally considered acceptable. Hallux valgus is mild with an angle of 16–25°, moderate with an angle of 26–35° and severe with an angle of greater than 35°. The common term for hallux valgus is 'bunion' from which the term 'bunionette' (also known as tailor's bunion) is derived. This describes a prominence lateral to the fifth metatarsal head secondary to a varus angulation of the fifth proximal phalanx with respect to the fifth metatarsal.

Deviation of the cartilaginous surface of the first metatarsal can be identified by construction of the *proximal articular set angle* (PASA) which may be relevant in planning hallux valgus surgery. This angle is between a line representing the limits of the articular cartilage on the first metatarsal head and a perpendicular to the longitudinal axis of the first metatarsal (normal PASA <10°). A deviation in the shaft of the first proximal phalanx is occasionally responsible for the valgus deformity seen in a hallux when the first metatarsophalangeal joint alignment is normal and can be identified by drawing the *distal articular set angle* (DASA). This angle is between a line representing the articular surface of the first proximal phalanx and a line perpendicular to the longitudinal axis of the phalangeal shaft (normal DASA = 0–6°).

The *hallux interphalangeal angle* is formed between the longitudinal axes of the proximal and distal phalanges of the hallux. A normal angle is less than 10°. A larger angle indicates an interphalangeal joint valgus deformity which is sometimes referred to as 'terminal valgus' or hallux interphalangeus.

Lateral view

The *calcaneal inclination axis* is a line along the inferior surface of the calcaneus connecting the most inferior point of the calcaneal tuberosity with the most distal inferior point of the calcaneus at the calcaneocuboid joint (Fig. 12.10). The *calcaneal inclination angle* is between the calcaneal inclination axis and the

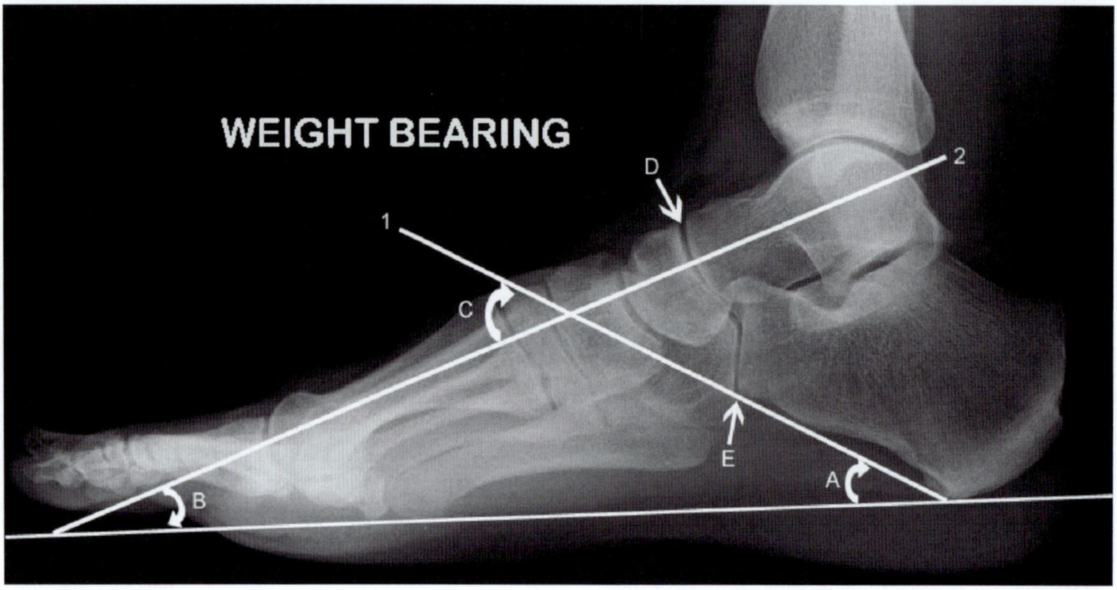

Figure 12.10 Alignment lateral view. Line 1 – calcaneal inclination axis. Line 2 – midline axis of talus. Angle A – calcaneal inclination angle. Angle B – talar declination angle. Angle C – lateral talocalcaneal angle. Arrows D and E – the cyma line.

supporting surface and reflects the height of the foot framework (Fig. 12.10). Measurements of 10–20° would be considered low, 20–30° medium and >30° high. The measured angle varies according to whether the foot is abnormally pronated or supinated and clinical judgement is important.

The *talar declination angle* is the angle between a bisection through the body and neck of the talus and the supporting surface (normal approximately 21°) (Fig. 12.10). A continuation of the midline talar axis should bisect the first metatarsal shaft. If the first metatarsal axis extends downwards compared with the talar axis, i.e. the first metatarsal is steeper in relation to the horizontal, the talar declination angle decreases and the line falls above the first metatarsal. This indicates that the longitudinal arch is high and there is a *cavus foot* (pes cavus). Conversely, if the talar axis extends downwards compared with the first metatarsal axis, the talar declination angle increases and the line falls below the first metatarsal. This is indicative of a low to flat longitudinal foot arch or a *planus foot* (pes planus).

Another method for assessing cavus or planus is measuring the *angle of the longitudinal arch* between the calcaneal inclination axis and a line which extends along the undersurface of the fifth metatarsal (normal 150–170°). Cavus is present with an angle of less than 150°. In planus the angle is increased approaching 180°. The *lateral talocalcaneal angle* is between the calcaneal inclination axis and the midline axis of the talus (normal 35–50°) (Fig. 12.10). *Boehler's angle* is measured between a line drawn along the superior margin of the subtalar joint and a line drawn along the posterior superior border of the calcaneus (normal 20–40°).

Calcaneus and equines are used to express a relationship between the tibial axis and the calcaneus. Normally the undersurface of the calcaneus is a bit higher anteriorly than posteriorly. If the anterior calcaneus extends lower than the posterior, or if they are at the same level, an *equinus calcaneus* is present. If the anterior calcaneus extends more upwards than normal, above the rest of the upper surface of the bone, a *calcaneus calcaneus* is present.

The sinus tarsi is seen as a radiolucent area that lies above the sustentaculum tali and between the anterior and posterior subtalar facets. The subtalar facets and the sinus tarsi become obscured in a pronated foot (where the great toe moves down and the little toe assumes the higher position) and more visible in a supinated one (where the great toe moves up and the little toe assumes the lower position on the lateral view).

The talonavicular and calcaneocuboid joints together produce a superimposition on a lateral X-ray known as the *cyma line* (Fig. 12.10). These curved joints together form a reverse 'lazy S' as an intact curve in a normal foot. In a pronated foot the 'S' becomes broken as the talonavicular joint moves anterior and plantar to the calcaneocuboid joint and the reverse occurs in a supinated foot.

In a severely pronated foot the talus and navicular plantarflex and exert a downward force on the posterior aspect of the medial cuneiform, resulting in a *naviculo-cuneiform fault*. In such cases the intermediate cuneiform, not normally visible, may be seen protruding above the medial cuneiform. Less commonly, a *calcaneocuboid fault* may be seen in a high-arched foot. In this situation the cuboid may become partially displaced under the anterior plantar process of the calcaneum. In a supinated foot the metatarsals become more clearly outlined. In a pronated foot the superimposition of the metatarsals becomes more complete, and it may only be possible to clearly distinguish the first metatarsal.

The hallux should normally lie in line with the metatarsal, being neither dorsiflexed nor plantarflexed. The lesser metatarsophalangeal joints are occasionally visible and it may be possible to detect dorsal subluxation or dislocation.

Anatomical variation

Accessory ossicles are unfused secondary ossification centres and are commonly seen in association with all the major bones in the foot. They are usually asymptomatic but a small proportion may give rise to symptoms, particularly following trauma or sporting activity and may need to be considered in a differential diagnosis or differentiated from a fracture. An ossicle has a well-defined sclerotic margin and the adjacent bones are normal. A recent fracture fragment is tender with at least one edge where the sclerotic margin is absent and one of the adjacent bones has an irregular margin indicating the site of origin of the avulsed fracture fragment.

Os trigonum

This ossicle is a secondary epiphysis, found on the posterior aspect of the trochlear surface of the talus, which fails to fuse to the talus in about 8–15% of the population. The os trigonum can give rise to posterior ankle pain when it is compressed between the posterior tibia and posterior calcaneus during forced plantar flexion, as occurs in certain sports such as football and tennis, and with other activities such as ballet or yoga. This is referred to as the os trigonum syndrome or posterior impingement.

Os tibiale externum

The accessory navicular bone may cause pain for several reasons. Painful degenerative changes may occur between the accessory ossicle and navicular, a painful bursa can develop in the soft tissues superficial to the ossicle and there is a higher incidence of tibialis posterior tendon tears or dysfunction. The incidence of the bone in radiographic studies is 2–20%.

Os vesalianum

This ossicle is a secondary epiphysis at the fifth metatarsal base and must be differentiated from an avulsion fracture. Generally, a fracture will have a longitudinal orientation and an irregular outline, compared with the transverse orientation and smooth contour of the ossicle.

Os peroneum

This lies within the peroneus longus tendon in the peroneal groove of the cuboid. It is the commonest accessory bone present in up to 26% of the population. It can be injured with repeated ankle sprains or following a forced dorsiflexion injury.

Hallux sesamoids

The medial and lateral sesamoids should appear as two smooth ovoid structures approximately 0.5 cm proximal to the articular surface of the first metatarsal head. Sesamoids may be symptomatic for several reasons: fractures, osteonecrosis, inflammation (sesamoiditis), infection and involvement in degenerative or inflammatory joint disease (Fig. 12.11). In a case of developing hallux valgus, the sesamoids progressively move laterally, eventually ending up in the

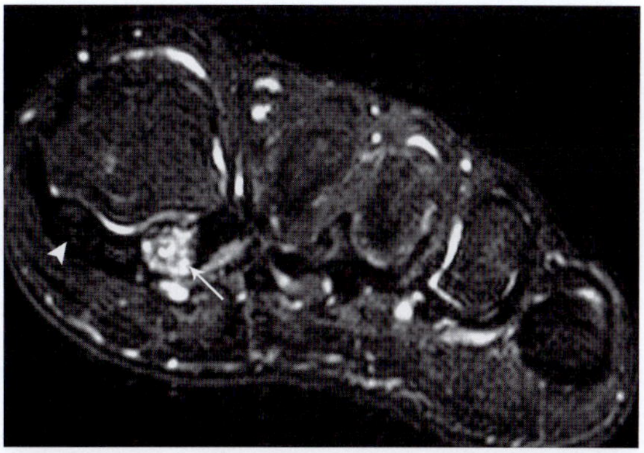

Figure 12.11 Sesamoiditis. Coronal short tau inversion recovery (STIR) MR image. High signal within the lateral sesamoid (arrow) is consistent with inflammation or sesamoiditis. Compare with the normal marrow signal of the medial sesamoid (arrowhead).

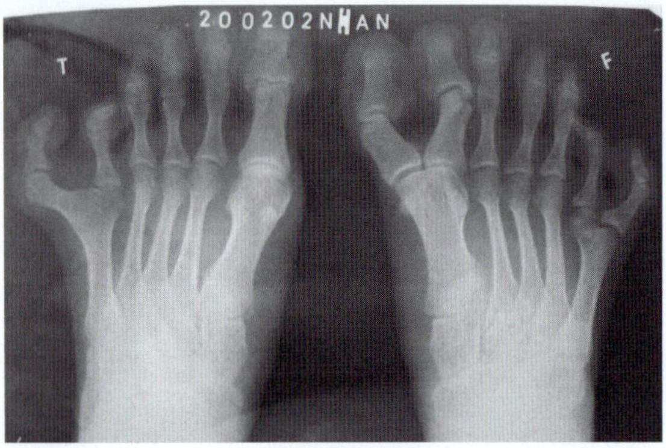

Figure 12.12 Polydactyly. Dorsiplantar radiograph. Polydactyly with additional fifth digit bilaterally and additional first digit on the left.

interspace between the first and second metatarsals. Sesamoids may be bipartite or multipartite and occur under any of the other metatarsophalangeal or interphalangeal joints.

Polydactyly is the presence of additional phalanges or complete digits (Fig. 12.12). **Brachydactyly** is due to partial failure of development of a metatarsal or phalangeal segment leading to shortening of the digit. **Congenital aplasia** is complete failure of development of a segment and is rare (Fig. 12.13).

Tarsal coalitions may be fibrous (syndesmosis), cartilaginous (synchondrosis) or osseous (synostosis) and are thought to represent failure of proper segmentation of the tarsal bones. Coalitions occur in about 6% of the population, may be bilateral and result in restricted subtalar joint motion. The more common forms are calcaneo-navicular and talocalcaneal, which usually occurs at the middle facet of the subtalar joint. Calcaneo-navicular coalition is usually well seen on oblique views (Fig. 12.14A). Talocalcaneal coalition may be associated with a prominent talar beak arising from the dorsal aspect of the head or neck of the talus. Suspected tarsal coalitions may be confirmed with CT or MRI (Fig 12.14B). Limited subtalar joint motion results in increased stresses elsewhere in the tarsus and this may result in bone marrow oedema adjacent to the coalition on MR images.

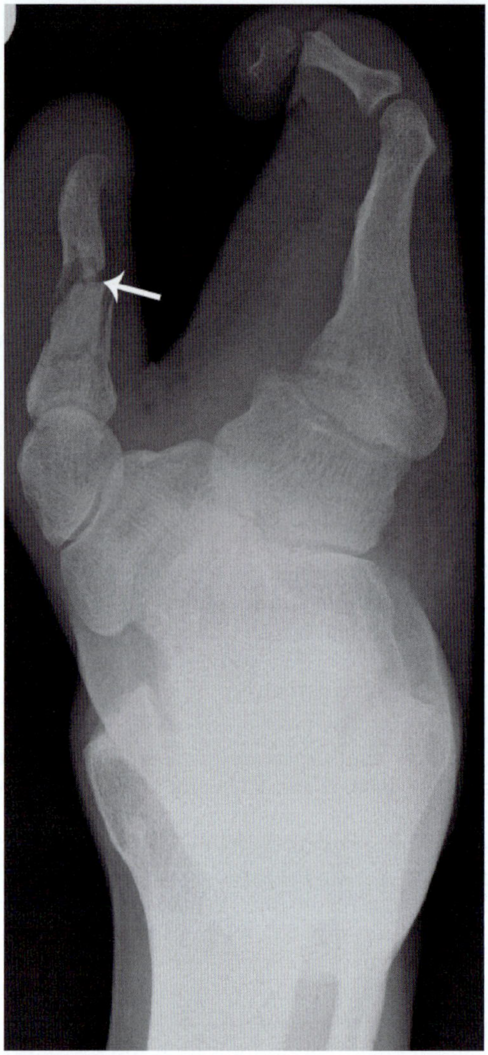

Figure 12.13 Congenital aplasia. Dorsiplantar radiograph. Congenital aplasia with a fracture of the medial digit (arrow).

Bone density

Bone is in a constant state of change with new bone formation by osteoblasts normally being balanced by the resorptive activity of osteoclasts. These activities are governed by the endocrine system and are also altered by chemical and vitamin factors in the blood, diet, malabsorption from the gut, disease and by physical forces to which the bone is subjected. The appearance of decreased density of bone on an X-ray is known as osteopenia. This is a generic term that includes both osteoporosis and osteomalacia. Osteoporosis is diminished bone quantity in which the bone is otherwise normal. Osteomalacia is normal bone quantity but the bone itself is abnormal in that it is not normally mineralised. It is often not possible to distinguish between osteoporosis and osteomalacia on plain radiographs. The radiographic finding of increased bone density is called osteosclerosis.

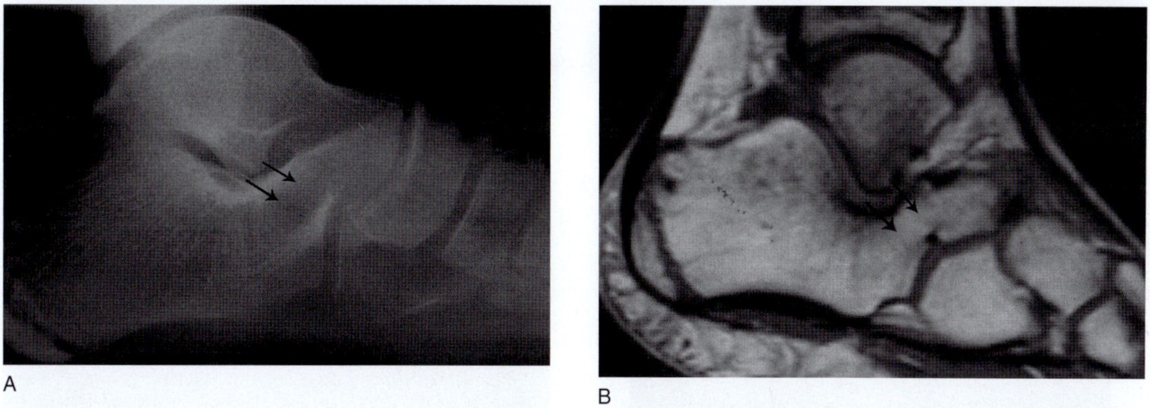

Figure 12.14 Osseous calcaneonavicular coalition. **A** Lateral radiograph. **B** Sagittal T1-weighted MR image. There is union of the anteromedial corner of the calcaneus with the navicular (arrows) consistent with an osseous coalition.

Osteoporosis

The commonest cause of osteoporosis is primary osteoporosis which is most commonly seen in postmenopausal women. Up to 30% of postmenopausal women will develop osteoporosis, which is largely preventable with hormone replacement therapy. Secondary osteoporosis is seen with a large number of underlying diseases which cannot usually be accurately distinguished by looking at a radiograph. More common causes include renal disease, long-term steroid use and endocrine disorders such as hyperthyroidism and Cushing's syndrome (increased levels of cortisol either secondary to hyperactivity of the adrenal glands or a pituitary adenoma).

Decreased bone density confined to a region of the appendicular skeleton is referred to as regional osteopenia. The most common cause is **disuse osteoporosis** which occurs following a period of disuse of a limb such as with immobilisation of fractures. The osteoporosis usually appears after 8 weeks of immobilisation and reverses when stress and function return. Another cause of localised osteopenia is complex regional pain syndrome (**Sudeck's atrophy**), which is mediated via a neurovascular mechanism usually following trauma. There is pain and soft-tissue swelling which are out of proportion to the injury and radiographic evidence of irregular mottled osteoporosis distal to the injury site. **Regional migratory osteoporosis** is a disease of unknown aetiology that typically occurs in middle-aged men and is characterised by pain and localised osteoporosis which migrates from one joint to another.

The main radiographic finding in osteoporosis is decreased bone density with thinning of the cortex. There is accentuation of primary trabeculae with thinning of secondary trabeculae and an increased incidence of fractures with delayed healing. Bone density may be assessed on plain radiographs, but bone loss of up to 30% can occur before radiological changes are apparent. Some scientific methods that may be used for the evaluation of bone density by radiologists include:

- dual energy X-ray absorptiometry (DEXA) – used on the spine and femoral neck
- single-photon or dual-photon absorptiometry (SPA or DPA) – measures bone density in the forearm
- quantitative computed tomography (QCT) – used on the spine
- ultrasound – may be used to indicate the bone density of the calcaneum.

Osteomalacia

In osteomalacia, there is a failure of the osteoid tissue to mineralise. The commonest causes of osteomalacia are renal osteodystrophy and disorders of vitamin D metabolism. A distinctive radiographic feature is Looser's zones, which are areas of unmineralised osteoid that may develop insufficiency fractures, and tend to occur in the pelvis and scapula. The trabecular pattern is often coarse and indistinct. Osteomalacia in children is called rickets. Rickets causes characteristic enlarged and irregular epiphyseal plates with splayed metaphyses and bowing of the bones from bone softening (Fig. 12.15). As in adults, the commonest cause is renal disease, although other

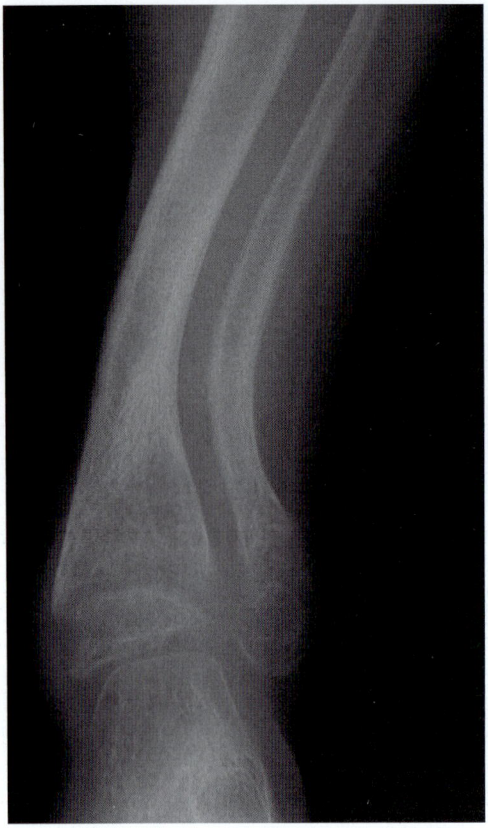

Figure 12.15 Rickets. AP radiograph. Rickets is characterised by decreased bone density with splayed metaphyses, enlarged irregular epiphyseal plates and bowing of the distal tibia and fibula.

causes such as biliary disease and dietary insufficiencies are seen.

Hyperparathyroidism

Hyperparathyroidism occurs from excess parathyroid hormone and is due to hyperplasia of the parathyroid glands (primary type), persistent stimulation due to low serum calcium levels (secondary type) or an adenoma (tertiary type). Parathyroid hormone causes increased bone resorption by osteoclasts which leads to osteoporosis and osteomalacia.

The classic radiographic sign of hyperparathyroidism is subperiosteal bone resorption which is most commonly seen on the radial aspect of the middle phalanges of the hand but can be seen in any long bone in the body. Other radiographic features include distal phalangeal tuft resorption, soft-tissue calcification, osteosclerosis typically involving the vertebral end plates giving rise to the 'rugger jersey

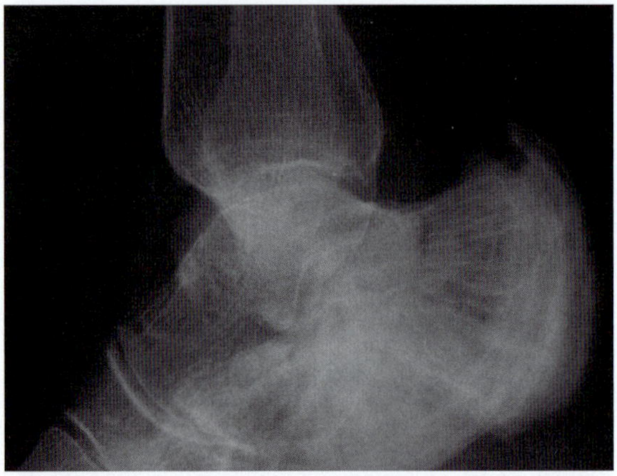

Figure 12.16 Paget's disease. Lateral radiograph. Paget's disease of the calcaneum, appearing dense and enlarged with a coarse trabecular pattern and thickened cortex.

spine' and brown tumours which are lytic expansile bone lesions.

Osteosclerosis

Many disorders have been reported to cause osteosclerosis and only the more common entities are covered.

Renal osteodystrophy is a constellation of musculoskeletal abnormalities that occur with chronic renal failure. Osteosclerosis is one of the more common manifestations occurring in up to 20% of patients. Other features are those of hyperparathyroidism, osteomalacia and soft-tissue calcification.

Myelofibrosis is caused by progressive fibrosis of the marrow in patients over 50 years of age. This leads to a generalised increase in bone density with anaemia, splenomegaly and extramedullary haematopoiesis.

Paget's disease is a common disorder of unknown origin which can involve the entire skeleton or isolated bones, including the bones of the feet. The disease causes excessive bone resorption followed by haphazard new bone formation and remodelling. The bones are enlarged and appear dense with a coarse trabecular pattern and thickened cortex (Fig. 12.16). Although the bones are enlarged and appear dense on X-ray they are of poor quality and microfractures are common. Paget's disease predisposes to an increased incidence of sarcoma, although less than 1% progress to malignancy.

Metastatic bone disease with diffuse sclerotic deposits may rarely mimic osteosclerosis. Primary tumours are usually carcinoma of the breast and prostate. Radiolucent components of the metastasis and cortical destruction may be present.

Osteopetrosis (Albers–Schönberg disease or marble bone disease) is a rare hereditary disorder causing extremely dense bones throughout the skeleton. A characteristic finding is a 'bone in bone' appearance seen in the vertebral bodies, which contain a small replica of a vertebral body inside it. Densely sclerotic endplates give the appearance of 'sandwich' vertebrae. Although the bones are dense they are more susceptible to shear forces and may fracture more easily.

Increased fluorine ingestion (fluorosis) over many years may result in the laying down of new bone inside the medullary cavity of long bones, leading to a sclerotic appearance. Ligamentous calcification, particularly of the sacrotuberous ligament, may be present.

Cartilage

Cartilage is radiolucent and normally not visualised on plain radiographs. The condition of articular cartilage has to be assessed by the relationship of the adjacent bones in the joint. A healthy joint will show smoothly outlined joint surfaces evenly separated by a 1–2 mm black space which represents the cartilaginous surfaces. Diseased cartilage results in irregularity and narrowing of the joint space which may become malaligned. There may be full thickness articular cartilage loss with complete loss of joint space. Occasionally the joint space may be increased in the presence of a joint effusion or early synovitis. Calcification of articular cartilage is known as chondrocalcinosis and is seen in osteoarthritis, the crystal deposition arthropathies such as gout and calcium pyrophosphate dihydrate deposition disease, haemochromatosis and hyperparathyroidism.

Soft tissue

On a normal X-ray, the soft-tissue outline of the foot will be delineated and fat may be distinguished from adjacent soft tissues but there is little other soft-tissue detail.

Soft-tissue mass

A soft-tissue mass may cause distortion of the soft-tissue contours and an area of increased density in comparison with the adjacent soft tissues (Fig. 12.17). Calcification within a mass may be the only radiographic clue that a lesion is present. Occasionally a long-standing soft-tissue mass may result in erosion and displacement of adjacent bones. A radiograph taken at a lower energy will show more soft-tissue detail and if an X-ray is specifically requested for a suspected soft-tissue lesion, this should be stated on the request form.

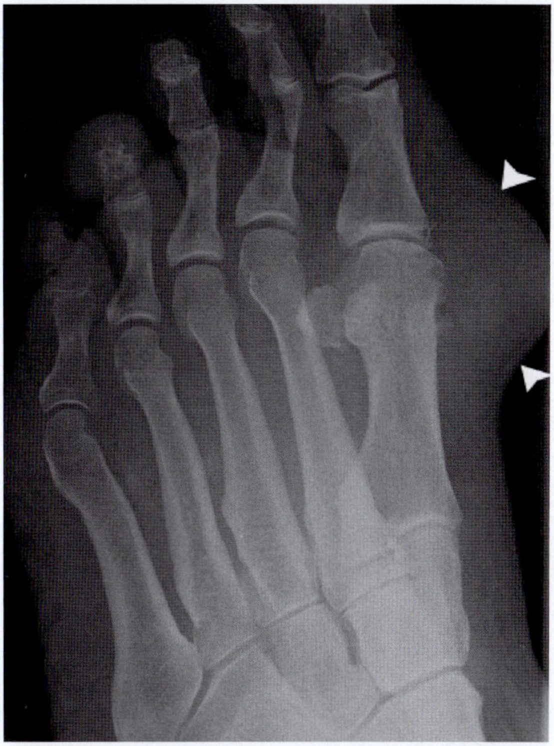

Figure 12.17 Soft-tissue mass. Dorsiplantar oblique radiograph. A soft-tissue mass (arrowheads) at the level of the first metatarsophalangeal joint corresponded to a ganglion.

Calcification within soft tissues

Calcification within soft tissues is visible on plain radiographs and may be indicative of a variety of diseases. Vascular calcification has a linear 'worm-like' appearance and is commonly seen in diabetes (termed Mönckeberg's sclerosis), particularly between the first and second metatarsals along the course of the dorsalis pedis artery. Similar changes may also be seen arteriosclerosis and hyperparathyroidism. Bursae may undergo degenerative calcification which is most common at the first metatarsophalangeal joint (Fig. 12.18). Calcification within the muscles following trauma results in myositis ossificans which characteristically has dense peripheral calcification. Neoplastic calcification may be the only indication of a soft-tissue mass such as a haemangioma, soft-tissue chondroma or synovial

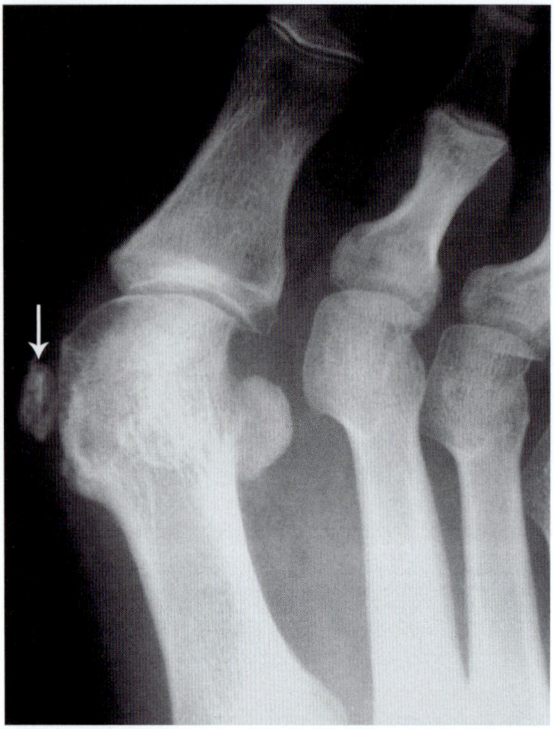

Figure 12.18 Soft-tissue calcification. Dorsiplantar radiograph. Calcification of a bursa (arrow) adjacent to the medial aspect of the first metatarsal head with hallux valgus.

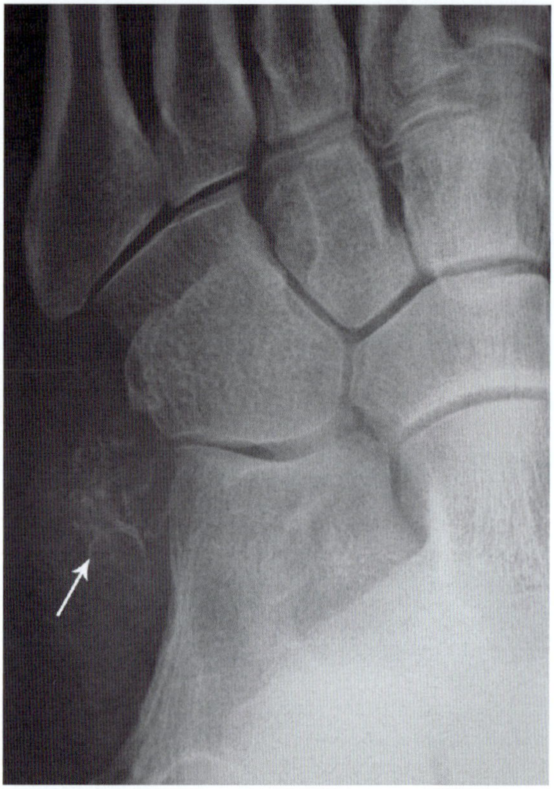

Figure 12.19 Soft-tissue calcification. Dorsiplantar oblique radiograph. Calcification within the soft tissues (arrow) at the level of the calcaneocuboid joint was the only radiographic evidence of a soft-tissue chondroma.

sarcoma (Fig. 12.19). Soft-tissue calcification may be present in various collagen vascular diseases such as scleroderma and dermatomyositis as well as metabolic disorders such as hypercalcaemia and gout where the urate crystals deposited in the skin become calcified.

Gas within the soft tissues

Gas within the soft tissues secondary to a penetrating injury or infection by gas producing organisms may be seen as radiolucent locules within the soft tissue (Fig. 12.20).

Other imaging modalities

Magnetic resonance imaging

Generation of magnetic resonance image

MR images are obtained by placing the part under investigation into a strong magnetic field and passing pulsed radiofrequency signals through the field. Between the pulses, the protons (hydrogen nuclei) alternately relax and realign and emit a characteristic radiowave of their own. These signals can be detected and recorded, and computers are able to build a picture of the spatial relationships, density and tissue distribution of the protons. Soft tissues vary in their water content, and hence concentrations of hydrogen nuclei, according to both their nature and whether or not inflammatory changes are present, and the resultant signals therefore vary. MR appearances are described in terms of signal intensity which refers to the strength of the radiowave that a tissue emits. The strength of this radiowave determines the degree of brightness of the imaged structures. A bright (whiter) area in an image is said to demonstrate high signal intensity, whereas a darker area is said to demonstrate low signal intensity. Detailed high-resolution images of soft tissue and bone marrow are generated as thin 'slices' through the body part which can be obtained in sagittal, coronal and axial planes using

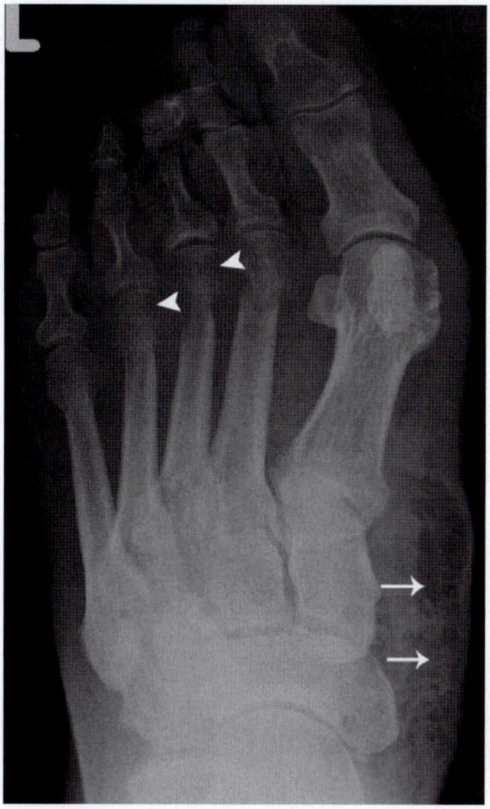

Figure 12.20 Osteomyelitis and gas gangrene. Dorsiplantar radiograph. Osteomyelitis with radiolucency and cortical destruction of the third and fourth metatarsal heads (arrowheads). Gas is present in the adjacent soft tissues which tracks along medial aspect of the foot (arrows).

different imaging sequences. The main MR imaging sequences used are T1-weighted which provides good anatomical detail; T2-weighted which provides good contrast for evaluation of pathological processes and STIR (short time inversion recovery) in which the signal from fat is suppressed. Different tissues display different signal intensities on T1- and T2-weighted images, some of which are given in Table 12.2.

Indications

See Box 12.5.

MR images are excellent for identifying oedema and inflammation, as the water content of the tissues is increased. MRI is particularly sensitive in demonstrating bone marrow oedema as seen with osteonecrosis, osteomyelitis, stress fractures, trabecular microfractures and marrow replacement disorders such as metastatic disease. The STIR sequence (a fat-suppression technique) is highly sensitive in detecting marrow pathology. Fat in healthy bone marrow normally returns high signal on T1- and T2-weighted images. With the STIR sequence, the signal from normal marrow fat is suppressed and appears black. Diseased marrow fails to be suppressed and is clearly seen as a white area (Fig. 12.21).

IMAGES

Bone marrow pathology is usually detected with MRI long before plain radiographs become positive. MRI provides excellent soft-tissue contrast resolution with depiction of tendon, ligament, muscle and nerve pathology. In patients with an arthropathy, joint effusions, synovitis and erosions may be seen before

Table 12.2 Magnetic resonance imaging signal intensities of various tissues relative to skeletal muscle

Tissue	**Image**	
	T1-weighted	*T2-weighted*
Cortical bone, tendons, ligaments, plantar fascia, fibrocartilage, scar tissue	Low	Low
Muscle, nerves, hyaline cartilage	Intermediate	Intermediate
Fat, lipomas	High	Intermediate–high
Fluid	Low–intermediate	High
Tumours (generally)	Low–intermediate	High
Haematoma (acute, subacute)	Intermediate–high	High
Haematoma (chronic)	Low	Low

Box 12.5 Magnetic resonance imaging: indications

- Bone marrow
  - Osteonecrosis
  - Osteomyelitis
  - Stress fractures
  - Trabecular microfractures
  - Bone tumours
  - Coalitions
- Soft-tissues
  - Soft-tissue tumours
  - Sinus tarsi syndrome
  - Plantar fasciitis
  - Tendon dysfunction
  - Ankle ligaments
- Joints
  - Arthropathy
  - Cartilage
  - Osteochondral fractures
  - Intra-articular bodies
- Bone and soft tissue tumours
  - Tumour characterisation
  - Intra-osseous and soft-tissue extent
  - Compartmentalisation
  - Neurovascular involvement
  - Intra-articular extension
- Post surgical follow-up

plain radiographic changes are apparent. MRI is a good technique for evaluating articular cartilage, osteochondral fractures (e.g. talar dome) and in detecting and localising loose intra-articular osteocartilaginous bodies. Intra-articular structures are better demonstrated if they are separated by means of capsular distension which can be achieved with an intra-articular injection of contrast material which is usually performed under fluoroscopic guidance. The resultant magnetic resonance arthrography (MRA) images are similar to those obtained of a joint with a pre-existing joint effusion. MRI is used for the preoperative evaluation of bone and soft-tissue tumours. MRI may further characterise the tumour and delineate both its intra-osseous and soft-tissue extent. Compartmental and neurovascular involvement and intra-articular extension are well shown with the multiplanar images obtained. MRI is important in post-operative follow-up to assess for residual or recurrent tumour.

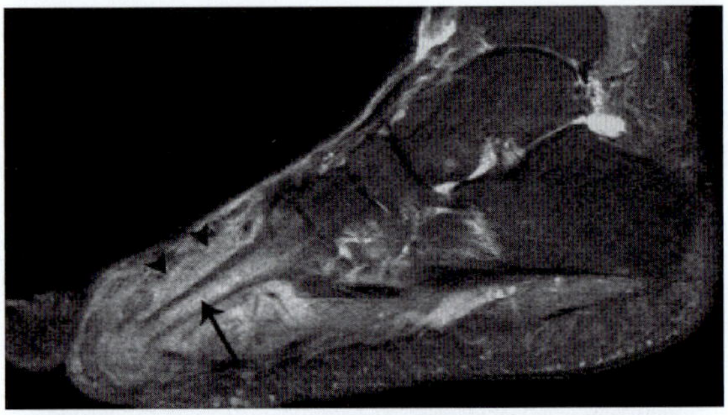

Figure 12.21 Osteomyelitis. Sagittal STIR magnetic resonance image. Osteomyelitis of the second metatarsal is seen as increased signal within the shaft (arrow, compare with the normal suppressed marrow signal in the hindfoot). A high signal inflammatory mass is present in the adjacent soft tissues (arrowheads).

Limitations

Although MRI is sensitive in detecting abnormalities of bone marrow, further osseous detail is limited and MRI is less helpful for assessing periosteal new bone formation, bone fragments and fractures. Some patients get claustrophobic in the MR scanner and patients with metalwork such as cardiac pacemakers and surgical clips cannot be subjected to the strong magnetic field. Metallic objects such as ferromagnetic surgical clips result in focal loss of signal with distortion of the image. MRI is the most expensive imaging modality and examinations can be time intensive.

Normal magnetic resonance imaging anatomy

Tendons

Tendons are generally best evaluated on axial images where they are depicted in cross-section (Fig. 12.22). IMAGE The flexor tendons, located on the medial side of the ankle, are often remembered using the mnemonic 'Tom, Dick and very nervous Harry'. Running from medial to lateral, 'Tom' represents the **t**ibialis posterior tendon; '**D**ick' is the flexor **d**igitorum longus tendon; '**a**nd **v**ery **n**ervous' are the posterior tibial **a**rtery, **v**ein and **n**erve; and '**H**arry' corresponds to the flexor **h**allucis longus tendon. Tibialis posterior is approximately twice as large as the adjacent medial tendons, measuring about 6 mm in diameter. The tendons are surrounded by separate tendon sheaths and pass through the tarsal tunnel together with the neurovascular bundle posterior to the medial malleolus and deep to the flexor retinaculum. The peroneal tendons are located on the posterolateral aspect of the ankle and are held in place as they pass posterior

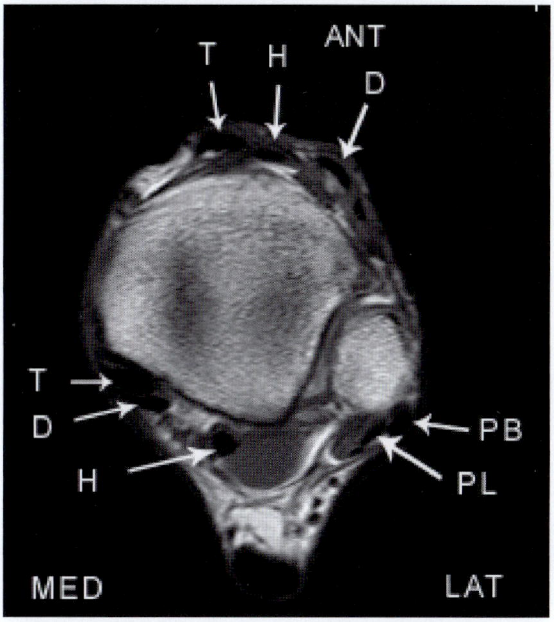

Figure 12.22 Normal ankle tendons. Axial T1-weighted magnetic resonance image. The tendons along the medial aspect of the ankle (MED) are tibialis posterior (T), flexor digitorum longus (D) and flexor hallucis longus (H). The tendons on the lateral aspect of the ankle (LAT) are peroneus brevis (PB) and peroneus longus (PL). The tendons found anterior to the ankle (ANT) are tibialis anterior (T), extensor hallucis longus (H) and extensor digitorum longus (D).

to the lateral malleolus by a connective tissue band termed the peroneal retinaculum. The brevis tendon is usually located anterior to the longus. The tendons found anterior to the ankle, from medial to lateral, are **t**ibialis anterior, extensor **h**allucis longus and extensor **d**igitorum longus and the order of the tendons may be remembered using the mnemonic '**T**om **h**ates **D**ick'.

Ligaments

The medial collateral ligament complex (deltoid ligament) lies deep to the medial flexor tendons. The lateral ankle ligaments include the anterior and posterior talofibular ligaments which are best seen on axial images running from the tip of the fibula to the talus just below the level of the tibiotalar joint. The calcaneofibular ligament runs obliquely from the tip of the fibula to a small tubercle on the lateral side of the calcaneum beneath the peroneal tendon sheath and may be traced over several axial MR images.

Box 12.6 Computed tomography: indications

- Fractures
  - Fracture characterisation
  - Fracture fragments
  - Fracture union
  - Stress fractures
- Bone tumours
  - Tumour characterisation (matrix calcification, nidus in osteoid osteoma)
  - Intra-osseous extent
  - Cortical breach
  - Computed tomography guided biopsy
- Coalitions
- Joints
  - Osteochondral defect
  - Intra-articular ossific bodies
  - Pre-operative joint fusion assessment

Computed tomography

Generation of computed tomography image

The patient lies on the CT table and is moved slowly through a hole in a circular scanning gantry containing a mobile X-ray generator and detectors. The X-ray tube rotates completely around the patient in a plane determined by the radiographer. The X-rays generated are absorbed or attenuated to various degrees depending on the density of the tissues being imaged. The remaining unabsorbed or unattenuated X-rays pass through the tissue and are picked up by an array of detectors and processed by a computer. The CT computer software converts the X-ray beam attenuations of the tissue into an image which is digitised and fed to a visual display screen. Tissue with a high attenuation such as normal cortical bone appear white, tissue with a low attenuation such as air appears black and soft tissues with an intermediate attenuation are variations of grey. The images produced are in fact slices through the body representing a thickness of 0.1–1.5 cm of body tissue. Usually 1.5–2 mm contiguous axial sections are obtained through the foot and ankle which can be used to create multiplanar sagittal and coronal reformats as well as three-dimensional reconstructions.

Indications

See Box 12.6.

The major use of CT is the identification of bone-based pathology as CT images give excellent bone detail. In trauma, CT is valuable in characterising complex fractures, detecting small intra-articular fracture fragments and assessing the state of fracture union. Multiplanar reconstructions are particularly helpful in pre-operative planning of dislocations and fractures. CT plays a significant role in bone tumours by further characterising the lesion, clearly delineating the intra-osseous extent of the tumour and any cortical breach. A biopsy of a bone lesion may be performed under CT guidance which allows precise placement of the biopsy needle within the lesion. Other bone pathology such as stress fractures and coalitions are well demonstrated. In joint-based pathology, CT is useful to define osteochondral defects, loose intra-articular ossific bodies and in pre-operative planning of joint fusions.

Limitations

CT images may be viewed with bone or soft-tissue windows, however, soft-tissue discrimination is poor in comparison with MRI. Metalwork for example, prostheses or various rods and screws will produce significant artifact. The radiation dose may be high when a large volume of contiguous and overlapping sections are obtained.

Ultrasound

Generation of ultrasound image

Ultrasound (US) examinations involve using reflections of pulsed sound waves to detect differences between soft-tissue interfaces. Whenever the directed pulsing of sound waves encounters an interface between tissues of different density, reflection or refraction occurs. The sound waves reflected back to the US transducer are recorded and converted into images. US provides a real-time image that may be obtained in any scan plane by simply rotating the transducer. Thus imaging may include transverse or longitudinal images and any obliquity can also be produced. Most of the structures that surround the foot are superficial and higher frequency transducers of 7.5–12 MHz are used, which give high resolution images but less penetration. US appearances may be described in terms of echogenicity. Brighter areas such as cortical bone, calcium and fat are said to be echogenic or hyperechoic. Darker areas such as fibrous or scar tissue are described as hypoechoic. Some tissues such as fluid produce no echoes and are completely black and referred to as anechoic.

Box 12.7 Ultrasound: indications

- Tendon dysfunction
  - Tendinopathy
  - Tenosynovitis
  - Tendon rupture
  - Tendon subluxation
- Plantar fasciitis
- Ligament injury
- Soft-tissue masses
- Morton's neuroma
- Tarsal tunnel syndrome
- Joints
  - Effusion
  - Synovitis
- Ultrasound guided procedures
  - Aspiration
  - Injection
  - Biopsy

Indications

See Box 12.7.

Ultrasound has an important role if patients present with symptoms localised to a particular area of the foot. If symptoms are more diffuse, MRI may be more appropriate for more complete assessment and in particular to assess bone and joint surfaces.

Ultrasound provides excellent images of the ankle tendons and dynamic scanning with movement of the foot is useful to assess for tendon subluxation and confirm full-thickness tendon tears. Plantar fasciitis is well shown and injuries of the lateral ankle ligaments may be detected. One of the most useful features of ultrasound is the ability to differentiate solid from cystic soft-tissue mass lesions. Although ultrasound may not be able to confirm a specific diagnosis, a purely cystic lesion can be assumed to be benign. An extension of ultrasound is Doppler imaging, which can detect and measure blood flow and this has an important role in assessing the vascularity of mass lesions. US may be used in the detection of Morton's neuromas and mass lesions within the tarsal tunnel resulting in neural compression. In joint-based pathology, a joint effusion seen as compressible black anechoic fluid can be differentiated from synovial hypertrophy, which has a bright echogenic appearance. In active synovitis, increased blood flow is demonstrated in the synovial tissue with Doppler imaging. Various procedures such as aspirations, injections and biopsies may be performed under US guidance.

Limitations

US images are transient and are thus observer-dependent. The bones and joint surfaces are not well visualised, in particular the talar dome and subtalar joint.

Nuclear isotope scanning

Generation of isotope image

Nuclear isotope scanning detects the distribution of a radioactive agent that is injected intravenously into the body. It relies on the fact that an inflamed or pathologically active area of the skeleton has increased blood flow and bone activity with resultant increased isotope uptake. The radiopharmaceuticals most commonly used in bone scanning are phosphate markers, labelled with technetium-99 which has a short 6-hour half-life and is a pure gamma emitter. Following the injection, the patient is positioned under a scintillation camera which detects the distribution of radioactivity in the body by measuring the interaction of gamma rays emitted from the body with sodium iodide crystals in the head of the camera. The radioactivity is converted into light photons, multiplied and enhanced electronically before being displayed on a screen. The images consist of a pattern of dots forming the osseous outline, with the greatest concentration of dots in the area of greatest isotope uptake. Images are obtained in multiple projections and may include the entire skeleton or selected parts.

Isotope scanning usually involves 3 phases: Phase 1 or blood flow images are taken every 3 or 5 seconds for the first minute and demonstrate the immediate distribution of radioactive tracer into the bloodstream. Phase 2 or blood pool images are obtained 1–3 minutes following the injection and give an indication of blood perfusion into the area before being taken up by bone. The most intense uptake in phases 1 and 2 occurs in areas with increased blood flow. Normally the patient will then return 2–4 hours later for phase 3 or static bone scan images which demonstrate isotope uptake into bone. Increased uptake in phase 3 is seen in areas with increased osteoblastic activity and active bone turnover.

Indications

See Box 12.8.

Box 12.8 Isotope bone scan: indications

- Tumours
  - Multiple lesions
  - Radiographically occult lesions
- Fractures
  - Stress fractures
  - Insufficiency fractures
  - Occult fractures
- Infection
- Prosthetic loosening
- Metabolic bone disease
- Arthritis

A major advantage of skeletal nuclear isotope scanning over other imaging modalities is its ability to image the entire skeleton at once. A bone scan may confirm the presence of bony pathology at an early stage and demonstrate the anatomical distribution of disease by assessing its mineral turnover compared with adjacent normal bone.

Skeletal scintigraphy is useful in localising bone tumours particularly when multiple lesions are present such as with metastases, multifocal tumours and skip lesions. It is also important in localising small lesions such as an osteoid osteoma which may not always be visible on the plain radiograph. In most instances, bone scans cannot distinguish between benign and malignant lesions as increased blood flow with subsequent increased isotope deposition and osteoblastic activity occurs in both conditions. Bone scans are helpful in the early diagnosis of stress and insufficiency fractures when plain radiographs appear normal. Skeletal scintigraphy is very sensitive in detecting early and occult osteomyelitis. In chronic osteomyelitis, imaging with gallium-67 citrate is more accurate than technetium-99 phosphate in highlighting active osteomyelitis and thus in detecting response to treatment. Isotope uptake may be negative in areas of rampant bone infection with destruction. Increased isotope uptake around a joint prosthesis more than 12 months after the joint replacement surgery is suspicious for prosthetic loosening or infection. Bone scans may be helpful in demonstrating the extent of skeletal involvement in metabolic bone disease and the distribution of arthritic changes in arthritis.

Limitations

Scintigraphy is highly sensitive in detecting pathology; however, it is not specific and frequently it is

Box 12.9 Fluoroscopy: indications

- Intra-operative
  - Fracture reduction
  - Hardware placement
- Bone biopsies
- Joint injections

impossible to distinguish the various processes that result in increased isotope uptake.

Fluoroscopy

Generation of fluoroscopic image

Fluoroscopy uses X-rays to cause fluorescence on a screen, most commonly containing caesium iodide. Resultant images are intensified and fed to a display monitor or camera to provide real-time instant images.

Indications

See Box 12.9.

Fluoroscopy has an important role intra-operatively to assess osseous alignment such as fracture reduction, positioning of joint fusions or osteotomies and also in the placement of hardware (e.g. pins, screws, plates and prostheses). It is useful to guide percutaneous bone biopsies and joint injections, including arthrography and therapeutic injections.

Limitations

The radiation dose is dependent on the screening time and exposure parameters. Modern fluoroscopes can take a series of time-delayed images which, while not a moving picture, are adequate and significantly reduce the radiation dose.

Radiological assessment of specific bone pathology

Infection (diabetic foot)

VIDEO

Infection may be blood-borne, an extension from an adjacent soft-tissue infection or secondary to a direct entry wound such as surgery or a compound fracture. Acute bacterial infections caused by organisms such as *Staphylococcus aureus* and *Haemophilus influenzae* are most common. Occasionally diseases such as tuberculosis and fungal agents result in bone and joint infections.

The initial signs of infection are often delayed on plain radiographs, which usually show normal findings for up to 10 days following the development of infection. One of the first X-ray signs is soft-tissue oedema with increased soft-tissue swelling and density and obliteration of normal soft-tissue planes. The infection spreads first into the medullary bone and has an ill-defined radiolucent hazy, appearance (Fig. 12.20). It does not cross the epiphyseal growth plate in children. The infection then spreads laterally penetrating through the cortex, and the pus produced elevates and strips the periosteum. The first visible osseous change will often be the subperiosteal reaction, which lifts the periosteum and gives a fuzzy outline to the bone (Fig. 12.23). As the periosteum is elevated and stripped from the cortex, there is disruption of the periosteal vascular supply with resultant cortical necrosis. The necrotic bone is seen as a dense area of sclerosis and is known as a sequestrum which may be a focus of continuing infection. In some cases, a layer of periosteal new bone encapsulates the necrotic sequestrum producing a sclerotic osseous shell referred to as an involucrum. The pus may penetrate the periosteum and periosteal new bone to decompress into the adjacent soft tissues with abscess formation. External migration of necrotic bone with subcutaneous and skin breakdown results in a sinus track from the infected bone to the skin surface.

If treatment is inefficient a chronic walled-off abscess containing debris and sometimes a sequestrum may form and can persist for years. Known as a Brodie's abscess, this appears as a radiolucent ovoid area surrounded by reactive sclerosis usually seen in the long bone metaphyses.

MRI is highly sensitive in detecting osteomyelitis allowing an early diagnosis and differentiation from soft-tissue infection. The infected bone marrow results in low signal intensity on T1-weighted sequences, replacing normal high signal fatty marrow, and high T2-weighted and STIR signal (Fig. 12.21). MR imaging establishes the extent of bone marrow and soft-tissue involvement, the presence of septic arthritis and defines necrotic bone, abscess cavities and sinuses. MRI is important in the investigation of the diabetic foot to differentiate osteomyelitis from neuropathic changes. Osteomyelitis tends to occur at pressure points where soft-tissue ulcers develop such as the first and fifth metatarsal heads, calcaneal tuberosity, malleoli and distal toes. There is high signal on STIR images in the adjacent soft tissues from cellulitis, abscess formation and sinus tracts. Neuropathic changes always involve joints, most commonly the

IMAGES

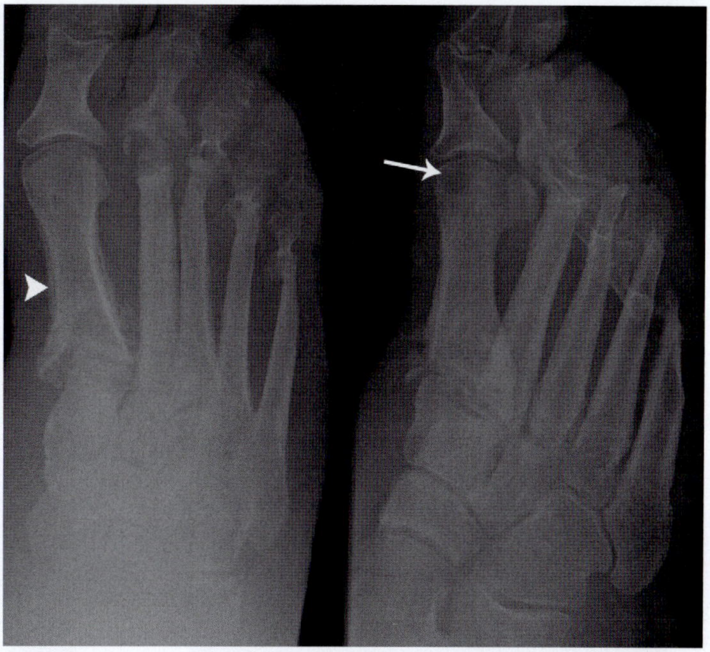

Figure 12.23 Osteomyelitis and rheumatoid arthritis. Dorsiplantar and dorsiplantar oblique radiographs. Osteomyelitis of the first metatarsal with a periosteal reaction along the metatarsal shaft (arrowhead) and radiolucency within the metatarsal head (arrow). An advanced erosive arthropathy of the metatarsophalangeal joints with destruction of the lesser metatarsal heads is secondary to rheumatoid arthritis.

tarsometatarsal joints, and there is often joint destruction, subluxation and bone fragmentation with little adjacent soft-tissue abnormality. In the diabetic foot 80% of Charcot's arthropathy occurs at the tarsometatarsal or Chopart joints, 10% involve the calcaneus and 5% relate to the ankle or forefoot.

Osteochondrosis

Osteochondrosis, also known as osteochondritis, is a condition of defective bone formation in the epiphysis or apophysis of a growing skeleton. The cause is thought to be due to a vascular disturbance to that part of the bone which is possibly trauma related but sometimes associated with endocrine dysfunction. It occurs in several sites in the foot, as well as other locations including the femoral epiphysis (Perthes' disease), lunate (Kienböck's disease) and the tibial tubercle (Osgood–Schlatter disease). In all the conditions there is sclerosis, flattening, irregularity and possibly fragmentation of the epiphysis. Revascularisation occurs over a period of months and the epiphysis remodels, sometimes with residual deformity. The conditions are self-limiting and the clinical importance relates to the functional importance of the joint involved. In the foot the common conditions are as follows:

Freiberg's disease occurs at the metatarsal heads, usually the second or third, at the age of about 12–14 years. Widening of the joint space may be noted due to the 'eggshell crush' degeneration that occurs in the metatarsal head. In late stages, the remodelled head is flattened and sclerotic and may result in secondary osteoarthritis (Fig. 12.24).

Köhler's disease occurs in the navicular bone in the 2–10-year age range, and 70% of cases are in males. There is a familial incidence. The navicular becomes sclerotic and collapses into a disc shape which is clearly seen on the lateral view.

Sever's disease is thought to be caused by excessive traction on the calcaneal apophysis. It usually occurs posteriorly due to traction from the Achilles' tendon but can occur on the plantar aspect due to traction from the plantar fascia/intrinsic foot muscles. It usually occurs in the 8–12-year age range and may be bilateral. The apophysis of the calcaneum appears irregular and sclerotic. These features may, however, be a normal finding in an asymptomatic child and a diagnosis of Sever's disease cannot be made with any certainty on radiographic evidence alone.

Other rarer conditions are **Iselin's disease** of the fifth metatarsal base and **Buschke's disease** of the cuneiforms.

Trauma

Plain radiographs are the mainstay of imaging in trauma. At least two radiographic views at 90° to each other must be taken of any suspected injury site.

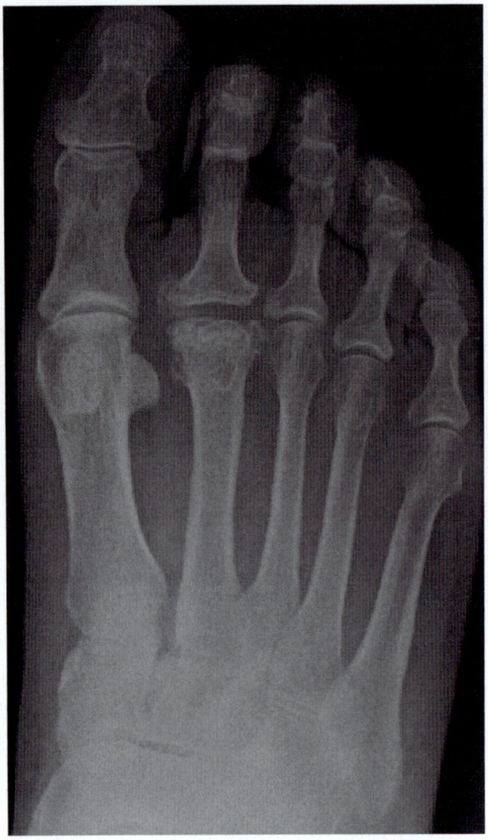

Figure 12.24 Freiberg's disease. Dorsiplantar radiograph. Flattening and sclerosis of the second metatarsal head with secondary widening of the second metatarsophalangeal joint space consistent with Freiberg's disease.

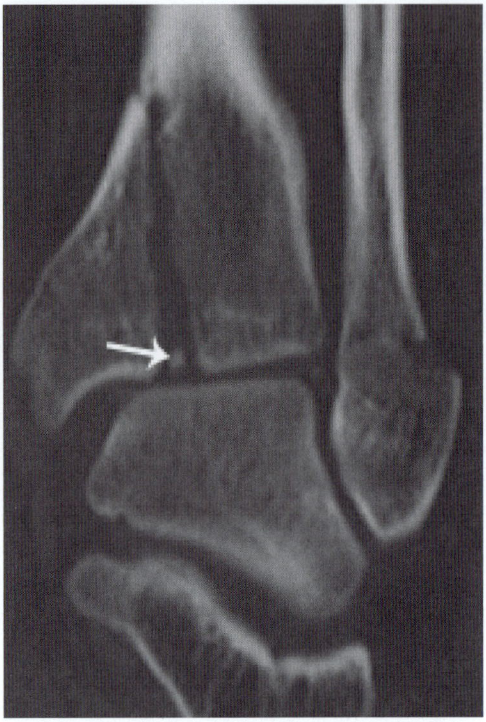

Figure 12.25 Intra-articular fracture. Coronal computed tomography (CT) reformat. A coronal CT image through a Pilon fracture clearly shows a distal tibial fracture extending to the tibiotalar articular surface. A small bone fragment is situated in the distal aspect of the fracture (arrow). A distal fibular fracture is present.

A high percentage of fractures are only seen on one view and will therefore be missed unless two views are routinely obtained. Once a fracture is identified, the rest of the radiograph should be carefully searched for associated dislocation, additional fractures and foreign bodies.

Fractures can be classified as follows:

- Simple fracture – this is not fragmented and there is no penetration through the skin. There may be displacement and angulation of the fractured bone ends.
- Comminuted fracture – this is splintered or fragmented.
- Compound fracture – this is where the skin has been breached by fractured bone.
- Complicated fracture – there is associated trauma or infection involving adjacent muscles, tendons and blood vessels.
- Impacted fracture – in this the fracture fragments are forcibly driven into each other.
- Intra-articular fracture – this involves an adjacent articular surface (Fig. 12.25).
- Greenstick fracture – this is common in children and occurs when the bone is bent but only one side of the cortex breaks.
- Stress fracture – this is produced as a result of repetitive stresses on bone. Common sites are the tibia, fibula, calcaneum, navicular and metatarsals secondary to sporting activity such as long distance runners or with marching and prolonged standing (see Ch. 15). A stress fracture may appear as a linear band of sclerosis with periostitis (Fig. 12.26). However, the fracture initially may be so fine that it is missed until a later stage when bony callus can be seen around the site. Suspected stress fractures can be confirmed by demonstrating increased isotope uptake at

bone scintigraphy, a subtle fracture line with early periosteal thickening on CT (Fig. 12.27) and a linear low signal fracture line surrounded by bone marrow oedema on MRI (Fig. 12.28).

- Pathological fracture – this occurs at the site of a pre-existing osseous abnormality such as osteoporosis or a bone tumour.
- Avulsion fracture – this occurs when a chip of bone is pulled away from the parent bone by a tendon or ligament attachment. Care must be taken to differentiate an avulsion fracture from an accessory ossicle. Clinical correlation is important as fractures are tender and accessory ossicles are usually asymptomatic.
- Salter–Harris fracture – this involves the epiphyseal plate and the classification can be remembered using the mnemonic SALTR: **S**lip of the physis is type 1, fracture **A**bove the physis is type 2, fracture **L**ower than the physis is type 3, fracture **T**hrough the physis is type 4 (Fig. 12.29) and a **R**ammed physis is type 5.

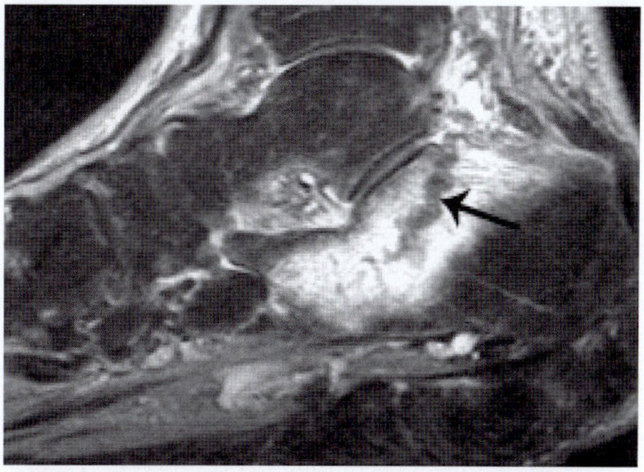

Figure 12.28 Calcaneal stress fracture. Sagittal STIR magnetic resonance image. A calcaneal stress fracture is seen as a low signal line (arrow) surrounded by high signal marrow oedema. The plain radiograph findings appeared normal.

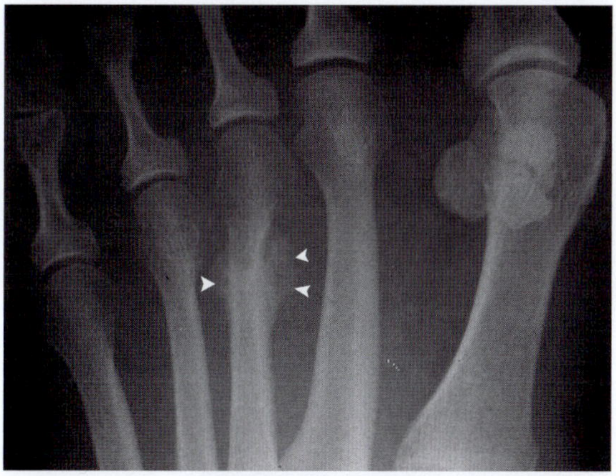

Figure 12.26 Metatarsal stress fracture. Dorsiplantar radiograph. There is a stress fracture of the distal third metatarsal shaft with sclerosis and periosteal new bone formation (arrowheads).

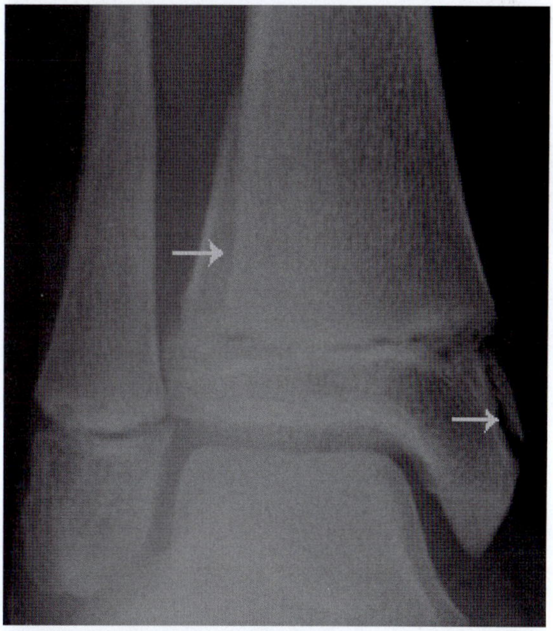

Figure 12.29 Salter–Harris type 4 fracture. Anteroposterior ankle radiograph. A fracture extending through the distal tibial metaphysis, epiphyseal plate and epiphysis (arrows) is in keeping with a Salter–Harris type 4 fracture.

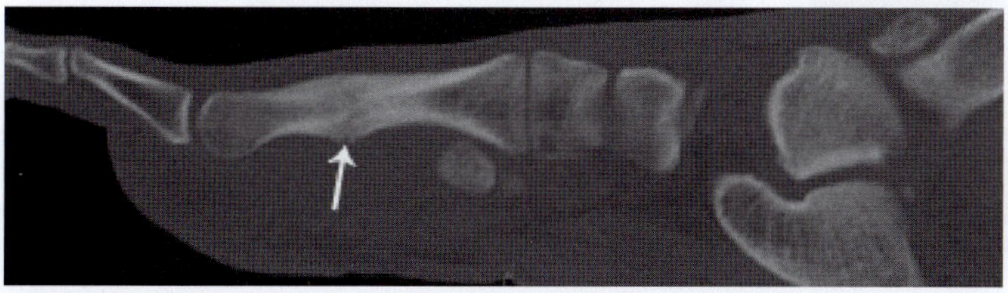

Figure 12.27 Metatarsal stress fracture. Sagittal computed tomography reformat. A metatarsal stress fracture is clearly depicted (arrow) with surrounding sclerosis and periosteal thickening.

Certain parts of the foot are prone to specific types of fracture:

- The Weber fracture classification is used to describe malleolar fractures. A medial malleolar fracture may be associated with a proximal fibular fracture referred to as Maisonneuve's fracture. Unless anticipated, these fractures may go undetected as they are too proximal to be included on routine ankle radiographs.
- The talar neck may fracture following contact with the distal tibia with forced ankle dorsiflexion. This may lead to disruption of the blood supply to the proximal portion of the talus with avascular necrosis of the talar dome (**Fig. 12.30**).
- Calcaneal fractures are common following a fall from a height and 75% are intra-articular and/or comminuted (**Fig. 12.31**). If Boehler's angle is less than 20°, a compression fracture of the calcaneum should be diagnosed. A sclerotic line may be the only evidence of an impacted calcaneal fracture.
- A Chopart fracture is a fracture/dislocation through the midtarsal joint (calcaneocuboid and talonavicular).
- A Lisfranc fracture is a fracture/dislocation of the tarsometatarsal joints. This injury may be missed radiographically when the dislocation is minimal. A key to normal alignment is that the medial border of the second metatarsal should always line up with the medial border of the intermediate cuneiform on the AP view and the

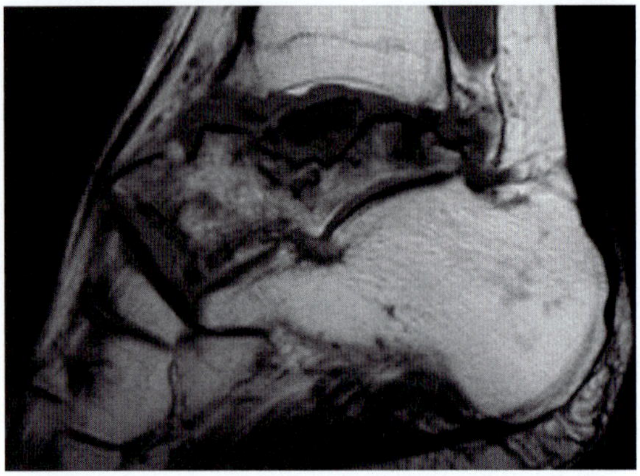

Figure 12.30 Avascular necrosis of the talar dome. Sagittal T1-weighted MR image. Sclerosis, collapse and fragmentation of the talar dome is consistent with avascular necrosis, which was secondary to a previous talar neck fracture.

Figure 12.31 Calcaneal fracture. **A** Axial computed tomography (CT). **B** Three-dimensional (3D) CT reconstruction. There is a comminuted calcaneal fracture (arrows). The peroneal tendons are seen on the 3D reconstruction (arrowheads).

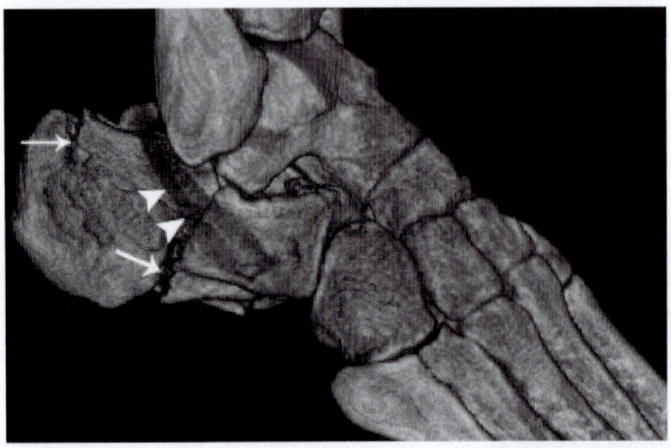

B

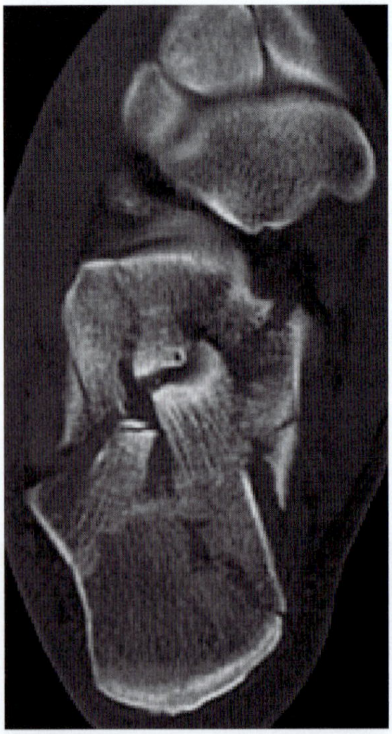

A

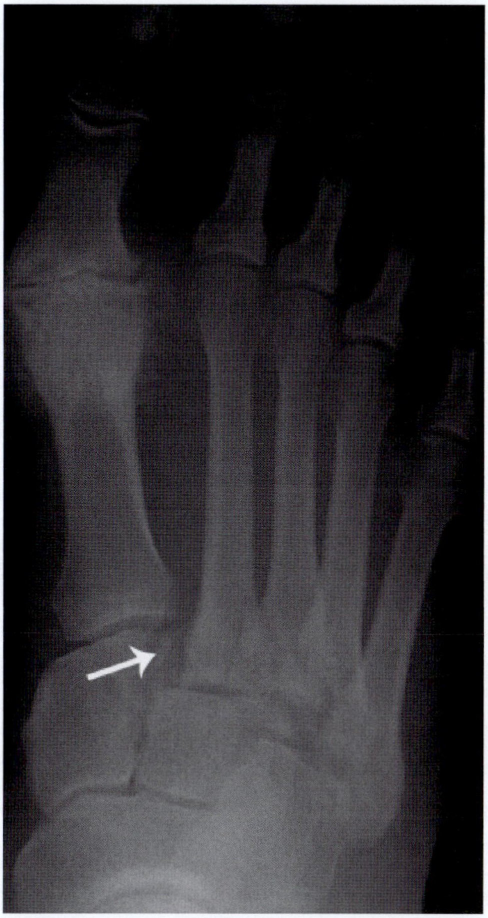

Figure 12.32 Lisfranc fracture. Dorsiplantar radiograph. A medial Lisfranc fracture is present with a small bone fragment between the medial cuneiform and the base of the second metatarsal (arrow). The medial border of the second metatarsal lies lateral to the medial border of the intermediate cuneiform. There is first metatarsophalangeal osteoarthritis with loss of joint space, subarticular sclerosis and cyst formation with marginal osteophytes.

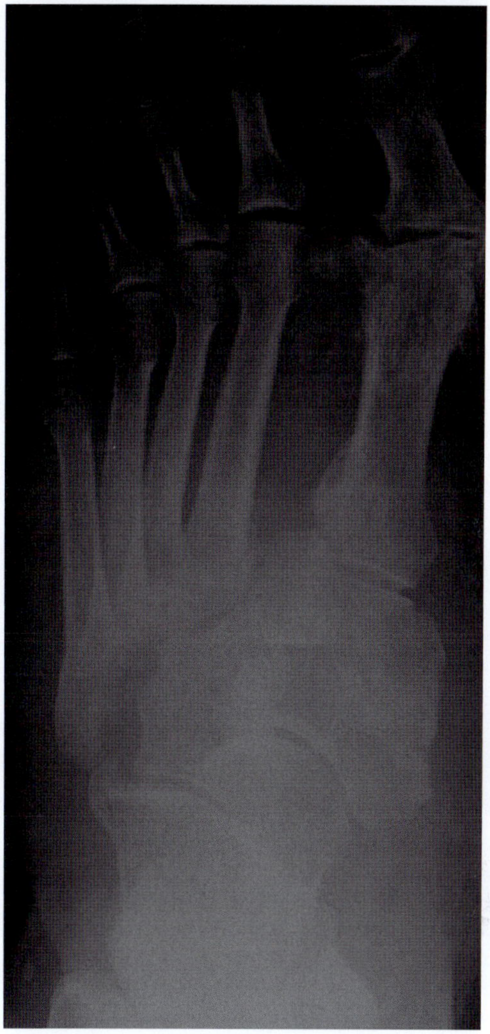

Figure 12.33 Lisfranc fracture/dislocation. Dorsiplantar radiograph. There is an extensive Lisfranc fracture/dislocation. The intermediate cuneiform has subluxed distally between the first and second metatarsals.

medial margin of the third metatarsal should line up with the medial margin of the lateral cuneiform on the oblique view (Figs 12.32, 12.33).

- An avulsion fracture of the base of the fifth metatarsal (by the peroneus brevis tendon insertion) must be differentiated from a normal unfused apophysis. A fracture line lies transverse to the long axis of the metatarsal whereas an apophysis lies parallel to the long axis of the metatarsal (Fig. 12.34). Jones's fracture should not be confused with an avulsion injury. It is situated in the diaphysis of the fifth metatarsal distal to both the tarsometatarsal joint and the articulation between the fourth and fifth metatarsals.
- Ankle pain following injury – in a small percentage of cases following an ankle sprain, symptoms persist beyond the expected timeframe of around 6 weeks and further imaging usually with plain radiographs and MRI may be helpful. Residual instability, syndesmotic injury, missed or ununited fractures, osteochondral defects, sinus tarsi syndrome, impingement syndromes

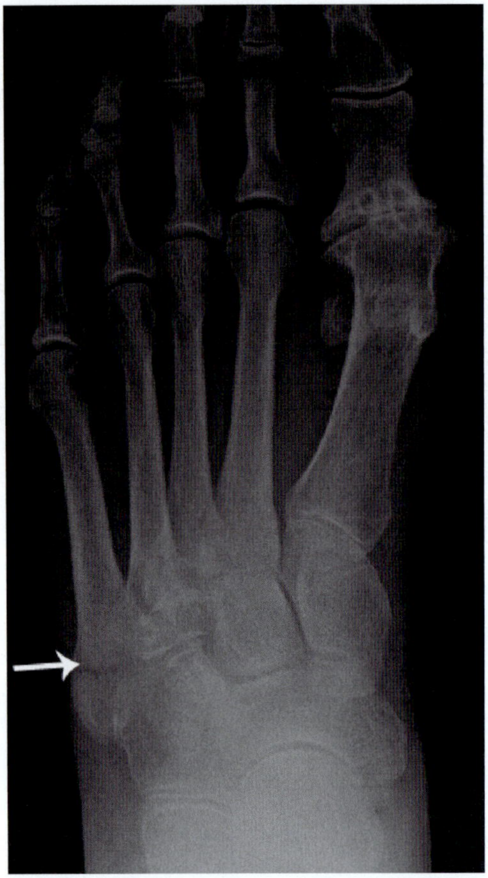

Figure 12.34 Fracture base of fifth metatarsal. Dorsiplantar radiograph. A fracture through the base of the fifth metatarsal lies transverse to the long axis of the metatarsal shaft (arrow). There is first metatarsophalangeal joint osteoarthritis.

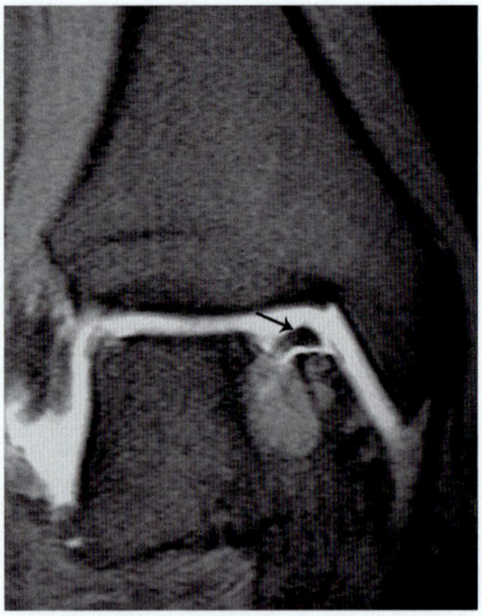

Figure 12.35 Osteochondritis desiccans of the talar dome. Coronal T2-weighted magnetic resonance image. There is an osteochondral fragment involving the medial aspect of the talar dome (arrow). Joint fluid extending between the fragment and the talus and cystic change in the underlying talus indicate that the fragment is unstable.

and secondary osteoarthritis are common causes of persistent pain.

Osteochondritis desiccans describes partial or complete detachment of an osteochondral fragment usually involving the medial corner of the talar dome. Appearances may be subtle on plain radiographs with a tiny step or irregularity of the talar dome on the AP projection. MR imaging is sensitive and shows osteochondritis desiccans as a focal area of low signal in the subarticular portion of the talar dome on T1-weighted images. On T2-weighted images, if high signal is seen surrounding the dissecans fragment, in the bone at the bed of the fragment or throughout the fragment, it is most likely an unstable fragment (Fig. 12.35). MR imaging may be useful in localizing the fragment if it becomes displaced and lies in the joint as a loose body.

Sinus tarsi syndrome is characterized by lateral foot pain and the feeling of hindfoot instability. The sinus tarsi is the space that lies between the talus and the calcaneus and opens up in a cone-like configuration to the lateral aspect of the ankle, beneath the lateral malleolus. It is filled with fat and several ligaments which give some hindfoot stability. In sinus tarsi syndrome, the ligaments are disrupted and the sinus tarsi contains inflammatory tissue or fibrosis, depending on the chronicity of the changes. On MR imaging, the high signal fat in the sinus tarsi is obliterated on T1-weighted images and associated tears of the lateral collateral ligaments are often present.

Impingement syndromes are quite common around the ankle. They are chronic traumatic injuries where soft tissue is repeatedly trapped between the bones of the ankle joint. The commonest are anterior, posterior and anterolateral impingement. Anterior impingement is usually obvious on the lateral plain radiograph with an osseous spur arising from the anterior inferior margin of the distal tibia. MRI is useful in confirming posterior impingement by demonstrating marrow oedema in an os trigonum or prominent posterior stieda process, which impinges between the dorsal tibia and posterior talus on

Table 12.3 Differential diagnosis of bone tumours

	Benign	*Malignant*
Unfused skeleton	Enchondroma Osteochondroma Fibrous cortical defect Simple bone cyst Aneurysmal bone cyst Osteoid osteoma	Osteosarcoma Ewing's sarcoma
Fused skeleton	Enchondroma Giant cell tumour	Chondrosarcoma Metastasis

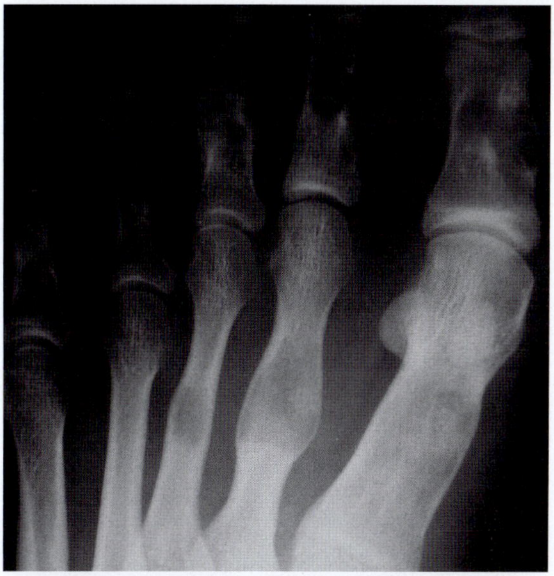

Figure 12.36 Enchondromas. Dorsiplantar radiograph. Multiple well-defined radiolucent lesions in the proximal phalanges and second and third metatarsal shafts are consistent with enchondromas. Some of the enchondromas are expansile with cortical thinning.

plantar flexion. Anterolateral impingement is primarily a clinical diagnosis.

Bone tumours

The radiological diagnosis of bone tumours requires the expertise of a radiologist. A misdiagnosis could prove fatal to the patient. A complete classification of tumours with radiological features is beyond the scope of this chapter and only the more common lesions are discussed here. It is useful to consider the age of the patient and decide whether the lesion has a benign or malignant appearance to help with the differential diagnosis (Table 12.3).

Benign bone tumours

Benign bone tumours are characterized by a well-defined, often sclerotic margin. An expansile lesion may result in cortical thinning, but there is no cortical destruction. Occasionally a periosteal reaction is present which appears uniform and solid.

Enchondroma

These benign cartilaginous tumours are caused by the development of embryonic cartilage cells within the shafts of long bones. They are often found within the diaphyses of the metatarsals and phalanges. The tumour is radiolucent and expansile with cortical thinning and may have internal calcification. Pathological fractures can occur. Enchondromas may have a malignant tendency, particularly multiple enchondromatosis or Ollier's disease (Fig. 12.36).

Osteochondroma

This is a cartilage capped exostosis which is seen on plain radiographs as a bony outgrowth (Fig. 12.37). The cartilaginous component is invisible on plain radiographs unless calcified. Rarely, the cartilage cap may undergo transformation to a malignant chondrosarcoma and a thickness of more than 2 cm is suspicious. This is usually assessed on MR imaging, however, the thickness of the cartilage cap is also well seen with ultrasound. Pedunculated subungual exostoses on the distal phalanx of the hallux are common and usually have a cartilaginous cap, classifying them as osteochondromata.

Fibrous cortical defect

This is a common lesion in the unfused skeleton found in 20% of growing children. It is caused by fibrous tissue from the periosteum invading the underlying cortex that may be related to a subclinical injury. It is usually seen as an incidental finding on plain radiographs as a small radiolucent lesion with a sclerotic border in the cortex of a long bone metaphyses (Fig. 12.38). Larger lesions (>2 cm) that expand into the medullary cavity are referred to as **non-ossifying fibromas**.

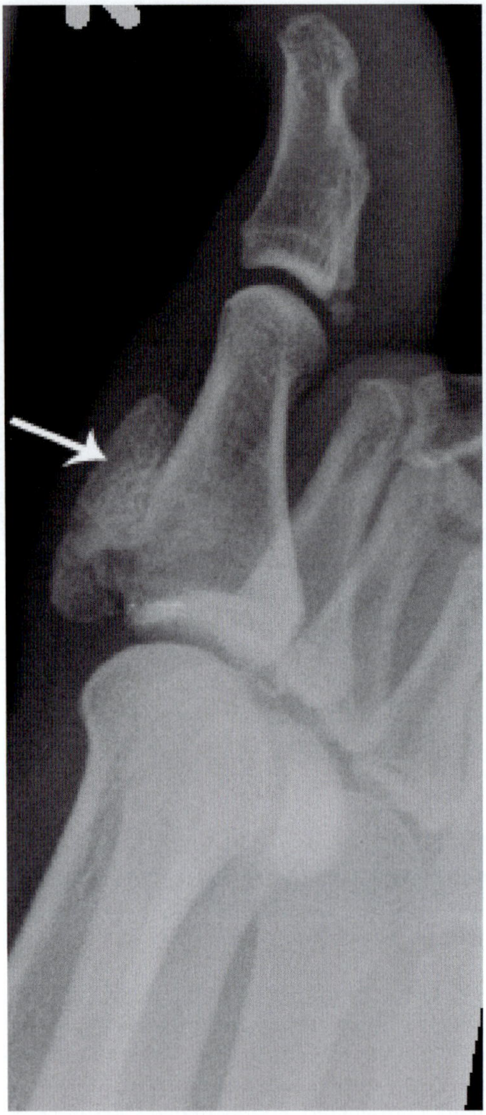

Figure 12.37 Osteochondroma. Dorsiplantar oblique radiograph. An osteochondroma arising from the dorsal aspect of the first proximal phalanx (arrow).

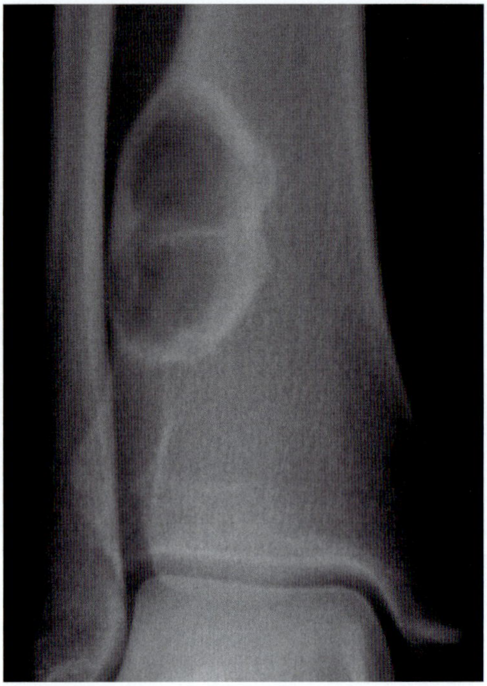

Figure 12.38 Fibrous cortical defect. Anteroposterior ankle radiograph. A fibrous cortical defect is seen as a radiolucent cortically based lesion with a well-demarcated sclerotic margin in the lateral aspect of the distal tibia.

Solitary (simple) bone cyst

This is a cyst of unknown origin containing clear or serosanguinous fluid, occurring in the unfused skeleton. It may occur in the long bones of the foot and the calcaneum where it is seen as a well-demarcated radiolucent intramedullary lesion with cortical thinning (Fig. 12.39). It may present with a pathological fracture.

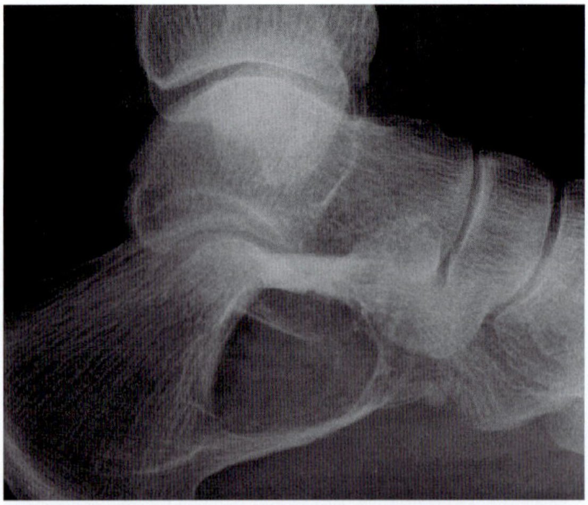

Figure 12.39 Simple bone cyst. Lateral radiograph. A large well-defined radiolucent lesion in the anterior aspect of the calcaneum is consistent with a bone cyst.

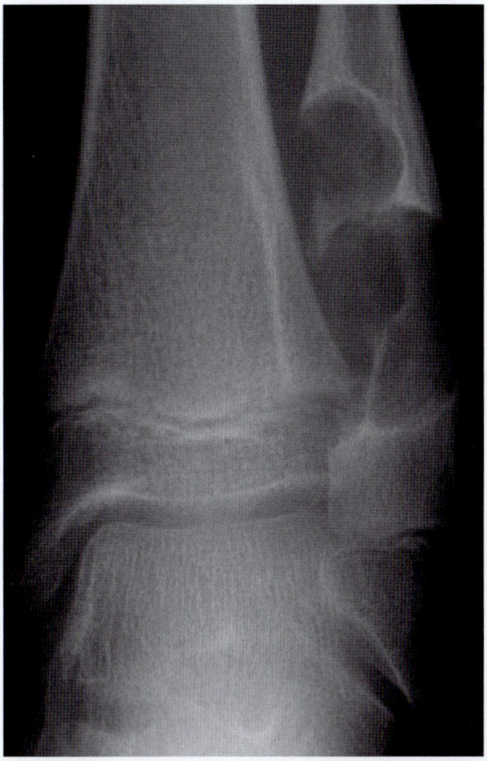

Figure 12.40 Aneurysmal bone cyst. Anteroposterior ankle radiograph. A loculated expansile radiolucent lesion in the distal fibula of an unfused skeleton with a thin cortical shell, which was histologically confirmed to be an aneurysmal bone cyst.

Aneurysmal bone cyst

A sponge-like cyst with blood-filled spaces and fibrous septa, this may arise as the result of a vascular anomaly. It tends to occur in patients under the age of 30 years in the long bone metaphyses. The lesion is radiolucent and rapidly expansile with a thin cortical shell (Fig. 12.40). On MR imaging, aneurysmal bone cysts typically have internal septations with fluid-fluid levels indicating internal bleeding.

Osteoid osteoma

This occurs most often in young patients who may complain of severe pain at night and at rest with dramatic relief with aspirin. Radiologically it exhibits an ovoid radiolucent nidus up to 1 cm in diameter surrounded by an area of sclerosis with periosteal thickening (Fig. 12.41). The sclerosis may mask the radiolucent nidus on plain radiographs which is readily seen on thin CT sections. The differential diagnosis includes a Brodie's abscess.

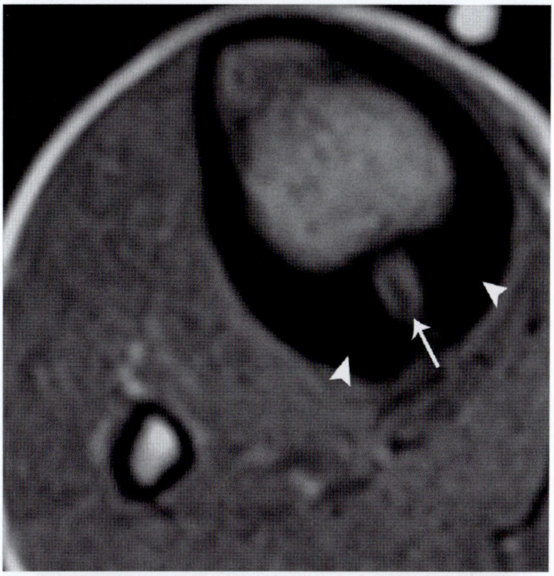

Figure 12.41 Osteoid osteoma. Axial T1-weighted magnetic resonance (MR) image. The cortically based nidus (arrow) of a distal tibial osteoid osteoma is clearly depicted on this MR image with adjacent periosteal thickening (arrowheads).

Giant cell tumour

These tumours occur primarily in the fused skeleton in an eccentric epiphyseal location. The lesion is usually radiolucent with a well-defined but non-sclerotic margin (Fig. 12.42). They may be expansile with cortical thinning and rarely the cortex is breached. Approximately 15% of giant cell tumours are malignant.

Malignant bone tumours

Malignant tumours typically have an ill-defined margin and 'moth-eaten' appearance. There may be cortical destruction and a periosteal reaction which has a lamellated ('onion-skinned') or spiculated ('hair on end' or 'sunray') appearance. An adjacent soft-tissue mass is often present.

Osteosarcoma

Although this is the commonest primary malignant bone neoplasm, it is not common in the foot. It typically occurs in the unfused skeleton, but it may occur in an older people, usually secondary to Paget's

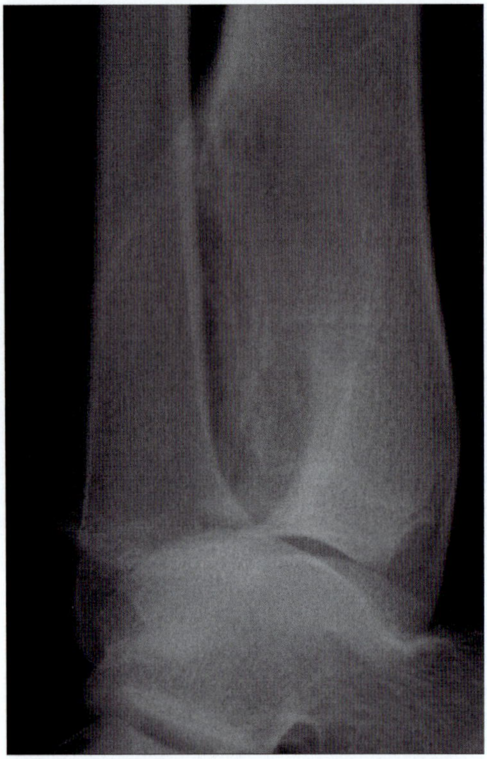

Figure 12.42 Giant cell tumour. Lateral radiograph. A radiolucent expansile lesion eccentrically situated in the distal tibia of a fused skeleton extends to the articular surface consistent with a giant cell tumour.

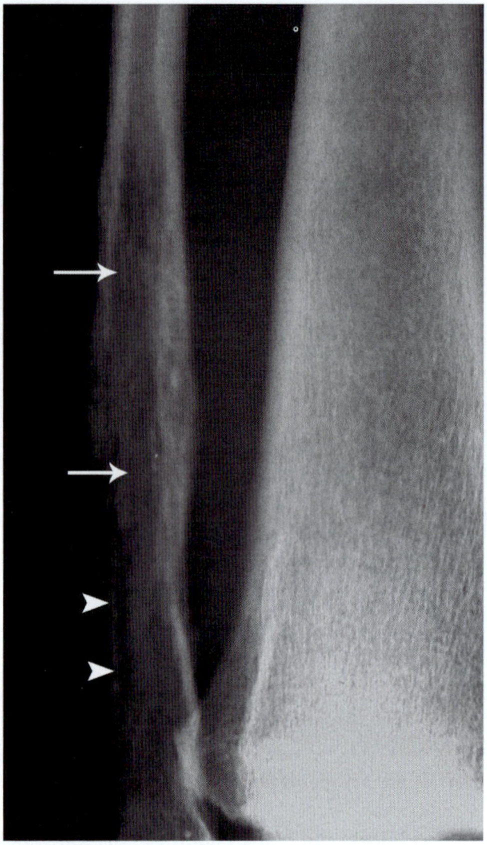

Figure 12.43 Ewing's sarcoma. Anteroposterior radiograph. Ill-defined permeative infiltration of the distal fibula (arrows) with loss of the lateral cortex (arrowheads) was histologically consistent with a Ewing's sarcoma.

disease. Radiographically, there is an ill-defined often mixed lytic and sclerotic lesion within the shaft of the bone. As the tumour osteoid becomes mineralised, there is increasing sclerosis and new bone formation which may have a 'cloud-like' density. An aggressive periosteal reaction may be present and a wedge of ossified tissue can form under the periosteum, called Codman's triangle.

Ewing's sarcoma

This occurs in the unfused skeleton and is seen as an ill-defined, permeative (multiple small radiolucencies) lesion which extends along the diaphysis of a long bone or within a flat bone. A spiculated periosteal reaction and cortical penetration may be present (Fig. 12.43). Osteomyelitis can have a similar radiographic appearance.

Chondrosarcoma

These cartilaginous tumours are rare in the foot but have been noted in the calcaneum. These tumours occur in the fused skeleton in the 50–70 year age group. Radiologically they have a varied appearance but usually contain calcification which may have a 'popcorn' or 'snowflake' appearance indicative of their cartilaginous origin (Fig. 12.44).

IMAGES

Metastases

Secondary bone metastases need to be considered in the differential diagnosis of any lytic lesion in a patient over the age of 40 years. Bone metastases may also be sclerotic, most commonly prostate and breast metastases. Thyroid and renal metastases produce expansile lesions. Metastases to the foot are most commonly from a primary lung carcinoma (Fig. 12.45).

IMAGES

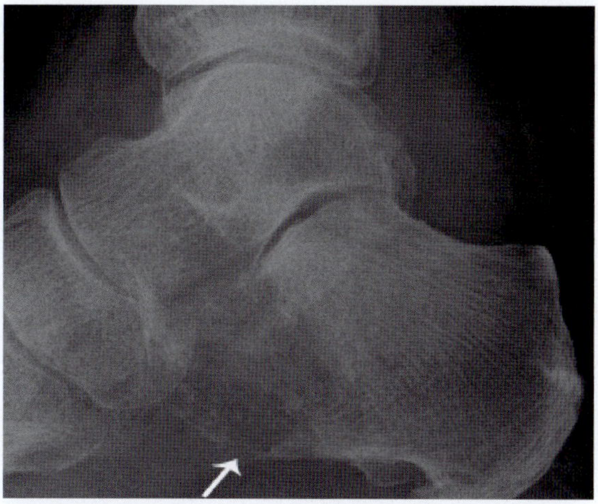

Figure 12.44 Chondrosarcoma. Lateral radiograph. A radiolucent lesion in the anterior aspect of the calcaneum with destruction of the inferior calcaneal cortex (arrow) was histologically confirmed to be a chondrosarcoma.

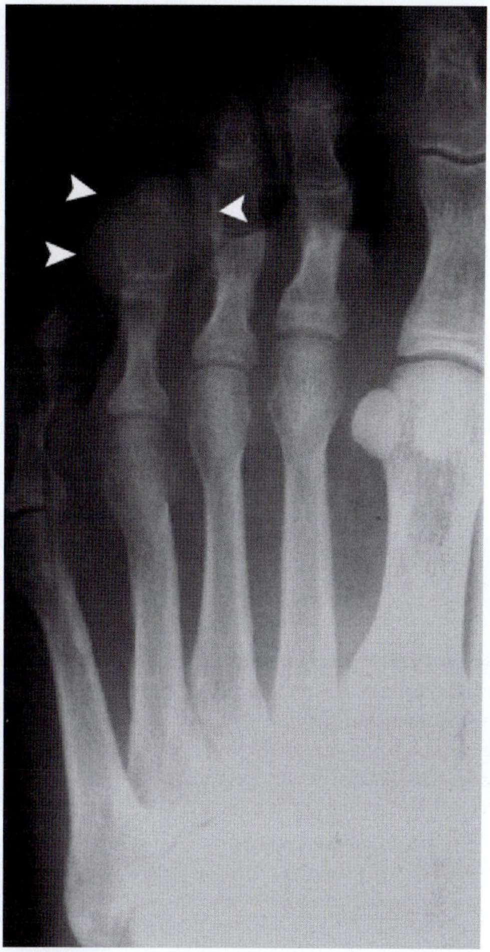

Figure 12.45 Metastases. Dorsiplantar radiograph. A radiolucent lesion expands the fourth middle phalanx with cortical destruction and a large associated soft-tissue mass (arrowheads). Histological examination confirmed metastasis from a primary lung carcinoma.

Radiological assessment of specific joint pathology

Arthritis

Rheumatoid arthritis (connective tissue disorders)

Rheumatoid arthritis is a connective tissue disorder of unknown aetiology that can affect any synovial lined joint. It classically involves the metatarsophalangeal joints in a bilaterally symmetrical fashion. Early radiographic changes are soft-tissue swelling, joint effusions and periarticular osteoporosis. As the synovial pannus invades the cartilage and bone there is progressive joint space narrowing and loss of the bony cortex with periarticular erosions. Generalised osteoporosis and foot deformities develop with characteristic abduction deformities of the digits that progress to gross subluxations and dislocations in severe cases (Fig. 12.46). Midtarsal and rearfoot involvement occurs in long-standing cases.

In juvenile disorders such as Still's disease there may be epiphyseal overgrowth and early fusion with delayed long bone growth and 'spindling' of the digits. Other connective tissue disorders that attack the joints include scleroderma and systemic lupus erythematosus which produce similar radiographic features, although erosions are generally not present. Soft-tissue calcification is a characteristic finding in scleroderma.

MRI is highly sensitive in detecting synovitis and bone erosions in patients with early rheumatoid arthritis. Recent advances in ultrasound with improved visualisation of the small distal joints have resulted in ultrasound becoming a more widely available low-cost imaging technique that is also sensitive in detecting early synovitis (Fig. 12.47). US can differentiate hypervascular synovitis from fibrous pannus by demonstrating increased vascular flow with Doppler imaging in active synovitis. This may be used to monitor disease activity and thus assess therapeutic response. US can also detect tenosynovitis and bone erosions before the latter become evident on plain radiographs.

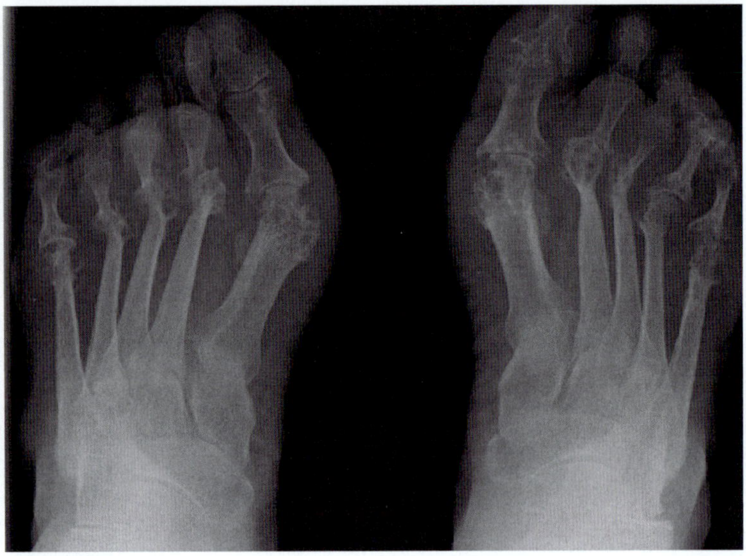

Figure 12.46 Rheumatoid arthritis. Dorsiplantar radiograph. An arthropathy involving predominantly the metatarsophalangeal joints in a symmetrical fashion is characterised by periarticular erosions, loss of joint space and subluxation of the proximal phalanges typical of rheumatoid arthritis.

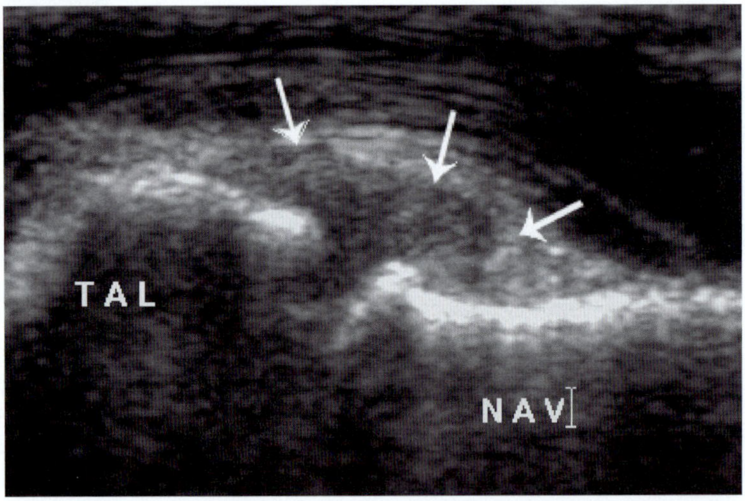

Figure 12.47 Rheumatoid arthritis. Longitudinal ultrasound image. A longitudinal ultrasound image across the talo (TAL)-navicular (NAV) joint shows a mass of synovitis extending beyond the confines of the joint (arrows).

Osteoarthritis

The earliest radiographic features of osteoarthritis are related to degeneration of the cartilage with irregularity and narrowing of the joint space. The damaged cartilage may become calcified (chondrocalcinosis). There is increased subarticular sclerosis with the formation of subchondral cysts. Osteophytes or bony outgrowths develop at the periphery of the joint and can attain considerable size, limiting joint motion and resulting in pain and pressure symptoms (Figs 12.48, 12.49). Bone density is usually maintained. In late stages of the disease, the joint becomes partially or fully ankylosed and the osteophytes may fracture, causing loose bodies within the joint capsule.

Gout

Gout is a metabolic disorder that results in hyperuricaemia and leads to urate crystals being deposited in various sites, especially the joint cartilage. The first metatarsophalangeal joint is commonly involved, and this is called podagra. It takes several years for gout to cause radiographically evident disease. The classic radiographic findings are well-defined

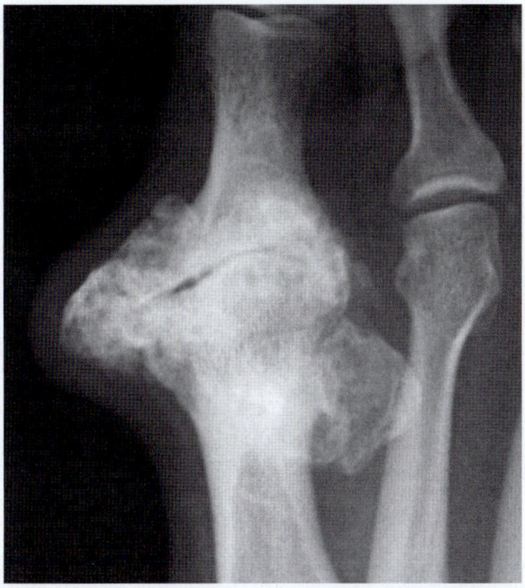

Figure 12.48 Osteoarthritis. Dorsiplantar radiograph. This case of hallux rigidus shows loss of the first metatarso–phalangeal joint space, subarticular sclerosis and lateral osteophytes.

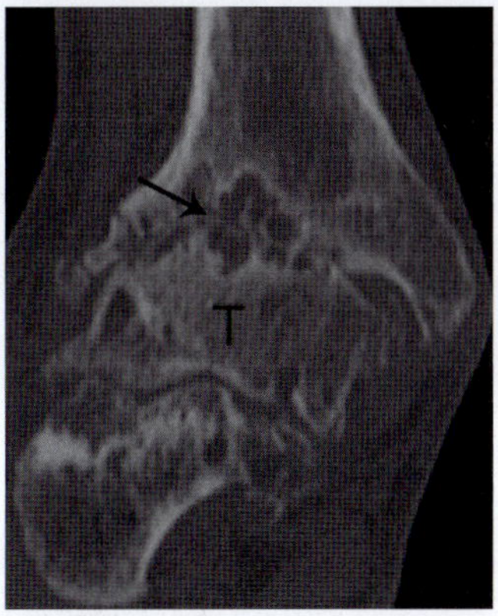

Figure 12.49 Osteoarthritis. Coronal computed tomography reformat. Advanced osteoarthritis of the tibiotalar joint (arrow) with complete loss of joint space and subchondral cyst formation. There is valgus tilt of the talus (T).

erosions often with sclerotic borders which have a 'punched-out' or 'rat bite' appearance and overhanging margin (Fig. 12.50). Chondrocalcinosis is often present. Joint space and bone density are preserved until late in the course of the disease. Deposition of urate crystals in the soft tissues are known as tophi and lead to periarticular lobulated soft-tissue masses.

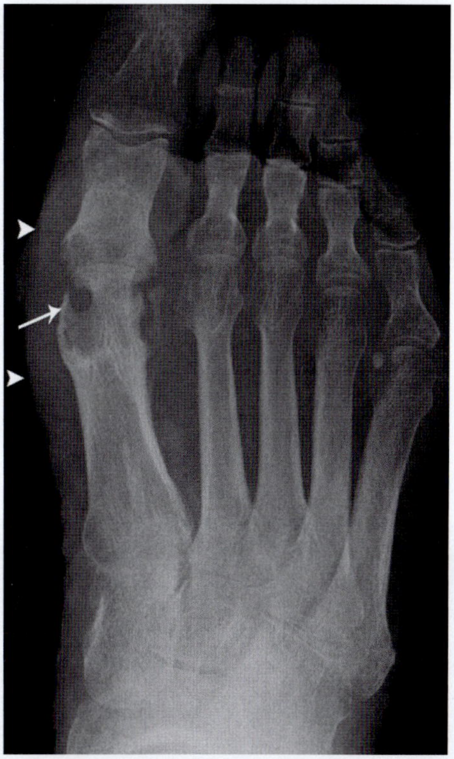

Figure 12.50 Gout. Dorsiplantar radiograph. Gout of the first metatarsophalangeal joint characterised by loss of joint space and a well-defined 'punched-out' erosion with an overhanging margin (arrow). There is adjacent soft tissue swelling (arrowheads).

Sero-negative spondyloarthropathy

This group of diseases, which includes ankylosing spondylitis, psoriasis and Reiter's syndrome, are linked to the HLA B27 antigen complexes. They usually involve the interphalangeal joints in an asymmetrical distribution. Soft-tissue swelling may lead to 'sausage digits'. There is loss of joint space and rather ill-defined erosions with proliferative new bone formation and periostitis (Fig. 12.51). Severe forms may progress to ankylosis across joints. A fairly common finding is fluffy new bone formation and inflammation at the calcaneal insertion of the Achilles tendon and plantar aponeurosis with erosions at the superior posterior calcaneal margin. Paravertebral ossification leading to ankylosis of the spine and sacroiliitis is common.

Neuropathic or Charcot's joint

Charcot's joint is a traumatic arthritis due to loss of sensation and proprioception in the affected limb. It

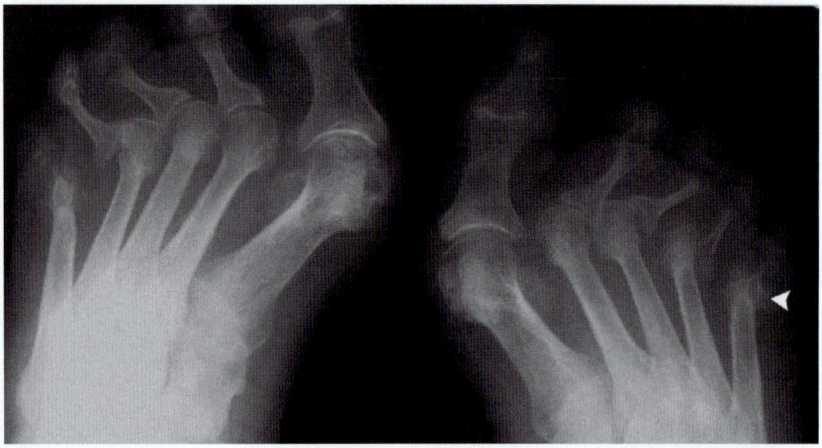

Figure 12.51 Psoriatic arthropathy. Dorsiplantar radiograph. Arthropathy of the metacarpophalangeal and interphalangeal joints with poorly demarcated erosions, fluffy new bone formation (arrowhead) and preservation of bone density is consistent with a psoriatic arthropathy.

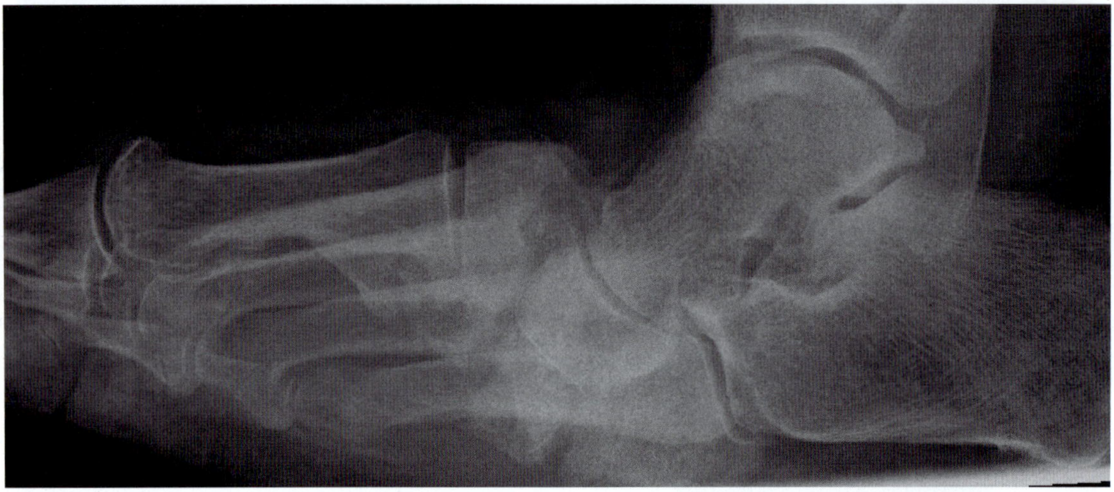

A

Figure 12.52 Neuropathic joint. **A** Lateral radiograph. **B** Bone scan. There is destruction of dense tarsal bones with dislocation and deformity in this diabetic patient consistent with a neuropathic foot. Corresponding increased isotope uptake is present in the region of the tarsus on the bone scan.

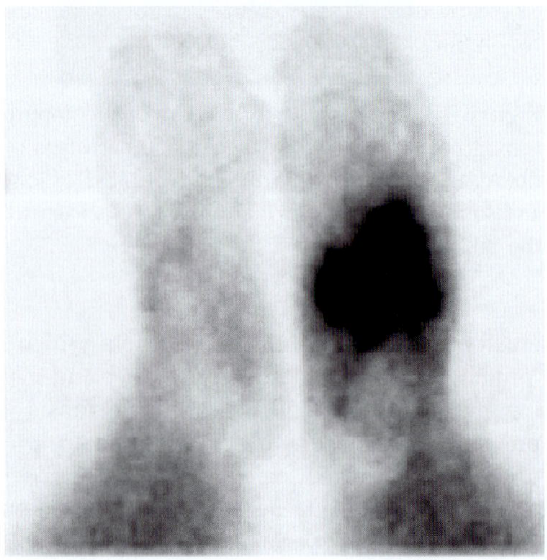

B

is most commonly seen in diabetes and typically involves the tarsometatarsal joints. The radiographic features may be remembered by the following five Ds (Fig. 12.52):

IMAGES

- Destruction of the joint – which is often severe
- Dislocation
- Debris – which is made up of heterotopic new bone and loose bodies
- Deformity
- Dense sclerotic subchondral bone.

Synovial osteochondromatosis

This condition occurs mainly in young or middle-aged men. Multiple metaplastic cartilaginous bodies form within the synovial membranes of a joint and subsequently may become ossified. These osteocartilaginous bodies may remain attached to the synovium or become true loose bodies within the joint. The radiographic appearance is of multiple calcified intra-articular bodies, accompanied by a joint effusion. In chronic cases, there may be pressure erosion of the adjacent periarticular bone.

Pigmented villonodular synovitis

This condition is most commonly seen in young men and is characterised by villous nodular proliferation of the synovium with haemosiderin deposition. This results in dense soft-tissue swelling around the effected joint with subsequent subarticular pressure erosion of the adjacent bone. The joint space is preserved until fairly late in the course of the disease and there is no calcification. MRI demonstrates the masses of synovial tissue in the joint which contain foci of low signal on all imaging sequences representing the haemosiderin deposits.

Radiological assessment of specific soft-tissue pathology

Soft-tissue masses (Table 12.4)

Ganglion cysts

VIDEO

A ganglion is a mucoid cyst which usually arises from an underlying joint, tendon or ligament. Ganglia are usually anechoic at ultrasound and the lesion may be seen to communicate with a tendon or joint capsule via a neck of varying length and width (Fig. 12.53A). On MR images, a ganglion usually demonstrates homogeneous low T1-weighted and

Table 12.4 Common soft-tissue tumours of the foot and ankle

Benign	Ganglion cyst Morton's neuroma Haemangioma Lipoma Plantar fibromatosis Foreign body granuloma Nerve sheath tumour Giant cell tumour of the tendon sheath Soft-tissue chondroma
Malignant	Synovial sarcoma
Soft tissue tumour mimickers	Accessory soleus and peroneus quartus muscles

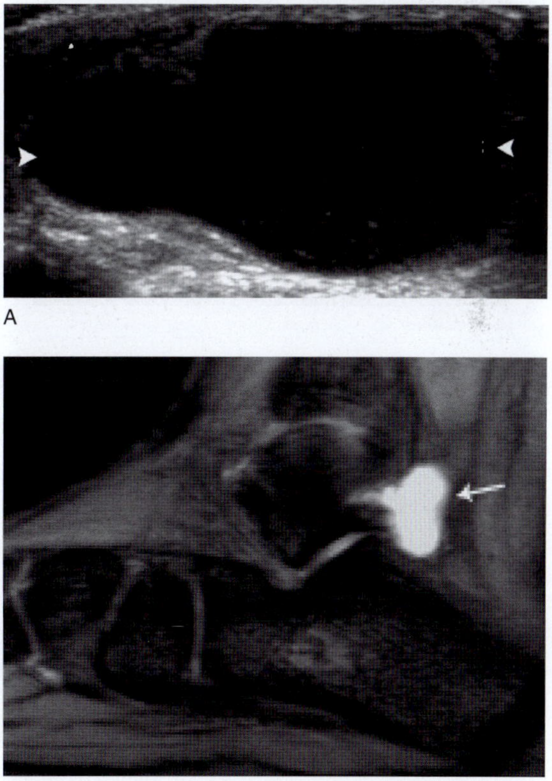

A

B

Figure 12.53 Ganglion. **A** Ultrasound (US) image. The ganglion is seen as an anechoic or black mass at US (between arrowheads) confirming its cystic nature. **B** Sagittal T2-weighted magnetic resonance image. A ganglion posterior to the talus returns uniform high T2-weighted signal (arrow).

high T2-weighted signal (Fig. 12.53B). In certain locations such as the tarsal tunnel, ganglia may cause signs and symptoms of neural compression.

Morton's neuroma

Morton's neuroma is thought to be secondary to chronic entrapment of the plantar digital nerve with subsequent fibrous degeneration of the nerve. The usual location is in the second or third intermetatarsal spaces and there is often adjacent intermetatarsal bursitis. A Morton's neuroma is visualised as a teardrop-shaped soft-tissue mass between the metatarsal heads that is hypoechoic on US and returns low MR signal because of the fibrosis present (Fig. 12.54). On US, a Morton's neuroma may become more obvious by gently squeezing the metatarsal heads as they appear to bulge from between the metatarsal heads and occasionally this can be accompanied by a palpable click, called Mulder's click. Once identified, the Morton's neuroma can be injected under ultrasound guidance.

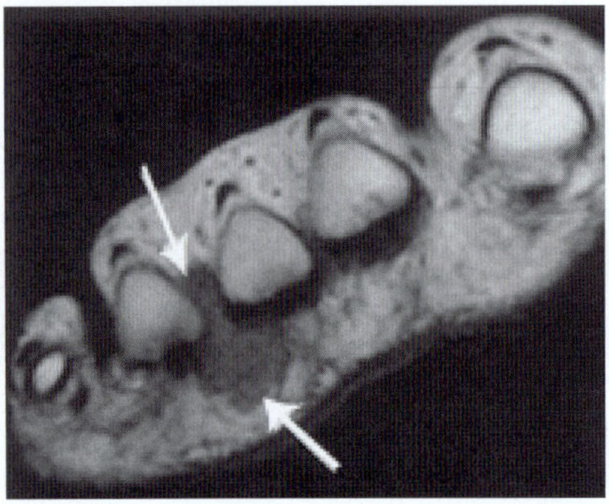

A

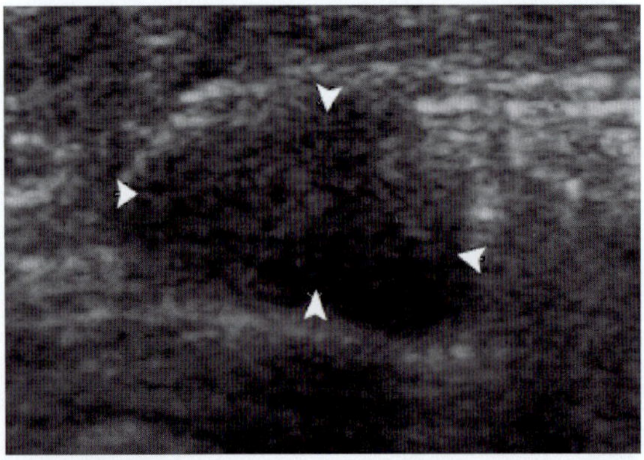

B

Figure 12.54 Morton's neuroma. **A** Axial T1-weighted MR image. A Morton's neuroma is seen as a low signal mass (between arrows) within the normal high signal fat in the third intermetatarsal space. **B** Longitudinal ultrasound image. A neuroma is seen as a hypoechoic mass (between arrowheads) replacing the more echogenic fat within the interspace.

Haemangioma

Haemangiomas are lesions characterised by the presence of vascular channels of various sizes. A soft-tissue haemangioma may contain calcified phleboliths which can be seen on plain radiographs. US is an excellent modality for demonstrating the fatty matrix of the lesion with multiple serpiginous vessels in which blood flow can be detected with Doppler imaging. Other highly vascular lesions may mimic haemangiomas, and MRI should be done if the diagnosis is in doubt.

Lipoma

Lipomas are common benign masses composed of fatty tissue. A lipoma is seen at US as a well-defined uniform echogenic mass. On MRI, a lipoma returns high T1-weighted and T2-weighted fat signal and suppresses on fat saturation or STIR sequences (Fig. 12.55).

Plantar fibromatosis

Plantar fibromatosis is a benign proliferation of fibrous tissue which forms single or multiple discrete nodular thickenings of the plantar fascia. Plantar fibromas are well depicted by US as a well-defined hypoechoic mass superficial to, but intimately related to, the plantar fascia, which itself may be distorted or displaced by the lesion. The nodules appear as low to intermediate signal intensity masses on all MR imaging sequences (Fig. 12.56).

Nerve sheath tumour

Nerve tumours can be divided into neurofibromas and neurilemomas (also known as schwannomas). Neurofibromas are embedded inside the nerve with nerve fascicles traversing them whereas neurilemomas arise at the periphery of the nerve and usually grow eccentrically. A nerve sheath tumour is seen at US and MRI as a well-defined solid fusiform-shaped mass related to the neurovascular bundle. In some cases the nerve is clearly seen entering the lesion at one end and leaving at the opposite edge creating a 'string sign' which is considered pathognomonic. At US, compression of the mass with the transducer can produce peripheral tingling.

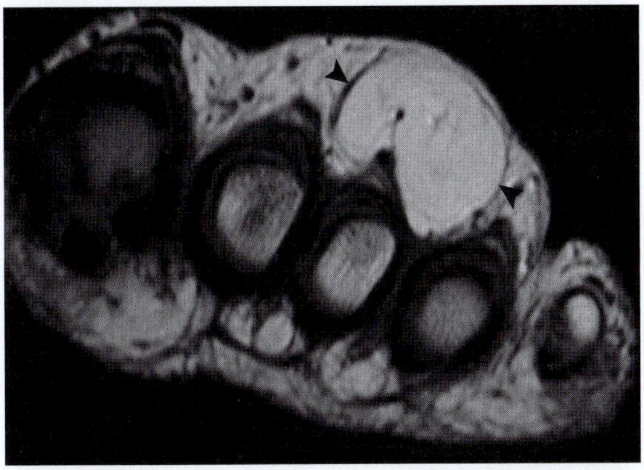

A

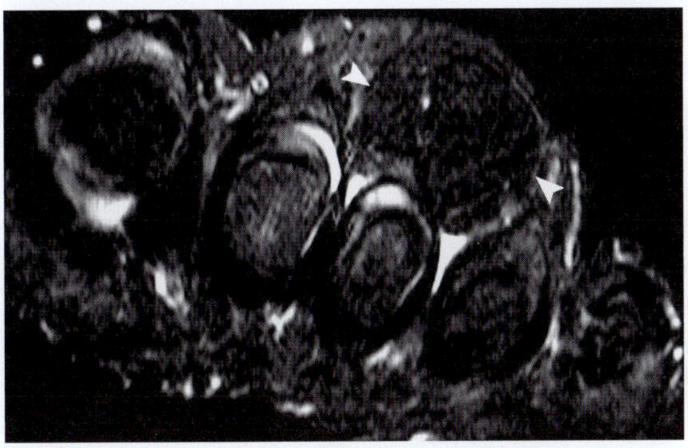

B

Figure 12.55 Lipoma. Axial T1-weighted (**A**) and axial STIR (**B**) magnetic resonance images. A lipoma in the dorsal subcutaneous tissues (between arrowheads) returns high T1-weighted signal and suppresses on the STIR sequence confirming its fatty nature.

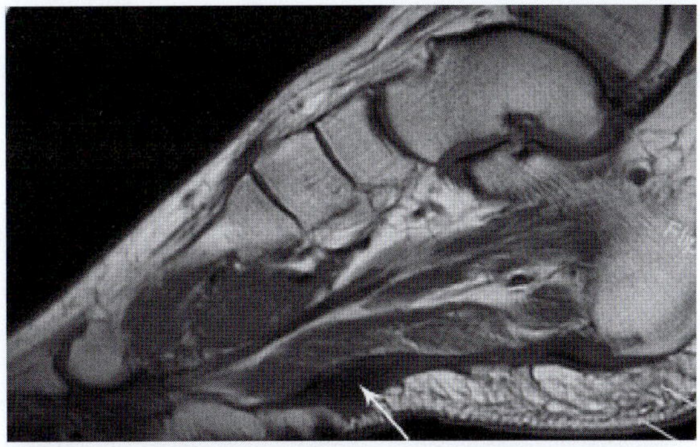

Figure 12.56 Plantar fibroma. Sagittal T2-weighted magnetic resonance image. A plantar fibroma (arrow) is seen as a localised low signal intensity mass arising from the plantar fascia.

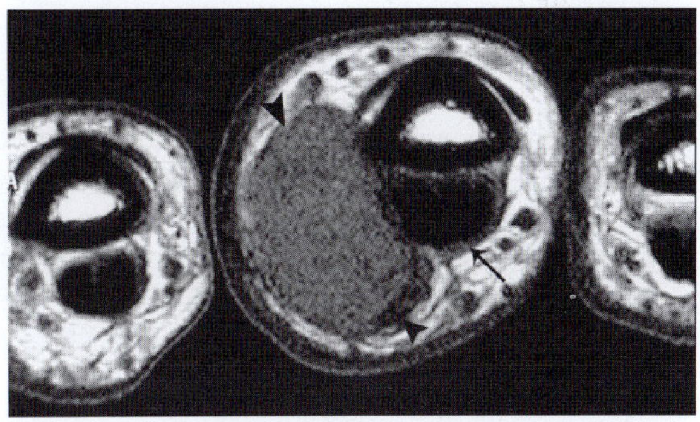

Figure 12.57 Giant cell tumour of tendon sheath. Axial T2-weighted magnetic resonance image. A histologically confirmed giant cell tumour of the tendon sheath (between arrowheads) is closely related to the flexor tendon (arrow) and returns low T2-weighted signal due to internal haemosiderin.

Giant cell tumour of tendon sheath

Giant cell tumours of the tendon sheath are a localised extra-articular form of pigmented villonodular synovitis. As they contain haemosiderin, giant cell tumours return low signal on all MR sequences which is useful in narrowing the pre-biopsy diagnosis (Fig. 12.57). US shows a giant cell tumour of the tendon sheath as a well-defined solid hypoechoic mass intimately related to the tendon sheath; the mass usually demonstrates internal vascularity with Doppler imaging.

IMAGES

Soft-tissue sarcoma

Up to 16% of synovial sarcomas occur in the foot, and it is the most common malignant soft-tissue tumour found in the foot. This is an extra-articular soft-tissue mass that may show scattered calcification in approximately 50% of cases on plain radiographs. There are no specific radiological features of this tumour; it may be infiltrative with adjacent bone destruction but can also appear well defined (Fig. 12.58). Other sarcomas seen around the ankle are liposarcomas and malignant fibrous histiocytomas.

Tendons

Achilles tendon

Achilles tendon is formed by the confluence of the gastrocnemius and soleus tendons and inserts into the os calcis. The normal tendon measures about 7 mm in the anteroposterior dimension and has a flat or concave anterior margin on axial images. On MR

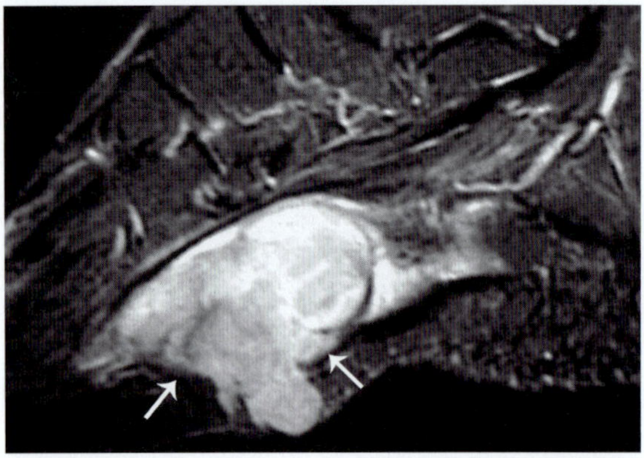

Figure 12.58 Synovial sarcoma. Sagittal STIR magnetic resonance image. An aggressive lobulated soft-tissue mass invades the plantar fascia (between arrows) to extend into the superficial tissues along the plantar aspect of the foot. Histology was consistent with a synovial sarcoma.

imaging, tendons show uniformly low signal intensity on all sequences. At US, the linear parallel pattern of echogenic tendon fibrils can be seen.

Tendinopathy

A thickened Achilles tendon with a convex anterior contour is indicative of a tendinopathy. The tendon may contain partial tears that are seen as linear areas of hypoechogenicity on US and high signal on T2-weighted MR images (Fig. 12.59). Doppler imaging may demonstrate increased vascularity, particularly along the anterior surface of the tendon. The seronegative arthropathies may result in inflammation of the distal Achilles tendon close to its calcaneal insertion. Distal Achilles tendinopathy may also be seen in Haglund's syndrome where a bony protrusion from the posterior superior margin of the calcaneum impinges on the anterior surface of the tendon.

Figure 12.59 Achilles tendinopathy. **A** Sagittal T2-weighted magnetic resonance (MR) image. **B** Longitudinal ultrasound image. Thickening of the mid Achilles tendon is consistent with a tendinopathy (between arrowheads). An intratendinous tear is seen as a linear area of hypoechogenicity on ultrasound and high signal on the MR image (arrow).

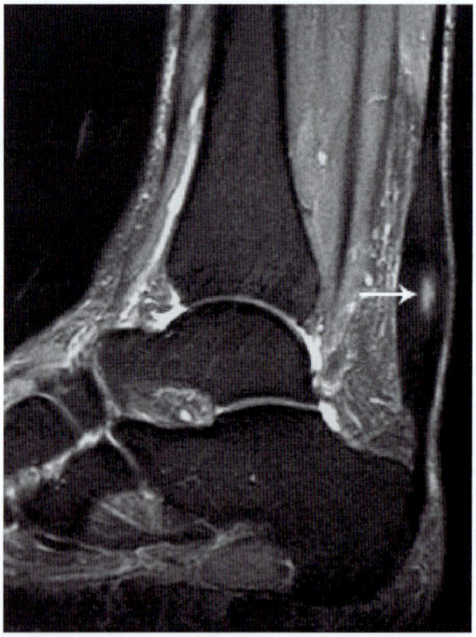

A

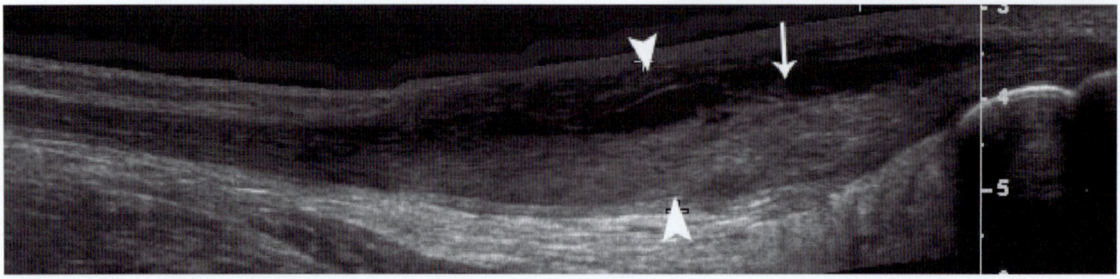

B

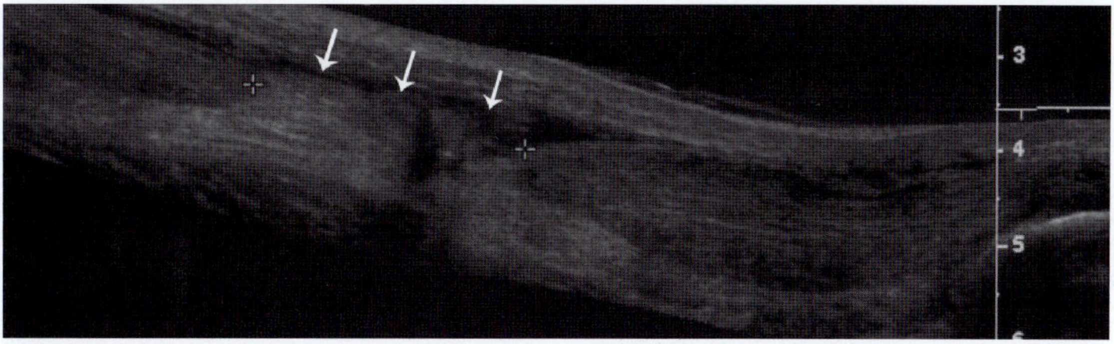

Figure 12.60 Achilles tendon rupture. Longitudinal ultrasound image. Interruption of the normal tendon fibres (arrows) is consistent with an Achilles tendon rupture. The torn tendon ends are retracted (tendon ends demarcated by crosses).

Tendon rupture

Rupture of Achilles tendon most commonly occurs in the mid-portion of the tendon, about 5–6 cm above its insertion. Rupture may also occur at the musculotendinous junction or least commonly, as an avulsion, either from the tendon insertion itself or as an avulsion fracture. US is useful in confirming the diagnosis of Achilles tendon rupture by demonstrating interruption of the normal tendon fibres (Fig. 12.60). The tendon gap is often filled with fluid or haemorrhage. Scanning during dynamic tendon movement with gentle plantar and dorsiflexion of the patient's foot will show discontinuity of movement between the tendon ends and will often open a gap in the tendon that has been previously difficult to see. Approximation of the tendon ends with plantar flexion is important if conservative management is being considered.

Medial and lateral ankle tendons

Tendinopathy

Tendinopathy is seen as an enlarged tendon with loss of the normal fibrillar pattern on US and areas of increased internal signal on T2-weighted MR images (Fig. 12.61). Longitudinal tears which may be present within the tendon are usually seen at the level of the malleoli but may propagate variable distances proximally and distally.

IMAGES

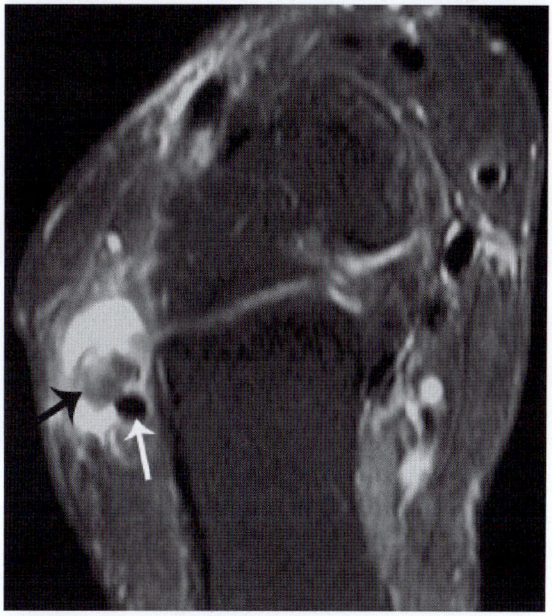

Figure 12.61 Tendinopathy. Axial T2-weighted magnetic resonance image with fat saturation. The peroneus brevis tendon is enlarged and of increased signal intensity consistent with a tendinopathy (black arrow). Fluid is present surrounding the tendon. Compare with the normal peroneus longus tendon (white arrow).

Tenosynovitis

Tenosynovitis is seen on US as hypoechoic fluid within the sheath surrounding the tendon (Fig. 12.62A). Areas of solid synovial thickening are hyperechoic and may have internal vascularity with Doppler imaging. US guided steroid injections into the tendon sheath may be considered if the tendon is normal. If the tendon is abnormal, it is generally felt that injection into the tendon sheath should be avoided as it may predispose the deranged tendon to rupture. On MR imaging, tenosynovitis is best seen

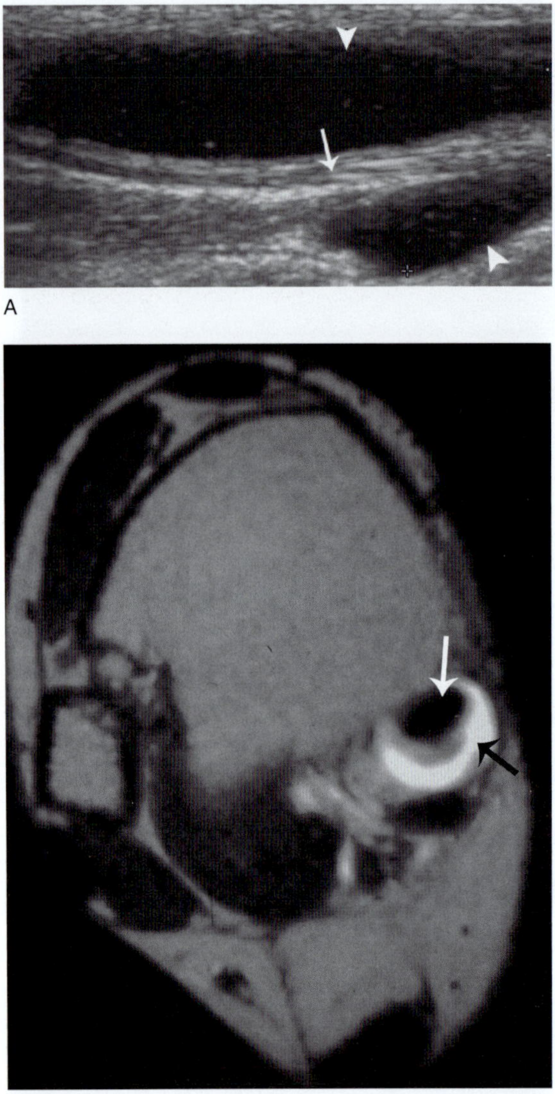

A

B

Figure 12.62 Tenosynovitis. **A** Longitudinal ultrasound image. **B** Axial T2-weighted magnetic resonance (MR) image. The tibialis posterior tendon (white arrows) is surrounded by fluid seen as high signal on the MR image (black arrow) and hypoechoic fluid in the tendon sheath (arrowheads) on ultrasound.

on T2-weighted images with high signal fluid in the tendon sheath surrounding the low signal tendon (Fig. 12.62B). The tendon sheath of flexor hallucis longus communicates with the ankle joint in 20% of people and fluid surrounding the tendon may thus have no significance if an ankle joint effusion is present.

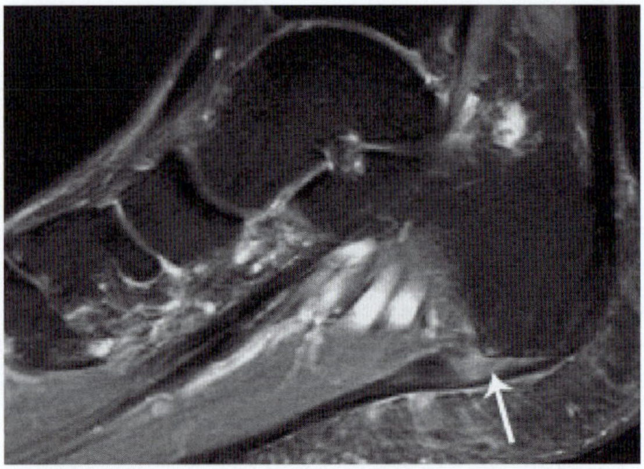

Figure 12.63 Plantar fasciitis. Sagittal STIR magnetic resonance image. The plantar fascia is thickened and returns high signal near its calcaneal insertion (arrow) in keeping with plantar fasciitis.

Tendon subluxation

Rupture of the peroneal retinaculum, with or without an associated fibular fracture, can result in anterior subluxation of the peroneal tendons. US scanning during inversion and eversion of the foot easily confirms the diagnosis of tendon subluxation.

Plantar fascia

The plantar fascia is normally less than 4 mm thick and can be traced from its origin on the undersurface of the calcaneum, along the entire plantar aspect of the foot, where it diverges to join the deep fascia beneath the metatarsal heads.

Plantar fasciitis

Plantar fasciitis is the inflammation of the plantar fascia at its calcaneal attachment, which is seen to be thickened on imaging, measuring greater than 4 mm. The thickened hypoechoic fascia is easily seen at US which can be used to guide injections into the perifascial tissue to help reduce patient's symptoms. On MR imaging, the inflamed plantar fascia returns a high signal on T2-weighted and STIR images (Fig. 12.63). High signal fluid surrounding the fascia and oedema in the adjacent calcaneal bone marrow are common findings.

Ligaments

Among the ankle ligaments, tears occur most commonly in the anterior talofibular ligament. Anterior talofibular ligament tears are seen on US as disrup-

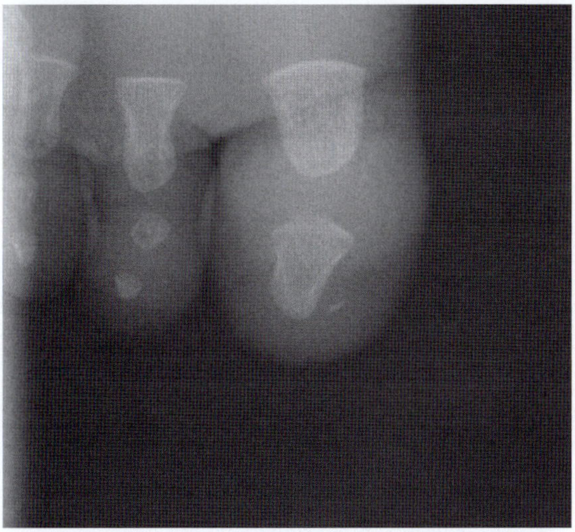

Figure 12.64 Foreign body. Dorsiplantal radiograph. A radiopaque foreign body is present. Medial to the first distal phalanx.

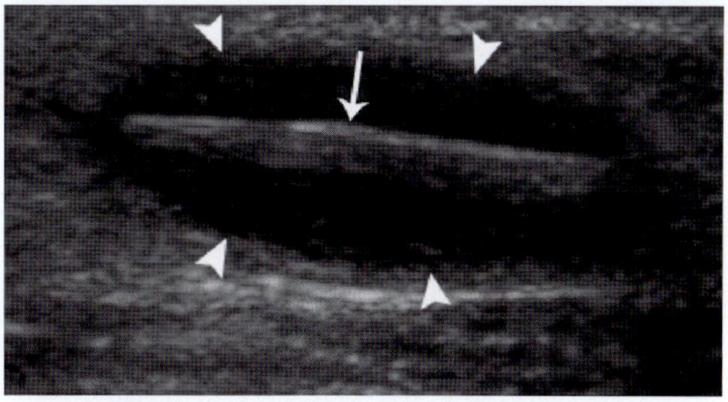

Figure 12.65 Foreign body. Longitudinal ultrasound image. A linear echogenic foreign body (arrow) is surrounded by hypoechoic inflammatory tissue (arrowheads) forming a foreign body granuloma.

tion of the normal organised ligamentous structure which becomes a hypoechoic mass anterior and inferior to the fibula. Varus stress can increase the sensitivity of the examination. On MR imaging, an acute tear is seen as a discontinuous low signal ligament with surrounding oedema and fluid extending anterior to the ligament. A chronic tear may show discontinuity of the ligament, but scarring often occurs so that the ligament appears intact but irregular and thickened.

Foreign bodies

Injuries from foreign body penetration are common in the foot. Radiopaque material will be seen as areas of increased density on X-ray (**Fig. 12.64**). More than one view is often necessary to locate the foreign body. Most foreign bodies such as glass, plastic, thorns and wood splinters are not radiopaque and cannot be seen on radiographs. Small foreign bodies may migrate from the site of entry through the skin to a more distant site. US is an excellent technique for identifying foreign bodies, which are seen as echogenic structures surrounded by hypoechoic inflammatory tissue (Fig. 12.65).

IMAGES

Conclusion

Diagnostic imaging has an important role in the assessment of foot and ankle pathology. The imaging technique needs to be tailored to the clinical question and relevant clinical information is essential. The plain radiograph is the most important initial imaging modality and should always be available for comparison if other radiological techniques are used. MRI is an excellent technique where symptoms are diffuse and the diagnosis is uncertain as it can exclude most clinically relevant pathologies. MRI is particularly sensitive in demonstrating bone marrow pathology and provides excellent soft-tissue contrast resolution. Computed tomography gives high-quality bone detail and is valuable in characterisation of bone-based pathology. US is an excellent tool for imaging focal soft-tissue abnormalities and allows dynamic real-time scanning which is useful in guiding interventional procedures. Doppler imaging can detect and measure blood flow in areas of active inflammation and vascular mass lesions. Nuclear isotope scanning is highly sensitive in detecting pathology anywhere in the skeleton, however, it is not specific. Fluoroscopy is important in guiding interventional procedures. In the light of the diagnostic imaging findings, practitioners may direct their knowledge, skills and clinical findings to complete the clinical diagnosis and plan appropriate treatment.

Further reading

Backhaus M, Kamradt T, Sandrock D et al 1999 Arthritis of the finger joints: a comprehensive approach comparing conventional radiography, scintigraphy, ultrasound and contrast enhanced magnetic resonance imaging. Arthritis Rheum 42:1232–1245

Bedi D G, Davidson D M 2001 Plantar fibromatosis. Most common sonographic appearance and variations. Journal of Clinical Ultrasound 29:499–505

Berkowitz J F, Kier R, Rudicel S 1991 Plantar fasciitis: MR imaging. Radiology 179:665–667

Berquist T 2000 Radiology of the foot and ankle, 2nd edn. Lippincott, Williams & Wilkins

Bontrager K L 1993 Textbook of radiographic positioning and related anatomy, 3rd edn. Mosby Year Book, pp 190–197

Buckwalter K A, Rydberg J, Kopecky K K et al 2001 Musculoskeletal imaging with multislice CT. Pictorial essay. American Journal of Roentgenology 176:979–986

Cardinal E, Chhem R K, Beauregard C G et al 1996 Plantar fasciitis: sonographic evaluation. Radiology 201:257–259

Chatha D S, Cunningham P M, Schweitzer M E 2005 MR imaging of the diabetic foot: diagnostic challenges. Radiology Clinics of North America 43:747–759

Cheung Y, Rosenberg Z S, Magee T et al 1992 Normal anatomy and pathologic conditions of ankle tendons: current imaging techniques. Radiographics 12:429–444

Christman R 2003 Foot and ankle radiology. Churchill Livingstone, St Louis, USA

Clark K C 1986 Positioning in Radiography, 11th edn. William Heinemann Medical Books, pp 89–107

Conaghan P G, Wakefield R, O'Connor P et al 1999 The metacarpophalangeal joints in early arthritis: a comparison of clinical, radiographic, MRI and ultrasonographic findings. Annals of Rheumatic Diseases 28 (Suppl)

Craig J G, Amin M B, Wu K et al 1997 Osteomyelitis of the diabetic foot: MR imaging – pathologic correlation. Radiology 203:849–855

Gentili A, Masih S, Yao L et al 1996 Pictorial review: foot axes and angles. British Journal of Radiology 69:968–974

Greenspan A 2004 Orthopaedic imaging. A practical approach, 4th edn. Lippincott Williams Wilkins, Philadelphia, pp 17–37, 293–311

Greenspan A, Stadalnik R C 1997 A musculoskeletal radiologist's view of nuclear medicine. Seminars in Nuclear Medicine 27:372–385

Gumann G 2004 Fractures of the foot and ankle. Elsevier Saunders, Philadelphia, USA

Helms C A 1995 Fundamentals of skeletal radiology, 2nd edn. W B Saunders Philadelphia, p 7–55, 111–145, 146–160

Kang H, Ahn J, Resnick D 2002 MRI of the extremities. An anatomical text. W B Saunders, Philadelphia, USA

Lin J, Fessell D P, Jacobson J A et al 2000 An illustrated tutorial of musculoskeletal sonography. American Journal of Roentgenology 175:637–645, 1313–1321

Lin J, Martel W 2001 Cross sectional imaging of peripheral nerve sheath tumours: characteristic signs on CT, MR imaging and sonography. American Journal of Roentgenology 176:75–82

Llauger J, Palmer J, Monill J M et al 1998 MR imaging of benign soft tissue masses of the foot and ankle. Radiographics 18:1481–1498

Love C, Din A S, Tomas M B et al 2003 Radionuclide bone imaging: an illustrative review. Radiographics 23:341–358

Morrison W B, Schweitzer M E, Wapner K L et al 1994 Plantar fibromatosis: a benign aggressive neoplasm with a characteristic appearance on MR images. Radiology 193:841–845

Oestreich A E 1990 How to measure angles from foot radiographs: a primer. Springer Verlag, pp 1–48

Pham H, Fessell D P, Femino J E et al 2003 Sonography and MR imaging of selected benign masses in the ankle and foot. American Journal of Roentgenology 180:99–107

Quinnn T J, Jacobson J A, Craig J G, et al 2000 Sonography of Morton's neuromas. American Journal of Roentgenology 174:1723–1728

Raby N, Berman L, de Lacey G 2005 Accident and emergency radiology: a survival guide. Elsevier Saunders 216–235

Rosenberg Z 2001 Magnetic Resonance Imaging: update on the foot and ankle. 9(3) Clinics of North America

Rosenberg Z S, Beltran J, Bencardino J T 2000 MR imaging of the ankle and foot. Radiographics 20:153–179

Schneck C D, Mesgarzadeh M, Bonakdarpour A et al 1992 MR imaging of the most commonly injured ankle ligaments II: ligament injuries. Radiology 184:507–512

Sobiesk G A, Wertheimer S J, Schulz R et al 1997 Sonographic evaluation of interdigital neuromas. Journal of Foot and Ankle Surgery 36:364–366

Steinbach L S 1998 Painful syndromes around the foot and ankle: magnetic resonance imaging evaluation. Topics in Magnetic Resonance Imaging 9:311–326

CHAPTER

13

Laboratory tests

A Percivall

Indicates figures on DVD, including colour

Chapter contents

Introduction

This chapter provides an overview of laboratory tests which can be performed on tissue and fluid samples from the lower limb. The tests of most relevance are:

- microbiology
- urinalysis
- blood analysis – haematology, biochemistry and serology
- histology.

These tests have a vital role in enabling the practitioner to understand the nature of local and systemic-related pathologies affecting the lower limb. Data from these tests can be used to:

- aid the diagnostic process
- enable a definitive diagnosis to be made in situations where there may be several possible diagnoses
- measure the disease process in relation to normal parameters
- reveal occult disease processes that might affect therapeutic and treatment options
- enable implementation of effective treatment.

The accuracy of any laboratory test is determined by its sensitivity, specificity, predictive value and efficiency. Sensitivity indicates how often a positive test result is obtained from a patient with a particular disease, whereas specificity indicates the number of negative results from patients without a particular disease. Predictive values of positive test results give a measure of the frequency of the disease among all patients who test positive for that disease. The efficiency of a test indicates the percentage of patients correctly diagnosed with a particular pathology.

Some of the tests can be undertaken in the clinic (near-patient testing) but most require the use of laboratory services. Because of the expense, ethical issues regarding testing, and possible inconvenience related to some of the tests, it is important that they are only used where appropriate.

Microbiology

Indications for microbiology

Practitioners often request microbiological analysis to determine which particular organism is causing an obvious infection. However, the process can often be wasteful of both time and resources. Organisms found and identified in the laboratory usually fall into two categories: they either reflect the normal microbial flora or they fall outside this group and may be considered pathogens. It must be remembered that some normally resident organisms have the propensity to cause disease when found in abnormal sites. Conversely, just because a normal resident organism has been isolated at an abnormal site, it may not be the causative agent of the disease as commensals often contaminate samples sent to the laboratory. Further, the distinction between a pathogenic organism and a non-pathogen is often imprecise, e.g. where a person is a 'carrier' of a disease. This has led to the adoption of two basic rules:

- Never without good reason dismiss a microbe as a contaminant because it is not an 'accepted' pathogen.
- Never without good reason accept a microbe as the *necessary* cause of a disease merely because it is an 'accepted' pathogen.

Microorganisms are classified into four main groups: viruses, protozoa, bacteria and fungi. In podiatry, with the exception of some superficial mycoses, most infections are caused by bacteria. Some viral infections of the foot do occur: the main protagonist is the human papilloma virus (HPV), which gives rise to plantar warts or verrucae.

As with other forms of laboratory testing, microbiological testing should only be considered when it is likely to serve a useful purpose. The circumstances where it is applicable are:

- when the results of testing may influence the choice of treatment and result in more effective treatment for the patient
- if the results will help identify sources of infection that need to be traced.

Sampling techniques

Specimen types

Specimens may be divided into two groups: those from normally sterile sites and sites containing a normal resident flora. The differentiation is important since samples taken from normally sterile sites need to be inoculated into enrichment media. The media provides nutrients that will allow rapid growth (or amplification) of the organisms so that enough will be available for identification. Specimens taken from sites which have resident flora will, in contrast, need to be inoculated into media containing selective agents which will suppress the growth of any commensal organisms that might mask a potential pathogen.

Ideally, when microbiological information is needed, an appropriate specimen is taken from the correct site. The specimen is transported immediately to the laboratory where it is processed quickly using the best tests, which are then correctly reported; these results are returned to the originator where they can be properly interpreted at a time when the information is relevant. Thus, it is important that the results of the work done in the laboratory are a true reflection of that specimen. Reasons for failure to report an organism originally present in a specimen are shown in Box 13.1.

It is imperative to use reputable laboratories that employ strict internal standards and where reagents and media are performance-tested using standard organisms. If this procedure is adhered to, failure to report pathogens often rests with the sampling technique employed by the requesting practitioner. It is essential to follow certain guidelines (Box 13.2) in order to obtain quality samples.

Even if the guidelines given in Box 13.2 have been adhered to, in order to be effective the laboratory requires good clinical information about the patient. It is imperative that the site of the suspected infection is stated. The symptoms should be included on the clinical history section and it is important to

Box 13.1 Reasons for failure to report an organism originally present in a specimen

- A delay in examination
- The amount of specimen was insufficient
- The amount of medium into which the specimen was inoculated was insufficient
- The medium used for inoculation was of doubtful quality or unsuitable for the growth of the organism present
- The incubation time of the inoculated medium was too short or the wrong conditions were provided
- Too few colonies were examined or the organism was not recognised

Box 13.2 Guidelines to obtain good-quality specimens

- The sample should be taken from the actual site of an infection or from where it is suspected
- Skin should not be cleaned with an antiseptic prior to taking the sample
- Strict aseptic technique must be followed to reduce the risk of the sample becoming contaminated by the microbiological flora of either the patient or the person taking the sample
- Many pathogenic organisms are surprisingly delicate. Unless special measures are taken they do not survive for long away from the body. This means it is often vital that specimens are transported to the laboratory without delay
- If some delay in transporting specimens is anticipated, it is important that steps are taken to prevent significant growth of contaminating organisms that can grow at room temperature and swamp the genuine pathogen. Suppression is normally achieved by refrigeration or inclusion of an inhibitor in the transport medium.
- It is important that sufficient sample is supplied so that the laboratory may use different methods for culture analysis of the sample and thus maximise the chances of providing meaningful results
- If at all possible, samples should be taken prior to the commencement of antibiotic therapy. A drug may suppress a pathogen sufficiently to thwart isolation and identification, without actually working well enough to allow the patient to recover
- It is often desirable for practitioners to wait for the initial results from the laboratory before starting antibiotic therapy. The results allow practitioners to choose a narrow-spectrum drug that they can be confident will do the job. However, if a life-threatening infection is suspected, then a broad-spectrum antibiotic should be prescribed without delay
- Specimens taken for microbiological analysis are by their very nature likely to contain pathogenic organisms and should, therefore, be treated with care
- Good documentation is vital to ensure that samples are not mixed up, lost or subject to inappropriate tests
- It is vital that there is dialogue between the practitioner taking the sample and the laboratory staff. For more unusual organisms the microbiologist may be able to provide advice about the most appropriate methods of sampling and transportation.

note recent treatment with antibiotics. Is there anything in the patient's history or in the clinical features (e.g. colour of pus, cellulitis) that may provide a clue as to the type of organism that is causing the problem? Without this sort of detailed information, valuable time and resources may be wasted in inappropriate analyses. There is provision for all these data on the laboratory request form, which also has an integral bag for the inclusion of the specimen (Fig. 13.1).

Apparatus for obtaining specimens

Containers

Strong leakproof sterile containers of adequate size, conforming to the relevant British Standards specification, must be used to transport specimens from source to laboratory. These British Standards pay attention to minimising the health hazard from leakage, aerosol formation or spread of airborne particles when opening containers holding specimens.

Containers range from 6 ml 'bijou' bottles, with screw caps suitable for body fluids, transport media and biological cultures, to large 300 ml bottles suitable for early morning urine samples and sanitary specimens. Whatever container is used, it must be clearly labelled in indelible ink with sufficient space for name, address, date and nature of specimen together with the time the specimen was taken. The label should have a water-resistant back.

Swabs

Bacteriological swabs are often made from a pledget of Dacron (Terylene) attached to the end of a holder made from wood, plastic or metal, the whole of which is sterilised before use. Cotton wool pledgets can be used, but they may release lipoproteins, which can harm some fastidious bacteria. Swabs are the instrument of choice for collection of samples where microbial contamination or infection is suspected. Sterilised swabs with or without transport media are available commercially (Fig. 13.2).

Collection of samples

Wounds and mucosal surfaces

If a large quantity of pus is present this may be drained and sent to the laboratory; otherwise, a swab should be taken. Great care should be taken to avoid contamination with the normal flora from surrounding healthy tissue. It is important that a sample is taken from the base of the wound (Fig. 13.3). If the

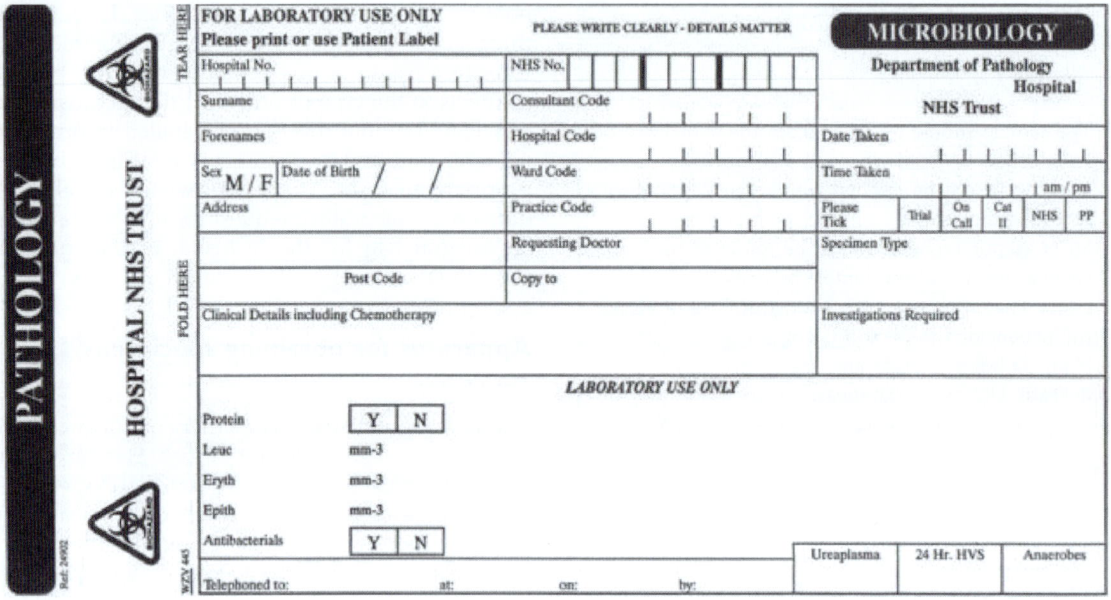
PATHOLOGY

HOSPITAL NHS TRUST

TEAR HERE

FOLD HERE

FOR LABORATORY USE ONLY
Please print or use Patient Label

PLEASE WRITE CLEARLY - DETAILS MATTER

MICROBIOLOGY
Department of Pathology
Hospital
NHS Trust

Hospital No. | NHS No.
Surname | Consultant Code
Forenames | Hospital Code | Date Taken
Sex M / F | Date of Birth / / | Ward Code | Time Taken am / pm
Address | Practice Code | Please Tick | Trial | On Call | Cat II | NHS | PP
Requesting Doctor | Specimen Type
Post Code | Copy to
Clinical Details including Chemotherapy | Investigations Required

LABORATORY USE ONLY

Protein Y N
Leuc mm-3
Eryth mm-3
Epith mm-3
Antibacterials Y N

Ureaplasma | 24 Hr. HVS | Anaerobes

Telephoned to: at: on: by:

Ref: 24902

WZV 445

Figure 13.1 Laboratory request form.

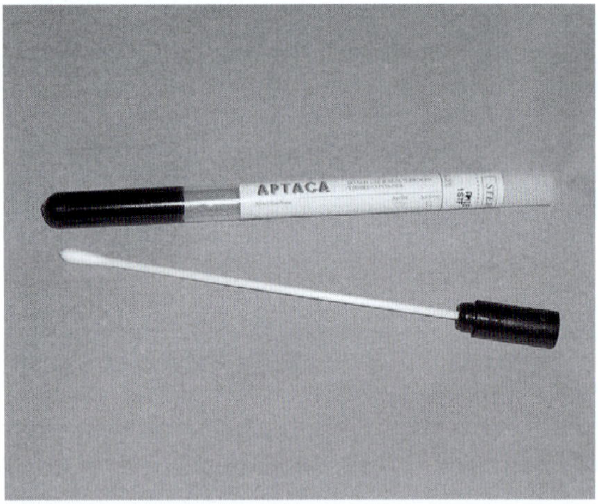

Figure 13.2 Example swab.

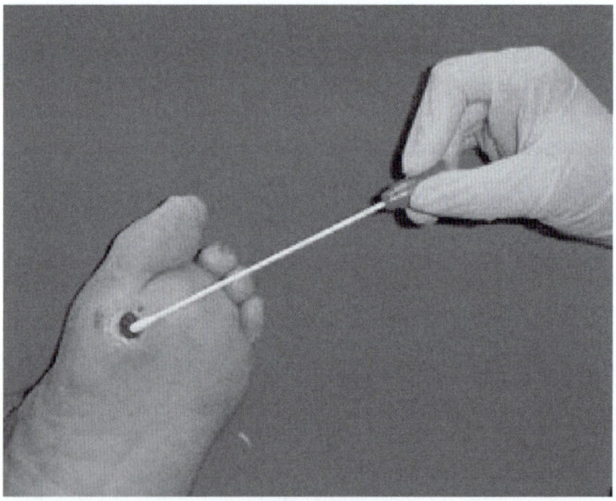

Figure 13.3 Taking a wound swab.

swab is taken from the superficial edges, the flora of the adjacent skin could contaminate it. Swabs are placed into tubes containing a semi-solid transport medium, which prevents them from drying out.

Skin

For mycological (fungal) investigations, nail clippings or skin scrapings from the edge of the lesion, taken with a blunt scalpel, can be placed in either a purpose-designed packet which has a black/dark blue inner surface to help identify the sample (Fig. 13.4), or a clean, dry plastic container.

Once the sample has been obtained it should be sent directly to the laboratory. Accompanying the sample will be a laboratory request form. Accurate information will enable the laboratory staff to carry out the most appropriate tests and investigations quickly, and thus provide the clinician with the results without delay. Laboratory request forms vary, but it is important that the following information is

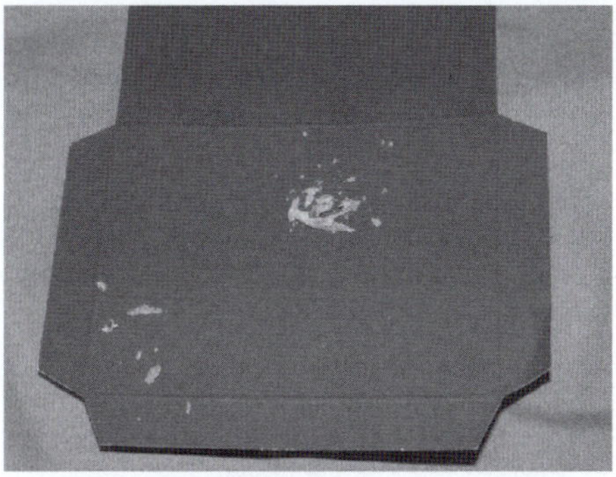

Figure 13.4 Fungal nail clippings on blue paper.

IMAGES

included:

- The patient's name.
- The ward name or place where the sample was taken.
- The patient's date of birth – resident flora change with age and it is therefore helpful to the laboratory staff in their investigations.
- Date of admission to hospital – useful for infection control staff to monitor nosocomial infection.
- Site of infection – be as specific as possible, it will help laboratory staff distinguish commensals from pathogenic flora.
- Antibiotic therapy – even small amounts of antibiotic inhibit the growth of micro-organisms in the laboratory.
- Date and time of collection of the specimen – microorganisms survive or multiply at varying rates and, thus, this information is important when the sample is cultured.
- Specimen type and investigation requested – remember most swabs look the same when they arrive in the laboratory, therefore state clearly what the specimen is. State whether the sample is for microculture and sensitivity (MC&S), for virology or serology.
- Biohazard status – if suspected, then the sample should not only be marked as such but should be transported in double-wrapped specimen bags.

Laboratory examination

When samples containing suspected bacterial or fungal pathogens are sent to the laboratory, the most appropriate methods for investigation will be carried out. The methods used fall into the following categories:

- direct examination – macroscopy and microscopy
- culture
- biochemical tests
- sensitivity testing
- serology and antigen testing
- pathogenicity testing in animals.

Macroscopy

Direct examination of the sample may give clues to the presence of infection or other factors. Turbid cerebrospinal fluid or the presence of pus in urine is immediate evidence of infection. The foul smell of anaerobic organisms may be detected in pus. Macroscopy will also show if there has been any contamination of the specimen, for example if the swab smells of disinfectant, rendering the sample useless. Most specimens will, however, need to be examined under a microscope.

Microscopy

Although it is possible to examine specimens directly as an unstained preparation, more information can be obtained by staining the organisms present. However, there are often only a few organisms present and although these can be concentrated in some samples by, for example, centrifuging cerebrospinal fluid, it is usual to stain organisms obtained after culture. The use of microscopy on non-cultured specimens is most valuable when the sample has been obtained from a normally sterile site and thus the presence of any organism indicates infection.

The most widely used stain is Gram's stain: gentian violet in Gram's stain binds to the cell wall of Gram-positive organisms and resists decolorisation with methanol or acetone. Those cells decolorised and stained with a counterstain, to make them visible, are classified as Gram-negative bacteria. The Gram stain immediately separates most bacteria into two groups and this together with other factors significantly aids diagnosis (Fig. 13.5). The other commonly used stain is the Ziehl–Neelsen stain for acid-fast bacteria such as *Mycobacterium* spp.

Staining and subsequent microscopy can be rapidly done and is often more valuable than culture – it can take up to 8 weeks to obtain a culture result in mycobacterial disease – to give a presumptive diagnosis of potentially life-threatening diseases. Other microscopic techniques such as dark ground, immunofluorescence and electron microscopy are used in specific cases, the last being especially useful for viruses.

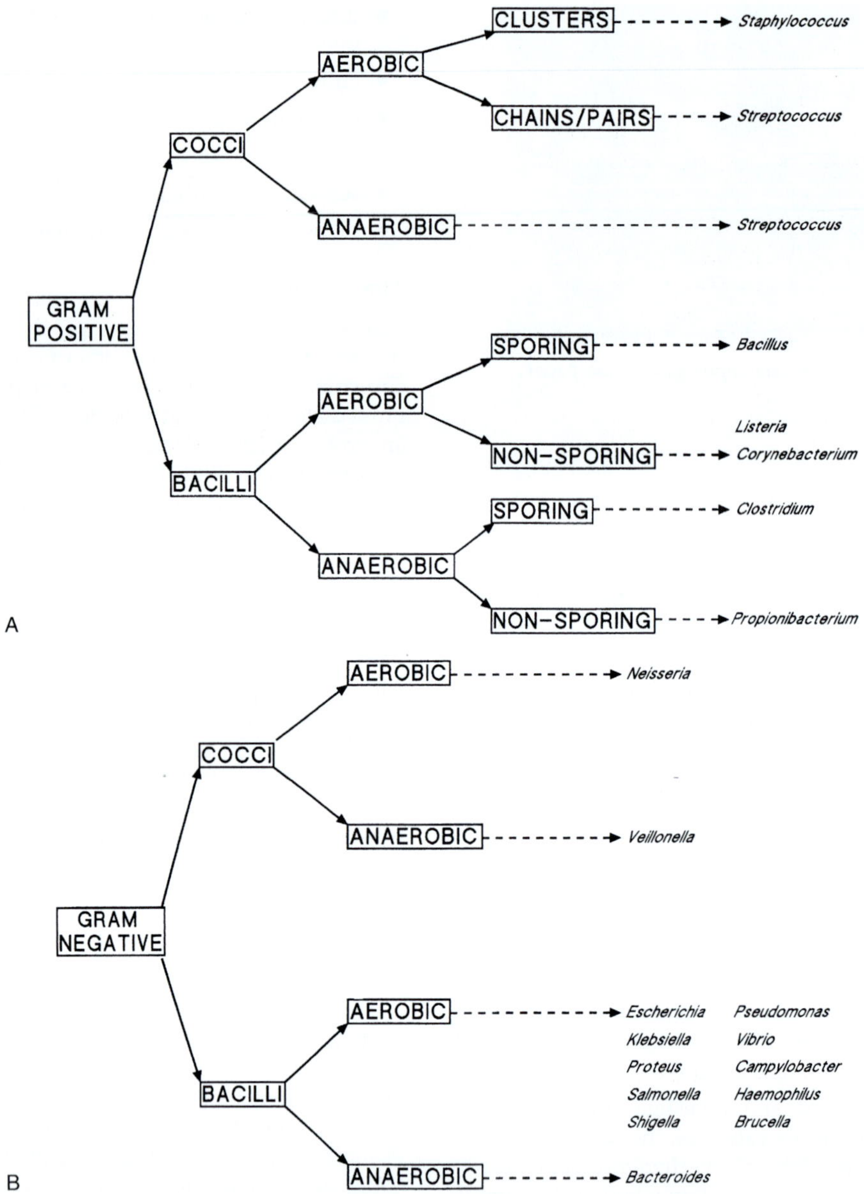

Figure 13.5 Bacteria classified by staining, shape and use of oxygen. **A** Gram-positive bacterial. **B** Gram-negative bacteria.

Fungal hyphae and spores can often be seen under the light microscope: skin scrapings with suspected dermatophyte infection are mounted on a slide, cleared with 10% potassium hydroxide and stained with lactophenol blue. This simple procedure can often be done by the clinician without recourse to the laboratory, thus giving an instant diagnosis. Culture of these specimens can take 2–3 weeks. Many patients will have been prescribed a topical antifungal medicament based on the clinical features of the disease which, if caused by a dermatophyte, should be well on the way to resolution by the time the results are reported.

Culture

Culture allows either the amplification of organisms initially present only in small numbers or selection of organisms from mixed inocula. Media for cultivation of bacteria and fungi must be capable of satisfying all their nutritional requirements and provide appropriate conditions which satisfy any factors which may affect their metabolism such as temperature, pH, osmolarity, oxygen, carbon dioxide and radiation.

Culture media fall into the following classes:

- Synthetic or defined media – prepared entirely from organic or inorganic chemicals such that the exact composition is known and is repeatable on any occasion.
- Routine media – prepared from a mixture of digested or extracted animal or plant protein, such as beef or soya bean. They are usually supplemented with accessory growth factors and the pH adjusted to 7.4.
- Enrichment media – usually routine media with specific additions such as whole blood, serum or additional sugars, for the growth of more exacting organisms.
- Selective media – routine media to which has been added selectively inhibitory chemicals that suppress or kill all but a few types of (known) organisms.
- Indicator media – routine media with the addition of substances which change the appearance of the media when a particular organism grows on it: for example, haemolysis of red blood cells by haemolytic bacteria.

Identification of microorganisms

Bacteria

It is first necessary to isolate the microorganism in pure culture before carrying out identification tests. This is usually achieved by streaking or spreading the initial inoculum on the surface of solid selective media to produce isolated colonies of the desired organism. A colony is then selected and may need subculturing in routine or enriched media to restore normal growth before examination. Table 13.1 lists the bacterial pathogens typically found in the lower limb. The process of identification usually involves the following steps.

Morphology

Stained microscopic mounts are examined for size, shape, cell aggregates, the presence of spores, etc. Hanging drop mounts of living organisms are examined for motility and special techniques can be applied for the examination of capsules and flagellae.

Staining reaction

The Gram stain is the most important of the staining reactions and, in conjunction with the morphology, is often enough to narrow the field considerably. Staining with malachite green will show the bacterial spores in *Bacillus* and *Clostridium* spp., the position of which in the cell can determine the species.

Cultural characteristics

The size, shape and colour of colonies on solid media are sometimes helpful in diagnosis but are not sufficiently stable enough to be of routine value. However, the ability of an organism to grow on different media, including the stimulatory effects of added substances such as glucose, whole blood or serum, can be significant, e.g. the degree of haemolysis of blood incorporated into the media is used to differentiate streptococci. Alpha-haemolytic streptococci such as *Streptococcus pneumoniae* produce colonies which are surrounded by a green ring, whereas *Strep. pyogenes*, a beta-haemolytic bacterium that is responsible for human throat infections, grows with a clear ring around it where the blood cells have been completely lysed (**Figs 13.6, 13.7**). These characteristics of colony growth of bacteria are accompanied by observations of the optimum temperature and pH ranges for growth and any pigment that may be produced. The gaseous requirements of organisms can also be diagnostic. Some bacteria are obligate aerobes (e.g. *Bordetella*), but others (e.g. *Pseudomonas aeruginosa*), which usually use molecular oxygen, are capable of using nitrate if cultured anaerobically. Anaerobes are either facultative (i.e. they can grow either aerobically or anaerobically) or obligate. Other factors such as the ability to grow in the presence of antibiotics, bile salts and high salt concentration should also be noted.

Biochemical reactions

The ability of organisms to use particular substrates with a detectable end product, such as sugars, is a widely tested function. A range of these biochemical tests are available, including fermentation patterns, catalase, oxidase and nitrate production, and are, perhaps, the most useful aids to identification. For example, if a positive identification of Gram-positive cocci has been made, a catalase test can be done to aid further diagnosis. Staphylococci and streptococci are both commonly found cocci. Staphylococci are catalase-positive and are able to produce bubbles of oxygen when incubated with hydrogen peroxide.

Table 13.1 Bacterial pathogens found in infections of the lower limb

Bacterium	*Gram reaction*	*Atmosphere*	*Morphology*	*Notes*
Staphylococcus aureus	Gram-positive	Aerobe	Coccus	Most frequent cause of foot infections. Able to form an enzyme which coagulates citrated plasma: therefore the infection tends to remain localised. Commonest pathogen in foot sepsis and osteomyelitis
Streptococcus pyogenes	Gram-positive	Aerobe or anaerobe	Coccus	All strains are beta-haemolytic. Produce enzymes which help break down surrounding connective tissue and thus aid spread. May lead to cellulitis, lymphangitis and lymphadenitis. May be prime organism responsible for necrotising fasciitis
Pseudomonas aeruginosa	Gram-negative	Aerobe	Bacillus	Gives rise to blue–green pus and produces a pungent odour. May be found in paronychia alongside *Candida albicans*
Escherichia coli	Gram-negative	Aerobe	Bacillus	Usually found in gut but may be present in mixed infections and can be found alongside *Candida albicans* in paronychia
Klebsiella spp.	Gram-negative	Aerobe	Bacillus	Found in the gut but may be present in mixed infections
Proteus spp.	Gram-negative	Aerobe	Bacillus	Found in the gut but may be present in mixed infections
Corynebacterium minutissimum	Gram-positive	Aerobe	Bacillus	Responsible for erythrasma and pitted keratolysis
Clostridium welchii	Gram-positive	Anaerobe	Bacillus	Responsible for gas gangrene

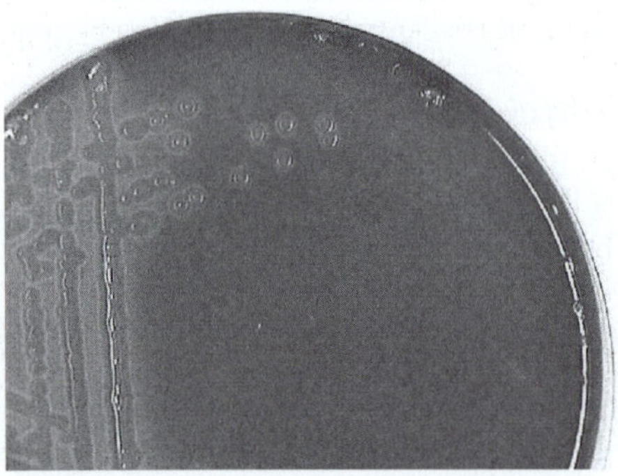

Figure 13.6 Alpha-haemolytic streptococci (*S. pneumoniae*).

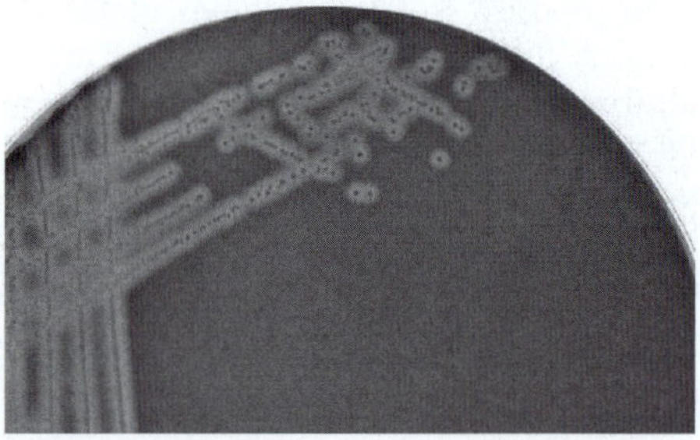

Figure 13.7 Beta-haemolytic Streptococci (*S. pyogenes*).

Streptococci, which are catalase-negative, do not react in this way and no oxygen is produced. This may help identify, say, a colony of staphylococci, but it does not help with identification of the species within the genus. A mannitol fermentation test may be able to determine if the colony consists of *Staphylococcus aureus* or *Staph. epidermidis*, since *Staph. aureus* tests positive, whereas *Staph. epidermidis* does not. Ready-made kits for multiple biochemical analyses are freely available commercially to enable complex tests to be carried out simultaneously with remarkable accuracy. All help to build a pattern of the metabolic activity of the organism, which – together with the information gained from microscopic and cultural examination – may be sufficient to identify the organism.

Sensitivity testing

Once the organism has been identified, the susceptibility of the organism is often predictable. However, not all organisms have predictable resistance patterns and, thus, testing for sensitivity to particular antibiotics is required. Perhaps the most common method used to test antibiotic sensitivity is disc diffusion. A Petri dish is inoculated to produce a lawn of the test organism and an antibiotic-impregnated disc containing a range of antibiotics at concentrations comparable with therapeutic plasma levels is placed on the surface of the lawn (**Fig. 13.8**).

Inhibition of growth around the disc indicates the organism is sensitive to the antibiotic. Although this test indicates sensitivity of the organism, it does not show the lowest concentration (minimum inhibitory concentration, MIC) at which the antibiotic will inhibit growth of the microorganism. Although a relationship between MIC and successful outcome of antimicrobial chemotherapy cannot be clearly established, it is considered the most useful guide to the efficacy of antimicrobial therapy. Several methods of obtaining the MIC are available, and recently commercial test strips of paper with antibiotic incorporated along its length in increasing concentration have simplified the test. These test strips are put on a lawn inoculum of the test organism and the point at which the growth meets the test strip corresponds to the MIC (**Fig. 13.9**). From these figures the minimum bactericidal concentration (MBC) can be determined; this is defined as the lowest concentration that prevents growth after subculture to an antibiotic-free medium. These figures are required where accuracy of dose is important, e.g. in treating the immunocompromised patient.

Serological and bacteriophage testing

It is often possible to identify bacteria by determining their antigenic composition. This can be achieved by incorporating suspensions of the organism in a series of standardised solutions of purified antibodies. Where agglutination occurs, it can be inferred that the organism possesses a specific antigen against which that antibody was originally prepared. Bacteriophages are also highly specific in their lytic action of bacteria. Thus, stock preparations of known phages can be used in a similar way to antisera, allowing precise identification of variants within species, e.g. staphylococci.

Animal tests

The identification of pathogenic organisms may require the use of animal inoculation but is only of

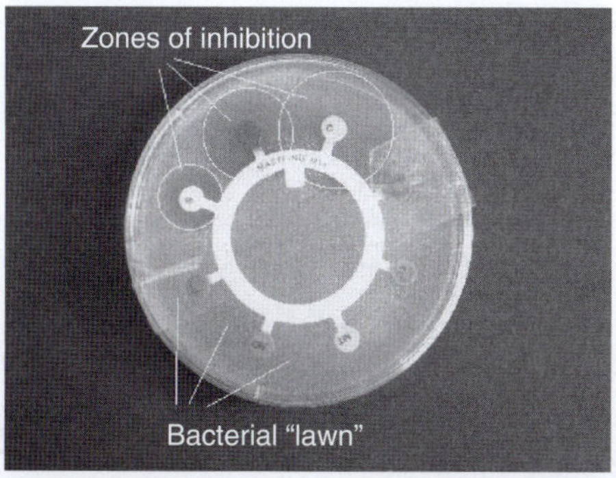

Figure 13.8 Bacterial lawn showing zones of inhibition.

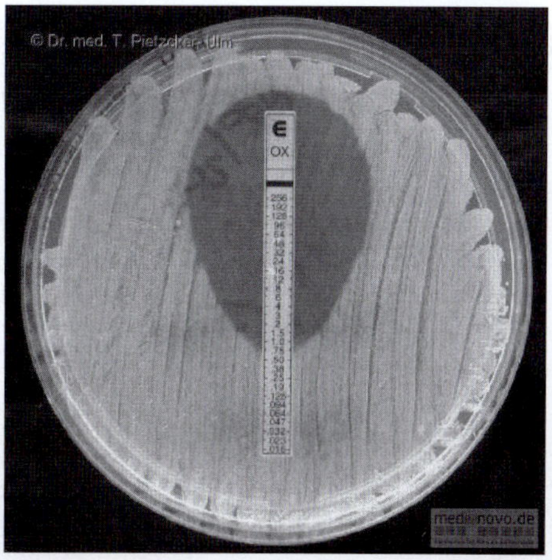

Figure 13.9 Antibiotic test strip demonstrating minimum inhibitory concentration (MIC).

value if the inoculum produces highly specific symptoms or lesions in the sensitive laboratory animal.

Fungi

Fungal infection is common in podiatric practice and is usually diagnosed on the basis of its clinical presentation. Where an infection is suspected, scrapings from the active periphery of a skin lesion or full-thickness clippings of nails together with subungual debris should be taken and inoculated on and into Sabouraud's agar, which is selective for fungal growth. The plates should be incubated at 25–28°C. Colonies of *Candida* spp. often appear overnight or in a day or two; dermatophytes take 1–3 weeks to appear. Species identification depends on the rate of growth, colony appearance and microscopic appearance of the fungus, in particular the fungal spores – both micron and macroconidia. Sporulation of dermatophytes usually occurs within 5–10 days of inoculation. Table 13.2 lists the fungi responsible for fungal infections affecting the feet.

Viruses

Unlike bacteria and fungi, viruses cannot be grown on artificial media and usually require tissue culture, chick embryo culture or inoculation into laboratory animals. Much work is in progress to simplify viral identification. The processes are complex and outside the scope of this chapter.

Although newer techniques for the detection and identification of microorganisms, such as detection of antigens, antibodies and polymerase chain reaction studies, help in the overall armamentarium available to the practitioner, culture still remains the gold standard against which all these newer techniques are measured. The best non-culture tests have specificities and sensitivities in the order of only 85–90%, even in the hands of experienced staff.

It should always be remembered that because of the skill and costs involved in culturing and carrying out the exacting tests to identify organisms, the practitioner must take care to ensure that correctly taken specimens are sent to the laboratory. This will help speed the result and thus allow appropriate, efficient and, more importantly, effective treatment to be delivered to the patient.

Urinalysis

The kidneys play an important part in the maintenance of homeostasis, one of their functions being the excretion of waste and foreign substances through the formation of urine. Water accounts for 95% of the total volume of urine; the remaining 5% consists of electrolytes, cellular metabolites and exogenous substances such as the excretion products of drugs. The amount of fluid drunk and the amount lost through perspiration, respiration and defecation modify the

Table 13.2 Fungi responsible for fungal infections of the feet

Fungus	*Features*
Trichophyton rubrum	Affects skin and nails; 85% of cases of onychomycosis thought to be due to *T. rubrum* Can affect skin and hair in a number of ways. Diffuse dry scaling tinea on the soles is usually due to *T. rubrum*
Trichophyton mentagrophytes	Affects skin and nails. Can cause a range of skin responses but is especially associated with vesicle eruption; 12% of cases of onychomycosis due to *T. mentagrophytes*
Epidermophyton floccosum	Affects skin in a variety of ways but is especially associated with vesicle eruption Rarely causes onychomycosis
Scopulariopsis brevicaulis	Secondary pathogen. Produces a dark green–black discoloration
Candida spp.	A yeast, of which *Candida albicans* is the most common pathogenic species. Affects skin and nails. In nails it is often responsible for paronychia

amount of urine produced. The average daily output of urine for an adult is 1200 ml.

If a disease alters the body's metabolism or kidney function, traces of substances not normally present (or normal constituents in abnormal amounts) may appear in the urine. Many early disease states can be detected by urinalysis before they become clinically obvious and it therefore has a useful role in the assessment of patients. Assessment of a patient's urine can be made both in the clinic and in the laboratory. Testing is non-invasive and cost-effective, and urine specimens are easily obtained. Clinical assessment is commonly performed, allowing the practitioner to obtain information about the health status of their patient rapidly.

Indications for urinalysis

Urinalysis may be used as an aid in the diagnosis of renal disease, hepatic disease and diabetes mellitus, all of which have relevance to the podiatrist. Diabetes mellitus can have widespread consequences for the lower limb. Renal and hepatic diseases may have serious systemic repercussions, which complicate diagnosis and affect the treatment of lower-limb problems. Urinalysis is particularly useful in the preoperative assessment of patients to screen for illnesses which may complicate or contraindicate elective procedures. Screening for a urinary-tract infection or the presence of bacteria in urine can also identify those patients at increased risk of developing post-operative wound infections.

Collection of the urine specimen

Urine specimens can be classified as a first-voided morning, random or timed sample. The first-voided morning specimen is the most concentrated of the day, and is the most specific for nitrates and proteins. The random specimen is the most convenient for patients to collect and is the most commonly used specimen. Timed specimens are combinations of urine voided over a specific length of time and are more applicable to the hospital environment.

Proper collection and prompt examination of urine is important for accurate analysis. The use of clean collecting vessels will minimise bacterial and chemical contamination. The patient is usually asked to provide a midstream specimen of urine (MSU), which should be less than 4 hours old at the time of testing. To collect the specimen, the patient should be instructed to first gently cleanse the opening to their urethra with water and begin to urinate into the toilet, subsequently inserting a clean container into the urinary stream to collect the sample. The container is removed from the urine stream and the act of voiding completed.

Clinical assessment

Physical examination of urine

Colour

Urine should be examined under good lighting against a white background. Normally, the colour of urine is yellow owing to a pigment called urochrome. The colour becomes deeper with increasing concentration, such as in the first void of the morning. Other changes in colour are seen, often due to the ingestion of certain medications or food (Table 13.3). The patient may be concerned about any change in their urine. Ascertain the circumstances surrounding the patient noticing the change in colour. Did the colour only appear after the urine contacted the container?

Table 13.3 Causes of colour change in urine

Colour	*Cause*
Red	Haematuria Haemoglobinuria Anthocyanin (in beetroot)
Orange-red	Rifampicin
Orange	Anthraquinones Dehydration
Yellow(++)	Bilirubin Riboflavin
Green	Biliverdin
Green–blue	Amitriptyline Resorcinol
Blue	Methylene blue
Brown	Urobilinogen Porphyria Metronidazole
Brown–black	Haemorrhage L-dopa Senna

Did the urine have to sit in the sun for hours before the colour appeared?

Clarity

The common terms used to describe urine are clear, hazy, cloudy, turbid or milky. Urine is normally clear. Suspended particles will give it a hazy or cloudy appearance. Turbid urine can be caused by the presence of a urinary tract infection, leucocytes, erythrocytes or parasitic disease. Prostatic fluid, blood, lipids or sperm can cause milky urine.

Odour

Freshly voided urine has little smell; stale urine may contain ammonium salts from the breakdown products of urea, producing an offensive odour. Infected urine has a foul smell; the odour worsens if the urine is left to stand. Ketones in the urine (ketonuria) produce a sweet pear-drop smell and suggest a ketoacidotic state that requires urgent medical attention.

Reagent testing

A variety of dipsticks are available for testing urine. Some are single-test based, such as Clinistix®, which tests for glucose; some are multi-test based, such as Multistix® 8SG which has eight reagent strips. To use a multi-test reagent, a reagent strip is taken from the bottle and completely immersed in the urine specimen. The strip is removed and excess urine wiped off on the rim of the specimen container. The strip is held horizontally (therefore not allowing chemicals to drip from one pad to another) and the colour of the test areas compared with the colour chart on the bottle, following the manufacturer's instructions.

Multi-test reagent test results are explained below.

Glucose

Glucose is not normally detectable in the urine. The presence of glucose in the urine may be due to elevated blood glucose levels (as in diabetes mellitus) or reduced renal absorption. A negative result is therefore normal. The test area will detect glucose at 7 mmol/l, and thus a positive result should be followed up with a blood glucose analysis to establish the cause of the glycosuria. The most common cause of glycosuria is diabetes mellitus. However, it is also seen with stress (as glycogen stores are mobilised from the liver) and secondary hyperglycaemia due to Cushing's syndrome, thyrotoxicosis or steroid use.

Bilirubin

The presence of bilirubin in the urine is indicative of hepatic or biliary disease. A positive result should be followed up – even trace amounts of bilirubin are sufficiently abnormal to require further investigation.

Ketones

Ketones (primarily acetone and acetoacetic acid) are breakdown products of fatty acid metabolism and are abnormal urinary constituents. Their presence may be due to starvation or uncontrolled diabetes mellitus. False-positive results are seen with certain medications such as metformin and insulin. A positive result in a diabetic patient requires urgent medical attention.

Specific gravity

This parameter tests the concentrating and diluting power of the kidney. The specific gravity of urine is normally between 1.012 and 1.030 and increases with glycosuria, proteinuria or infection. Decreased values are seen in diabetes insipidus, pyelonephritis and glomerulonephritis. A fixed value may indicate renal failure.

Blood

Haematuria is the presence of red blood cells (RBCs) in the urine. In microscopic haematuria, the urine appears normal to the naked eye, but examination under a microscope shows a high number of RBCs. Gross haematuria can be seen with the naked eye. Most of the causes of haematuria are not serious, for example exercise may cause haematuria for 24 hours and blood is often found in the urine of menstruating females. However, the condition can be associated with serious renal or urological disease and/or urinary tract infection. A positive result will require a medical opinion.

pH

Normal urine is slightly acidic, with a pH of 5–6. Values are lowest after an overnight fast and highest after meals. Strongly acid urine may indicate starvation or uncontrolled diabetes mellitus. Recheck the glucose and ketone test results if this is the case. Very high (alkaline) values suggest infection and warrant further investigation.

Protein

Normal urine contains small amounts of albumin and globulin, not normally detectable by the reagent strip. A negative result does not therefore rule out abnormal proteinuria. A positive result indicates renal disease, urinary tract infection or hypertension, and requires confirmation.

Urobilinogen

Although normally present in urine, elevated levels of urobilinogen indicate liver abnormalities or haemolytic anaemia. A positive result requires an urgent medical opinion.

Nitrite

The presence of nitrites requires their conversion from nitrates by Gram-negative bacteria. A negative test does not rule out infection since Gram-positive cocci will not produce nitrites. Also note that the urine must also be retained in the bladder for several hours to allow the reaction to take place. A positive result confirms a urinary-tract infection and requires further analysis.

Leucocytes

The presence of leucocytes and other components of pus in the urine, pyuria, is an indication of bladder or renal infection. A negative result where clinical symptoms are present would require microscopy and culture. A positive result confirms a urinary-tract infection and also requires further analysis to identify the infecting organism.

Laboratory assessment

Microscopy

A small amount of the collected specimen is centrifuged at 5000 rpm for 5 minutes and the sediment re-suspended in a few drops of urine and mounted on a glass slide:

- **Erythrocytes**: more than 5 erythrocytes per high power field is abnormal.
- **Leucocytes**: more than 5 leucocytes per high power field may indicate bacterial infection or renal disease.
- **Epithelial cells**: these are derived from the cellular lining of the genitourinary tract, and small numbers of epithelial cells may be found in urine. A large number is an abnormal finding.
- **Casts**: casts result from the precipitation of protein, cells and debris inside the renal tubules. They are so named because their shape represents a 'cast' of the lumen of a tubule. Hyaline casts are formed from Tamm–Horsfall protein and may be found in normal patients but are more frequently seen in sufferers of hypertension, congestive heart failure or renal disease. Granular casts are composed of protein and tubular cells and indicate renal tubular disease. Red cell casts suggest disease associated with bleeding and white cell casts are an indicator of acute pyelonephritis.
- **Crystals**: crystals may be found in patients with urinary stones but are found in the urine of normal patients as well. Formation of crystals varies with the pH; urate crystals can be found in acid urine and phosphate crystals can be found in alkaline urine. Cystine crystals are found in patients with cystinuria and oxalate crystals may be present in patients with oxalate stones.

Culture

A urine culture is used to estimate the number of bacteria present in urine and to identify the exact organism present. Urine is an excellent culture medium and is easily contaminated from the genitourinary tract. At room temperature, contaminants will grow rapidly unless the urine is plated or refrigerated promptly. Urine cultures are obtained from patients suspected of having a urinary-tract infection, and should be collected taking extra care to follow the MSU method as described above. Cultures that demonstrate multiple organisms have usually been contaminated during collection.

Blood analysis

Blood is the fluid component of the vascular system and constitutes about 8% of the total body weight – approximately 5–6 litres in men and 4–5 litres in women. It comprises plasma (55%), a watery liquid that contains dissolved substances, and formed elements (45%), which are the cells and fragments (Table 13.4). The principal functions of blood are:

- transportation of heat, hormones and metabolites (such as oxygen) around the body
- help in the regulation of pH and temperature
- protect the body through clotting mechanisms, the action of white blood cells and antibodies.

Indications for blood analysis

Blood tests can aid in the diagnosis of the following, all of which are relevant to the practitioner dealing

Table 13.4 Components of blood

Plasma (55% of blood)	*Formed elements (45% of blood)*
Water (91.5% of plasma)	Red blood cells (RBCs)
Solutes (8.5% of plasma)	White blood cells (WBCs)
Protein	Neutrophils (40–75%)
Albumin	Lymphocytes (20–45%)
Globulin	Monocytes (2–10%)
Fibrinogen	Eosinophils (1–6%)
Electrolytes	Platelets
Respiratory gases	
Enzymes	
Hormones	
Digestion products	
Waste	

with the lower limb:

- anaemias, e.g. from an altered erythrocyte count
- infections, e.g. from a raised leucocyte count
- systemic inflammation, e.g. from a raised C-reactive protein (CRP) or erythrocyte sedimentation rate (ESR)
- metabolic disorders, e.g. raised serum glucose and ketone levels
- clotting disorders, e.g. from an abnormal platelet count
- hormonal disorders, e.g. from a high level of serum thyroxine
- immunology-related disorders, e.g. in seropositive arthritides.

The use of routine blood sampling in asymptomatic patients is questionable. Many studies of routine biochemical screening prior to surgery have revealed less than 1% of abnormality in unsuspected cases. In cases where abnormality was detected, the results of the tests made no difference to the anaesthetic or surgical management of the patient.

Blood screening can be useful in detecting certain haematological diseases such as sickle-cell anaemia and thalassaemia. Both conditions can have implications for the management of lower-limb problems, especially surgical management. When surgical intervention is planned it may be worthwhile to screen those at particular risk for these conditions. Blood tests are also indicated for surgical patients with a history of thrombosis or clotting disorders. However, in general, patients without clinical signs of systemic disease are unlikely to produce grossly abnormal results. Significant liver disease, for example is almost certain to produce jaundice. The appearance of bilirubin in the urine offers a cheap alternative screening test. Initial detection of diabetes can be reliably performed on a urine sample, which also has the benefit of revealing proteinuria and unrecognised renal impairment.

Collection of the blood sample

There are several ways in which blood samples may be obtained. An autolet with a disposable needle can be used to produce a small drop of blood from a pinprick. It is usual to prick the distal pulp of the thumb and is the method by which diabetic patients perform daily monitoring of their blood sugar levels.

For laboratory-based tests, a greater quantity of blood than that obtained from a pinprick is required. It is important that the person taking the sample has appropriate and current qualifications – a phlebotomist is a technician who has been trained to take samples of blood. Blood samples are taken from a vein, usually in the forearm, using a tourniquet above the elbow to force blood to accumulate in the vein. A needle is inserted into the vein and this needle fitted to a syringe or a vacutainer (an evacuated tube).

To ensure appropriate stability of the sample, containers that contain an appropriate additive are used. Many samples must be prevented from clotting and therefore an anticoagulant is added. The anticoagulant of choice is the dipotassium salt of ethylenediamine tetra-acetic acid (EDTA). Where an infection is suspected, two or more samples may be taken. One type of container used to transport the blood sample facilitates testing for the presence of aerobic organisms; another type facilitates testing for the presence of anaerobic organisms.

Whether you take the sample yourself or refer to a hospital it is essential you provide the laboratory undertaking the tests with relevant information. The patient's hospital number or laboratory number, if there have been previous tests, will enable current results to be compared with previous test results. Many laboratories produce cumulative results which give an indication of patient progress. Normal ranges vary in pregnancy; for this reason it is vital to provide this information on the request form (Fig. 13.10).

Blood can be analysed in a variety of ways. Analysis may focus on the cellular content (haematology),

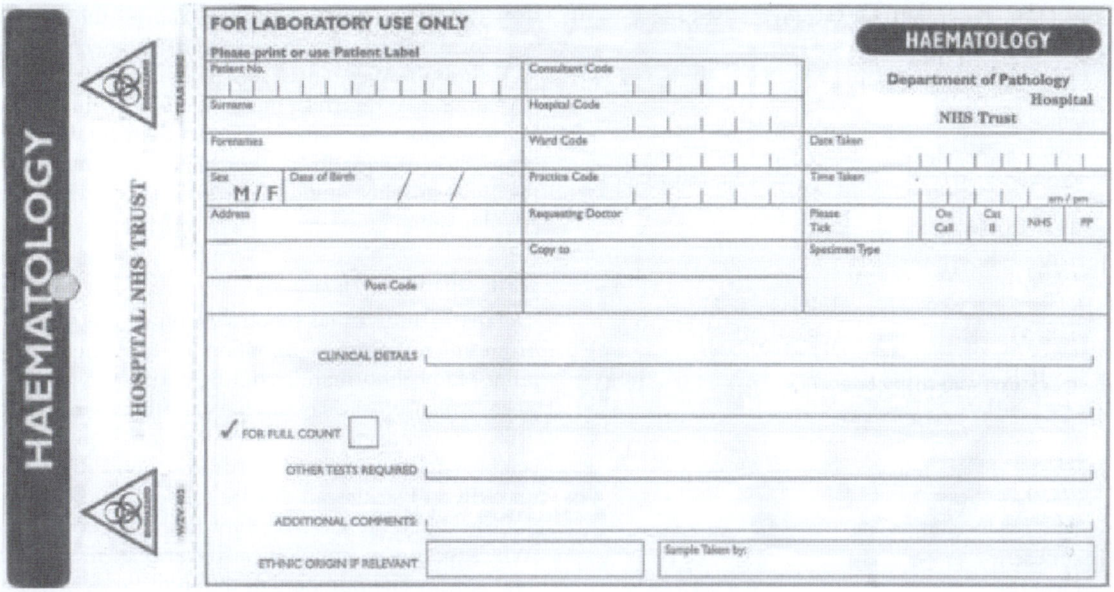

HAEMATOLOGY

HOSPITAL NHS TRUST

FOR LABORATORY USE ONLY

Please print or use Patient Label

Patient No.

Surname

Forenames

Sex M / F | Date of Birth / /

Address

Post Code

Consultant Code

Hospital Code

Ward Code

Practice Code

Requesting Doctor

Copy to

HAEMATOLOGY

Department of Pathology
Hospital
NHS Trust

Date Taken

Time Taken am / pm

Please Tick | On Call | Cat II | NHS | PP

Specimen Type

CLINICAL DETAILS

✓ FOR FULL COUNT

OTHER TESTS REQUIRED

ADDITIONAL COMMENTS

ETHNIC ORIGIN IF RELEVANT

Sample Taken by:

Figure 13.10 Haematology request form.

chemistry (biochemistry) or immunological aspects (serology) of blood.

Haematology

Haematological investigation generally follows a sequence of diagnostic steps:

- The full blood count
- The blood film
- Inflammatory tests
  - Erythrocyte sedimentation rate (ESR)
  - Plasma viscosity
  - C-reactive protein
- Clotting studies.

The full blood count

A full blood count (Table 13.5) includes basic data on RBCs, white blood cells (WBCs), haemoglobin concentration and mean cell volume (MCV). In the laboratory, automated blood count machines perform the analysis:

- Normally, more than 99% of the formed elements are RBCs. The percentage of total blood volume occupied by the RBCs is called the packed cell volume (PCV) or haematocrit, expressed as the percentage of total blood volume packed by centrifuge in a given volume. The PCV is reduced in all types of anaemia; a haematocrit measurement of less than 30% is probably detrimental to surgical intervention.
- The **haemoglobin concentration** reflects the oxygen-carrying capacity of the blood. It is reduced in all forms of anaemia and is increased in polycythaemia.
- **RBC indices** are arithmetic ratios derived from the RBC count, PCV and haemoglobin concentration. The most useful of these ratios is the MCV, which is a measurement of the haematocrit divided by the RBC count. It is low, less than 82 fl, with microcytic anaemia and greater than 100 fl with megaloblastic anaemia. The mean cell haemoglobin (MCH) is the haemoglobin concentration divided by the RBC count; the mean cell haemoglobin concentration (MCHC) is the haemoglobin concentration divided by the PCV.
- The **WBC count** can be decreased (leucopenia) or increased (leucocytosis). Leucopenia can result from a viral infection, ingestion of certain drugs (especially antineoplastics) and radiation. Leucocytosis can result from acute bacterial infection, leukaemia, acute haemorrhage and tissue necrosis.
- The **platelet count** provides quantification of thrombocytopenia but gives no indication of platelet function.

Table 13.5 Normal haematological values

Factor	*Value*
Haemoglobin	
Men	130–180 g/l
Women	120–160 g/l
Erythrocytes: red cell count (RCC)	
Men	$4.5–6.5 \times 10^{12}$/l
Women	$3.8–5.8 \times 10^{12}$/l
Leucocytes: white cell count (WCC)	$4.0–11.0 \times 10^{9}$/l
Mean cell volume (MCV)	78–98 fl
Packed cell volume (PCV)/ haematocrit	
Men	0.40–0.54%
Women	0.35–0.47%
Mean cell haemoglobin (MCH)	27–32 pg
Mean cell haemoglobin concentration (MCHC)	300–350 g/l
Thrombocytes	$150–400 \times 10^{9}$/l
Reticulocytes (adults)	$10–100 \times 10^{9}$/l
Differential WCC:	
Neutrophil granulocytes	$2.5–7.5 \times 10^{9}$/l
Lymphocytes	$1.0–3.5 \times 10^{9}$/l
Monocytes	$0.2–0.8 \times 10^{9}$/l
Eosinophil granulocytes	$0.04–0.4 \times 10^{9}$/l
Basophil granulocytes	$0.01–0.1 \times 10^{9}$/l
Erythrocyte sedimentation rate (ESR) (<60 years of age)	<20 mm/h
C-reactive protein (CRP)	8 μg/ml
Prothrombin time (PT)	11–13 seconds
Activated partial thromboplastin time (APTT)	27–36 seconds
Bleeding time	1–4 minutes

- The **reticulocyte count** measures those early forms of RBC with inclusion fragments of the endoplasmic reticulum. The count quantifies the rate of erythropoiesis: increased numbers of reticulocytes reflect increased formations of RBCs, as seen in haemorrhage or haemolysis; a low number suggests nutritional deficiency or leukaemia.

The blood film

Details of individual blood cell types are obtained from microscopic examination of a stained blood film. Many abnormalities in RBC morphology can be seen. Anisocytosis is excessive variation in the size of RBCs, poikilocytosis is excessive variation in their shape, spherocytosis demonstrates round RBCs, and the RBCs of sickle-cell disease are long and bent.

The differential WBC count is a reflection of 100 WBCs that are morphologically examined in a peripheral smear. The numbers of different types of WBCs are expressed as a percentage of the whole (see Table 13.5). A left shift denotes a decrease in neutrophil segmentation, which is a sign of increased turnover and demand for WBCs most commonly seen in acute bacterial infections.

Tests for inflammation

- **ESR** is the rate of fall of RBCs in a column of blood. The ESR increases with age and is higher in females than in males. A raised ESR reflects an increase in the plasma concentration of proteins and is indicative of diseases associated with malignancy, infections and inflammation.
- **Plasma viscosity** is used by some laboratories instead of an ESR. As with the ESR, the level of viscosity depends on the concentration of proteins, but is the same in males and females, and increases only slightly with age.
- **C-reactive protein** (CRP) is synthesised in the liver and can be detected in the blood within 6 hours of an inflammatory response. This test is replacing the ESR due to its greater sensitivity.

Clotting studies

- The **prothrombin time** (PT) determines the amount of prothrombin in the blood. Test reagents are added to a sample and the time taken for the blood to clot noted. It provides a laboratory measurement of the extrinsic blood coagulation pathway. The PT is prolonged by deficiencies in fibrinogen, prothrombin and factors V, VII and X but remains normal in patients with haemophilia A and B, or platelet deficiencies. It is commonly used to monitor patients taking warfarin.

- The **activated partial thromboplastin time** (APTT) provides a laboratory measurement of the intrinsic blood coagulation pathway and is the best single screen for disorders of coagulation. The APTT is prolonged by deficiencies in fibrinogen, prothrombin and factors V, VIII, IX, X and XII, and in patients with haemophilia A and B, or platelet deficiencies.
- The **thrombin time** (TT) measures the clotting (fibrin formation) time of a sample of blood following the addition of a small amount of thrombin. The most common cause of a prolonged TT is the presence of heparin.
- The **bleeding time** is the time required for cessation of bleeding from a small skin puncture, usually of the ear lobe. As the droplets of blood escape, touching the wound with filter paper blots them. When paper no longer stains, the bleeding has stopped. It is a standard assay that measures the effectiveness of platelet plug formation. The bleeding time is increased if platelet function is abnormal, e.g. patients who are suspected of having a qualitative platelet disorder such as von Willebrand's disease or patients on aspirin therapy.

Biochemistry

Arterial blood gas studies are the best single determination of lung function, referring to the determination of arterial oxygen and carbon dioxide tensions and the pH. Indications for blood gas studies include the assessment of preoperative lung function, documentation of pulmonary disease and continuing assessments of cardiopulmonary diseases. Serum chemistry assays useful in the diagnosis or monitoring of many metabolic, renal and fluid/electrolyte abnormalities are detailed below.

Urea and creatinine are dependent on the kidney for excretion: therefore, their measurement is an index of renal function. Urea, an end product of protein metabolism, is synthesised in the liver, and is the principal nitrogenous constituent of urine. In pathologies that affect renal function, its serum concentration rises. Azotaemia is defined as increased nitrogenous substances in the blood and is characterised by a blood urea nitrogen (BUN) level greater than 20 mg/100 ml. The BUN : creatinine ratio is 10:1 in normal individuals; in patients with acute renal failure both BUN and creatinine levels rise and the ratio may be unchanged. The BUN level alone is increased in patients with renal disease, gastrointestinal haemorrhage or increased protein metabolism. The BUN level is decreased in patients with severe cirrhosis, inadequate protein intake or in pregnancy.

The concentration of **creatinine** in the serum has a linear relationship to glomerular filtration, making it a more sensitive indicator of renal disease than BUN. Creatinine levels rise in patients with renal disease, gigantism, acromegaly and increased dietary intake from roasted meats.

The normal range for **uric acid** is 3.5–7.2 mg/dl for males and 2.6–6.0 mg/dl for females. Elevated serum uric acid is not a reliable diagnostic test for gout. However, acute gout never occurs in patients who have a serum uric acid level in the lower half of the normal range. The test can give rise to false negatives and positives. In the first few attacks, when it is often difficult to diagnose, the serum acid level is often below the higher level. Despite these sensitivity issues serum uric acid levels are used to monitor treatment.

Sodium levels are increased in patients with dehydration, primary aldosteronism, Cushing's syndrome and with some diuretic drugs. Sodium levels are decreased in fluid retention (seen in congestive heart failure), with unreplaced body fluid loss (vomiting, diarrhoea) and in Addison's disease. Sodium is the principal cation of extracellular fluid. Concentration of **chloride** tends to follow sodium to maintain electrical charge equilibrium.

Potassium levels may be increased (>5.5 mmol/l) (hyperkalaemia) in patients with renal failure, mineralocorticoid deficiency, acidosis, massive tissue necrosis and with high-dose penicillin. Hypokalaemia may occur in patients with chronic diarrhoea, primary/secondary aldosteronism, Cushing's syndrome or with diuretic drugs.

The measurement of **carbon dioxide** provides a differential diagnosis in the change of blood pH, acidosis or alkalosis. The carbon dioxide level is higher in respiratory alkalosis (pulmonary emboli, asthma or liver disease), with metabolic acidosis (diabetic ketoacidosis), with decreased excretion of hydrogen ions (renal failure) and with increased loss of alkaline fluids (chronic diarrhoea).

Blood glucose

Blood sugars bind non-enzymatically to proteins forming stable covalent linkages. The measurement of glycated derivatives of haemoglobin and plasma proteins has provided a reliable index of long-term blood glucose control in patients with diabetes. In normal individuals a small percentage of the haemoglobin molecules in RBCs become glycosylated, i.e. chemically linked to glucose. Glycosylated haemoglobin (GHb) can be separated from normal HbA by electrophoresis into three fractions: HbA_{1A}, HbA_{1B} and HbA_{1C}. Usually only HbA_{1C} is quantitated, and gives a measure of mean blood sugar over the preceding 2 months. The percentage of glycosylation is proportional to time and to the concentration of blood glucose. Therefore, poorly controlled diabetes will have a greater percent of GHb. Testing blood glucose levels is an important part of wound assessment in patients with diabetes as demonstrated in Case history 13.1.

Case history 13.1

A 55-year-old neuropathic patient with insulin-dependent diabetes and a history of ulceration beneath the metatarsophalangeal joint of his plantar-flexed first metatarsal, presented at the multi-disciplinary clinic with a further breakdown to the area with signs of infection. Previously he had responded well to debridement, redistributive padding and flucloxacillin therapy which was given to him for this episode. A week later the wound was showing some signs of resolution but not as well as in the past. A swab was taken from the base of the wound and sent to the laboratory for culture and sensitivity and also for possible methicillin resistant *Staph. aureus* (MRSA) involvement. Blood tests were performed to determine his plasma viscosity, HbA_{1C}, and inflammatory markers. Treatment continued as before.

A week later the wound healing had progressed little but not worsened and the results from the laboratory showed contamination of the wound with MRSA but blood tests revealed a normal C-reactive protein level indicating no systemic infection, with a raised HbA_{1C} indicating poor glycaemic control. A course of topical mupirocin to be applied every 24 hours was implemented and the other treatment therapy continued. His insulin dosage was altered by the endocrinologist in light of the poor HbA_{1C}. Ten days later the wound was showing excellent signs of resolution and the mupirocin and flucloxacillin were stopped with weekly cleansing and redistribution therapy continued. A swab was taken from the base of the wound and again sent for culture and sensitivity. The results from this showed the wound was clear of infection. A new insole was manufactured for the patient and introduced into his footwear on resolution of the ulceration 4 weeks later.

The glucometer uses a small sample of blood to test blood glucose levels. Glucometers vary slightly in design; all come with instructions for use. It is essential that the practitioner follows the manufacturers' guidelines, regularly cleans the equipment and takes care to calibrate the equipment prior to use. The glucometer gives the amount of glucose in the blood, in millimoles per litre, as a digital readout. A normal reading is within the range of 4–8 mmol/l (non-fasting) and 3–5 mmol/l (fasting). Glucometers have been known to give false-positive and -negative readings. This is usually due to inadequate cleaning, poor calibration or failure to follow the manufacturers' guidelines when carrying out the test.

Serology

Conditions associated with unclear causes of joint pain in the foot and lower limb pose a concern for the practitioner, especially where the metatarsophalangeal, interphalangeal, ankle or subtalar joints are involved. Seropositive arthritides can be a cause of this type of joint pain. Serum analysis for the presence of rheumatoid factor can be helpful in these instances. Rheumatoid factors are autoantibodies found in the serum, usually of the immunoglobulin M (IgM) class, which are directed against human IgG. Either the latex or Rose–Waaler tests can detect their presence. Their presence may indicate rheumatoid arthritis (in 80% of cases), systemic lupus erythematosus (in 50% of cases), systemic sclerosis (in 30% of cases), Sjögren's syndrome (in 90% of cases), polymyositis (in 50% of cases) or dermatomyositis (in 50% of cases).

Histology

Histopathology is the examination of tissues or cells for the presence or absence of changes in their structure due to abnormal condition. It provides a useful method for clarifying or confirming a diagnosis and gives an insight into how a disease originates, progresses and is influenced by therapy. The preparation of thin slices or sections of the tissues, which are coloured differentially by the use of various stains, makes this study possible. Tissue and body fluids (other than blood and urine) can be removed from the lower limb for histological examination.

Indications for histological examination

The indications for histological analysis are:

- when a lesion does not have a clear clinical diagnosis and resists treatment, e.g. neuroma
- when there is no exudate which can be cultured for the presence of pathogens; in this case, a sample of tissue is needed for microbiological purposes and for identification of cellular changes
- where tissue has an abnormal appearance and malignancy is suspected
- where the lesion fails to heal, e.g. inclusion cyst, pyogenic granuloma (see Ch. 8, Fig. 8.28).

Sampling techniques

The range of tissues from the lower limb that can be removed for histological analysis are given in Table 13.6. Various methods can be used to remove tissue or fluid for investigation. The technique used will depend on the site and the amount that needs to be removed. A wide range of investigations can be performed on tissues taken from the body. Samples should be collected in such a way as to pre-empt the method to be used. The practitioner should therefore decide at the outset which investigations are required. Appropriate collection and storage techniques are vital to preserve the sample.

Most techniques require local analgesia. In the case of tissue it is generally advisable to remove a

Table 13.6 Tissues which can be removed from the foot for histological analysis

Epithelial	Keratinised stratified epithelial tissue (skin) Stratified cuboidal epithelium (sweat glands/secretory function) Multicellular exocrine glands: Coiled tubular eccrine and apocrine (sweat) Branched acinar holocrine (sebaceous)
Connective	Mesenchymal found in adult tissue below skin and blood vessels Loose areolar: subcutaneous layer of skin and blood vessels, nerves associated with fibroblasts, macrophages, mast cells and various fibres Adipose: under weightbearing surfaces, joints and bone marrow Dense collagenous: common to fascia, aponeuroses, tendons, ligaments Elastic and reticular: less abundant in feet Hyaline and fibrocartilage: chondrocytic cells associated with joints, especially distal metatarsal ends, fibrocartilage submetatarsals, between bones and tendons Osseous (bone): made of compact (outer), cancellous (inner) and cellular components associated with regeneration
Muscle	Skeletal: striated, contractile form attached between bones; mainly intrinsic form in feet in four layers
Nerve	Cell body and axons Neuroglia: found at sites of tumours
Synovial membranes	Loose connective tissue: line structures and secrete synovial fluid, tendon lining, bursae, do not contain epithelial cells
Tissue repair	Stroma: supporting connective tissue restoration; active repair or scar tissue due to fibroblasts or keloid (overactivity) Scab/fibrin plug: sealing wound Granuloma: active repair tissue

section of surrounding healthy tissue as well as the abnormal tissue; this allows the pathologist to make comparisons between normal and abnormal tissue.

Sources for histological diagnoses can be either tissue or cell preparations. Tissues can be obtained by biopsy (shave, punch, needle or excision), from resected organs (partial or complete) or via autopsy. Cell preparations include fluid aspirates, smears, brushings and fine needle aspirates. In podiatric practice it is primarily tissues that are sampled and sent to histopathology. Some examples of biopsy are given below.

Biopsy

Shave

A shave biopsy can be achieved by introducing an endoscope into the body. This procedure is used when it is necessary to remove a piece of tissue from a deep structure, e.g. synovial membrane from a joint.

Punch

A punch biopsy (incisional biopsy) involves the removal of a small section of abnormal tissue. The procedure is not as extensive as excisional biopsy but is still open to complications such as deep infection. A punch, which consists of a cylinder with a sharp, fine cutting edge, is used. The punch is pushed through epithelial tissue and a small section of epithelial and/or connective tissue is removed. A trephine is a similar instrument to a punch but much more sturdy. It is used for punching holes in bone. In these cases a larger access hole is necessary. Bone samples should, wherever possible, have clear radiographs attached to assist the determination of the general appearance of the lesion. The advantage of punch biopsy lies in the small area of tissue removed. Normal tissue is not usually included. The depth of tissue sampling will depend upon the pressure applied. Punch biopsy is likely to be used where large areas have been affected and treatment cannot be undertaken at the same time. Unlike excisional biopsy it is purely a diagnostic procedure. When skin biopsy is performed it is essential to create an unobtrusive scar. In the foot, tissue around digits may require a section of bone to be removed in order to achieve closure. A surgeon specialising in the foot and ankle should be consulted to reduce the risk of ischaemia.

Needle

Aspiration is the technique used to withdraw fluids from the body, e.g. synovial fluid. Examination of synovial fluid can be very useful when examining for the presence of uric acid crystals (gout), infection or bleeding into a joint space. Where uric acid crystals are suspected the sample of synovial fluid should be placed in absolute alcohol or placed directly on to a slide. Bursae can be aspirated. This usually leads to a temporary relief of symptoms.

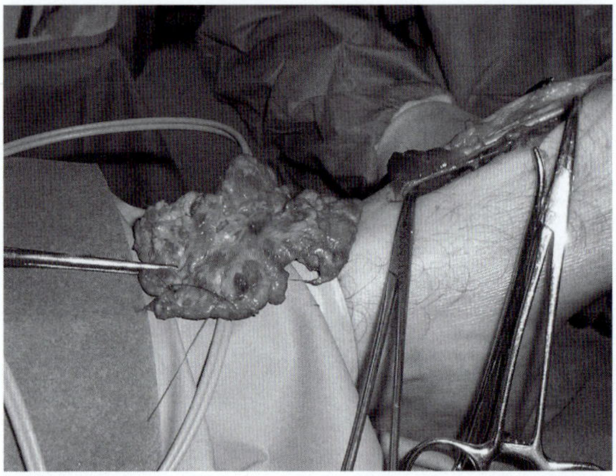

Figure 13.11 Giant cell tumour resected from the dorsum of the foot.

IMAGES

Resection

Partial

Partial resection or excisional biopsy involves the removal of all the abnormal tissue plus a section of the surrounding normal tissue. This procedure permits examination of the abnormal tissue as well as, hopefully, providing treatment at the same time. It is a surgical technique which requires high standards of asepsis. A scalpel is used to incise and then dissect the abnormal tissue and some surrounding normal tissue from the site. Haemostasis should be carefully performed (Fig. 13.11) to prevent unnecessary complications. Tissue from skin down to muscle, ligaments and tendon will require careful repair. Ganglion formation must be removed in total as it has a high recurrence rate. The gelatinous mass is difficult to retrieve. The thin translucent membrane should be included wherever possible. Thicker membranes suggest that they have undergone longer periods of deep trauma.

Complete

Whole parts, such as amputated feet, toes and excised rays, can be sent to the pathology department. Analysis of whole anatomy takes a good deal longer due to the time required to separate and fixate tissues. Bone needs to undergo a decalcification process.

Transportation and storage

Laboratory personnel will discuss the best mode of collection to ensure that an appropriate sample for testing is achieved. Specimens labelled urgent are unwelcome unless requested during or following surgery where a quick result is necessary, e.g. in the case of a suspected malignancy. Even small samples will take 24 hours to fix before the tissue can be usefully analysed.

All specimens should be clearly marked with the patient's name, hospital number, site and the date/time that the sample was taken. A full history of the patient is essential. High-risk cases should be identified with a separate 'high risk' label. The specimen should be sealed in a plastic bag, the request form remaining outside.

As with microbiological samples, damage can be sustained by using an incorrect method of transportation. Most tissue samples are placed in a screw-cap container containing normal buffered formalin (NBF) solution. Formalin itself constitutes a hazard, especially if spilt on living tissue. Samples for frozen section should be transported dry. They will be damaged if they come into contact with formalin. Frozen sectioning provides rapid results, usually within 5–10 minutes, and is used where results are urgently required: often when the patient is still on the operating table, when the result of the test will decide the course of action to be taken.

Tests and interpretation of results

These fall into several categories depending upon the nature of the lesion and/or suspected pathology. Slides of tissue are produced for microscopy. Often, staining techniques are used in order to show up changes more distinctively.

The main purpose of histological examination is to assess whether the tissue or fluid sample differs from what is normal. Abnormal cellular findings, e.g. changes to the nucleus, may indicate malignant changes. Chronic inflammation may be evident because of the presence of lymphocytes, plasma cells and macrophages. Abnormal findings may relate to the presence of giant cells, a characteristic feature produced by foreign bodies. This is a common feature in the foot.

Scarring and inflammatory changes may tether down tissue, which can account for some pain syndromes seen in the lower limb. These syndromes are difficult to diagnose accurately other than by exploratory procedures. Nerves fall under this category. They can show marked changes, involving abnormal blood vessels, as in the case of neuromas. Nerve conduction tests may provide evidence of damage prior to surgical investigation in the lower limb.

Summary

This chapter has covered the indications for the use of a range of near-patient and laboratory-based tests, appropriate sampling techniques, the principles of testing and interpretation of results. Emphasis has been placed on starting with the simplest tests prior to using more specific and sophisticated investigations.

The use of laboratory tests can never replace good interview and assessment techniques. Tests should be used economically and wisely to support treatment, confirm diagnosis or rule out a suspected malignancy. Results should be acted on to ensure that effective treatment is provided.

Further reading

Axford J 1996 Medicine. Blackwell Science, Oxford

Bayer Diagnostics Urinalysis – the inside information

Blandy J 1998 Lecture notes on urology, 5th edn. Blackwell Science, Oxford

Hanno P M, Wein A J 1994 Clinical manual of urology. McGraw-Hill, New York

Hoffbrand A V, Pettit J E 1993 Essential haematology. Blackwell Scientific, Oxford

Karlowicz K A 1995 Urological nursing – principles and practice. W B Saunders, Philadelphia

Kumar P, Clark M 2005 Clinical medicine, 6th edn. W B Saunders, Philadelphia

Murray P, Pfaller M, Rosenthal K 2005 Medical Microbiology 5th edn. Mosby, Edinburgh

Philpott-Howard J 1996 Microbiology. In: Hooper J, McCreanor G, Marshall W et al (eds) Primary care and laboratory medicine. ACB Venture Publications, London

Quinn G 1995 Laboratory blood tests in podiatry. British Journal of Podiatric Medicine and Surgery 7(2):24–27

Robinson S H, Reich P R 1993 Haematology, 3rd edn. Little, Brown and Company, Boston

Stokes E J, Ridgeway G L, Wren M W D 1993 Clinical microbiology, 7th edn. Edward Arnold, UK

Tortora G J, Grabowski S R 2000 Principles of anatomy and physiology, 9th edn. John Wiley and Sons, New York

Part 4

Specific client groups

CHAPTER 14

Assessment of the paediatric patient

P Thomson

Chapter contents

Introduction

When assessing the paediatric patient it is important to appreciate that during the early years of life the lower limbs undergo many physiological changes as the child passes through numerous developmental milestones. The practitioner needs to be familiar with these normal changes as they will influence management decisions. These variations in lower-limb position and function can often concern the parent and confuse the inexperienced practitioner.

Areas of concern can often be recognised by seeing the child walk. Observation of the child's gait will provide vital clues to potential underlying pathology. Furthermore, in evaluation of the restless child, scrutinising stance and gait is valuable as hands-on examination time is often reduced. Whereas a well-structured, systematic and holistic approach to assessment is encouraged, to ensure vital information is not omitted, an opportunistic approach may be desirable in cases of non-compliance. To prevent pathology in later life, it is essential to identify, as early as possible, any problems that might need specialist treatment.

This chapter considers the normal development process, presents an overview of factors which should be taken into consideration when assessing the child and reviews the assessment findings of specific conditions that arise in the lower limb of children.

Normal development

Normal development covers a wide spectrum of values and, although it is age related, there is variation within this as well. Even between healthy siblings there may be what appear significant differences. However, with time it is probable that such differences will have equalised out. The skill for the practitioner lies in deciding whether a presentation is pathological or likely to cause pathology in later life, or it is normal. In order for the practitioner to make objective decisions it is important that they has a good understanding of normal development and the approximate age by which certain milestones should be reached (Table 14.1). The developmental stage of the child, as measured by neurological maturation, will influence both their posture and gait.

Table 14.1 Developmental milestones

Age	*Milestone*
Birth	Head control absent. Flexion to upper and lower limbs.
2/12	Can rise up onto forearms and can extend head to look up.
5/12	May take major proportion of weight when supported in standing.
6/12	Rolling from prone to supine
7/12	Can sit unsupported
9/12	Begins to crawl and can stand momentarily holding on to furniture
1 year	Can walk supported by one hand. Can squat with wide base of support
15/12	Can walk, kneel and stand up unaided. Can climb stairs on all fours
2 years	Climbs stairs two feet per stair. Can run and jump
3 years	Can run and hop and falls less frequently
4 years	Can walk downstairs one foot per step
5 years	Can skip with both feet

Abridged from Thomson & Volpe (2001).

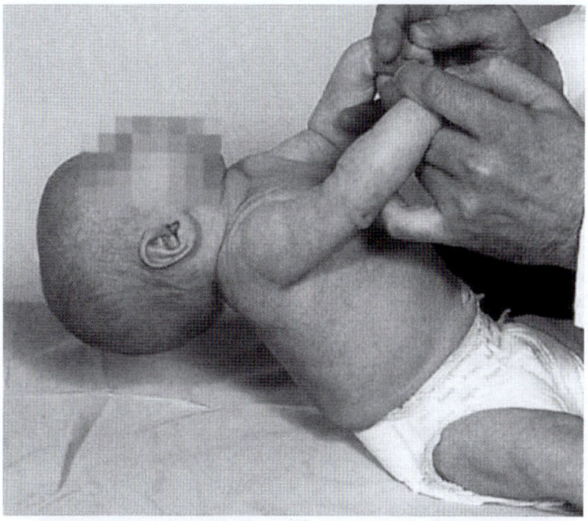

A

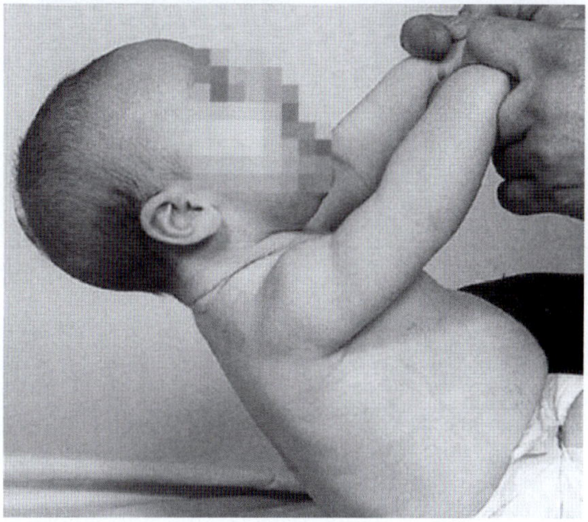

B

Figure 14.1 **A** Newborn with little muscle strength and head lag. **B** With maturity, although the distal muscles still have little power, the neck muscles have developed enough strength to keep the head in alignment with the spine.

Early posture

Neurological maturation is cephalic to caudal in direction. Hence, strength is first seen in the neck muscles (Fig. 14.1). At 6–7 months most babies will sit unassisted and attempt to crawl by 9–12 months. They will start to pull themselves up into a standing position and stand holding on to furniture (cruising) at 9–12 months, but they frequently fall backwards into a sitting position. By 12 months the child should be able to stand alone briefly and may possibly walk alone; 97% of children start to walk between 9 and 18 months. Of the remainder only 6% are neurologically compromised (Luder 1988). The early walker has an immature spinal curvature, that is 'C' shaped (in the sagittal plane) as opposed to 'S' shaped in the adult. The child will have a wide base of gait for stability, with the arms flexed and held high for balance and no arm swing (Fig. 14.2). The base of gait will become narrower as the child gains confidence and develops a heel-to-toe gait from 3 years of age.

Determinants of gait

Gait is closely associated with maturation of the central nervous system (CNS) and encompasses the essential developmental milestones, based on six

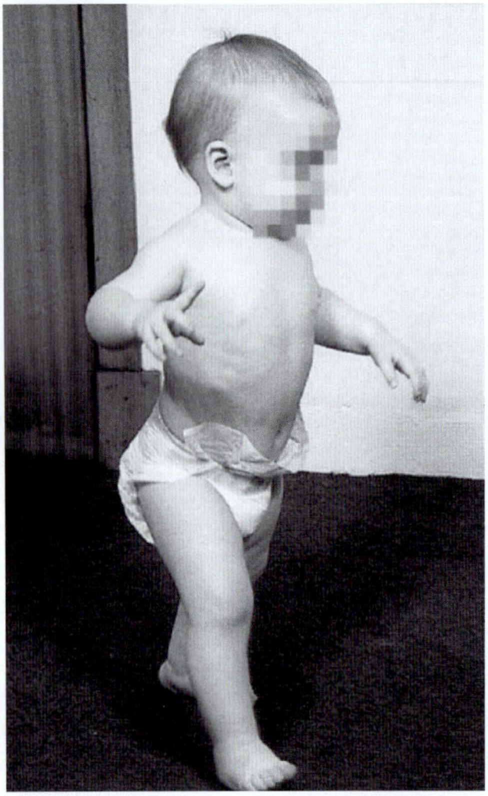

Figure 14.2 Gait of an early walker. Wide base of gait with arms flexed and held high.

components affecting walking. The various components (see Ch. 10, section B) commence from the time the child first starts to walk and continue to the age of 6+. Learning skills, balance and physiological changes all contribute to the process of maturity, assisting the young child to eventually walk in an adult fashion. If all these develop normally, by the sixth year there is little to differentiate the child's gait from that of the adult.

Early gait

On average a child will start to walk independently at about 1 year of age, although some will be later than this. If a child has shown no desire to walk by 18 months, investigation is required. At this stage the base on which the child balances will be wide. Cadence is relatively high (approximately 180 strides/min) (Volpe 2001) and single leg support and stride length short. There is no reciprocal arm swing/contralateral footstep. There is weakness of the ankle dorsiflexors causing a foot drop and a slapping flat-foot strike. The foot neither supinates nor pronates. There is little frontal or sagittal plane movement at the pelvis. The child thrusts their head, the heaviest single component of the body, downwards to increase speed and upwards and backwards to reduce velocity.

Two years of age

The child's gait will have refined considerably. The foot is still not capable of supinating at toe-off; however, the pelvis is beginning to rotate in all three body planes and the leg demonstrates signs of internal rotation at heel contact. The frontal plane position of the knees is valgus. The net result is a much smoother gait. Although velocity control is improved, the arms still do not swing in coordination with the legs.

Three years of age

The 3-year-old still demonstrates high cadence. However, it may be observed that the heel-strike is near normal and the child can balance on a much narrower base. Reciprocal arm swing can be seen to be developing by this age.

Four years of age

Gait is no longer apropulsive; heel-lift and the associated subtalar joint supination are apparent for the first time. Leg and pelvic rotations are now completely developed, although arm swing is still not fully coordinated with leg movement.

Six+ years of age

Cadence has now reduced to approximately 140 strides/min and gait is now indistinguishable to that of an adult. According to Volpe (2001) walking velocity, reduction base of gait (determined by pelvic span divided by ankle spread), duration of single leg support and cadence are the major factors distinguishing the immature gait of the toddler from that of the adult.

Growth and development

Growth of feet in children is synchronised with the body and not the limb. The foot normally doubles in length at the first and fifth month in utero. From birth to 4 years of age it doubles in size again, but after 4 years the growth rate decreases markedly.

At birth many of the bones of the foot are still cartilaginous and therefore not visible on X-ray. Only bone cells with a calcium and phosphate mineral composition are readily identified on X-ray film. As the diaphyses are apparent before birth, metatarsals and phalanges can be seen on plain X-ray, albeit as rather poorly defined areas. The calcaneus and talus are clearly visible on X-ray. The short bones of the midtarsus are also already formed at birth, although the navicular and cuneiforms are rather imprecise (lateral appears first at 3–6 months) and can take another 2–3 years to have a functional calcific appearance. The sesamoids of the first metatarsal appear around 8–10 years of age (Ch. 12).

Most books on anatomy will have a useful and comprehensive timetable of ossification for the bones of the lower limb, therefore these will not be considered here. When reading X-rays, knowledge of the position of the epiphyses is desirable to avoid misinterpretation, for example, the first metatarsal base is the site of the epiphysis, whereas the epiphysis of the other metatarsals is located at the metatarsal head. However, of special interest is the epiphysis of the styloid process at the base of the fifth metatarsal. The epiphysis runs parallel with the longitudinal axis of the bone and is often misdiagnosed as a fracture. Fractures in this area tend to lie at 90° to the axis (Fig. 14.3). Knowledge of ossification is also important for providing effective treatment at the most appropriate time (e.g. metatarsals ossify around 14–16 years in females and 16–18 years in males). It is also useful to remember that in children some bones may appear

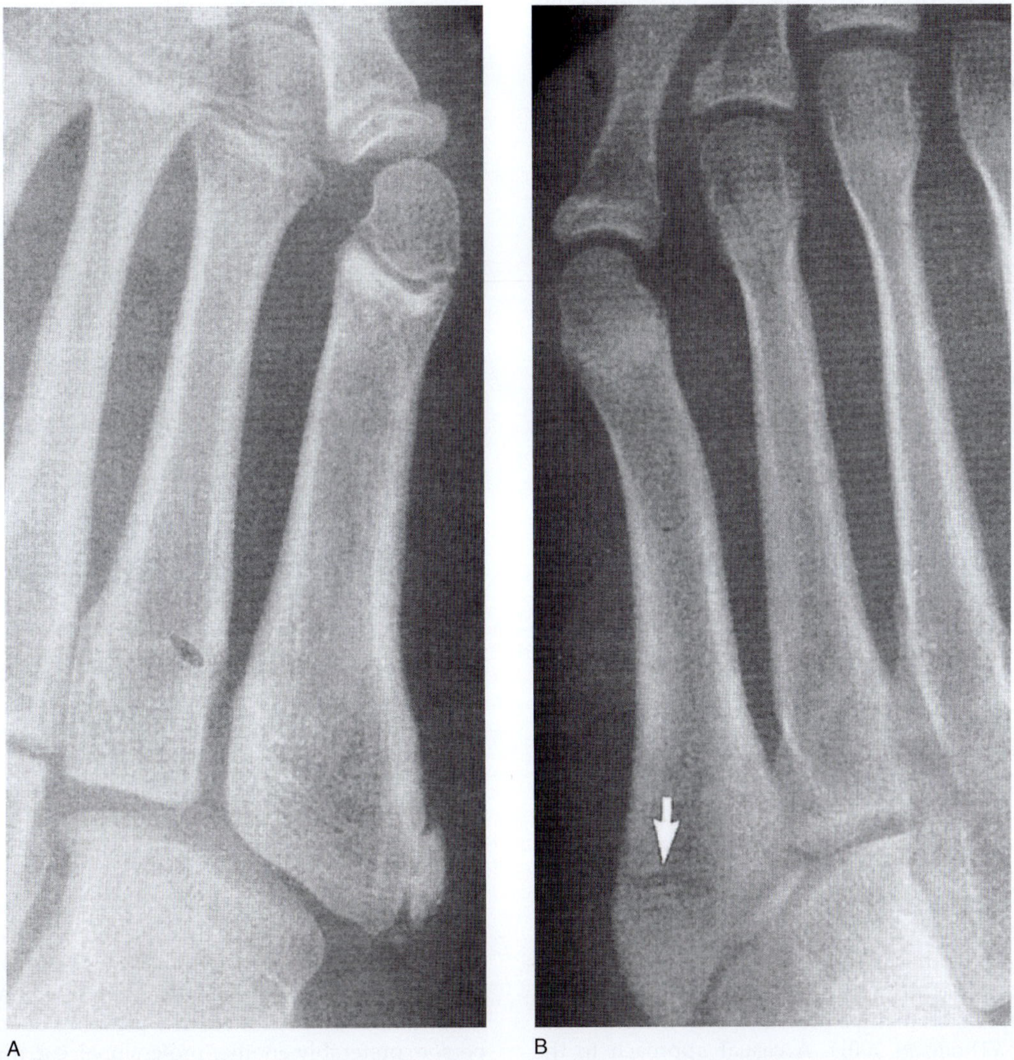

Figure 14.3 **A** Normal epiphysis of the styloid process at the base of the fifth metatarsal. **B** Fracture.

to be oriented differently from those of the adult foot. The lower limb continues to grow in length and girth until the age of 19–20 years in males. Females tend to mature earlier and therefore growth usually ceases around 15–17 years.

The assessment process

Assessment can be divided into two areas: history taking and examination.

Initiating the process

It is unusual for a child to complain of a foot problem. However, parents are often concerned about the manner in which their child is walking or are unhappy about the shape, position or size of the lower limb or foot. Parents' observations or opinions will often be based on what they, or another family member, consider to be normal. It is the role of the practitioner to identify whether there is an abnormality. Commonly, reassurance that the presentation is part of normal development is all that is required. Throughout the developing years there are recognisable features which confirm normal trends, therefore an holistic approach to examination is indicated. Such an approach requires taking a detailed family history. Treatment should be needed only if an abnormality is progressive and can be halted. When the condition does not warrant immediate treatment, careful monitoring alone may be appropriate to ensure the child develops normally.

General considerations

It is essential that the practitioner creates a relaxed and pleasant environment for the assessment. A number of factors may influence the paediatric consultation:

- First impressions
- Previous encounters with medical intervention
- Psychological development
- The waiting room
- Time
- The child's relatives.

A child needs time to settle and questions should always precede 'hands-on' examination. Watching, listening and adopting an 'open' posture all convey the impression that the practitioner is interested and caring (Thomson 2001). A casual approach to the practitioner's dress may also be desirable as children who have suffered discomfort at a previous medical consultation may associate a white coat with a bad experience. Research suggests that doctors who dress more casually are perceived to be more friendly (Brandt 2003). To a frightened child such perceptions may make the difference between a consultation that has gone well and one that has been fraught for all parties concerned. When children can relate to the practitioner, they may be more willing to cooperate.

It must also be remembered that children between the ages of 6 months and 3 years undergo 'stranger anxiety' and a child might become distressed when approached by a stranger. It may be that under these circumstances the consultation process needs to be prolonged until the child feels comfortable enough to cooperate with the examination. At the other end of the age spectrum adolescents may be more cooperative but less communicative. They may also be embarrassed about the changes that are happening to them physically. Therefore great sensitivity may be required when requesting articles of clothing be removed for the examination (Thomson 2001). Time may also be a great restraint. However, a little time spent getting to know the child is never time wasted. The use of toys and other distracters may also be helpful.

Interviewing

Several cognitive aspects about children are worthy of consideration as they may influence the interview process:

- Limited attention span
- Influence of immediate events
- Limited experience (black and white)
- Egocentrism
- Non-conceptual.

It is important to build a rapport with both the child and parents and not to alienate or talk down to the child. This helps develop the cooperation of the child to examination and compliance of both child and parent(s) to the treatment plan. Questions should be relevant and all explanations should be clear and free of jargon.

It may be easier to interview the parent while the child is playing. Watching the child at play allows evaluation of motor coordination and posture. It is important that during any assessment the child is chaperoned, as any misinterpretation of the physical exam cannot be permitted. The presence of another person, preferably another professional, e.g. nurse or care assistant, but at the very least the parent, will allow a third party to bear witness to events. During the examination it is also reassuring for the patient if the practitioner explains that they are about to touch a limb or hip and gives a reason why, in language appropriate for the child's age. In young children, it is preferable that the parent undress the child in order to aid the process and to lower any anxiety for the child. The parents should be requested, prior to attending, to dress the child in easy-to-remove clothing.

A flexible approach to questioning may be necessary in cases of difficult children. If the child is uncooperative, do not hesitate to temporarily abandon the examination or reschedule the appointment for a time when the child is less tired or irritable. Bereavement or a seriously ill sibling may be the reason for inappropriate behaviour especially in young children who are unable to express their fears or emotions any other way (John 2001). The practitioner may have to alter their approach in order to get the best from such consultations.

One aspect of paediatric management is an ability to reassure the parents (Meadow 1992). Importantly, the practitioner should always address the parents' concerns. Cause and treatment should be explained using plain language and any existing parental anxiety should not be exacerbated by giving a list of all possible complications. Similarly, the use of terms such as chronic, progressive, delay or tumour should be avoided unless the diagnosis is to have a fundamental impact on the life of the child and of the family and support is available. While it is wise to avoid raising expectations of treatment, always try to end the consultation on a positive note.

History taking

To obtain a good history a structured systematic approach should be adopted. Such an approach will reduce the possibility of omitting relevant information. In particular, attention should be paid to the following areas:

- Perinatal history (pregnancy and delivery)
- Neonatal history
- Post-neonatal history
- Developmental milestones
- Family history
- Previous consultations.

The child's age and presenting symptoms will influence the emphasis placed on the different aspects of the past medical history. In patients with congenital disorders such as talipes equinovarus, metatarsus adductus, calcaneovalgus and torsional problems, it may be useful to concentrate on the perinatal history.

Perinatal history

Pregnancy

It is important to determine whether the pregnancy was normal. Once again it is obligatory to be fastidious in obtaining a full relevant history. There is a 2% increase in postural problems among first-born children born to young women with tight abdominals (Dunn 1974). Widhe (1997) reported an incidence of 4% foot deformities among 2400 newborns examined. Therefore it is important to record the child's position in the family. Similarly the mother's medicine history during this period needs to be investigated. For example, methotrexate or phenytoin (an anti-epileptic drug), and high doses of vitamin A, are known to be teratogenic during the first trimester of pregnancy. This trimester is a period of organogenesis where organs and systems are developing. Any insult at this stage may have major consequences for the still-developing fetus. Certain questions will be easy to get answers to. Some questions, especially regarding non-prescribable or social drugs, may be reserved for cases in which visible signs of abnormality are evident. Smoking by the mother has been reported to cause intra-uterine growth retardation (IUGR) and excessive alcohol intake can delay intellectual development. In the worst cases, the child may be born with fetal alcohol syndrome. The practitioner must elicit such information without creating anxiety or appearing to be judgemental. However, such an avenue of exploration requires considerable tact. History of complications such as threatened miscarriage, antepartum haemorrhage or toxaemia need to be recorded as does known exposure to infections that have been proven to cause abnormality in the child (e.g. measles, chicken pox). It is important not to alarm the parent as incidental findings are rarely conclusive. The majority of babies encountered are healthy.

Delivery

The mother should be asked about the nature and duration of her labour. Was the delivery uneventful, full term (40 weeks) or premature (gestational age less than 37 weeks)? Muscle tone is diminished in premature babies compared with those who reach full term and they also have an increased predisposition to developmental dysplasia of the hip (DDH). Incidence of hip dislocation is higher among malpositioned fetuses (breech position) or when there are twins. In a recent study of children born with congenital postural deformities (Mikov et al 2005) foot deformities were the most common deformity (78%), and in this study group over 17% were breech presentations (compared with 0.7% in the control). A caesarean section is often indicated in cases of malposition, large fetal size or fetal distress. Therefore, although having a caesarean delivery may lessen the trauma and potential injury for the child that is inherent via the vaginal route, the practitioner must be alert to the reasons why this was procedure was chosen, i.e. was it elective or an emergency. Non-elective surgery may have been necessary because the child was anoxic in utero and this knowledge may be significant in cases where there is evidence of poor posture, poor coordination or other example of impaired motor function.

Neonatal history

At birth, babies undergo several tests to determine their APGAR score (Apgar 1953). This routine procedure is performed at the first (index of asphyxia) and fifth (index of neurological residua or death) minute after birth. It is used to evaluate the cardiovascular, respiratory and neurological status of the neonate:

- **A**ppearance – colour
- **P**ulse – indication of heart rate
- **G**rimace – plantar aspect of the foot is stimulated to provoke the child to cry
- **A**ctivity – muscle tone
- **R**espiratory effort

A baby's response to each test is rated on a scale of 0–2. A score of 10 is the maximum and is rarely achieved; a low score below 6 especially at the second test is a reason for concern and may indicate some form of long-term neurological deficit (Table 14.2).

Post-neonatal history

This mainly relates to feeding problems in the early months, which may influence normal growth and development.

Developmental milestones

Knowledge of the normal developmental milestones (see Table 14.1) is important for the recognition of suspected neurodevelopmental disorders. When neurodevelopmental delay is suspected, detailed questions on the following are indicated:

- Head control
- Ability to sit alone
- Ability to crawl
- Ability to stand, walk, run
- Ability to hop on one foot, tandem walk
- Ability to walk up and down stairs
- Result of 8-month hearing test
- Ability to comprehend and obey simple commands.

However, it must be remembered that the older the child at consultation the less reliable will be the ability of the parent to recall such information with any accuracy. Some parents may bring their Child Development Record book to the consultation. The book details the child's progress and the involvement of other professionals in the child's care to date; however, this is not always available.

Family history

A family history of the presenting condition may provide vital information about the cause and the prognosis of the complaint. Information concerning

Table 14.2 Apgar scoring system

Points	*2*	*1*	*0*
Colour	Completely pink	Pink with blue extremities	Blue or white
Heart rate	>100 bpm	<100 bpm	Absent
Respiration	Crying lustily	Shallow and irregular	Absent
Muscle tone	Active movement	Some flexion of extremities	Flaccid
Reflex irritability	Cough	Grimace	Nil

From Thomson & Volpe (2001).

siblings with similar problems and what the success (or otherwise) of any interventions should be noted. It is helpful to ascertain if any family traits exist, and these may be usefully represented by constructing a pedigree chart (Ch. 5). In genetically determined conditions, e.g. immune-deficiency states, neurodegenerative disease or muscular dystrophy, enquiries about second-degree and third-degree relatives may be worthwhile.

Previous consultations or advice

This should be noted as it may affect the parent's perceptions of the outcome of the child's foot problem. It must be stressed that the majority of paediatric problems are usually normal developmental variations, rarely requiring anything more than explanation and reassurance.

Examination

Once a clear history has been taken, the child is examined. The younger the child, the more expedient the process needs to be. Tests which require the child to be lying down may be perceived by the child as threatening (e.g. hip examination) and should be left until last. The examination should consider the following points:

- Observation of gait and posture
- General walking capability
- Symmetry of body
- Obvious deformity
- Muscle bulk and wasting
- Joint motion
- Vascular and skin quality
- Footwear.

First impressions are useful and the practitioner should start with a general observation of the child walking, sitting and playing, and how they interact with their parents. When assessing children, the focus is usually on the locomotor system, therefore in most children only a brief assessment of vascular, neurological and dermatological systems is necessary. Further detailed examination should be performed in cases where the presenting problem, history or initial assessment indicates the presence of a significant problem. Tests should only be used to clarify an otherwise unclear diagnosis. The parts of the examination process that are of particular relevance to the examination of the child are described below.

Neurological assessment

Neurological assessment implies motor and sensory evaluation. In the UK all neonates are examined by a paediatrician after delivery; midwives and health visitors undertake follow-up tests during the early years of development. Most neurological abnormalities will be detected during this stage. Reflexes are an important method for determining normal muscle development and innervation in the neonate. Certain involuntary (primitive) reflexes disappear after 1 year of age. Reflexes present during the first year of life are summarised in Table 14.3. The formal neurological examination of an infant will include an evaluation of the primitive reflexes, muscle tone/power, coordination (hand/eye) and posture in relation to development. Neurological examination of the older child should emphasise evaluation of superficial/deep reflexes, muscle tone/power (stand on tiptoes/heels) and coordination (heel-to-toe walking, balancing on one leg, hopping). This is one area where a working knowledge of the developmental milestones is essential as it makes a nonsense of the examination to ask a 3-year-old to skip with both feet when they do not have the neurological maturity to be able to carry out the instruction.

All practitioners should be mindful of skeletal and gait abnormalities which indicate a neuromuscular disorder, e.g. Charcot–Marie–Tooth disease (Case history 14.1), Duchenne's muscular dystrophy and Friedreich's ataxia. In some cases late walking may be due to neurological dysfunction undetected at birth or to DDH. Neurological tests should be carried out if an abnormality is suspected in such cases (Ch. 7).

Case history 14.1

A mother diagnosed with Charcot–Marie–Tooth disease brought her son to the clinic for assessment. She reported that he seemed to limp when he was tired. Gait analysis revealed a mild high-stepping gait and marked inverted heel-strike. The child presented with mild forefoot valgus and a tight posterior muscle group. The foot demonstrated early signs of cavoid syndrome. Neurological tests revealed stocking distribution of hypoaesthesia and diminished reflexes. Muscle tone and bulk were reduced and the lateral compartment of the leg demonstrated early signs of peroneal muscular atrophy.

Diagnosis: The child has early clinical features of Charcot–Marie–Tooth disease.

Table 14.3 Reflexes associated with development

Reflex	*Description*
Oral reflex	If a finger is placed in a baby's mouth, the baby will automatically suck and swallow. Failure to suck may indicate a cerebral problem later leading to motor dysfunction in the lower limb
Moro reflex	This reflex (startle reflex) disappears by 5 months. The infant is held in a supine position with one hand supporting the head and neck. By sudden slight dropping of the examiner's hand supporting the head a response is elicited. The normal response is for babies to spread their arms away from their chest with hands open and fingers spread apart followed by a movement of the arms towards the centre of their chest as if in an embrace. The legs are flexed. Failure to respond suggests weakness. Asymmetry may indicate lower spinal lesion if one leg affected. Hyperactivity suggests CNS infection and reverse Moro. Where the baby extends limbs with external rotation, this indicates basal ganglia disease
Grasp reflex	Palmar or plantar response up to 9 months. An object is placed in the palm and the fingers automatically flex to grip the object. The foot would be similarly stimulated in the area behind the toes. Failure to respond suggests CNS weakness, depending on symmetry of reflex
Plantar reflex	This is achieved by firmly stroking the lateral sole of the baby's foot and extending the movement across the ball of the foot. A normal response in a child under 1 year is extension of the hallux. An abnormal response indicates dysfunction of the upper motor neurones
Placing and stepping/ walking reflex	If you touch the anterior aspect of either upper or lower limb (anterior tibia) against the edge of an examination couch the child will lift the limb to place the foot/hand onto the surface of the couch. Alternatively, place the dorsum of the foot beneath the table top to attain the same response. This occurs in the newborn up to about 4 weeks of age. If the baby is gently held above a surface with the soles lightly contacting the surface this will elicit a stepping/walking motion. This response is present until 8 weeks of age. Absence may indicate brain damage
Tonic neck reflex	When the baby is supine and not crying, the head will be turned to one side and the arm on the same side will be extended. The other knee will often be flexed. In normal babies, passive rotation of the head will increase upper body muscle tone on the side to which the head is turned. This reflex present up to 3 months
Patellar and ankle	Results should be similar to normal adult tendon reflex

Musculoskeletal assessment

Walking is perhaps the most sensitive indicator of a child's neuromuscular status. It is an ability that is refined with age and with practice, yet many parents are dissatisfied with their child's style of gait. Parents seek advice less frequently before their children walk. In those cases the complaint usually relates to the shape or the position that a foot or the toes are adopting. Once again it is vital to differentiate normal development from true abnormality.

Musculoskeletal assessment can be subdivided into three parts:

- Gait analysis
- Weightbearing assessment
- Non-weightbearing assessment.

The examination process outlined in Chapter 10 can be used with children as well as adults; however, the following specific points should be noted.

Gait analysis

The principles of gait analysis in the paediatric examination are the same as those for an examination of an adult patient (see Chs 10, 11). However differences do exist and these are fundamentally due to the child's changing gait as they mature. The examiner must familiarise themselves with the changes in order to identify a pathology when it exists. Gait analysis starts from the walk from the waiting room to the surgery and this initial contact enables the practitioner to gain a general impression of lower-limb function. Capturing the child unawares may reveal many clues to the problem which may be hidden when under the glare of the formal examination. It is also an opportunity to observe the child wearing shoes in order to evaluate the effect of the footwear on lower limb mechanics. Formal gait analysis should be done with the child barefoot and in shorts. This allows the position of the lower limb, especially the knees to be assessed. An evaluation should be made as to whether the child's gait is appropriate for their age. As with all patients it is important to observe the child from head to toe, taking note of any signs of asymmetry of posture. The head should be level in the frontal plane. In very young children the head is positioned slightly ahead of the body and may tilt downwards in the sagittal plane to improve forward momentum as the child chases their centre of gravity. Symmetry of facial features and head size should also be evaluated. The shoulders should be aligned and a child over 6 years should have symmetry of arm position (same distance from the body) and symmetrical arm swing. In static stance the arms should hang level; if they appear uneven when fingers are straightened this may suggest a corresponding shoulder drop. If shoulders are level and there is no evidence of scoliosis then anisomelia of the arms may be present. When one arm is held close to the body in a flexed position a neurological assessment is indicated in order to rule out an upper motor neurone lesion, e.g. as in hemiparesis or cerebral palsy (Fig. 14.4).

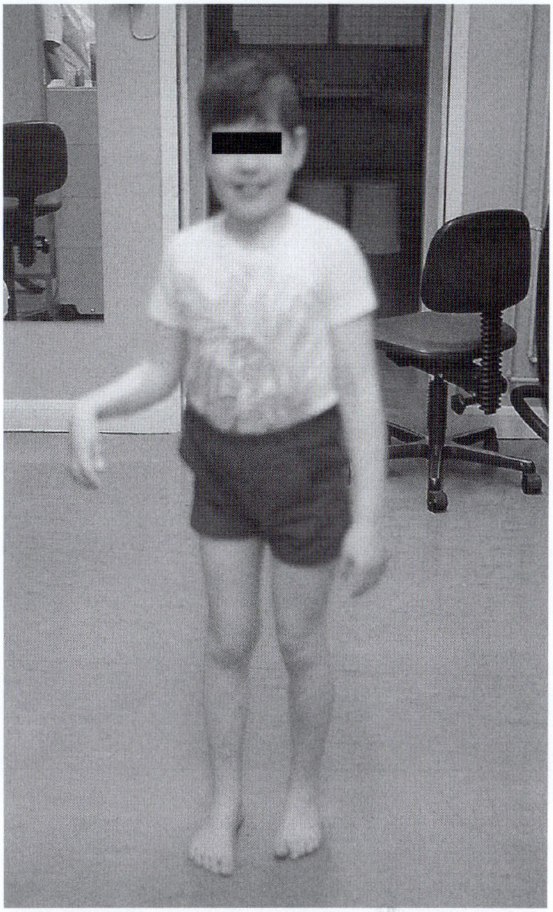

Figure 14.4 An 11-year-old boy with cerebral palsy. Right-sided spasticity and ankle equinus.

Asymmetry at the level of the pelvis during walking may indicate pathology associated with a scoliosis or a limb-length discrepancy, although it should be remembered that small discrepancies of up to 1 cm are common and usually transient in children. Nevertheless weightbearing and non-weightbearing examination of the spine should be performed in order to exclude a true pathology that should be referred for an orthopaedic opinion. Gluteal muscle weakness or paralysis associated with hip disorders will cause a distinct lateral lurch in gait (Trendelenburg's gait) as the fulcrum for the muscle is lost.

Equinus may be apparent during gait. In children up to 4 years it is not uncommon to observe toe-walking. Abnormal intoeing or out-toeing should be noted. A limp if suspected needs further investigation (see later section on limping), and the presence of a scissoring gait, indicative of spastic adductors, warrants closer neurological examination.

Weightbearing assessment

Spine

It is important to check the spine for shape, deformity and movement. Check for normal skin covering and absence of dimpling at the base of the spine over lumbar vertebrae 3/4. Dimpling, or the presence of a tuft of hair at the base of the spine may indicate spina bifida occulta (Figs 14.5, 14.6). Note whether scoliosis, kyphosis or lordosis is present and whether it is a functional or fixed deformity. A fixed deformity is usually due to bony abnormality (structural), whereas a flexible (functional) deformity is due to soft-tissue contracture. Fixed spinal curvatures are retained when sitting and flexing the spine, especially scoliosis. Scoliosis is a frontal plane deformity but there may be signs of vertebral rotation, causing a kyphotic or humped appearance in the sagittal plane. Progressive thoracolumbar problems can impair pulmonary function and in time may lead to strain on respiration.

Marked scoliosis in children, especially where epiphyses are still open, must be considered potentially progressive. Such patients should be referred for a specialist opinion. Lordosis is increased forward curvature in the sagittal plane and commonly affects the lumbar vertebrae. The lordotic curvature varies among races, and African Caribbeans having a larger lordotic curvature than Asians and Caucasians. Early walkers also seem to have an increased lumbar lordosis but this is due to a protruding abdomen.

Hips

Trendelenburg's sign may be useful in detecting hip weakness. Trendelenburg's test is a measure of normal muscle action between the pelvis and greater trochanter (gluteus medius). If the mechanism fails, it is deemed positive (see Ch. 10, section A).

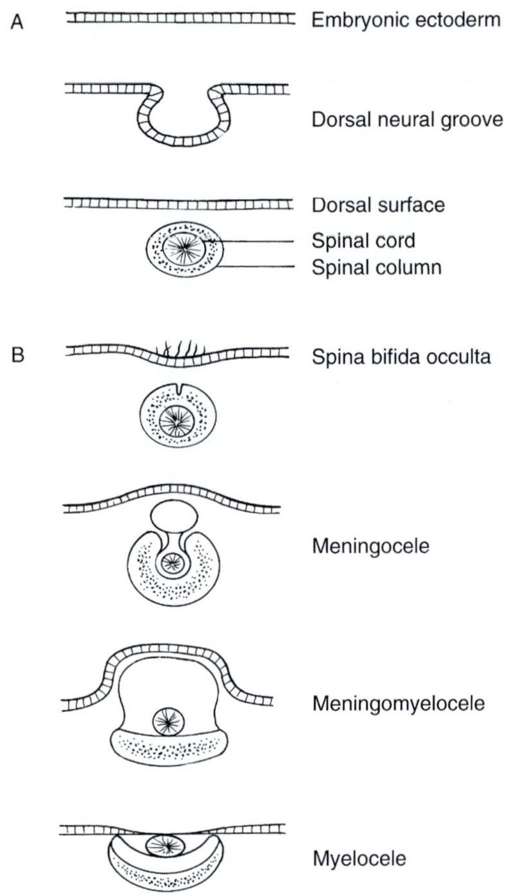

Figure 14.5 **A** Normal development of the neural tube and spine. **B** Classification of spinal dysfunction.

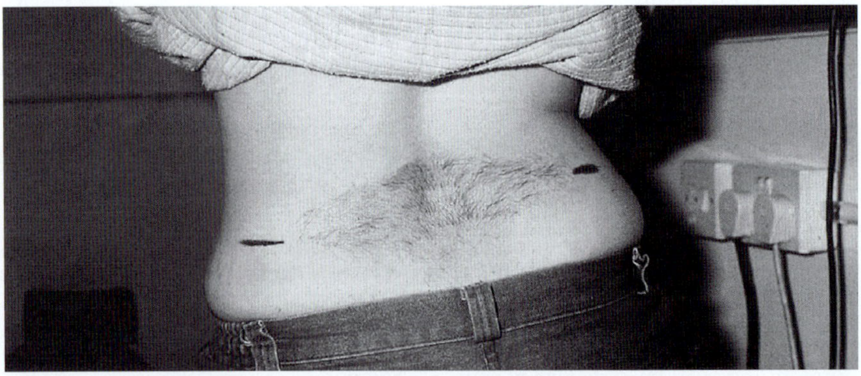

Figure 14.6 Hair at the base of the spine, associated with spina bifida occulta.

Non-weightbearing assessment

Very young children may be best examined on a parent's lap. The lower limb is examined for pain, swelling, obvious deformity and signs of weakness. Both limbs should appear the same regarding position, muscle bulk and tone. There should be symmetry in ranges and direction of joint motion on each side. Ranges of motion change with development, i.e. the younger the child the greater the range of motion. Quality of motion should be smooth and unhindered. The limbs should be warm and the temperature gradient symmetrical. The limbs should be examined for dislocations, fractures, soft-tissue masses and enlargement of bony areas. A visual estimation of limb length should be made at the level of the malleoli, with the legs together.

Pelvis and hips

Altered function of the gluteal muscles due to hip dysplasia will cause a change in the shape of the buttocks. As a result the gluteal fat folds will not appear level. This is the so-called 'anchor sign' in which the central crease forms the shaft of the anchor and the two gluteal folds at the inferior edge of the buttocks form the arms the anchor. If the arms of the 'anchor' are not level this implies asymmetry (Fig. 14.7). When performing tests on the hips of children, the practitioner must avoid damaging the blood supply to the femoral head. At birth the head of the femur lies superficially in the acetabulum, which gives the appearance that the thigh is externally rotated on the pelvis. As the child develops, the head of the femur goes deeper into the acetabulum, which in turn allows the limb to internally rotate. In a normal neonate there is a ratio of 2:1 external to internal hip rotation. With development, the amount of external rotation reduces as the amount of internal rotation increases to the point where a normal adult value shows equal internal and external rotation of 45° in each direction (Table 14.4). When undertaking formal hip examination it is important to evaluate flexion/extension, abduction/adduction and internal/external rotation in both hip-flexed and hip-extended positions (see Ch. 10, section A). This should be followed by assessment of hamstring tightness (Fig. 14.8). The lengths of the tibiae and femurs can be compared using the Allis/skyline test (see Fig. 10A.28). A limb-length discrepancy in an infant may be indicative of hip dislocation. However, the examiner must be vigilant to the possibility of bilateral dislocation, where there will be symmetry.

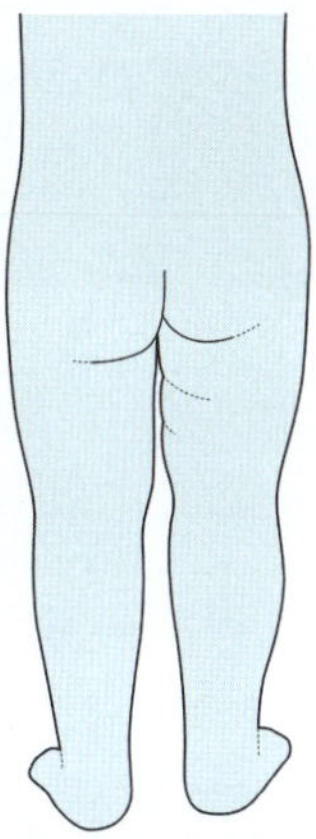

Figure 14.7 The anchor sign. Note asymmetry of gluteal folds and asymmetrical creases in the leg.

In the neonate, ligamentous laxity may be present, together with instability of the hip. This is associated with circulating maternal hormones, in particular, relaxin, a polypeptide produced by the corpus luteum. Correct technique in hip examination is paramount in order to prevent iatrogenic dislocation or avascular necrosis of the femoral head. Nerves lying posterior to the hip joint, particularly the sciatic

Table 14.4 Average range of motion at hip

Age	*Total range*	*Neutral position*	*External*	*Internal*
Birth	100°+	30° external	70°+	0–30°
6 months	90°	30° external	50–60°	30°
18 months	90°	10° external	40–50°	35–45°
6 years	90°	Patella in frontal plane	45°	45°

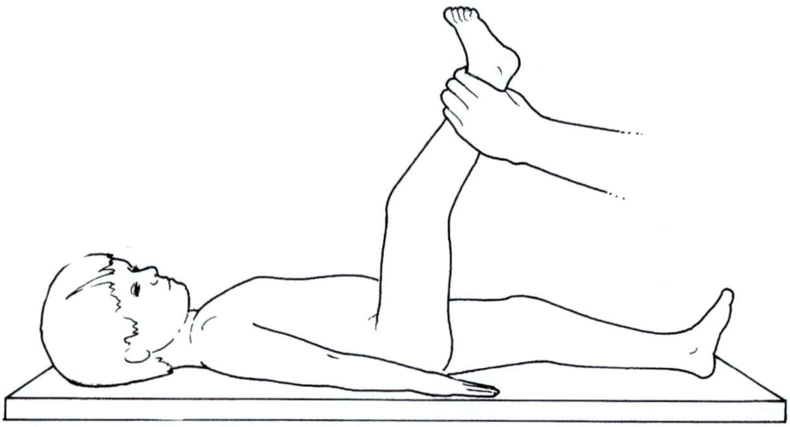

Figure 14.8 To determine hamstring tightness the child is laid supine and the hip flexed to 90°. The knee is also flexed to 90° and then extended. A minimum of 70° extension is required from this position.

Table 14.5 Frontal plane alignment of the knee

Birth	*Genu varum 15–20°*
2–5 years	Straight
4–6 years	Genu valgum 5–15°
6–12 years	Straight
12–14 years	Genu valgum 5–10°
14–16 years	Straight

nerve, are subject to trauma in posterior hip dislocation. Damage to the nerve may lead to motor and sensory loss.

Knees

During childhood the knee undergoes a swing in the frontal plane from varus to valgus and then back towards neutral as shown in Table 14.5 (Beeson 1999). Bow legs (genu varum) occur normally between birth and 2 years of age (Fig. 14.9). Physiological genu valgum (knock knees) is commonly seen between the ages of 3 and 6 years (Salenius & Vankka 1975). At 4 years of age girls tend to be more knock-kneed than boys (Heath & Staheli 1993). Children usually outgrow physiological genu valgum by the age of 8 years (Beeson 1999). Some authors have suggested that a second episode of genu valgum may occur between 12 and 14 years of age (Laporta 1973); this is mainly seen in girls due to the pubertal effects of growth (Cahuzac et al 1995).

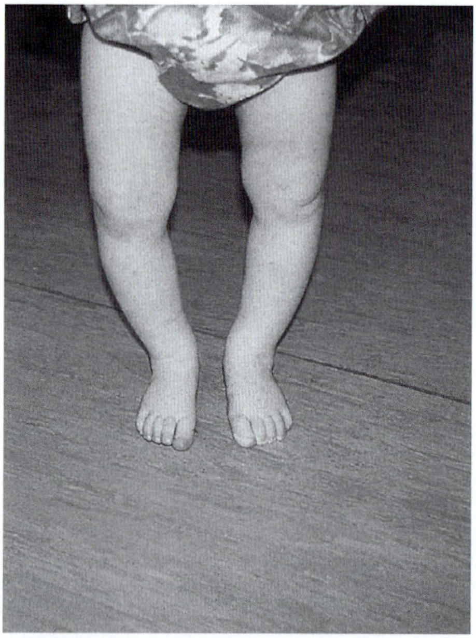

Figure 14.9 A 16 month-old girl with tibia varum.

Knee position can be assessed with the child either lying supine or standing. In the supine position the child's knees or ankles are placed together with the legs parallel to the examination couch. The distance between the medial femoral condyles of the knees and medial malleoli of the ankles can then be measured with a tape measure.

The child should be observed from the side for genu recurvatum (hyperextension). This deformity occurs in the sagittal plane. In very early childhood, genu recurvatum may be present but should reduce with development as the knee ligaments tighten. If reduction does not occur the patient should be tested for ligamentous laxity (Harris & Beeson 1998).

The range of transverse plane motion in the knee should be equal in both directions and be minimal by the age of 4 years. In the newborn 20–30° of total motion may be available (Kilmartin 1988). The amount of rotation of the tibia on the femur should reduce by 10° at 3 years of age and at 6 years of age should show minimal movement.

Table 14.6 Malleolar position (MP) and tibial torsion (TT) at various ages

Age	*TT*	*MP*
Birth	0	0
1 year	6	3–4
2 years	12	6–8
6 years	22	18–20

Patellae

The patellae may be up to 30° externally rotated at birth. In young children it is considered normal for the patellae to be externally rotated, but by 5 years of age the patellae should face forwards. This optimal positioning of the patellae depends on normal hip development. The change of direction of motion and range of motion (ROM) at the hip, femoral torsion and reduction of external position of the femoral head allow the patellae to face anteriorly. These changes may continue until 10 years of age.

Tibiofibular segment

The tibiae should appear symmetrical. Signs of excessive frontal plane bowing should be noted and conditions such as Blount's disease and rickets ruled out. The calf muscles should be assessed for tone, bulk and symmetry. Exaggerated lateral calf muscles with forward facing patellae may suggest medial genicular position.

The tibia and fibula twist with normal development. At birth it will be apparent that the malleoli are on the same level in the frontal plane. As development ensues, the distal end of the tibia twists externally (tibial torsion). The lateral malleolus moves to a more posterior position. There is axial rotation of the tibia and fibula as well as twisting within the bone itself. Malleolar position will reach an adult value around 6 years of age with a position of approximately 18° external rotation (Table 14.6). This represents a true external tibial torsion of around 25° (Elftman 1945, Lang & Volpe 1998).

Ankle

In the newborn there is approximately 50° dorsiflexion and 30° plantarflexion at the ankle. The ROM at this joint decreases with development. Any limitation of ankle joint ROM needs further evaluation (see Ch. 10, section B). There should be no deep creasing anterior to the ankle; if present, this may indicate a fixed dorsiflexed ankle (calcaneovalgus deformity). Where persistent toe-walking exists, neurological pathology needs to be distinguished from habitual causes.

Foot

Careful examination of each joint followed by assessment of forefoot to rearfoot alignment is indicated. The rearfoot must be examined with the ankle, the forefoot with the midtarsal joint and the toes with the metatarsophalangeal joints. Documenting the shape of the weightbearing foot is also important.

Rearfoot

The calcaneus will have a relatively low calcaneal inclination angle in the sagittal plane. In the neonate the neutral position of the calcaneus is 8–10° varus. The talus undergoes valgus rotation until 6 years. The angle of declination of the talus increases, which helps bring the foot from its supinated embryonic position to its more pronated adult position. At birth the forefoot may be slightly inverted, but this reduces with normal development. The young child has a relatively narrow heel in relation to the breadth of the forefoot. The foot should have a straight lateral border. In a rectus foot a line bisecting the heel to forefoot will demonstrate equal parts medial and lateral to the line. In an adducted foot, the medial side will appear greater and, conversely, in the abducted foot the lateral side will appear greater (Fig. 14.10).

Forefoot

The midtarsus and metatarsus should be examined for frontal plane abnormalities as well as transverse abnormalities. The forefoot in the newborn is 10–15° inverted on the rearfoot (Tax 1985). Deformity distal to the metatarsals may be directly related to the metatarsals or may be an isolated deformity.

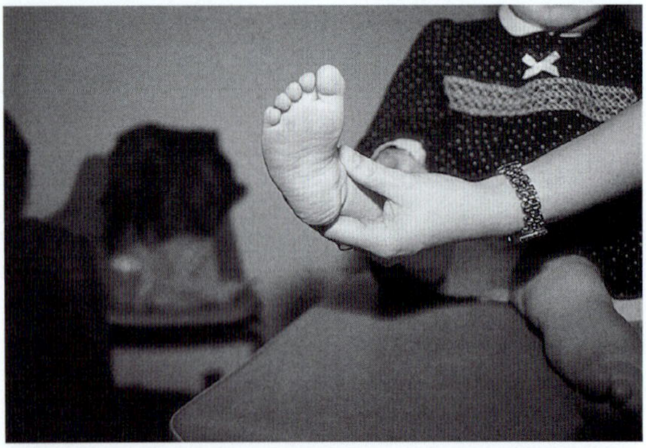

Figure 14.10 A line through the heel should bisect the forefoot through the second or third toe. In this patient the line passes lateral to the second/third toe demonstrating a mild metatarsus adductus.

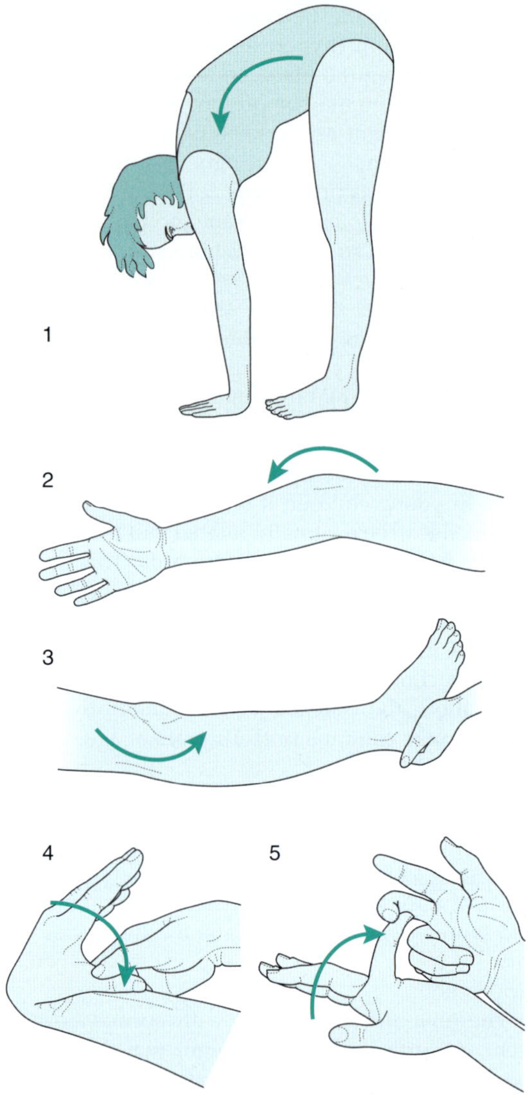

	Score Left	Right
1. Can you put your hands flat on the floor with your knees straight?	1	
2. Can you bend your elbow backwards?	1	1
3. Can you bend your knee backwards?	1	1
4. Can you bend your little finger back on to the front of your forearm?	1	1
5. Can you bend your little finger up to 90^0 (right angles) to the back of your hand?	1	1
	9	

Figure 14.11 Beighton's criteria. (Reproduced with kind permission of the ARC.)

Joint laxity

Lower limb joint pain in children may sometimes be associated with ligamentous laxity (Bulbena et al 1992). Such hypermobility can affect one joint or it may be generalised. Joint flexibility is in part determined by the shape of the articular surfaces and also the laxity in the ligaments and joint capsule; it may be quantified by using Beighton's criteria (Beighton et al 1989) (see below). Children with functional flat feet may also have hypermobility in other joints. Other typical presentations are children with a history of 'clicking' hips as babies or who now report 'clicking' joints, usually the ankle. They may also have a history of generalised 'growing pains'. Parents may also complain of the child being easily tired and wanting to be carried a lot. However, children with hypermobility may make very good gymnasts and dancers. Hypermobility itself may be seen to be a spectrum of joint mobility ranging from a generalised ligamentous laxity through to a benign hypermobility syndrome where, in addition to the above there may history of joint effusions, arthralgia or dislocations. There may be a link with other connective tissue disorders such as Ehlers–Danlos syndrome (Murray & Ferrari 2001).

Beighton's criteria

Beighton's criteria is a nine-point scoring system and centres on the ability of the patient to perform certain tasks (Fig. 14.11); points are awarded up to a maximum of 9. The patient is requested to:

1. Touch the floor with the palms of their hands, keeping their knees straight (1 point)
2. Hyperextend the elbows beyond 10° (1 point for each side)
3. Hyperextend the knee beyond 10° (1 point for each side)
4. Appose the thumb to the forearm on flexion of the hand and wrist (1 point for each side)
5. Hyperextend the metacarpalphalangeal joints to 90° or beyond (1 point for each side).

Children who get 4 or more points are considered to have ligamentous laxity (Murray & Ferrari 2001).

Footwear

Evaluation of the child's footwear and hosiery is important. Children's feet should be measured on a regular basis to ensure they have not outgrown their shoes. Footwear should be of the correct length, width and depth. Often parents present their children to clinic because they are concerned about excessive shoe wear. It is important to determine whether the shoe wear is normal or abnormal or, indeed, if the footwear is suitable for the purpose. For this, it is important to establish how long the shoes are worn each day, the level and type of activity the child engages in and the types of material the shoe is constructed from. Wear marks may be misleading, for example heavy toebox wear in a child using the foot as a bicycle break can be confused with a child who drags his foot due to a hemiparesis. When considering the use of orthotics in the management of any condition, the practitioner should bear in mind and reinforce to the patient that the first orthotic is the shoe itself (Ch. 9).

Conditions affecting the lower limb of children

Developmental dysplasia of the hip

DDH is usually detected shortly after birth, during routine examination of the neonate by the paediatrician with the help of Barlow's and Ortolani's tests (see below), which, although 100% specific, are at best only 60% sensitive (Paton et al 2005). Hence it is possible for the condition to be missed and not picked up until later in the child's development. Therefore it is good practice, when the opportunity arises to routinely check the child's hips for quality of motion and symmetry of ROM. The hips should move smoothly without resistance and with no discomfort to the child. The fact that hip dislocation is not always congenital has resulted in a change in terminology. Congenital dislocation of the hip (CDH) is now known as DDH, thereby reflecting the continuum of developmental dislocation over time (Coleman 1994, Novacheck 1996). DDH may have serious repercussions, leading to osteoarthritis, limb shortening and hip pain.

In a normal hip the quality of motion should be unimpaired when the hip is taken through its ROM. Various tests are used to establish the presence of DDH, although palpating for displacement of the femoral head may be all that is required. It should be noted that clinical examination may not reveal DDH. X-ray and ultrasound imaging can confirm a diagnosis.

Barlow's test

The baby is placed supine with hips and knees flexed. Thumb pressure is applied over the lesser trochanter with the middle finger of each hand over the greater trochanter. The femoral head is gently dislocated by moving the pressure on the hand backwards. Consequent release of pressure allows the head to slip back into position. A positive result indicates that the hips are unstable due to ligamentous laxity. The test becomes less useful as the child becomes older (Valmassy 1991). The wisdom of this manoeuvre is questionable, as the potential for avascular necrosis or neurological damage is increased by intentionally dislocating the hip joint.

Palmen's sign

This is similar to Barlow's test and performed in the same manner. It is a provocative test for a subluxable (but not dislocatable) hip. If the hip is subluxable, the examiner feels a give (but not a clunk) as the femoral head is displaced partially out of the acetabulum (Harris 1997).

Ortolani's manoeuvre

This is performed by flexing the hips to 90°. The middle fingers are again placed over the greater trochanter and the thigh is lifted and abducted. The hip can be relocated with a palpable (rather than audible) click. This test is reliable up to 6–8 weeks of age, but clicking can arise from ligaments moving, giving a false-positive result.

Limitation of hip abduction

This test is used when the infant's dislocated hips no longer reduce with Ortolani's manoeuvre (after 2 months). Abducting the hip with the thigh and knee flexed will be resisted on the dislocated side. This is due to contracted adductors. The anchor sign is abnormal.

Galeazzi's sign

The infant is observed supine with hips and knees flexed and with the feet placed flat on the couch. In normal limbs the level of the knees should be equal. If one knee is lower than the other this may indicate hip pathology on the low side. This is similar to the skyline test for checking the length of the femur and tibia.

Telescope (piston) sign

The hip may be out of the acetabulum but still mobile along the ala of the ilium. With the infant supine, the thigh in the sagittal plane and at right angles to the trunk, longitudinal traction may cause the head to slide up and down along the lateral side of the ala (Harris 1997).

Knee pain in the child

Complaints of significant, persistent knee pain are relatively uncommon in children, and usually children present with a limp or refusal to walk. The clinical history should attempt to localise the pain, determine what activities exacerbate the pain and what treatment has been provided to date. It is also useful to assess the psychosocial dynamics of the child and their family. All children between the ages of 5 and 15 years presenting with knee pain must also be evaluated for ipsilateral hip disorders (Davids 1996). A structured approach to knee assessment is essential (see Ch. 10, section A). Specific knee tests indicated in children are given below.

Patellar compression test

With the patient lying supine and the knee extended, the practitioner compresses the patella against the femoral condyles. If performed too vigorously it will cause pain, even in the normal knee. A more sensitive approach of gradually loading the kneecap is preferred and is less distressing for the patient.

Medial facet tenderness test

The patella is displaced medially and the practitioner palpates the posterior medial surface. Performing this test also determines whether there is any tightness of the lateral capsule tending to pull the patella laterally, increasing shearing forces on the posterior facets, which may damage the articular cartilage.

Quadriceps muscle bulk evaluation

The patient is asked to contract the quadriceps muscle group; the bulk of the vastus medialis muscle is assessed. Loss of muscle bulk can occur with chronic pain or poor mechanical function of the knee.

Muscle function

Quadriceps muscle strength and hamstring flexibility should also be assessed. The 90 : 90 test will determine hamstring tightness which, when present, will tend to flex the knee and increase patellofemoral compression forces.

Squatting test

The patient is asked to stand on both feet and then crouch down. Patients with severe pain will express discomfort; as the knee flexes the posterior surface of the patella is compressed against the femur. The degree to which squatting is restricted will indicate the severity of the condition.

Anterior knee pain can occur during adolescence (it is more common in girls). It is a recalcitrant problem which, in a minority of cases, can be disabling. The pain will be most intense during or after vigorous activity, although kneeling or sitting with a flexed knee for long periods ('cinema seat' sign) may also incite discomfort. A high 'Q' angle (see Ch. 10, section B) has been implicated as a precipitating factor. Internal femoral rotation, external tibial rotation and genu valgum are known to increase this angle. At certain stages of development an increased 'Q' angle will be normal when physiological knee valgus is present. The 'Q' angle should reduce to <15° by 6 years of age.

Osteochondritis dissecans, characterised by primary necrosis of subchondral bone, causes knee pain. The commonest site is over the lateral side of the medial femoral condyle. Osgood–Schlatter disease is a traction apophysitis affecting the tibial tubercle and is associated with patellar tendon strain. It predominantly affects boys between the ages of 10 and 14 years. Pain is anterior and below the knee. It is made worse by strenuous activity. Examination will reveal the presence of a prominent and tender tibial tubercle, and quadriceps wasting may be visible. Extending the leg against resistance exacerbates the symptoms. Radiographs may show fragmentation of the tibial tuberosity at the tendon insertion.

Abnormal frontal plane configuration of the knee

Parental concern about knock-knees or bow legs is a common presenting complaint.

Genu varum

Genu varum is normally present from birth until 2 years of age. If a child presents with bow legs at 3–4 years of age, further investigation and treatment may be necessary. A distance of more than 5 cm between the knees, at any age, is cause for concern and necessitates further investigation (Sharrard 1976). Rickets and Blount's disease are two conditions predisposing to genu vara with tibial vara.

Rickets will present as genu varum as well as anterior bowing at the junction of the middle and lower one-third of the tibia. Swelling of the wrists and ankles and bossing of the cranium is also seen in rickets. Radiological investigation will show the epiphyses to be widened and irregular, whereas the metaphyses will appear 'cupped' (see Ch. 12). Biochemical tests are performed to determine levels of vitamin D, calcium and phosphate, which may be low due to dietary deficiency, malabsorption, renal disease or hypophosphatasia. If biochemical tests prove normal, Blount's disease may be suspected.

Blount's disease is a condition in which the growth of the medial upper tibial epiphysis is affected. Cessation of the growth plate at this part will cause the tibia to develop a lateral varus tilt. This condition has an estimated incidence of 0.05 per 1000 live births and is due to the lateral side of the growth plate expanding faster than the medial side. Blount's disease is thought to be a combination of obesity and marked physiological bowing. This will have the effect of compressing the medial side of the growth plate, which causes further bowing of the tibia. The lateral epiphysis continues to expand as pressure is released. The medial epiphysis will appear fragmented on X-ray. Blount's disease may appear at any time between the ages of 18 months and 4 years. The patient should be referred for treatment as the condition will invariably progress without treatment. In the infant, Blount's disease is often severe with both knees affected. Arrest of the medial growth plate may also affect older children (between 6 and 13 years), in whom the deformity is usually unilateral and less severe than the infantile variety, though no less certain to progress without treatment. Unilateral tibia vara may contribute to limb-length discrepancy. Trauma, infection (McRae 1997) and fluorosis (Tachdjian 1972) can also result in marked genicular bowing.

Genu valgum

Genu valgum is normally present between 3–5 years of age and 12–14 years of age. In severe unremitting cases radiological examination should be used to rule out developmental or metabolic abnormalities of the epiphyses. Surgical correction may have to be considered, although this is rare. Unilateral knock knee should be investigated as it is almost always a pathological defect of the epiphysis associated with either trauma, osteomyelitis, tumour or developmental bone disturbance. Excessive subtalar joint pronation of the foot has been associated with genu valgum, as it throws body weight medial to the central axis of the foot and hence tends to force the foot into pronation. Conversely, excessive varus deformity of the forefoot may create frontal plane movement of the knee, in order to bring the entire forefoot into ground contact, resulting in genu valgum.

Popliteal angle in children

The popliteal angle is defined as the angle of the tibia to the femur when the hip is flexed and knee extended. The popliteal angle is measured to assess hamstring tightness in healthy children and hamstring contracture in cerebral palsy (Katz et al 1992). It is also used as an indicator of gestational age in infants. The mean angle in newborns is reported to be 27°, and it reduces to zero by the age of 11 months (Reade et al 1984).

Hamstring and, more specifically, medial hamstring shortening is a common cause of asymmetrical hip motion and subsequent intoeing. Diagnosis is made by flexing the hip to 90° and then attempting to extend the knee using the 90:90 test (see Fig. 14.8). In children under 10 years, less than 70% extension is unsatisfactory. Quality of motion is also evaluated while performing the 90:90 test. If the hamstrings resist the final 30° of motion, it is usual for the child to experience discomfort, which indicates an abnormal tightness. The medial hamstring tension can be tested by internally rotating the flexed upper thigh while gradually extending the knee. If, with internal rotation of the thigh, knee extension is limited and uncomfortable, then the medial hamstring is the principal cause of the complaint.

Children with tight hamstrings can assume a normal angle and base of stance; however, during gait, as the knee extends just prior to heel contact, the tight medial hamstring will abruptly rotate the leg internally. Such cases will also demonstrate a windmilling style of running, the lower leg being circumducted during the late swing phase of running in order to 'short-cut' around the extended knee position. Growing pains are common in children with such intoeing. Hamstrings should therefore be tested in any child with persistent nocturnal leg pains.

Intoe

The treatment of intoe is controversial, as it is considered by some to be a normal developmental condition that children outgrow whether they are treated or not (Fabry et al 1973, Svenningson et al 1990, Thackeray & Beeson 1996a, b). More research needs to be done in this area. However, when the child is constantly tripping and falling over and their normal activities are being affected, treatment is required. In addition, it is a common finding that if the child cannot achieve enough external rotation at the hip for the normal swing phase of gait, compensatory mechanisms come into play to circumnavigate this problem. Although intoeing was once thought to cause osteoarthrosis of the hip and poor sporting ability (Alvick 1960), it was subsequently shown to be unimportant in osteoarthrosis of the hip (Hubbard et al 1988).

When assessing the child with an intoe gait, it is important to decide at what level the problem lies. Intoe may originate at the level of the hip, thigh, knee, lower leg or foot (Fig. 14.12). It is generally accepted that the higher up the leg is the problem the greater the degree to which the child will intoe. It is important to remember that walking starts with swing phase. If the adductors are tight or if there is significant persistent femoral anteversion then this will have a greater influence on where the foot comes to rest and hence its relationship to the line of progression than if there is mild metatarsus adductus with normal external deflection of the leg during the swing phase. It is also important to note whether the intoe is constant or whether it varies with each step. If it is the latter, the practitioner may be confident that there will be a significant soft-tissue involvement – which should be looked for in the non-weightbearing part of the examination.

Assessment starts with gait analysis. The key to accurate diagnosis is the position of the patella. In children younger than 5–6 years the patella may be seen to lie in a slightly external position to the frontal plane. In the intoeing child, the patella will either point in the direction of progression or it will be internally rotated or 'squinting'. A squinting patella indicates that the cause of the gait defect is proximal to the knee joint. Severely adducted feet in the presence of a forward-looking patella occur in cases of internal genicular position, internal tibial torsion and metatarsus adductus.

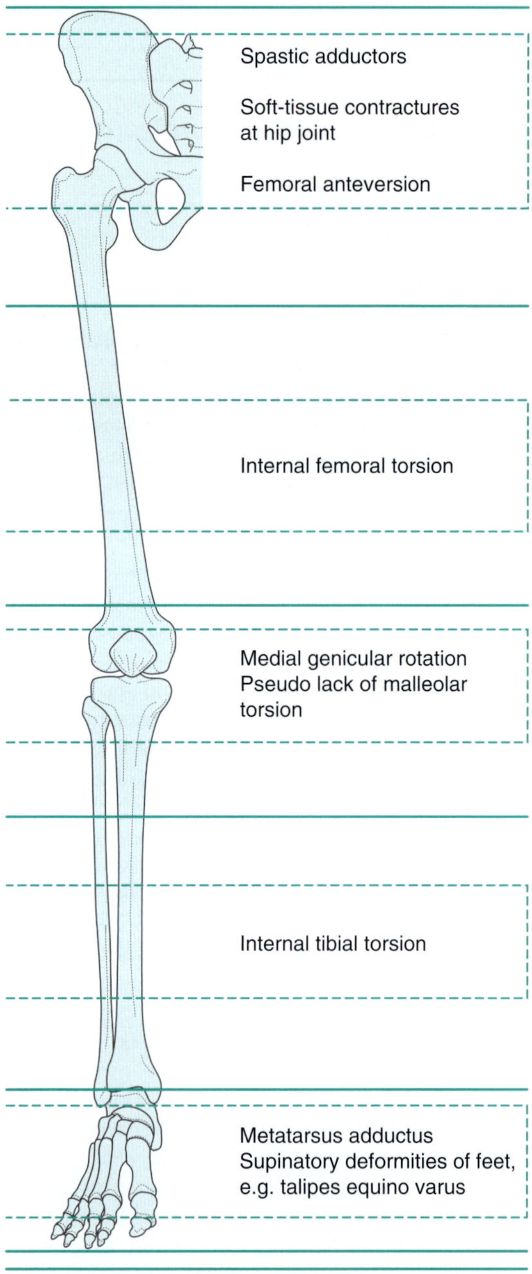

Figure 14.12 Transverse plane disorders. The examiner must decide at what level the disorder lies when treating intoe.

Following gait analysis, the ROM at the hip and knee joint and the position of the transmalleolar axis and forefoot should be assessed. The range of hip rotation is assessed with the knee and hip extended. The leg is brought to the neutral position where the patella is facing directly upwards (parallel with the frontal plane). While viewing the patella, the leg is internally and then externally rotated and the degree of rotation estimated. In children younger than 6 years it may be expected that there is a greater range of external to internal range of hip motion available. After this age equal amounts should be considered the norm (see Table 14.4). Therefore, any case where internal ROM is greater than external is abnormal. This movement should be repeated with the hip at 90°. Should the available external ROM increase in this position it may be assumed that the cause has been tight soft-tissue structures at the level of the hip, for example the iliofemoral and pubofemoral ligaments. By flexing the hip the practitioner has effectively relaxed these structures and allowed for the increased external rotation. When there is a true femoral torsion then changing position will not affect the internal: external ratio. It may be convenient at this point to enquire about sleeping and sitting positions that the child may have adopted. Any position where the child is likely to be found for long periods of time can affect hip ROM. If those positions encourage internal rotation of the hip this will not allow for any reduction in hip position due to soft-tissue contractures. A child who sleeps on their abdomen may adopt a position where the feet and legs are internally rotated against the mattress (Fig. 14.13). Likewise, a child who persistently sits in the reversed tailor or 'W' position will also encourage internal positioning of the hip in the frontal plane (Thomson 2001) (Fig. 14.14).

Tibial torsion and internal genicular position

Clinical diagnosis of internal tibial torsion is made by measuring the transmalleolar axis which is formed between the midpoints of the medial and lateral malleoli and the frontal plane. As previously mentioned this transmalleolar axis increases during the first few years of life from 0–4° at birth to 18–22° at age 6 (adult value). Many complex methods have been described for measuring tibial torsion (Reikeras & Hoiseth 1989). A quick clinical estimation is made by placing the thumb of each hand anterior to the malleoli; the medial malleoli should be one thumb's thickness anterior to the lateral malleoli (**Fig. 14.15**).

The incidence of internal tibial torsion has been reported to range from 1% to 40% (Hutter & Scott 1949, Michele & Nielson 1976). In some cases the transmalleolar axis will appear normal though it is apparent on gait analysis that the whole tibia is internally rotated on the knee. This condition is called internal tibial position or internal genicular position. An internal genicular position is an important cause of intoeing and is so similar to tibial torsion that it is quite likely to be misdiagnosed as such.

Internal genicular position only becomes a cause for concern for parents when a child starts to walk. Examination will reveal a normal transmalleolar axis but an abnormally high internal range of motion at

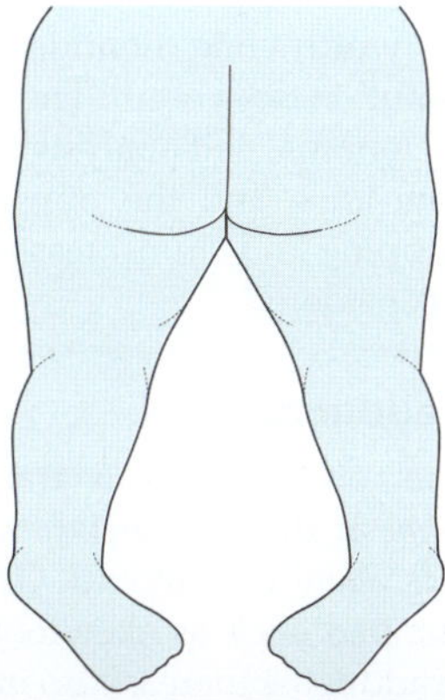

Figure 14.13 Lying prone for long periods of time such as when sleeping with the legs internally rotated will encourage internal rotation at the level of the hip. Note also internal rotation of the feet.

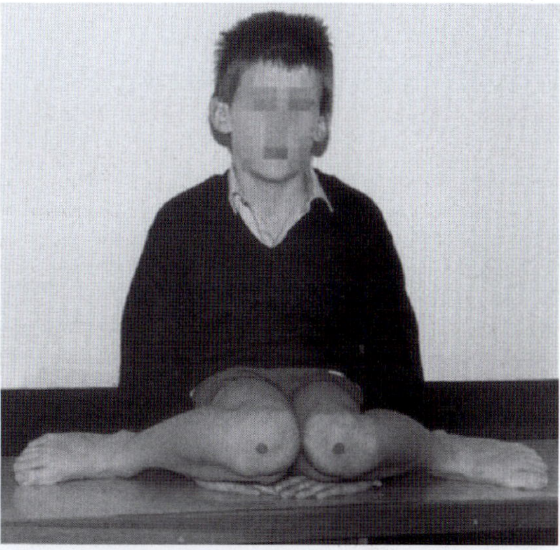

Figure 14.14 Reversed tailor or 'W' sitting position. Note internal position of femur.

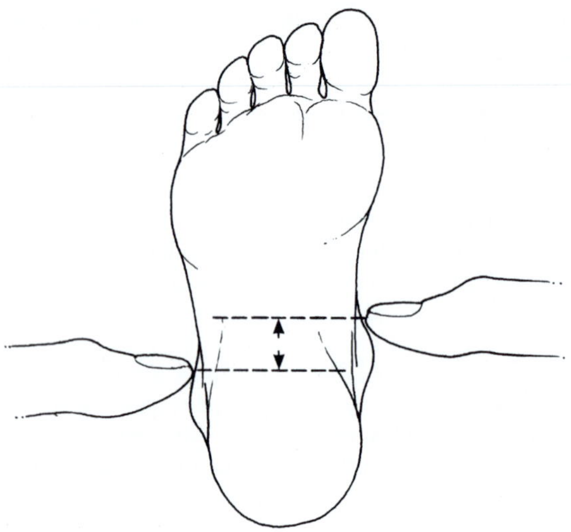

Figure 14.15 Check malleolar position by placing the thumbs on the anterior surface of the malleoli. There should be one thumb's thickness difference between the medial and lateral malleoli.

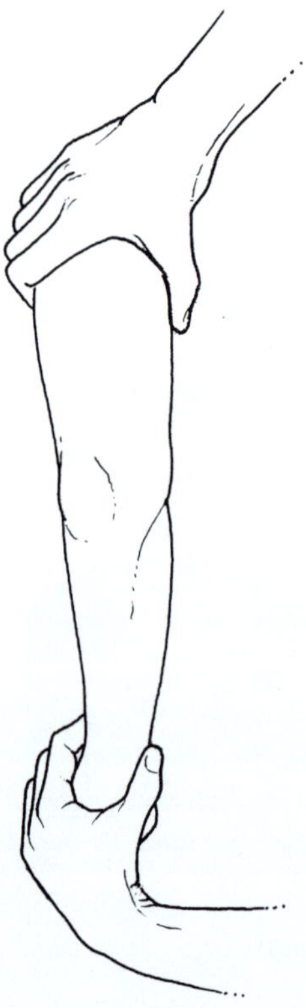

Figure 14.16 Internal tibial position is estimated by rotating the tibia internally and externally on the knee joint.

Case history 14.2

A 2-year-old child presented with an adducted angle of gait and tibial varum. Examination revealed a normal tibial angle for the child's age; however, during gait the tibiae appeared bowed. Clinical findings revealed a forward-facing knee, with normal range of motion at the hip. Transverse motion at the tibial–femoral interface revealed excessive motion on medial rotation. An intoeing gait pattern was evident and an exaggerated bulging of the gastrocnemius muscle on the lateral side of the leg observed due to the internal position of the leg. This gave a false impression of tibial varum.

Diagnosis: Medial genicular position.

the knee (Case history 14.2). This is estimated by stabilising the thigh and grasping the foot and rotating the tibia internally and then externally (Fig. 14.16). Normally a small but symmetrical ROM of 10–20° will be evident. In cases of internal genicular position, 45° or more of internal rotation may be present. External rotation usually remains no more than 10–20°, although in some cases it is completely absent.

The prognosis for internal genicular position and internal tibial torsion without treatment is good provided that there are no persistent external forces encouraging the deformity and preventing normal external rotation, for example excessive kneeling. It tends to resolve spontaneously around 5–6 years of age. Its significance lies in the fact that it can cause frequent tripping. There is also evidence that it may be a factor associated with the development of osteoarthrosis of the knee (Turner & Smillie 1981). For that reason it is worthwhile monitoring the child to ensure that resolution does occur. The patient should be seen every 6 months, gait analysis performed and the ROM at the knee and the transmalleolar axis measured. If tripping and clumsiness is severe, treatment must be considered.

Metatarsus adductus

True metatarsus adductus is a transverse plane deformity arising at the tarsometatarsal (Lisfranc's) joint. The heel is usually in neutral. Other variations have been described such as skewfoot, in which in addition to the adductus there is also inversion of the forefoot and eversion of the heel, and metatarsus varus, in which there is also adduction of the metatarsals and inversion of the forefoot but the heel may be inverted. Certain authors consider all of these to be the same condition demonstrating varying degrees of complexity and severity (Fagan 1992) and others that the more complex variations are in fact the result of compensatory mechanism from untreated simple metatarsus adductus (Wan 2006).

The aetiology is uncertain. Intra-uterine moulding is a much vaunted explanation and may account for a few cases in which the fetus is large and constrained in its tight container especially when associated with oligohydramnios and where the legs are crossed and one foot tightly trapped against the tibia of the other leg. Other researchers have demonstrated contractures of abductor hallucis or abnormal insertion of tibialis anterior to be possible causes. There may also be a genetic link. The main clinical features are:

- a concave medial border
- a convex lateral border
- a prominent styloid process
- increased metatarsus primus adductus angle.

These features are best seen when holding the child's foot in the cleft of the examiner's second and third fingers (**Fig. 14.17**).

Other clinical signs can help confirm the diagnosis, including wrinkling of the skin in the medial longitudinal arch as a consequence of bunching of the metatarsal bases, a dorsal plantar crease medial to the first metatarsal cuneiform joint, a high arch profile created by adduction of the forefoot on the rearfoot and, if the child is walking, a marked tendency to lateral weightbearing. Internal tibial torsion and abnormal knee position may also occur in combination with metatarsus adductus.

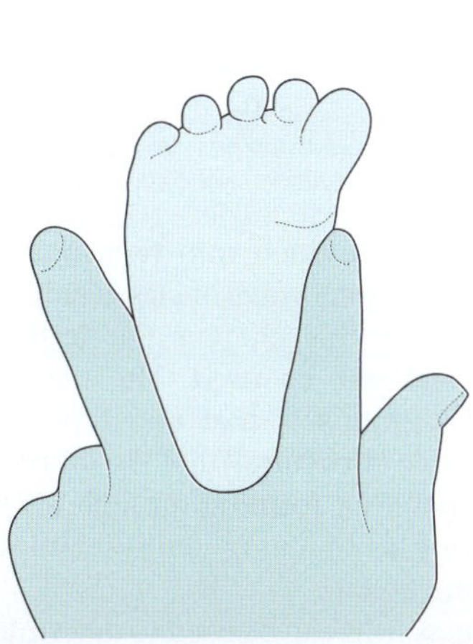

Figure 14.17 Holding the child's foot in the 'V' of the examiner's second and third finger allows for a quick and simple evaluation of the degree of metatarsus adductus.

Metatarsus adductus resolves spontaneously in more than 90% of cases (Staheli 1993). Ponsetti & Becker (1966) found that only 11.6% of their patients required treatment. Rushforth (1978) in an 11-year follow-up of 83 children, also found that 86% demonstrated complete resolution of the deformity. However, others contest the premise that leaving nearly 12% of patients with a deformity is acceptable and advocate a proactive approach (Valmassy 2001, Wan 2006). Metatarsus adductus may be categorised as mild, moderate or severe (Table 14.7). Assessment of the foot's flexibility is the practitioner's primary objective as this will dictate the management pathways (**Fig. 14.18**). If the foot can easily be corrected and the adductus position is mild, the prognosis for spontaneous resolution is excellent. As the deformity becomes more marked there is often a corresponding increase in rigidity. Clinical features of calcaneal eversion, medial talonavicular joint bulging and 'humping' of the dorsolateral midfoot indicate that spontaneous correction is unlikely.

Uncompensated metatarsus adductus presents as a high-arched supinated foot and the older child may complain of a painful styloid process, skin lesions under the fifth metatarsophalangeal joint, incipient hallux abducto valgus and problems with footwear fitting (Valmassy 2001). Accordingly, prognosis is less favourable and treatment should be instigated as soon as possible. Another significant finding on assessment is the presence of a vertical crease overlying the medial cuneiform. The vertical cuneiform crease presents only in the more severely affected feet.

Radiographic examination can assist the evaluation of metatarsus adductus in cases of skew- or Z foot where rearfoot involvement exists. This complex variant of metatarsus adductus presents an everted rearfoot with plantarflexed and adducted talus. Several charting techniques have been developed to measure metatarsus adductus and its variants (Berg 1986). Important X-ray findings include an increased metatarsus angle, metatarsal base superimposition, hypoplasia of the medial cuneiform and metatarsus primus adductus (Valmassy 2001).

Table 14.7 Classification of metatarsus adductus

Mild	Flexible, passively correctable
Moderate	Semi-flexible/reducible
Severe	Rigid

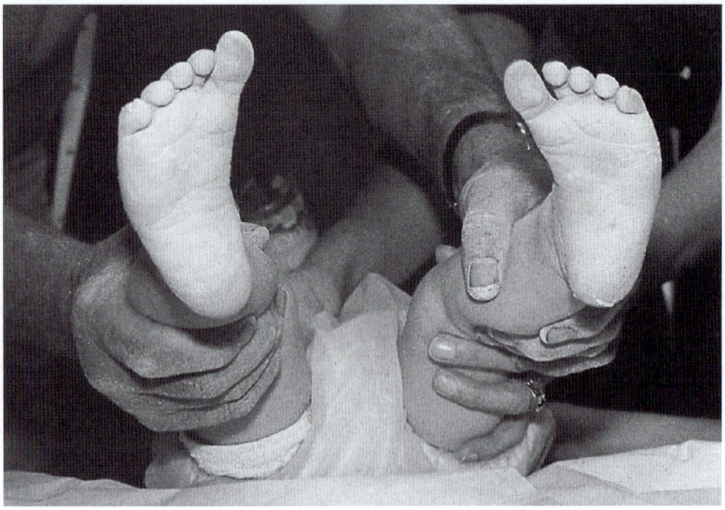

Figure 14.18 A C-shaped curvature of the lateral border of the foot is the hallmark of metatarsus adductus. This 2-year-old boy responded poorly to treatment as the deformity was quite rigid. The early management of metatarsus adductus is desirable.

In order to ensure consistent and reliable diagnosis, all other causes of adducted gait, including internal femoral rotation, internal tibial torsion, genicular position, compensation for a forefoot valgus and hallux varus (Jiminez 1992), must be ruled out. It is important therefore to note any element of these conditions which may be superimposed upon the metatarsus adductus, as management of more than one condition may be necessary.

Congenital talipes equinovarus (clubfoot)

In congenital talipes equinovarus (CTEV), the adductus of the forefoot occurs at the midtarsal joint and not at the tarsometatarsal joint. There are four components to the deformity: equinus, inversion of the rearfoot, and adductus and pronation of the forefoot. The most severe deformities, however, occur in the rearfoot. The talus is abducted and the calcaneus is in equinus. The calcaneus is also inverted, whereas the navicular is displaced medial to the head of the talus. The posterior and medial soft tissues, including tibialis posterior, flexor digitorum longus and triceps surae, are also shortened and atrophied, forming a 'pipe stem' shape to the leg.

CTEV is difficult to correct and there is a high incidence of recurrence. It is well documented that it is easier to correct a clubfoot deformity in the first few days of life than after even a few weeks (Ponsetti 1992). Assessment of the clubfoot should address the relative severity of each of the four components of the condition. The plantarflexed first metatarsal component is critical but usually yields well to manipulative correction. The equinus and inversion components of the rearfoot and the adduction of the forefoot at the talonavicular joint are more resistant to correction (Ponsetti 1996). Internal tibial torsion may also occur with clubfoot and must also be corrected.

No matter how effective the initial treatment is, clubfoot will always result in shortening of the foot, reduced calf muscle circumference and reduced ankle and subtalar joint motion. Medial displacement of the navicular and abduction of the talus on the calcaneus may also persist. In less well corrected clubfeet, poor gait and abnormal forefoot loading results in plantar callus and shoe-fitting difficulties. Ilizarov's technique is occassionally used for the correction of persistent deformities (Wallander et al 1996).

Flatfoot

Flatfoot may be divided into two main categories, and there are various ways of classifying flatfoot. For the purposes of this chapter the terms structural and functional will be used. The main distinction between the groups is that one type is rigid and non-correctable (structural) and the other type is flexible and capable of forming an arch either by non-weightbearing or by being gently manipulated into position (functional).

Three quick tests can be used to determine whether the flatfoot is rigid or flexible. For a baby or very young child the 'Dangle' test may be appropriate. In this test the child is lifted off the ground and the feet allowed to dangle in mid air. The natural response is for the feet to invert and an arch may be observed. The second test is the so-called Jack's test which is based on Wicks' windlass mechanism, where on weightbearing the hallux is manually dorsiflexed. If the flatfoot is of the functional type then the foot will supinate and the medial longitudinal arch will form. The third test involves simply asking the child to stand on tip toe, which causes the heels to invert and form an arch. This manoeuvre is not possible in a structural flatfoot.

Causes of structural flatfoot

Tarsal coalition

This is uncommon. Due to the differences in ossification rates of the bones of the foot certain coalitions are more regularly found in certain age groups, for example talonavicular in 3–5 year-olds, talocalcaneo in the 8–12 year age group and calcaneonavicular in the 12–16 year-olds. There are three types of coalition, categorised by how the bones are connected. Coalitions may either be fibrous (syndesmosis), cartilaginous (synchondrosis) or bony (synostosis). Calcaneonavicular or talocalcaneo coalitions are the most common and account for over 90% of all cases (Fopma & Macnicol 2002, Kaushik 2005). Although they may be difficult to visualise in plain X-rays, initial investigation is usually by this method. However, computed tomography (CT) or magnetic resonance imaging (MRI) may be indicated when a syndesmosis or synchondrosis is suspected. Most authors recommend four X-ray views:

1. Weightbearing dorsiplantar
2. Lateral
3. 45° internal oblique
4. Harris–Beath posterior oblique (axial calcaneum view).

On occasions when the bar cannot be observed directly, changes to the surrounding structures such as talar beaking or narrowing of the talocalcaneo space should raise a high degree of suspicion. The so-called 'C' sign is an area of sclerosis outlining the medial talar dome and the posterioinferior sustentaculum tali. According to Fopma & Macnicol (2002) this observation is considered to have 86.6% sensitivity and 93.3% specificity for talocalcaneo coalitions.

Coalitions may be due to a failure of differentiation of embryonic mesenchyme leading to lack of joint formation or it may be secondary to intra-articular fracture, degenerative joint disease or infection. The incidence is 1–2% and 50% are bilateral. The condition is more common in males. Subtalar coalitions reduce motion at the subtalar joint to almost 0°. This leads to compensation at the midtarsal joint, lowering the medial longitudinal arch and shortening the peroneals resulting in the clinical features of:

- pain in the subtalar and midtarsal region alleviated by rest
- flatfoot, usually in marked valgus
- peroneal spasm.

These features are usually seen in the age group of 3–16 years.

It should be noted that in the absence of tarsal coalition a peroneal spastic flatfoot should be thoroughly investigated as, although it may be idiopathic, it may be associated with juvenile chronic arthritis, osteoid osteoma or osteochondral fracture (Harris et al 2004).

Vertical talus

In this congenital condition the plantar aspect of the foot is convex, the ankle and subtalar joints are rigid and the Achilles tendon is tight. Vertical talus is usually the result of some neural tube defect, neuromuscular disorder or chromosomal aberration. In such cases it is classified as teratogenic (Harris et al 2004). It may also exist with no obvious aetiology, and may then be labelled idiopathic congenital vertical talus. The full effect of the deformity is probably best assessed on X-ray where there can be seen an increased talocalcaneo (kite) angle (anteroposterior view), the talus lying parallel to the tibia and projecting below the first metatarsal. The calcaneus is in equinus and the forefoot dorsiflexed (lateral view). In addition there is disarticulation of the calcaneocuboid joint and a hypoplastic head and neck of talus. The subtalar facet of the calcaneus is abnormal and incomplete.

Talipes calcaneo valgus

The child presents with marked dorsiflexion at the ankle with little or no plantar flexion available. Often described as the 'up-and-out' deformity it is usually unilateral and affects approximately 1–3 per 1000 live births. It is commonly thought to be the result of intrauterine malposition (Silvani 1992). Clinical features include:

- calcaneus in valgus non-weightbearing
- talar head prominent on the medial aspect
- forefoot can touch the anterior leg
- Terdon Achilles not taught even at maximal dorsiflexion

- subtalar joint ROM normal
- foot abducted and dorsiflexed at the MTJ (the up-and-out component).

Causes of functional flatfoot

By definition, a functional flatfoot is a foot that functions with a flattened medial longitudinal arch but has sufficient form to retain an arch when non-weightbearing. Functional flatfoot is extremely common in children. 'Flatfoot' is a term used by both healthcare professionals and lay people. 'Excessive pronation of the foot' may be a more accurate term because, as well as a lowered medial longitudinal arch the flatfoot may also present the following clinical signs:

- Evidence of abduction of the forefoot on the hindfoot at the midtarsal joint (too many toes sign)
- Significant lowering of the medial longitudinal arch on weightbearing
- Plantarflexed and adducted talus
- Increased angle of gait
- Increased relaxed calcaneal stance position (excessive heel eversion)
- Decreased ankle joint dorsiflexion
- Helbing's sign
- Abnormal wear on shoes.

When considering whether to treat asymptomatic flat feet at least three of the above signs should be present. In addition, gait analysis should also be performed and five out of the following seven features should also be present. Otherwise it may be justified to continue to simply monitor the child.

Gait analysis

- Medial heel contact
- Subtalar joint pronation at heel-strike
- Reduced or negative re-supination
- Abductory twist
- Early heel lift
- Reduced propulsive gait
- Increased genu valgum beyond physiological norm.

A key aspect in the assessment of functional flat feet is to determine why the patient has attended for assessment. Common reasons for attendance are: foot or postural pain, parental concern, and withdrawal from sport or other social events because of clumsiness or from being unable to compete. These issues along with the clinical findings above are crucial in the decision to offer intervention.

Morley (1957) suggested that children under 5 years of age appeared to have flat feet because the medial longitudinal arch was filled with fat. Radiological studies of toddlers' feet have subsequently proved Morley wrong. All children under 5 years have a depressed medial longitudinal arch because of the low calcaneal inclination angle and the underdeveloped sustentaculum tali. It is only with external torsion of the tibia, in the first 5 years of life, that the calcaneus begins to assume its normal 20° angle of inclination and the medial longitudinal arch becomes apparent. However, in the neonate, fat deposits are retained for a short period and tend to be quite marked on the dorsum of the foot. This fat distribution does contribute to an immature foot shape, which disappears quite rapidly after the first 12 months.

Helbing's sign, described as a bowing of the calcaneal tendon as it inserts into the calcaneus, can sometimes be associated with excessive pronation. Helbing's sign is not always reliable because in some cases of excessive pronation it is not seen. This is so when the foot maximally pronates from a supinated position associated with rearfoot varus. Pronation can occur using the available range of subtalar joint motion, but the calcaneus may still remain in a relatively inverted position. This is commonly referred to as 'partially compensated rearfoot varus'. Marked eversion of the calcaneus will inevitably lower the medial longitudinal arch. With calcaneal eversion there will also be abduction of the distal end of the calcaneus, allowing the talus to assume a more adducted and plantarflexed position which can be seen clinically as medial bulging in the area of the talonavicular joint. Once congruency is lost at the talonavicular joint, progressive subluxation of the joint follows. As the talus adducts, the forefoot will assume an abducted position relative to the adducted rearfoot. This abnormality will manifest clinically as the 'too many toes sign'. When a normal foot is observed from the rear, it is possible to see the fifth and sometimes the fourth toe. In a pronated foot the third toe may be seen as well. The lateral border of the foot will be C-shaped with the concavity of the 'C' overlying the calcaneocuboid joint (see Ch. 10).

When evaluating the child's pronated foot the practitioner must consider other risk factors that may affect the foot in its overall development (Napolitano et al 2000). These contributing factors may influence

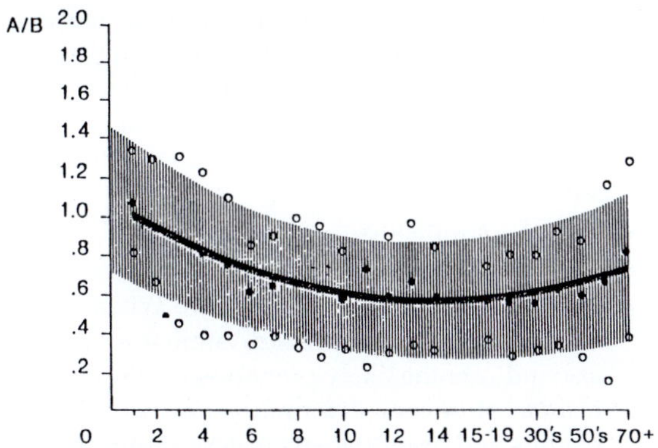

Figure 14.19 Staheli's table of normal arch index values. The mean value for the arch index and two standard deviations for each of the 21 age groups. The solid line shows the mean changes with age; the shaded area shows the normal ranges. The actual values for each age group are represented by solid circles for the mean and open circles for two standard deviations. (Reproduced by kind permission of the *Journal of Bone and Joint Surgery*.)

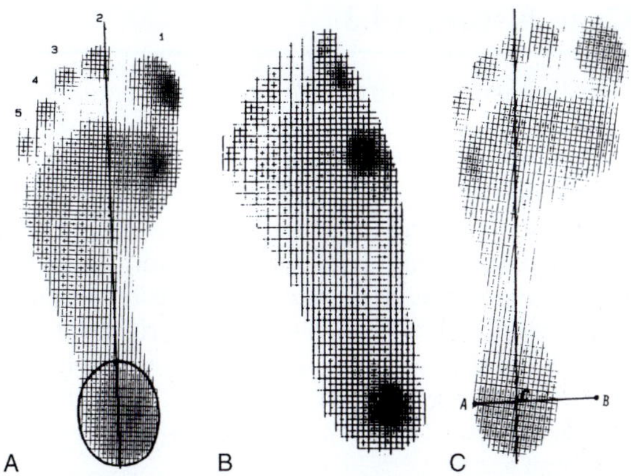

Figure 14.20 Rose's valgus index. Footprints to show diagnostic features. **A** The orientation of the heel – oval, in this case pointing towards the second toe. **B** The medial pressure pattern which is commonly found in flatfoot. **C** To show the measurements for calculation of the valgus index, which equals ½ *AB* – *AC* × 100/*AB* where *A* and *B* are vertically beneath each malleolus and *C* is the centre of the heel print. (Reproduced by kind permission of the *Journal of Bone and Joint Surgery*.)

the treatment plan. The risk factors include:

- obesity
- ligamentous laxity
- hypotonia (Down's syndrome)
- rotational deformities
- frontal plane tibial deformities
- equinus
- tarsal coalitions.

Objective assessment of the pronated (flat) foot is vital in order to measure how the patient's foot is changing with the passage of time or, indeed, how it is responding to treatment. Staheli & co-workers (1987) developed the arch index as an indicator of foot pronation (Fig. 14.19). They divided the narrowest point of the arch width by the widest point of the heel width to give an arch index value. Staheli recommended that their graph of normal values should be used to determine which children had an abnormality that required treatment. However, in practice, Staheli's normal limits have proved to be very wide. Moreover, the height of the arch alone is not a reliable indicator of excessive pronation of the foot as the arch is not flat in every pronated foot. Some patients will present with calcaneal eversion and talonavicular bulging, but the medial longitudinal arch may still be apparent.

Rose's valgus index (Rose et al 1985) takes into account the eversion of the foot relative to the leg and can be used in conjunction with Staheli's index to obtain more valid information about the degree of pronation (Fig. 14.20). Rose's technique measures the displacement of the medial malleolus relative to the weightbearing surface of the heel. The more the foot pronates, the greater the medial displacement of the malleoli.

The Rose and Staheli indices should be used to determine objectively foot position and arch height. Footprints should be repeated once yearly in an attempt to identify change. The decision as to which children require treatment should be based on an assessment of the magnitude of their symptoms, family history and the footprint indices. There are many other options in the measurement of a flatfoot posture and these are considered in detail in Chapter 10.

The patient with excessive pronation may suffer from chronic low-grade discomfort in the medial longitudinal arch, talonavicular area, or leg muscle pain, or even all three. The tibialis posterior muscle is particularly prone to causing discomfort where the foot is excessively pronated. This is because the excessive pronatory movement of the foot causes the muscle to work aphasically, leading to overuse. In many cases, such leg pain may be written off as untreatable 'growing pains'. However, the condition is responsive to conservative orthotic treatment (Case history 14.3).

Case history 14.3

Two brothers aged 8 and 10 years presented with excessively pronated feet in relaxed calcaneal stance with severe talonavicular bulging. Both boys experienced foot fatigue by the end of the day and pain in the styloid process. Their gait was excessively abducted and apropulsive. Jack's test and the tiptoe test were positive, demonstrating a flexible flatfoot. The posterior tibial tendon was anteriorly displaced over the medial malleoli, rendering it an inefficient invertor and plantarflexor of the foot. The peroneal muscles were contracted. Both boys scored 6 on Beighton's scale.

Diagnosis: Severe flexible flatfoot primarily caused by malposition of posterior tibial tendon and tightness of peroneal muscles and aggravated by ligamentous laxity.

Toe deformities

Hallux valgus

While not a common condition, juvenile hallux valgus is a significant foot problem. It begins as an isolated abnormality of the first metatarsophalangeal joint but as the condition progresses it affects the entire forefoot. Advanced hallux valgus is known to be associated with hammer second toe and crowding of the other lesser digits, widening of the forefoot leading to footwear-fitting problems, and plantar callosity and metatarsalgia.

A survey of 6000 9-year-olds found a 2% prevalence of hallux valgus (Kilmartin et al 1994). Although it is possible to detect hallux valgus in children younger than 9 years, the changes are often very subtle. On the other hand, in adolescents the condition may have already progressed to the point where it is involving the lesser toes. Therefore, 9 years is probably the optimum age for assessment and treatment.

The condition is known to be inherited (Johnston 1959), so children with the complaint are often presented by parents who are only too familiar with the long-term effects of 'bunions'. Diagnosis may be confirmed using the following three criteria:

- A first metatarsophalangeal joint angle in excess of 15° – this may be measured clinically with a digital goniometer or on a dorsoplantar weightbearing X-ray. If radiographs are taken, the first-second intermetatarsal angle should also be measured. An angle in excess of the normal 9° is known to be the forerunner of clinically apparent hallux valgus (Kilmartin et al 1994).
- Osteophytic thickening of the first metatarsophalangeal joint – visible thickening of the joint indicates hypertrophy of the metatarsal head caused by loss of congruency of the joint and subsequent early degeneration of the joint surface.
- A strong family history of the complaint – family history of hallux valgus, while not confirming diagnosis, must arouse suspicion. When hallux valgus is present in the child, family history may also indicate the likely prognosis for the child. A history of severe deformity affecting siblings, parents and grandparents is very significant.

Hypermobility may be a predisposing factor for juvenile hallux valgus; therefore, it would be beneficial to screen all children with hypermobility for hallux valgus (Harris & Beeson 1998). Pain is not usually a feature of hallux valgus until the deformity is more advanced. Pain can be associated with footwear irritation of the skin overlying the medial eminence. Because of the progressive nature of hallux valgus, once the diagnosis is made, assessment and review is likely to be a long-term commitment for both patient and practitioner. Dorsiplantar weightbearing radiographs will allow accurate assessment of the following:

- First metatarsophalangeal joint space
- Hallux valgus angle
- First-second intermetatarsal angle
- Medial eminence
- Osteophytic development
- Sesamoid position.

Radiographic changes are likely to be very subtle in the short term. Three-yearly X-ray reviews are therefore indicated. Objective clinical assessment can be made by taking a digital goniometer measurement of the first metatarsophalangeal joint angle. This value should be recorded after drawing around the weightbearing foot on a blank sheet of paper. When stored in the patient's records, this can provide a visual indication of the effectiveness of treatment. Because hallux valgus is usually a bilateral condition, both feet can be assessed in this manner even if at first only one foot is affected.

Lesser toe deformity

The following lesser toe deformities are common cause for parental concern:

- Adductovarus third, fourth, fifth toes
- Dorsiflexed second toe

- overriding fifth toe
- under-riding third and fourth toes.

Although the abnormal position is often real enough, the condition may be quite benign. It is essential that the practitioner applies the following criteria to determine which lesser toe problems require treatment:

- Is weightbearing on the apex of the toe rather than the soft plantar pulp? Apical weightbearing may lead to the development of painful corns and callus.
- Is the malposition of one toe likely to influence the position of an adjacent, otherwise normal toe? For example, a dorsiflexed second toe will lead to loss of buttress effect on the hallux, which will predispose to hallux valgus.
- Is the malpositioned toe likely to be irritated by footwear or cause footwear-fitting problems?
- Is the type of toe deformity likely to respond to conservative or surgical treatment?

Transverse and frontal plane deformities are resistant to conservative treatment. Sagittal plane deformities and even the sagittal plane component of complex digital deformities respond more favourably to conservative treatment. In children older than 9 years, conservative treatment becomes progressively less effective. In infants younger than 2 years, corrective devices are poorly tolerated and are technically difficult to make because of the size of the toes.

When treatment is indicated, conservative treatment should always be attempted first. Response to treatment may be monitored using anything from a Harris & Beath mat to a computerised pressure system. Apical weightbearing by the digits will be recorded as a very small area of digital contact, whereas adductovarus will often appear as the lateral side of the digit in contact with the mat. In overriding digits, toe purchase with the ground will be absent. Following treatment, the foot printing procedure should be repeated. Digital photographic records are also a convenient and effective means of recording progress which, in the short term may be subtle.

Causes of limping in children

Limping is abnormal, whether associated with pain or not. Few parents tolerate the problem for long before seeking medical help. The child who limps presents a diagnostic challenge, as there are numerous conditions that may result in limping (Table 14.8).

In young children physical signs rather than subjective symptoms will have a major role in determining aetiology. As communication is limited, thorough questioning of the parents is crucial. However, it is easy to make false conclusions, since pain may be influenced by psychological factors, subjectivity and referred pain (from the hip to the knee).

History

A detailed history is essential in reaching the correct diagnosis. The exact circumstances surrounding the onset and duration of the limp must be carefully and sympathetically explored. Therefore, several specific questions must be asked (Box 14.1).

An episode of trauma is frequently blamed as the cause of the limp. However, this may be misleading. Minimal trauma may fracture a pre-existing unicameral bone cyst or a bone weakened by a tumour. Similarly children diagnosed with osteogenesis imperfecta may have a history of fractures originating from the most minor of physical contact.

Limping after vigorous activity may be the first clue to an impending stress fracture. Rather than limp, the child may refuse to stand or walk and may ask to be carried. When pain is associated with the limp, the exact location and pattern should be explored with the child. The pattern of referred pain in children appears to be stronger than in adults (e.g. pain referred to the knee due to medial hip problems such as slipped capital femoral epiphysis (SCFE) or osteoid osteoma). The character of the pain may be helpful, such as the constant pain from infection or pain related to joint motion. Conditions that lead to demineralisation of bone frequently cause generalised pain, particularly in the weightbearing bones. Lower extremity pain and limping may be the first signs of systemic illness such as juvenile idiopathic arthritis (JIA).

The age of the child and the type of limp allows the examiner to focus in on the differential diagnosis (Beresford & Cleary 2005, Volpe 2001). Up to the age of 5 years, typical causes for a limp include DDH, infection, JIA, septic hip and fracture. The former is unlikely to present with pain as the primary complaint whereas pain is associated in the others and as a result the gait of the child with DDH would be expected to be lurching or Trendelenberg (T) in nature and the rest antalgic (A). Köhler's disease of the navicular (T, A), although rare, generally presents as a condition of 4–5-year-olds.

From age 5 to 11, Legg–Calvé–Perthes disease (T, A), JIA (T, A), transient synovitis (A) and Sever's apophysitis of the calcaneus (A) are the most common

Table 14.8 Limp relating to specific location

Location	*Possible causes*
Nervous system	
CNS	Cerebral tumour Cerebral palsy Spina bifida Spinal muscular atrophy
PNS/muscle	Poliomyelitis Friedreich's ataxia Muscular dystrophy Charcot–Marie–Tooth disease
Back	Trauma Acute appendicitis Herniated nucleus pulposus (slipped disc) Scheuermann's disease of the spine (osteochondritis of spine) Spondylolisthesis (forward displacement of vertebra on one distal to it)
Hip	Developmental dislocation of the hip (DDH) Slipped capital femoral epiphysis (SCFE) Transient synovitis of the hip Legg–Calvé–Perthes disease Trauma Coxa vara (provokes waddling gait) Trochanteric bursitis
Femur/tibia	Fracture (fractured femur may present as hip or knee pain) Blount's disease Limb-length inequality (short femur or tibia)
Knee	Osgood–Schlatter's disease (traction apophysitis) Osteochondritis dissecans Chondromalacia Haemophilia Sickle-cell anaemia Rickets Baker's cyst Referred pain from hip
Ankle/foot	Fracture/sprain Rickets (ankle) Osteomyelitis (calcaneus) Unicameral bone cyst (calcaneus) Sever's disease (traction apophysitis) Osteochondroses – Mouchet's or Diaz/Köhler's/ Buschke's/Freiberg's/Treve's disease Haglund's disease (osteochondrosis of accessory navicular) Iselin's disease (traction apophysitis) Accessory navicular – type II (Romanowsky & Barrington 1991) Tarsal coalition Embedded foreign body in foot Verruca Onychocryptosis Subungual exostosis
Miscellaneous	Septic arthritis (juvenile idiopathic arthritis) Angioleiomyoma Leukaemia Attention-seeking device Child abuse

Box 14.1 Questions a practitioner should consider when assessing a child with a limp

- Is the limp constant or intermittent?
- Is the limp only present in the morning, at the end of the day when the child is fatigued or is it present throughout the day?
- What is the posture of the lower extremity when the child is limping?
- What is the effect of climbing stairs or running?
- Did the limp start following vigorous activity?

conditions to appear in this age group. Finally, from 11 to 16 years of age, slipped capital femoral epiphysis (T, A), Osgood–Schlatter disease of the tibial tubercle (A), overuse injuries (A, T) and Freiberg's infraction of the second metatarsal head (A) would all be included in the differential diagnosis. Legg–Calvé–Perthes, Köhler's, and Freiberg's diseases are a group of disorders associated with trauma and altered vascular supply to bone (Caputo 1992, McCall 2001).

Physical examination of the limping child

Ideally gait assessment should be undertaken unassisted by the parent. Uncooperative children are best assessed when they think the examination is finished. Stiffness or limitation of motion in a single joint, forces the surrounding joints to compensate by increased movements. This results in an irregular or jerky gait, such as the forward thrust of the pelvis with a stiff hip or hiking the pelvis to swing through a stiff knee. Positional change may occur, such as external rotation of the foot to accommodate a stiff ankle and limited dorsiflexion or external rotation of the entire limb in SCFE. Sometimes it is helpful to accentuate the limp by asking the child to walk on their toes or heels. Listening to the gait can be informative: the slapping of the foot in drop foot, the scraping sound of spastic gait or the quick soft steps of an antalgic gait. Inspecting the shoes for abnormal wear is useful: increased toe wear in toe walkers, destruction of the medial shoe counter in severe abnormal pronation.

A non-weightbearing evaluation will help to clarify initial impressions about the limp. Joints should be examined individually and compared with the other side. Special attention should be given to joint stiffness, limited motion or to guarding. Marked changes to joint angle measurements indicate disease or injury and should not be attributed to immaturity. Joint stiffness frequently accompanies synovial swelling and/or joint effusion as seen in JIA, whereas laxity of a joint generally points to a ligamentous problem. In the hip, telescoping or pistoning are the classic signs of dislocation. A formal knee examination may be required to exclude knee pathology. Measurement of limb length is important, as limb shortening may be an early sign of a dislocated hip. Cutaneous changes should not be overlooked. Extra skinfolds, café-au-lait spots, erythema or heat may provide clues to diagnosis.

A complete neurological examination including evaluation of muscle function and strength is important. A neurological abnormality is frequently the underlying cause of many difficult to diagnose limp problems (e.g. the child with early Charcot–Marie–Tooth disease who presents with a mild cavus foot and toe clawing). Subtle variations in neurological function may only be noticeable with weightbearing or following vigorous activity. Trendelenburg's test is a valuable clue to limb stability. Most normal children over 4 years of age can sustain this position for a minimum of 30 seconds. Less time (delayed Trendelenburg's) may suggest weakness of the hip abductors or hip instability associated with acetabular dysplasia. Weakness of a specific muscle is usually due to a local problem (e.g. quadriceps atrophy accompanying a knee complaint), whereas weakness of muscle groups is usually associated with primary muscle diseases, systemic illness or neurological problems (Hensinger 1986).

Certain limping patterns are characteristically associated with weakness of specific muscles. Tightness or spasticity of the muscles and poor voluntary control are good clues to mild cerebral palsy. Similarly, running accentuates the flexion and posturing of the upper limb in a child with mild spastic hemiplegia. Rupture of the calcaneal tendon will lead to drop foot (see Thompson's test (Ch. 10). Hamstring inflexibility can result in a flexed knee gait with abrupt internal rotation of the leg at heel strike, particularly if the medial hamstrings are tight. Limited straight leg raise can be associated with hamstring inflexibility, but other causes such as discitis, spondylolysis or spondylolisthesis need to be excluded (Fields 1981). These usually give rise to back pain, which radiates laterally into the buttocks.

Special tests

The history and physical examination may be supplemented by a variety of radiological or laboratory tests, depending on the clinical assessment of the child. Due to the diffuse nature of pain patterns in children, a larger area may be exposed than might be chosen for an adult, for example radiographs of the hip and knee when a problem is suspected in the femur. Radiographs should include anteroposterior and lateral views of the area and comparison views of the uninvolved side. In acute osteomyelitis where bone changes may not be seen for 7–10 days an MR scan may be more helpful.

Laboratory studies include full blood count, differential count, erythrocyte sedimentation rate (ESR), blood cultures or direct aspiration. The ESR is normal in trauma, the osteochondroses and SCFE, whereas it is raised in osteomyelitis, septic arthritis, JIA and malignancy. Complex and invasive tests should be reserved for the more complicated cases.

Infections

Verrucae are endemic in children, particularly between 6 years of age and the late teens. The source of the viral infection is often hard to identify and advice will depend upon duration, symptoms, activities and attitude toward the problem. The presence of tinea pedis can be diagnosed from skin scrapings; teenage boys are particularly susceptible to fungal infections associated with hyperhidrosis.

Juvenile plantar dermatitis

Another seasonal condition is forefoot eczema or juvenile plantar dermatosis (see Ch. 8). The aetiology is uncertain but it is not thought to be a chronic contact dermatitis. A rash appears on the weight-bearing area of the foot. A pink, shiny or glazed appearance is noted with scaling. The skin thins and is inflexible, with resultant fissures forming. Differential diagnosis includes tinea pedis.

Psoriasis

Acute guttate psoriasis is the commonest form in the young and often related to a minor infection such as a streptococcal sore throat. The rash either subsides in about 6 weeks or progresses to plaque psoriasis (Beeson 1990). Plaque psoriasis mainly affects the extensor surfaces but occasionally the flexures. The latter may involve the interdigital webspaces and nail folds.

Vasospastic disorders

Vasospastic disorders used to be very common in children in poor economic and housing conditions, and their incidence has declined in recent decades. However, chilblains still occur in children who are exposed to extremes of temperature due to inadequate footwear and hosiery in winter or poor home conditions. They appear as red, blotchy, intensely itchy areas. Broken chilblains may become infected.

Dark mauve swellings around calf muscles, thighs and buttocks indicate erythrocyanosis. This affects overweight females in particular. Acrocyanosis, reddening of the hands and feet, may also occur in children. Both erythrocyanosis and acrocyanosis are indicative of poor blood supply and response to cold.

Juvenile idiopathic arthritis

JIA, previously known as juvenile chronic arthritis, is one of the most common chronic illnesses of childhood. It affects 1 in 1000 children (Malleson & Southwood 1993) and is a major cause of functional disability. The child with JIA may present with lower limb pain. Both forefoot and rearfoot deformities are common; however, the type of deformity is difficult to predict due to the influence of other joint deformities and the child's age when the disease is active (Beeson 1988). Treatment is based on maintaining a good lower limb position with splints/orthoses, maximum muscle strength, a full range of joint motion and appropriate footwear. A team approach in the management of this condition is paramount (Beeson 1995, Murray & Ferrari 2001).

Summary

Although the assessment process is similar, the skills required to assess the child do differ from those used to assess an adult. Assessment of the child requires sufficient knowledge of normal development and the ability to differentiate between self-limiting developmental conditions and significant, persistent abnormalities, and those that warrant further evaluation. The practitioner must have a working knowledge of normal developmental milestones in order to undertake a thorough assessment.

This chapter has primarily concentrated on common paediatric orthopaedic conditions of the lower limb. Pertinent vascular, dermatological and arthritic conditions that lead to patients seeking advice have been briefly considered. The practitioner must identify the cause of any pain and be vigilant for signs of neuromuscular deficit. In a well-resourced nation such as the UK, most severe problems associated with the foot and lower limb are detected at birth. However, all practitioners should be aware of problems that may have missed detection or which are relatively mild but may still lead to functional problems in later life.

References

Alvick L 1960 Increased anteversion of the femoral neck as a sole sign of dysplasia coxae. Acta Orthopaedica Scandinavica 29:301–306

Apgar V 1953 Evaluation of the newborn infant. Current Research in Anesthesia and Analgesics 32: 260

Beeson P 1988 Juvenile chronic arthritis: the foot. The Chiropodist 43:20–26

Beeson P 1990 The clinical significance for chiropodists of recent advances made in the pathology and treatment of psoriasis. British Journal of Podiatric Medicine 45:43–46

Beeson P 1995 Podiatric perspective: a case study of rheumatoid arthritis and a multidisciplinary approach. British Journal of Therapy and Rehabilitation 2:566–571

Beeson P 1999 Frontal plane configuration of the knee in children. The Foot 9:18–26

Beighton P H, Graham R, Bird H A 1989 Hypermobility of joints, Berlin, Springer

Beresford M W, Cleary A G 2005 Evaluation of a limping child. Current Paediatrics 15:15–22

Berg 1986 A reappraisal of metatarsus adductus and skewfoot. Journal of Bone and Joint Surgery (Am) 68:1185–1196

Brandt L 2003 On the value of an old dress code in the new millennium [commentary]. Journal of the American Medical Association 163:1277–1281

Bulbena A, Duro J C, Porta M et al 1992 Clinical assessment of hypermobility of joints: assembling criteria. Journal of Rheumatology 19:115–122

Cahuzac J P, Vardon D, Sales De Gauzy J 1995 Development of the tibiofemoral angle in normal adolescents. Journal of Bone and Joint Surgery (Br) 77:729–732

Caputo L J 1992 Miscellaneous developmental disorders. In: De Valentine S J (ed) Foot and ankle disorders in children. Churchill Livingstone, New York

Coleman S S 1994 Developmental dislocation of the hip: evolutionary changes in diagnosis and treatment [editorial]. Journal of Pediatric Orthopedics 14:1–2

Davids J R 1996 Pediatric knee: clinical assessment and common disorders. Pediatric Clinics of North America 43:1067–1090

Dunn P 1974 Congenital postural deformities: further perinatal associations. Proceedings of the Royal Society of Medicine 67:1174–1178

Elftman H 1945 Torsion of the lower extremity. American Journal of Physiology and Anthropology 3:255–265

Fabry G, Mcewan G D, Shands A R 1973 Torsion of the femur (a follow up study in normal and abnormal conditions). Journal of Bone and Joint Surgery (Am) 55:1726–1738

Fagan J P 1992 Metatarsus adductus. In: De Valentine S J (ed) Foot and ankle disorders in children. Churchill Livingstone, New York

Fields L 1981 The limping child: a review of the literature. Journal of the American Podiatric Association 71:60–64

Fopma E, Macnicol M F 2002 Tarsal coalition. Current Orthopaediatrics 16:65–73

Harris E J 1997 Hip instability encountered in pediatric podiatry practice. Clinics in Podiatric Medicine and Surgery 14:179–208

Harris E J, Vanore J V, Thomas J L et al 2004 Diagnosis and treatment of pediatric flatfoot. Journal of Foot and Ankle Surgery 43:341–373

Harris M-C R, Beeson P 1998 Generalised hypermobility: is it a predisposing factor towards the development of juvenile hallux abducto valgus? part 2. The Foot 8:203–209

Heath C H, Staheli L T 1993 Normal limits of knee angle in white children – genu varum and genu valgum. Journal of Pediatric Orthopedics 13:259–262

Hensinger R N 1986 Limp. Pediatric Clinics of North America 33:1355–1364

Hubbard D D, Staheli L T, Chew D E 1988 Medial femoral torsion and osteoarthrosis. Journal of Pediatric Orthopedics 8:540–542

Hutter C G, Scott W 1949 Tibial torsion. Journal of Bone and Joint Surgery 31:A511–518

Jiminez A L 1992 Hallux varus. In: Mcglamry D E, Banks A S, Downey M S (eds) Comprehensive textbook of foot surgery, 2nd edn. Williams & Wilkins, Baltimore

John A 2001 Psychological considerations in the child patient. In: Thompson P, Volpe R G (Eds.) Introduction to Podopediatrics. 2 ed. Edinburgh Churchill-Livinstone

Johnston O 1959 Further studies of the inheritance of hand and foot anomalies. Clinical Orthopedics 8:146–159

Katz K, Rosenthal A, Yosipovitch Z 1992 Normal ranges of popliteal angle in children. Journal of Pediatric Orthopedics 12:229–231

Kaushik S 2005 Computed tomography and magnetic resonance imaging of unusual causes of ankle pain. Australasian Radiography 50:1–11

Kilmartin T E 1988 Medial genicular rotation; aetiology and management. The Chiropodist 43:181–184

Kilmartin T E, Barrington N A, Wallace W A 1994 A controlled prospective trial of a foot orthosis in the treatment of juvenile hallux valgus. Journal of Bone and Joint Surgery 76:B210–214

Lang L M, Volpe R G 1998 Measurement of tibial torsion. Journal of the American Podiatric Medical Association 88:160–165

Laporta G 1973 Torsional abnormalities. Archives of Podiatric Medical Foot Surgery 1:47–61

Luder J 1988 Early recognition of cerebral palsy. Update 1955–1963

Malleson P N, Southwood T R 1993 The epidemiology of arthritis: an overview. In Southwood T R, Malleson P N (Eds.) Baillière's Clinical Paediatrics International Practice and Research. London Baillière Tindall

McCall I 2001 Radiological examination of the child's foot. In: Thomson P, Volpe R G (eds) Introduction to Podopediatrics, 2 edn. Edinburgh Churchill Livingstone

McRae R 1997 Clinical Orthopaedic Examination, Edinburgh Churchill Livingstone

Meadow R 1992 Difficult and unlikeable parents. Archives Diseases in Childhood 67:697–702

Michele A A, Nielson P M 1976 Tibiotalar torsion: bioengineering paradigm. Orthopedic Clinics of North America 7:929–947

Mikov A, Mikov I, Gajdobranski D 2005 Incidence and outcomes of breech presentation at term in newborns with congenital postural deformities. International Journal of Gynecology and Obstetrics 91:67–68

Morley A J 1957 Knock knees in children. British Medical Journal ii:976–979

Murray K, Ferrari J 2001 Rheumatic diseases of childhood and adolescence. In: Thomson P, Volpe R G (eds) Introduction to podopaediatrics, 2nd edn. Edinburgh, Churchill Livingstone

Napolitano C, Walsh S, Mahoney L et al 2000 Risk factors that may adversely modify the natural history of the paediatric pronated foot. Clinics in Podiatric Medicine and Surgery 17:397–417

Novachek T F 1996 Developmental dysplasia of the hip. Pediatric Clinics of North America 43:829–848

Paton R W, Hinduja K, Thomas C D 2005 The significance of at-risk factors in ultrasound surveillance of developmental dysplasia of the hip. Journal of Bone and Joint Surgery (Br) 87:1264–1266

Ponsetti I V 1992 Current concepts review: treatment of congenital clubfoot. Journal of Bone and Joint Surgery (Am) 74:448–454

Ponsetti I V 1996 Congenital clubfoot: fundamentals of treatment. Oxford University Press, Oxford

Ponsetti I V, Becker J R 1966 Congenital metatarsus adductus, the result of treatment. Journal of Bone and Joint Surgery (Am) 74:702–711

Reade E, Hom L, Hallum A et al 1984 Changes in popliteal angle measurement in infants up to one year of age. Developmental Medicine and Child Neurology 26:774–780

Reikeras O, Hoiseth A 1989 Torsion of the leg determined by computerised tomography. Acta Orthopaedica Scandinavica 60:330–333

Romanowsky C A J, Barrington N A 1991 The accessory ossicles of the foot. The Foot 1(2):61–7

Rose G K, Welton E A, Marshall T 1985 The diagnosis of flat foot in the child. Journal of Bone and Joint Surgery (Br) 67:71–78

Rushforth G F 1978 The natural history of the hooked forefoot. Journal of Bone and Joint Surgery (Br) 60:530–532

Salenius P, Vankka E 1975 The development of the tibiofemoral angle in children. Journal of Bone and Joint Surgery (Am) 57:259–261

Sharrard W J 1976 Intoeing and flat feet. British Medical Journal i:888–889

Silvani S H 1992 Congenital pes valgus. In: De Valentine S J (ed.) Foot and ankle disorders in children. Churchill Livingstone, New York

Staheli L T 1993 Rotational problems in children. Journal of Bone and Joint Surgery (Am) 75:939–949

Staheli L T, Chew D E, Corbett M 1987 The longitudinal arch. Journal of Bone and Joint Surgery (Am) 69: A426–428

Svenningson S, Tierjesen T, Auflem M 1990 Hip rotation and intoeing gait. Clinical Orthopedics and Related Research 251:177–182

Tachdjian M O 1972 Pediatric orthopedics, 2nd edn. W B Saunders, Philadelphia

Tax H 1985 Podopediatrics, Williams & Wilkins, Baltimore

Thackeray C, Beeson P 1996a In-toeing gait in children: a review of the literature. The Foot 6:1–4

Thackeray C, Beeson P 1996b Is in-toeing gait a developmental stage? The Foot 6:19–24

Thomson P 2001 History-taking and the physical examination. In: Thomson P, Volpe R G (eds) Introduction to podopaediatrics, 2nd edn. Edinburgh, Churchill Livingstone

Thomson P, Volpe R G (eds) 2001 Introduction to podopaediatrics, 2nd edn. Edinburgh, Churchill Livingstone

Turner M S, Smillie I S 1981 The effect of tibial torsion on the pathology of the knee. Journal of Bone and Joint Surgery (Br) 63:396–398

Valmassy R L 2001 Torsional and frontal plane conditions of the lower extremity. In: Thomson P, Volpe R G (eds) Introduction to podopaediatrics, 2nd edn. Edinburgh, Churchill Livingstone

Volpe R G 2001 Pediatric gait. In: Thomson P, Volpe R G (eds) Introduction to podopaediatrics, 2nd edn. Edinburgh, Churchill Livingstone

Wallander H, Hansson G, Tjenstrom B 1996 Correction of persistent clubfoot deformities with the Ilizarov external fixator. Acta Orthopaedica Scandinavica 67:283–287

Wan S C 2006 Metatarsus adductus and skewfoot deformity. Clinics in Podiatric Medicine and Surgery 23:23–40

Widhe T 1997 Foot deformities at birth: a longitudinal prospective study over a 16-year period. Journal of Pediatric Orthopedics 17:20–24

Further reading

Berkow R (ed) 1987 The Merck manual, 15th edn. Merck Sharp & Dohme Research Laboratories

Behrman R E, Vaughan V C 1987 Nelson textbook of pediatrics, 13th edn. W B Saunders, Philadelphia

Drennan J 1992 The child's foot and ankle. Ravens Press, New York

Ferrari J 1998 A review of the foot deformities seen in juvenile chronic arthritis. The Foot 8(4):193–196

Illingworth R S 1990 The development of the infant and the young child. Churchill Livingstone, Edinburgh

McCrea J D 1985 Pediatric orthopaedics of the lower extremity. Futura, New York

Pollak M 1993 Textbook of developmental paediatrics. Churchill Livingstone, Edinburgh

Sharrard M D 1979 Paediatric orthopaedics and fractures, Vols I and II, 2nd edn. Blackwell Scientific, London

Sheridan M D 1980 From birth to five years. Children's developmental progress, 7th edn. NFER-Nelson Publishing, Berkshire

Thomson P, Volpe R (ed) 2001 Introduction to podopaediatrics. Churchill Livingstone, Edinburgh

CHAPTER

15

Assessment of the sports patient

B Yates

Chapter contents

Introduction

With increasing numbers of people undertaking regular exercise there has been a corresponding rise in the number of sports injuries. In 1991 it was estimated that there were 5 million cases of exercise-related morbidity in the UK (Nicholl et al 1991). This equates to 1 in 10 people sustaining one injury each year. With the profile of sport in society increasing, and the incentive of high salaries for professional sports men and women, it is likely that the incidence of injury is now even greater among the general population. Podiatry has a significant part to play in the management of sports injuries, as the majority of these injuries occur in the lower limb. The commonest acute injury is the ankle sprain (Colville 1998, Ferran & Maffulli 2006); the commonest tendon injury is to the Achilles tendon (Jarvinen et al 2005, Marks 1999) and the most frequently seen joint pathology is patellofemoral syndrome (Tallay et al 2004, Walsh 1994). Podiatric intervention is often an integral component in the successful management of these and other lower-limb injuries.

Guiding principles

As with other areas of assessment it is essential to take an accurate history and perform a detailed examination. The majority of sports injuries seen by the podiatrist are chronic in nature due to overuse. As such they represent a diagnostic challenge due to the long injury period and compensation mechanisms which may have occurred as a result of the injury. Both of these factors can make it difficult to confirm the diagnosis of the injury and ascertain its aetiological factors.

The history and examination should be aimed at both diagnosing the injury and determining the presence or absence of intrinsic (personal) and extrinsic (environmental) risk factors associated with the injury. The identification of intrinsic and extrinsic risk factors can assist in making the diagnosis and guiding the management plan. It is important to gain as much information as possible about the injury. Information on the duration, nature, frequency and intensity of symptoms must be gained along with details of the injury mechanism, aggravating factors and previous treatment.

Clinical examination of the patient, which should include the whole musculoskeletal system, with a specific focus on the lower limbs and the injury site, should follow the standard examination protocol of observation, palpation and movement (see Ch. 10). When turning to the injury site it is imperative to know the anatomical structures of the region to make an accurate diagnosis. After observing the area for inflammation, erythema, ecchymosis, structural defects and malalignment the practitioner should physically examine the area. The purpose of the physical examination is to identify, isolate and then stress individual anatomical structures to try to reproduce the patient's symptoms. This should help enable the practitioner to identify whether the pathology is isolated to a specific tendon, ligament, bone, joint, muscle or nerve. A summary of the assessment process is given in Figure 15.1.

Role of the sports podiatrist

The podiatrist may be part of an interdisciplinary sports medicine team, a multidisciplinary sports medicine team or working as a sole practitioner. Central members of a sports medicine team are likely to include a sports physician, orthopaedic surgeon, physiotherapist and podiatrist. Other members of the team may include a general practitioner (GP), radiologist, osteopath, chiropractor, podiatric surgeon, masseur and professionals from the sports science disciplines such as an exercise physiologist, sports psychologist and nutritionist. Working in such a team is of obvious benefit to both practitioner and patient. The patient is likely to be treated more holistically, with appropriate intervention more readily available. For the practitioner there should be assistance in making an accurate diagnosis and being able to treat more of the aetiological factors of the injury (Case history 15.1).

Working as a sole practitioner is often more challenging. Assistance in making an accurate diagnosis through interdisciplinary discussion or access to specialist investigations such as magnetic resonance imaging (MRI), bone scans and intracompartmental pressure tests may not be available. It is important to develop a referral network with other healthcare practitioners to overcome these potential shortcomings and to be able to offer the patient more beneficial treatment plans. If such a network does not exist the practitioner may be required to provide treatment

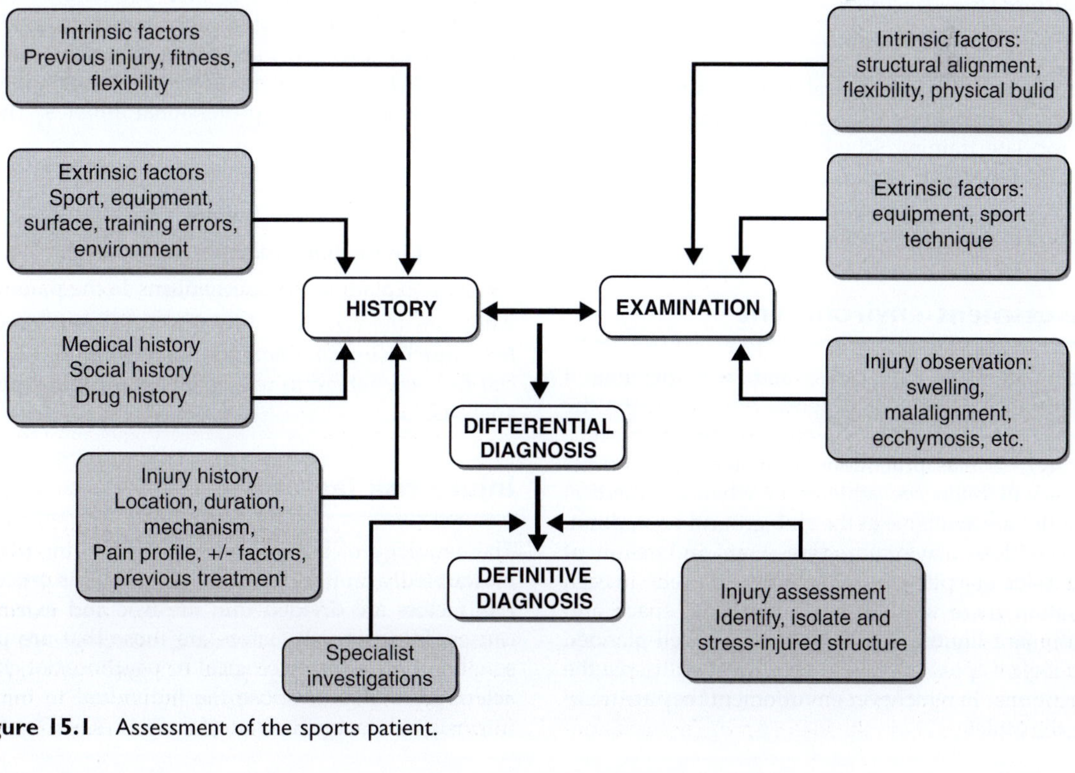

Figure 15.1 Assessment of the sports patient.

Case history 15.1

A 19-year-old female, elite cross-country runner with pain in her medial longitudinal arch was referred, by her coach, to a multidisciplinary sports medicine team. The pain had been present for 4 weeks and was gradually getting worse. The pain was centred around the navicular and the insertion of the posterior tibialis tendon was both prominent and painful. Base line X-rays were negative for a navicular stress fracture but demonstrated a type 2 os tibialis externum. A magnetic resonance imaging (MRI) scan was requested to examine the health of the tibialis posterior tendon and determine the presence of a stress fracture. The scan confirmed a navicular stress fracture and healthy tendon. She was treated with a short leg cast for 6 weeks followed by prophylactic orthoses to reduce pronatory compression forces on the navicular. She was also identified as being oligomenorrhoeic with only four menstrual cycles per year. This is known to be a risk factor for stress fractures (Tomten et al 1998). She was subsequently referred for dual energy X-ray absorptiometry (DEXA) scanning of her pelvis, spine and foot, which demonstrated reduced bone mineral density. She was therefore referred to a gynaecologist and sports nutritionist to address these imbalances. Three years on she is still competing at an elite level and has had no further stress fractures.

and advice using mechanical, physical and pharmacological modalities as well as giving advice on appropriate training schedules. Although this may not affect the treatment outcome, a practitioner must be aware of their limitations and refer to other practitioners where necessary.

Assessment environment

The practitioner may assess and treat the injured athlete in a variety of different environments: the majority are likely to be in a clinic or private practice setting, whereas practitioners involved with sports clubs will often see athletes in whatever medical facilities are available at the club ground or stadium. Some athletes may require assessment and treatment at the side of a pitch or track during an event. In each situation there will obviously be time, space and equipment limitations. A methodical, well-planned and logical approach to the assessment will assist the practitioner in whichever environment they are treating the athlete.

As with any biomechanical examination it is important to have an area to observe the athlete's gait. There should be a minimum of 5 m of uninterrupted non-carpeted surface. A flat bed couch is essential for a number of tests where the athlete must be able to lie fully prone, supine or on their side. There should be plenty of space on either side of the couch for the practitioner to undertake an assessment of the knee, thigh, hips and lower back. Tape, padding and temporary orthoses are useful adjuncts to diagnosis and should be available in all working environments.

It is important that the athlete wear clothing that permits an accurate examination. Shorts must be worn to allow assessment of the knees and observation of leg alignment and muscle bulk. Spare shorts of different sizes could be made available for patients who do not bring their own. Jumpers and jackets should be removed to assess the spine, hips and shoulder position. Assessment of the athlete's footwear – both sports footwear and general – is essential, as either or both can contribute to overuse injuries. Athletes should be advised to bring their sports shoes to all consultations.

Gait analysis equipment can be of great benefit in assessing the sports patient. The most commonly used equipment is a treadmill, with or without the use of a video camera. More specialist equipment such as force platforms, in-shoe pressure systems and digitised video gait analysis are discussed in detail in Chapter 11. Specialist equipment can be useful when assessing more complex sports injury cases or when treating professional athletes. These systems can:

- aid the diagnosis
- identify sporting technique
- assist in treatment planning
- help explain injury mechanisms to the patient.

Although the cost may prohibit most practitioners from purchasing such equipment, it would be beneficial to know where to refer patients for this type of analysis.

Injury risk factors

The aetiology of both acute and chronic injuries is undoubtedly multifactorial. To simplify this process, risk factors are divided into intrinsic and extrinsic causes. Intrinsic risk factors are those that are personal and are either biological or psychosocial characteristics that predispose the individual to injury. Intrinsic risk factors account for up to 40–60% of all

Table 15.1 Intrinsic and extrinsic risk factors associated with sports injuries

Intrinsic risk factors	*Extrinsic risk factors*
Age	Sporting equipment
Gender	Exercise surface
Previous injury	Sporting activity
Structural alignment	Sport position
Flexibility	Training errors
Physical fitness	Warm up and stretching
Physical build	Environmental factors
Psychological factors	
Systemic disease	

running injuries (Cavanagh & Kram 1990, James et al 1978). Extrinsic risk factors are independent of the person and are related to the type of sporting activity and the sporting environment. Extrinsic risk factors account for up to 80% of running injuries (McKenzie et al 1985). In the vast majority of chronic overuse injuries it is a combination of both intrinsic and extrinsic risk factors that have led to the condition (Kannus 1997). Of all risk factors for overuse injuries training errors are the most common and may be the decisive factor in 60% of the cases (Hreljac et al 2000). Table 15.1 lists the intrinsic and extrinsic risk factors for injury.

Intrinsic risk factors

Age

The age of an athlete can affect both the type of injury that may occur and the healing mechanisms that follow. Younger and older athletes tend to be more injury prone for a variety of reasons. There is generally less muscle mass and muscle strength in both of these groups compared with older adolescents and young adults. This can result in greater injury risk both in contact and endurance sports. Less protective sports equipment is available for children than adults, which can lead to greater injury risk from ground reaction forces and physical contact. The quality of coaches in children's teams is often lower than their adult counterparts, which may cause injury due to improper training and coaching supervision (Dalton 1992). Some studies have found that 70% of all sports injuries occur in children under 18 years (Hergenroeder 1998).

In children of all ages fractures are more common than ligamentous disruptions. Even the location of fractures varies with the age of the child. Adolescents tend to have fractures in the physeal areas, whereas preadolescents have more fractures in the diaphysis (Cantu & Micheli 1991). Certain bony injuries, such as the osteochondritides, can only occur in the young athlete. Also traction apophysitis of the calcaneus (Sever's disease), the fifth metatarsal (Iselin's disease), and of the tibial tubercle (Osgood–Schlatter's disease) only occur in children and adolescents, although rarely the symptoms may persist into adulthood in the case of Osgood–Schlatter's disease. Both traction apophysitis in the young athlete and musculotendinous injuries in the older athlete have been linked with reduced flexibility. It is known that reduced flexibility is more common in both groups (Anderson & Burke 1994, Gerrard 1993). Assessment of flexibility is therefore a key area when examining both children and older athletes with sports injuries.

Musculotendinous injuries are the commonest injury in the older athlete (over 40 years). This is due to a number of cellular changes which occur with increasing age. Changes in collagen cross-linking cause an increase in tendon stiffness and reduce the elasticity of the tendon. Similar change have also been seen in ligaments. This can result in a muscle being subject to earlier and prolonged loading in a movement cycle and being unable to undergo normal stretching, resulting in damage to the musculotendinous unit. The diameter, density and cellularity of the collagen fibrils are also diminished with advancing age, which results in reduced muscle mass and strength. Finally, the blood supply to tendons reduces with age, resulting in an increased risk of tendonitis, tendinosis or rupture (Sassmannshausen 2006, Strocchi et al 1991).

Overuse injuries in the older athlete may also develop due to a delayed physiological response to exercise. When a person starts an exercise programme there are gradual positive changes to the cardiovascular, neurological, endocrine and musculoskeletal systems. As a person becomes fitter the muscles become stronger and there is an increase in bone density. These normal adaptive changes are delayed in the older athlete and may cause musculotendinous injuries if the athlete increases their training volume too quickly. Older males are almost twice as likely to develop a sports injury as older females (Gerson & Stevens 2004).

Gender

Physiological differences between the sexes result in differences in athletic performance. For comparative body sizes women have a reduced cardiac output, blood volume, vital capacity and mean muscle mass when compared with males. Whether this increases the risk of injury in female athletes is uncertain. Studies involving civilian populations have not shown significant differences in injury rates between the sexes (Hootman et al 2002, Knowles et al 2006), except in children, where boys are twice as likely to be injured as girls (Bruns & Maffulli 2000). McQuillan & Campbell (2006) attributed this to football and found that if football was excluded from the analysis the rates of injury were the same for boys and girls. This is in contrast to studies involving military personnel in which injury rates among female recruits are between two and four times higher than among their male counterparts (Jones et al 1988, Ross & Woodward 1994, Yates & White 2004).

Perhaps of more significance than injury rates are the differences in the types of injury seen between males and females. Certain injuries are associated with certain sporting activities, for example posterior ankle impingement, which is most commonly seen in females participating in either dance or gymnastics. Pain from existing structural deformity or natural alignment may also occur in the female athlete. Hallux valgus is far more common in females and the joint or prominence can become painful due to the increased ground reaction and frictional forces of sporting activity. A valgus alignment of the knee is more common in females, and this can increase the strain on the medial soft-tissue structures of the knee during sport involving excessive knee flexion and rotation, for example, medial collateral ligament injuries in skiing. Patellofemoral syndrome is undoubtedly more common in females than in males, and this is probably due to a wider pelvis decreasing the mechanical efficiency and altering the muscle mechanics of the patellofemoral joint.

The incidence of stress fractures has also been reported to be higher in females. Early studies showed the female incidence to be 10 times greater than men (Protzman & Griffis 1977). Although more recent studies have not shown such a significant difference between the sexes it is generally accepted that female athletes are more prone to stress fracture than males, especially in the military. There are three common aetiological factors which may be responsible for this greater relative risk of stress fracture. These interlinking factors are known as the female athlete triad or unhappy triad and usually present as a combination of:

- amenorrhoea or menstrual irregularities (less than five menses per year)
- osteoporosis (due to menstrual abnormalities, hormonal imbalance, calcium deficiency or malnutrition)
- eating disorders (anorexia nervosa, bulimia nervosa, binge-eating disorders, anorexia athletica).

Although any of these factors can be present in the non-athletic female population, both amenorrhoea and eating disorders are more common among athletes. Some prospective studies have also demonstrated that stress fractures occurred more frequently in female athletes with low bone density (Bennell et al 1996) and also those with menstrual irregularities (Brukner & Bennell 2001, Rauh et al 2006).

It is generally agreed that females are more flexible than males. Whether this should affect injury rates between the sexes is unclear, but it has been reported that greater flexibility may predispose ligament injuries whereas inflexibility may predispose musculotendinous injuries. This would result in females being more prone to ligament injuries and males to musculotendinous injuries. Some evidence would appear to support this theory, as both anterior cruciate knee ligament injuries and lateral collateral ankle ligament injuries have been reported to be higher in females than in males undertaking the same activity (Almeida et al 1999, Griffin 1994) while Achilles tendon injuries are more common in males (Kannus & Jozsa 1991).

Previous injury

History of previous injury is a common finding when assessing the injured athlete. The relative risk of developing an injury when a history of a previous injury is present is two to three times greater than with a history of no injury. The majority of studies in this area have involved military subjects or runners. It is not surprising that a previously traumatised structure may be re-injured, as the athlete may frequently return to exercise too quickly or the underlying cause of the injury has not been addressed. The subsequent injury is often more severe than the previous injury. An example of this is seen in tibial stress fractures, where there is a history of previous exercise-induced shin pain in up to 50% of cases.

The subsequent injury does not necessarily occur at the same location as the previous injury. This may

Case history 15.2

A 26-year-old international male rugby player was diagnosed with right-sided Achilles tendinopathy. The pain in the tendon had been present for 2 months and had caused him to reduce his training volume. It had not improved with physiotherapy. The tendon was painful on palpation 4 cm proximal to its insertion and there was moderate swelling. There was a history of right-sided plantar fasciitis that had resolved 8 months ago with calf stretches, strapping and physical therapies. All non-weightbearing and static biomechanical parameters, including limb length, were the same for both limbs and calf flexibility was excellent in both limbs.

Dynamic video gait analysis with the athlete running on a treadmill demonstrated an earlier heel-lift on the right side. Video analysis taken prior to both injuries was used as a comparison and did not demonstrate an early heel-lift. It appeared that due to the previous plantar fasciitis the athlete had adapted his gait by an early heel-lift in an attempt to reduce the impact forces acting on the heel. This had resulted in excessive muscle activity of the calf muscle, inducing the tendinopathy. The athlete was successfully treated with gait re-education and a heel raise in his sports footwear, which was gradually reduced over a 3-month period.

suggest compensatory changes have occurred due to the injury or its treatment. These changes may be in proprioception or neuromuscular coordination resulting in excessive strain on adjacent or distant structures (Case history 15.2).

Structural alignment

The assessment of structural alignment must include an overall impression of the whole body, with a specific focus on the lower limbs and the injured area. The purpose is to assess and determine if the body's structure and function has caused or contributed to the injury. Biomechanical abnormalities may be identified, but their relevance to injury must be determined. It is also important to determine if any abnormality has occurred due to the injury rather than causing it (cause and effect). Although many studies have identified a biomechanical link with common overuse injuries there are also many studies which could not. It is therefore essential that the practitioner keeps an open mind when assessing a biomechanical causation for the patient's injury and explores all aspects of potential aetiology of the injury.

Structural alignment should be assessed with the patient non-weightbearing, weightbearing and dynamically. A thorough examination in all three components is essential if the practitioner is to gain a complete picture of the athlete's structure and function as it relates to the injury. This assessment should include examination of the joints, muscles and osseous alignment (Ch. 10, section A). The majority of podiatric interventions in sports injuries are related to the assessment and treatment of structural alignment and function that has caused or contributed to the injury.

Chronic or overuse sports injuries are usually due to the presence of one or both of the following situations:

- Normal structure and function but inadequate preparation or excessive demands placed on the tissues
- Abnormal structure and function with relatively normal demands placed on the tissues.

Although this is a rather simplistic view, it can be seen to be true in the majority of cases. If we consider two runners with patellofemoral syndrome: runner A runs over 160 km/week, running every day; runner B runs 32 km/week, running 3 times per week with 4 rest days. Apart from their injuries, they are both healthy and have taken 6 months to get to this weekly mileage. It should be clear that runner A is doing too much, too soon, and too frequently:

- running 160 km/week will often result in injury
- a running volume of 160 km/week in just 6 months has not allowed the tissues to undergo the normal adaptive processes required to meet these demands
- running every day does not allow adequate recovery time for the tissues, resulting in injury.

Other aetiological factors may also be present in runner A, but treatment will fail unless the errors of the training schedule are addressed. In the case of runner B, the aetiology of his injury is likely to be due to abnormal structure and function which has resulted in excessive patellofemoral joint reaction forces. His structural assessment should include examination of factors such as:

- muscle inflexibility (hamstrings, iliotibial band, quadriceps, lateral retinacula of the knee and calf muscles)
- muscle weakness (vastus medialis, gluteus medius, medial retinacula of the knee)

- patella malalignment or hypermobility (in frontal, transverse or sagittal plane)
- patella maltracking (during flexion and extension)
- excessive subtalar joint pronation
- frontal plane malalignment of the knee or tibia.

The presence or absence of these factors should assist the practitioner in identifying the aetiological factors and planning the most effective treatment (Witvrouw et al 2000).

Asymmetries between limbs may represent the obvious cause of a unilateral overuse injury. However, it is important to consider the role of other factors such as the type of activity, exercise surface, unilateral trauma and injury history. Any of these factors may cause a unilateral injury. If structural asymmetry is identified, then the practitioner must determine a biomechanical mechanism by which the asymmetry could have caused the overuse injury. If we consider stress fractures as an example, there is a strong association between stress fractures and limb-length inequality (Brukner et al 1999). Stress fractures tend to occur in the longer limb, and the greater the inequality the greater the incidence (Friberg 1982). The reasons for this are thought to be due to the biomechanical consequences of the limb-length difference, which results in a longer stance phase, skeletal realignment, greater osseous torsion and increased muscle activity of the longer limb. However, other studies have not shown any increase in injury risk when a limb-length inequality of >5 mm is present (Goss et al 2006).

Flexibility

Hypermobility due to increased muscle flexibility and ligamentous laxity has been associated with a greater risk of injury. Hypermobility is often determined by the Beighton score, which is based on a nine-point test designed to measure excessive joint movement (Ch. 14). This test has been used in a number of studies on flexibility and injury, which have generally shown that hypermobility is associated with a greater incidence of ligamentous injury. Rossiter & Galbraith (1996) found that hypermobility was present in 34% of military recruits with ankle and knee ligament injuries compared with 19% of control subjects. Increased flexibility, measured by the sit and reach test, in the absence of ligamentous laxity has not been shown to be a significant factor in injury prediction.

Generalised inflexibility due to muscle tightness has been linked to musculotendinous injury: while this is likely to be true, it has only been proved in one long-term prospective study to date (Witvrouw et al 2003). However, if a theoretical causal link can be made between the muscle inflexibility and the injury, then stretching of those muscles should be included in the treatment programme. Likewise, if hypermobility is present, then stretching should be avoided and athletes encouraged to perform specific stabilising exercises.

Stretching prior to activity in an attempt to reduce the risk of lower limb injury is contentious. Some large randomised controlled trials involving military recruits (Pope et al 1998, 2000) have shown no benefit in stretching while others have (Amako et al 2003). In two large systematic reviews of the literature neither set of authors could conclude on any significant benefit of stretching prior to sports participation (Fradkin et al 2006, Thacker et al 2004). This does not mean that injured athletes with muscle inflexibility should not be instructed to stretch, as this is an effective treatment modality. However, athletes are often questioned as to whether they stretch before and after activity and encouraged to do so if they do not. There seems little evidence to support this premise and failure to stretch before exercise should not necessarily be viewed as a risk factor to injury.

Physical fitness

Physical fitness is known to lower the risk of injury, as shown in a number of studies based on military and civilian populations (Neely 1998). This protective mechanism not only applies to practising a known sport but also to learning a new sport or athletic skill. The level of reduced risk varies among the studies, and is dependent upon the activity being undertaken and the fitness test used. Pope et al (2000) were able to demonstrate that the least-fittest group of their army recruits were 14 times more likely to sustain a lower limb injury than the fittest group. The fitness method used was the progressive 20 m shuttle run test, also known as the bleep test. This test is one of the most popular fitness tests used today.

When assessing injured athletes it is important to gauge their fitness level, as you may need to offer advice on a more appropriate training regimen. This is often the case for the novice athlete who enthusiastically embarks on an over-ambitious fitness programme. This will result in injury, as the musculoskeletal system is not prepared for such strenuous exercise. When an injury occurs, the athlete should be advised to modify their exercise regimen to prevent recurrence or further injury to other structures. This advice may include changing the method of exercise or reducing the intensity, frequency or duration of the exercise.

Physical build

The relationship of physical strength to injury is unknown. To avoid injury the musculoskeletal system must be able to cope with the physical demand of the sporting activity. Some evidence suggests that stronger athletes are more injury prone (Knapik et al 1992). The reasons for this are unclear, but it may be that the muscular forces generated by stronger athletes damage their joint structures and even the muscles themselves. It may also be that stronger athletes exercise at greater intensity or duration than weaker athletes, resulting in higher injury rates.

There is a correlation between strength imbalance and injury that is most frequently seen in the knee joint, where differences between hamstring and quadriceps strengths have been associated with cruciate ligament injuries. The role of strength differences between limbs has also shown a greater injury incidence on the weaker side. There is general agreement that strength differences greater than 10% can increase the injury risk to the weaker limb. These injuries may be acute, as with cruciate ligament injuries, or chronic, due to fatigue, for example tendinopathy, muscle strains and stress fractures. The role of limb dominance in injury incidence is less certain. Limb dominance in racket or ball sports is associated with different injury patterns. However, in sports that require equal stresses through both limbs there is no evidence to suggest limb dominance is a risk factor. Herring (1993) did not find any difference in injury incidence based on limb dominance in elite runners.

Anthropometric data such as height, weight, body mass index (BMI) and total body fat have also been examined as injury risk factors. In general, it is only the BMI that has been shown to be a positive indicator for injury risk. The BMI is determined by dividing the body weight in kilograms by the height of the patient in metres squared (kg/m^2). The normal BMI range is 20–25 with above 25 representing clinically overweight, above 30 clinically obese and below 20 representing underweight. As a general rule, the injury risk doubles for individuals who fall outside the normal BMI range.

Psychological factors

Psychological factors can play a significant part in both the development of a sports injury and the rehabilitation of the injury. Although there is no definite psychological profile of the injury-prone athlete, there are certain characteristics which may predispose the athlete to injury. Acute injuries may be more frequently seen in athletes who are extroverts with a low sense of responsibility. These athletes are natural risk-takers who may put themselves in injurious situations unnecessarily. The reasons for this type of sporting behaviour may be due to a daredevil attitude, poor decision making or an attempt to gain popularity with their peers, coach or supporters.

Chronic overuse injuries may be seen more frequently in athletes who demonstrate high levels of responsibility and dedication. These athletes will often train and play beyond the point of fatigue, resulting in small repetitive trauma to the tissues. This can cause chronic overuse injuries such as stress fractures, tendinopathy and muscle strains.

Other obvious psychological injury risk factors are stress and anxiety levels. Stress may come from the sport itself or other life stresses. Changes in personal circumstances, careers and relationships with family and friends can induce significant stress on an athlete. The athlete may then view sport as an escape or outlet to vent frustration, which can lead to poor decision making and injury. It is important to be aware of these factors when treating the athlete, as injury recurrence will be high if they are not addressed. This may mean liaising with the athlete's coach or team physician, so that an appropriate social support network can be provided.

The psychological response of the athlete to an injury can vary significantly. Most will go through a reaction of stress and grief. The grief response to an injury is like a minor or moderate version of losing a loved one. The severity of the injury and the importance of sport to the athlete will determine the level of the grief response. The grief response is characterised by three phases:

Phase 1 – shock

The immediate response to the injury may be one of sudden complete shock. The athlete may show signs of anger, disbelief and deny the existence of the injury. Rehabilitation of the athlete cannot begin until this phase is over.

Phase 2 – preoccupation

The athlete may demonstrate signs of depression and guilt about the injury, becoming isolated from other team members, family and friends. The athlete may also show signs of bargaining behaviour when undergoing treatment during this phase. Rehabilitation may begin during this phase, but real progress will not be achieved until the athlete enters the next phase.

Phase 3 – reorganisation

This is characterised by the athlete fully accepting the presence of the injury and demonstrating a renewed interest in the rehabilitation programme. The athlete is also likely to show a renewed interest in the sport and in relationships with family and team-mates. The practitioner should be aware of the various emotional states the athlete may demonstrate. This can help in formulating more appropriate treatment plans with one of the main aims being to guide the athlete to the final reorganisation phase.

Systemic disease

Practitioners must be aware that not all athletes are free from systemic disease or medical conditions. Cardiovascular, respiratory, endocrine, arthritic and neurological complaints are seen fairly frequently in the athletic population. The spur for many people to start to exercise may be the presence of hypertension, cardiovascular disease or obesity. Patients with systemic disease are often prescribed exercise programmes by other medical professionals such as general practitioners (GPs), medical consultants or physiotherapists. The role of exercise and sport is generally beneficial for patients with systemic disease as it can improve cardiovascular, respiratory and neurological function and help improve strength, flexibility and mobility. However, the exercise must be of the right type, intensity, duration and frequency to ensure medical complications do not arise. Practitioners should also be aware that undiagnosed systemic disease may be the underlying cause of the injury (Case history 15.3).

Patients with cardiovascular conditions such as peripheral vascular disease or hypertension must exercise with caution. Dynamic exercise increases the cardiac output, increases the blood flow to working muscles and causes peripheral vasodilation. The net result is a rise in systolic pressure in normotensive athletes. However, with hypertension there are rises in both systolic and diastolic pressures from already elevated baseline levels. This can elevate the blood pressure to dangerous levels, particularly if the athlete has moderate to severe hypertension, if the exercise intensity is too high or isometric exercise is performed.

In patients with vasospastic conditions or peripheral vascular disease, localised tissue hypoxia can result if the metabolic demands of the exercising tissues are greater than the blood supply can provide. It is also important to remember that certain sports

Case history 15.3

A 38-year-old male physical education instructor was referred by his GP with a 2-month history of localised pain in both forefeet. The patient was otherwise healthy and participated in a wide variety of sports both at work and socially. Both he and his GP were unsure of the nature of his pain and he had been referred for further investigation and orthotic treatment if appropriate.

A thorough medical history demonstrated no major illnesses, operations or a history of lower-limb injuries. There was no significant family medical history or social history. There was also no recent history of a change in exercise pattern or footwear. The pain was centred around the left fifth and right third metatarsophalangeal joints and tended to occur after activity. The pain was gradually getting worse. Moderate swelling was present at both joints, particularly in the right second interspace, with slight splaying of the second and third toes (Sullivan's sign). A list of differential diagnoses was considered, including stress fracture, capsulitis, synovitis, flexor digitorum longus tendinopathy, neuroma, bursitis, soft-tissue mass (right foot only), osteoarthritis and systemic joint disease. After a thorough clinical examination, osteoarthritis, stress fracture and tendinopathy were excluded. The examination of the joints caused pain and there were some neuritic symptoms in the right foot. The patient was given a local anaesthetic/cortisone injection into the webspace to exclude a Morton's neuroma and a temporary orthosis. The patient was also referred for X-ray.

On review the injection had not resolved the symptoms but the temporary orthosis had alleviated some of the pain. The X-rays revealed erosive changes in both metatarsal heads and the patient was subsequently diagnosed by a rheumatologist as having rheumatoid arthritis. The patient is currently taking disease-modifying drugs, wearing appropriate orthoses and continues to exercise. His exercise programme has been modified to avoid high-impact and contact sports.

This case demonstrates the importance of keeping an open mind when determining the diagnosis of an injury. Practitioners should consider all potential causes to avoid unnecessary or inappropriate treatment.

injuries are caused by cardiovascular changes such as acute and chronic compartment syndromes of the lower leg and foot, and popliteal artery entrapment syndrome. Exercise can also occasionally be the cause of cardiovascular pathology, such as effort-induced deep vein thrombosis or external artery endofibrosis (Bradshaw 2000).

Athletes with diabetes must monitor their blood glucose levels very closely, especially when starting or altering an exercise programme. Exercise increases the demand for glucose in the exercising tissues, resulting in a sharp drop in blood glucose levels. This can trigger a hypoglycaemic attack. Athletes will often have to reduce their dosage of insulin before exercise and should always have a ready source of glucose available when they exercise. It is important that patients with diabetes exercise to help reduce cardiovascular complications and limited joint mobility associated with the disease. Wolf (1998) demonstrated that patients with diabetes are at an increased risk of pedal stress fractures than patients without diabetes.

Neurological conditions such as upper or lower motor neurone lesions, hereditary motor and sensory neuropathies and nerve entrapments may occur in athletes. Patients with neurological disorders are often advised to exercise. Such patients may have altered sensation, altered muscle function and gait and a pes cavus foot deformity. These patients must be carefully assessed to ensure they undertake the appropriate exercise programme using appropriate supports as required. Avoidance of high-impact and contact sports is essential in neuropathic patients.

Extrinsic factors

Sporting equipment

The most important piece of sporting equipment in the assessment of lower-limb overuse injuries is the athlete's footwear. The athlete's shoes can assist in the diagnosis of the injury as they are often a contributory aetiological factor. They also represent an adjunct to treatment, as the practitioner will often modify the footwear or use it to accommodate an orthosis. In certain circumstances the practitioner may recommend changing the footwear completely. Recommending the right shoe for the patient is not easy. Sports shoe manufacturing is a multi-billion pound industry and company research data on shoe design and function are closely guarded secrets. Each company produces a number of different models for the same sport making it hard to know which is the best one. The most expensive model does not mean it is the best. The use of 'motion control systems' or special air or gel pockets to aid shock absorption is often used to market the brand as being better than that of the competition. The evidence to support such claims is often lacking.

The practitioner should appraise the athlete's shoe, identifying good and bad attributes and, if recommending a change in footwear, advise the athlete of what to look for when buying new sports shoes. To recommend one specific model for all patients will fail, as many patients will return dissatisfied if the injury does not resolve or complain that the shoe is uncomfortable. The aim for the practitioner is to ensure that the patient is exercising in a shoe that is:

- comfortable
- correct fit in length and width
- appropriate for the patient's sport
- does not show signs of excessive wear
- has appropriate tread, studs, spikes, cleats for the sport and exercise surface
- provides sufficient shock absorption, especially in the midsole
- provides appropriate motion control for the patient
- firm fastening
- lightweight.

Many sports shoes do not meet all of these criteria and can play a significant part in the development of an overuse injury. Worn shoes have been identified as risk factors in the incidence of a number of injuries such as stress fractures, exercise-induced leg pain, Achilles tendinopathy and patellofemoral syndrome due to a lack of shock absorption or motion control (Cheung et al 2006, Gardner et al 1988, Myburgh et al 1988, Taunton et al 2003). The shoe is the interface between the foot and the ground and must absorb significant ground reaction forces generated by sporting activity. As the shoe ages or becomes more worn, its ability to absorb these forces is reduced, resulting in increased forces being passed on to the musculoskeletal system. It has been estimated that the average running shoe loses 50% of its shock-absorbing capabilities after 480–800 km of running (Cook et al 1985). Old shoes may not only demonstrate signs of excessive wear but material degradation can also occur, which further reduces the shock-absorbing capabilities of the shoe. This is accelerated in cold climates (Dib et al 2005).

An uneven wear pattern on the sole of the shoe or the insole inside the shoe can give a guide to biomechanical abnormalities or sporting technique of the athlete. Excessive lateral wear of the rearfoot can indicate a varus alignment or strike pattern and may cause inversion ankle sprains or lateral foot and leg injuries. Excessive wear across the ball of the foot will cause a loss of traction and control, which may induce injury. Different wear patterns between the shoes may indicate different biomechanics or sporting technique. The most common example of uneven wear is limb-length inequality due to structural, functional or environmental factors.

The weight of the shoe is important to optimise performance: the heavier the shoe, the greater the muscle exertion and energy expenditure. This can cause fatigue in the lower leg muscles and therefore affect performance. Light running shoes may enhance speed but should only be worn for racing as they do not offer appropriate support or shock absorption.

The importance of comfort and correct fit cannot be overstated. Shoes that are too tight or narrow will obviously cause irritation, resulting in corns, calluses, subungual haematomas and other nail pathologies. It is common in kicking sports such as soccer and rugby that the athlete will wear a boot that is too small in order to get a better 'feel' for kicking the ball. This practice should be discouraged as it can often compromise foot function, cause clawing of the toes and exacerbate nail pathologies. Shoes that are too narrow or fastened too tightly can cause pain in the arch and neuritic pain in the forefoot during exercise. A shoe that is too long will allow excessive movement of the foot, resulting in friction blisters and heel slippage.

Exercise surface

The role that the exercise surface may play in the development of overuse injuries is a contentious issue. It was previously thought that athletes who exercise on hard unyielding surfaces such as concrete would have an increased incidence of osteoarthritis due to accelerated wear and tear of the joints. There is very little evidence to support this despite several long-term prospective studies. However, in athletics, harder synthetic track surfaces can increase performance but also increase the incidence of musculoskeletal injury. In athletes exercising solely on hard surfaces, increases in the incidence of medial tibial stress syndrome by 28% and Achilles tendonitis by 17% have been demonstrated (Nigg & Yeadon 1987).

Artificial grass was first used for sport in 1964 and has since become a major playing surface in a wide number of sporting activities. The injury profile of this surface is different from that of natural grass. Bowers & Martin (1976) identified an injury virtually unique to this surface. Turf toe is a hyperextension injury of the first metatarsophalangeal joint resulting in a sprain of the plantar capsuloligamentous structures. It is caused by shoes with a flexible sole in the forefoot bending excessively on a hard unyielding surface. It is primarily seen in American football but can occur in any sport played on artificial grass surfaces, such as AstroTurf.

Harder surfaces invoke greater ground reaction forces, which must be absorbed by the shoe and musculoskeletal system. The body absorbs these forces primarily through the joints and eccentric muscle activity. The harder the exercise surface, the greater the eccentric muscle activity (Richie et al 1993). Theoretically, exercising on harder surfaces should cause greater knee flexion, ankle dorsiflexion and greater or prolonged subtalar joint pronation to aid the absorption of the higher ground reaction forces. No biomechanical studies have shown this to date. There is, however, evidence that repetitive high-impact sports do increase the risk of lower-limb osteoarthritis particularly in the presence of previous injury (Conaghan 2002). This does not seem to apply to recreational running.

In addition to the hardness of the exercise surface, it is important to consider the friction and energy loss of the surface. Friction, or horizontal stiffness, is integral in acceleration and deceleration. Artificial athletic surfaces have greater friction than grass, allowing greater acceleration and deceleration. However, these greater frictional forces must be absorbed by the body and can result in increased injuries. These injuries may be to the musculotendinous units or the ligaments designed to limit joint movements such as the cruciate ligaments of the knee. Running on a treadmill is associated with far smaller tibial strain and loading than overground running which is suggestive that running injuries associated with reduced shock absorption (e.g. tibial stress fracture) could be significantly reduced by treadmill running (Milgrom et al 2003).

Energy loss of a surface is related to its elastic behaviour and deformation properties. Surfaces that deform when loaded are termed compliant and result in increased contact time. This increases cushioning as peak contact forces are reduced. However, it may reduce performance as the contact time is greater, resulting in slower acceleration. Exercising on softer surfaces can also alter joint positions. Consider an athlete running on sand. The greatest contact force occurs at heel-strike, so the sand will be maximally displaced at this time. This results in greater ankle dorsiflexion, requiring greater muscle activity of the calf muscles. Thus, exercising on softer surfaces may reduce injuries associated with high-impact forces but may lead to increases in muscle activity resulting in musculotendinous injury.

It is also important to consider the terrain and incline of the exercise surface. Uneven terrain such as grass will mean the body having to adapt to maintain ground contact and stability. These adaptive changes mainly occur in the frontal plane and can result in greater supinatory and pronatory moments within the foot and ankle. If these forces become excessive then frontal plane injury will result. The most obvious example of this is the inversion ankle sprain. Pronatory injuries can occur and usually involve the posterior tibial tendon. If an athlete exercises on uneven terrain with frontal plane movements of the foot and ankle limited by strapping, a brace or boots, then greater forces will be transferred to the knee. This can result in collateral ligament and cruciate damage. This injury pattern has been seen in skiing. Uneven terrain can also exist on surfaces which are perceived to be flat. The camber of roads is usually canted up to 14°. This can cause pronatory moments on one limb and supinatory moments on the other, resulting in an environmental limb-length difference.

The importance of exercising on an incline should not be overlooked. Both uphill and downhill running are associated with different joint angular relationships and muscle activity patterns. Uphill running requires greater ankle joint dorsiflexion and eccentric calf and hamstring muscle activity. Downhill running requires greater ankle plantarflexion and eccentric muscle activity of the foot dorsiflexors. This particularly affects the tibialis anterior muscle, which becomes active for longer and elongates further as it decelerates foot slap. Downhill running also increases the load on the quadriceps muscles and is known to exacerbate conditions such as patellofemoral syndrome and patella tendinopathy.

Sporting activity

The type of sport the athlete plays and the techniques they use are integral to the development of overuse injuries. Certain injuries are even named after certain sports or activities (Table 15.2). This does not mean that these injuries are unique to that particular sport, but they occur frequently due to the forces the anatomical structure has to absorb. Metatarsal stress fractures are not unique to military personnel who march, but this activity involves repetitive impact forces through the forefoot, which can result in a stress fracture. Patella tendinopathy is most commonly seen in jumping sports due to the high ground reaction forces (up to eight times body weight) that this activity produces. A significant component of these forces is absorbed by eccentric quadriceps activity, which can cause patella tendinopathy.

Table 15.2 Common injuries named after a sport

Injury name	*Definition*
Footballer's ankle	Anterior ankle impingement
Tennis leg	Rupture/tear of medial head of gastrocnemius
Fresher's leg	Exercise-induced shin pain
March fracture	Metatarsal stress fracture
Jumper's knee	Patella tendinopathy
Runner's knee	Patellofemoral syndrome
Golfer's elbow	Medial epicondylitis
Tennis elbow	Medial (forehand) epicondylitis, lateral (backhand) epicondylitis
Swimmer's shoulder	Rotator cuff pathology

It is important the practitioner has an understanding of the type of sport the athlete plays and its biomechanics. This will help the practitioner:

- understand the forces involved in the sport
- identify the structures at risk of injury
- determine the potential biomechanical mechanism of injury
- formulate the most appropriate treatment plan.

These four factors are all inter-related. Identifying the structures most at risk of injury requires knowledge of the forces involved in the sport. This knowledge is related to the biomechanical movements of that particular sport. Determining the biomechanical mechanism of injury is crucial to formulating the most appropriate treatment plan. Without this knowledge it is difficult to reduce or prevent the forces that caused the injury. Appropriate treatment planning must also take into account the limitations of the sport on the treatment. This will include the athlete's footwear and other sporting equipment. Some sports do not allow the use of mechanical supports as they may compromise player safety or give the athlete an unfair advantage.

It is also important to be aware of individual variation in sporting technique, which not only determines the athlete's skill and ability at a sport but can also predispose injury. Minor differences in sporting technique can have a significant effect on injury development. An example is in running techniques between forefoot and rearfoot strikers. Forefoot striking is associated with increased impact forces, a reduced stance phase and reduced subtalar joint pronation. These three factors combined could increase the forces being absorbed both in the forefoot and more proximally in the calf muscles, shin and knee.

The team position will also help determine the sporting technique of the athlete. The position played may be based on anthropometric characteristics, limb dominance and skill levels. Team position may be important to the practitioner, as the biomechanical movements and sporting techniques used by the athlete can vary. This will result in different injury profiles seen between positions: for example a prop forward and wing back in rugby, a wicket keeper and fast bowler in cricket, a linebacker and wide receiver in American football.

Training errors

As discussed earlier, athletes may do too much, too soon, and too frequently. Training errors are one of the commonest causes of chronic overuse injuries, and practitioners must identify these errors for successful treatment planning. Failure to do so will lead to a recurrence of the injury or development of other overuse injuries. To avoid injury athletes who wish to exercise regularly must find the correct balance of exercise intensity, duration and frequency. This will usually involve:

- participating in more than one sport
- combination of strength, flexibility and endurance training
- incorporation of rest days in the weekly training schedule
- periods during the year of greater training/sport levels, i.e. seasons
- variation in training methods to help maintain interest.

When athletes first begin to train they often overestimate their baseline fitness level. This can result in injury, as the musculoskeletal system is not physiologically prepared for this volume of exercise. Common injuries at this stage are muscle strains and exercise-induced leg pain (shin splints). Increasing the volume of exercise too quickly can also occur when an athlete is returning from injury or training for a specific competition that they are not prepared for.

Bones, like muscle, also undergo a normal physiological strengthening process during the early period of an exercise programme. This remodelling process is characterised by initial bone porosity due to osteoclastic channelling, which is then followed by osteoblasts laying down new bone matrix. The result is that the bone is initially weakened by exercise and then eventually strengthened beyond its pre-exercise level. This whole process usually takes 6 months and during the first 2 months the bone is especially prone to injuries such as stress fracture. This is one of the main reasons stress fractures are usually seen during the first 2 months of starting an exercise programme or significantly increasing the exercise level (Beck 1998).

Environmental factors

Changes in temperature, humidity and altitude can all affect performance and may increase injury risk. Practitioners providing treatment at endurance events should be particularly aware of the consequences of environmental factors. High temperatures and humidity levels can produce heat-intolerance illnesses including syncope, heat cramps, exhaustion and stroke. These are most frequently seen in athletes who have not fully acclimatised to the environment and become dehydrated and salt depleted.

Most cold-related sports injuries are seen in submaximal endurance sports such as marathon running or wilderness sports such as mountaineering and skiing. Cold climates reduce performance as the body must use energy stores for thermogenesis. Cold-induced injuries include chilblains, trench foot, frostbite and hypothermia. Pre-existing conditions, such as asthma, Raynaud's phenomenon and cold urticaria, can also be triggered by the cold.

High altitude ranges from 1500 to 3500 m above sea level. Above 1500 m, the maximum oxygen uptake by the body reduces by 10% for every 1000 m. This results in reduced performance at endurance events. The opposite is true for performance at short anaerobic events, due to lower air resistance. Illnesses associated with high altitude include acute mountain sickness, pulmonary oedema, cerebral oedema and retinal haemorrhage.

History taking

A significant part of the patient's initial consultation is likely to involve history taking. It is important to cover all relevant areas, otherwise vital clues may be missed, resulting in misdiagnosis or inappropriate treatment planning. The consultation will start with noting the patient's personal details. In addition to the patient's name, address, date of birth, GP, information on other healthcare practitioners treating the athlete should also be recorded. Recording the contact details of the athlete's coach(es) is useful, as communication between the coach and practitioner may assist in identifying risk factors and ensuring the athlete adheres to a treatment plan.

The history should cover the following areas:

- Medical history
- Social history
- Drug history
- Sport history
- Injury history.

Medical history

Taking an accurate medical history is essential in determining an athlete's suitability to perform a sport. As already discussed, poor physical fitness or systemic disease may predispose an athlete to injury. Diseases of the cardiovascular, respiratory, neurological, endocrine, gastrointestinal and genitourinary systems can affect performance and predispose injury. If medical conditions are identified, it is important to gain information about the onset, the type of symptoms experienced, the treating physician and the type of treatment. This information will help the practitioner to determine whether it is necessary to recommend participation in a different sporting activity or participation at a reduced level.

The history of any surgical procedures should also be recorded. Surgical procedures due to systemic disease or previous injury may have direct relevance to the assessment of the current injury. Information related to all surgical procedures is important as it provides an indication of the overall health status of the athlete and the athlete's healing capacity. Also, any recent operations that may have resulted in a reduced training programme and fitness level, which may have contributed to the current sports injury, need to be noted.

Both the patient and practitioner often overlook the role of nutrition in sports performance and injury. The practitioner should be aware of the nutritional requirements of athletic performance. Energy for exercise comes from carbohydrates, fats and, to a lesser extent, proteins. Muscle hypertrophy and skeletal development is reliant on proteins, vitamins and minerals. Homeostasis depends on water, fibre and minerals. A healthy diet will incorporate the right balance of these foodstuffs. Athletes will often manipulate this balance to enhance performance: e. g. carbohydrate loading prior to endurance events, protein supplements to increase muscle mass and anaerobic power. Manipulation of foodstuffs may not be detrimental as long as it does not increase one source at the expense of reducing another. However, if the practitioner is in doubt and suspects the athlete's diet is contributing to the injury then referral to a dietitian or sports nutritionist is warranted. Other indications for referral may include rapid changes in body weight, vitamin deficiencies and BMIs below 18 or above 27.

Accurate assessment of physical fitness is difficult without resort to specific exercise physiology tests. These tests are used to measure an athlete's ability to exercise aerobically or anaerobically. An impression of athletes' fitness can be gained from questioning them about their exercise programme, athletic performance, speed of recovery from exercise and injury history. Rapid increases in exercise intensity may not be associated with increases in physical fitness. Exercise at too low an intensity will also not produce improvements in fitness. As a general rule aerobic exercise must be performed at a level equivalent to 70–80% of the maximum heart rate. Exercising below this level will not produce significant improvements in fitness and exercise above this level may overstrain the cardiovascular system. A slow recovery from exercise may either be due to poor physical fitness or exercising at too high an intensity. Signs of a slow recovery may include laboured breathing post-exercise, severe fatigue or delayed-onset muscle soreness.

Social history

The social history of the athlete will involve questioning them regarding their occupation, dietary and alcohol habits and whether they smoke. High alcohol consumption, smoking and a poorly balanced diet may all predispose the athlete to injury due to their effect on physical fitness. A patient's occupation is often overlooked but may be a significant factor in both the aetiology of the injury and its management. It may be difficult for an athlete to truly rest an injured structure if their occupation involves heavy manual work or standing for prolonged periods. The social network of family and friends may be a cause of stress to the athlete. If these stresses become significant they may contribute to the development of injury. Questioning the athlete on these issues may be necessary if the practitioner suspects psychological stress as an aetiological factor in the injury.

Drug history

A thorough pharmacological history should include any current prescription only or over-the-counter medicines, previous medication and drug allergies. Current or past medication may indicate pathology not identified in the medical history. Drug allergies are obviously important, as they may contraindicate certain treatment options. Over-the-counter medicines may include nutritional supplements, homeopathic remedies, topical agents or pain medication. Pain medication is of particular importance, as it will mask some of the symptoms of the injury. This can result in the athlete and practitioner underestimating the severity of the injury, in addition to the potential long-term complications of such medication.

The use of pharmacological aids to enhance sporting performance is now more commonplace. Such practices are not confined to the elite level. The practitioner should be aware of the potential risks associated with pharmacological abuse, particularly their role in injury development. This is mainly confined to anabolic steroids, which can significantly increase muscle mass, muscle strength and the psychological drive to exercise. These drugs may cause injury due to the increased forces placed through the musculoskeletal system from the greater exercise intensity. There is also some evidence to suggest that continual long-term use causes weakening of collagen structures, resulting in injury to tendon, ligament and muscle. Other more serious long-term effects can include cardiomyopathy, liver damage and testicular atrophy. Abuse at the elite level is further complicated by athletes using masking agents, which may themselves be detrimental to health. Evidence on the effects of other ergogenic aids such as protein, vitamin and mineral supplements, creatine, caffeine, blood doping and human growth hormone is currently lacking. Although these aids are commonly used, their potential benefit to athletic performance has not been clearly proven.

Sport history

It is important to gain as much detail about the athlete's sporting history as possible. This should include the following:

- Type or types of sport
- Frequency (number of times/week)
- Duration
- Intensity
- Level.

The main sport the athlete participates in is of obvious importance but the practitioner should also focus on secondary sporting activities the athlete may undertake. These activities may be for interest or fitness but they can play a significant part in the development of an injury and should not be overlooked. Other factors to note would include the sports surface, footwear, limb dominance and sporting position.

The frequency, duration and intensity of sporting activity will help the practitioner determine if the athlete is over- or under-training: both can lead to injury. Over-training can cause overuse injury, as there is insufficient time for tissue replenishment and regeneration. Under-training can cause injury due to inadequate levels of fitness or strength. As a general rule, to improve cardiovascular fitness it is recommended to exercise three times a week for a minimum of 20 minutes each time at an intensity of 70–80% maximum heart rate.

The duration of activity is important: too short an exercise period will not produce the desired physiological improvement in fitness, and too long a period will cause fatigue and possible injury. Duration should also include how long the athlete has been participating in that particular sport, as this will impact on their fitness and skill level. When questioning athletes about their sporting activity, it is important to determine at what frequency, duration and intensity they were exercising when the injury occurred. The practitioner should pay particular attention to recent changes to the training schedule (Case history 15.4).

The level at which the athlete undertakes his sport is also important. This will help the practitioner determine the athlete's motivation to play sport and may also guide the treatment plan. Elite or professional athletes may find it harder to rest or modify their activity than novice athletes. Convincing a professional athlete to take time out from their sport is often very difficult and should involve collaboration with other members of the sports medicine team or coaching staff. These athletes are often more demanding of the practitioner and can present a management challenge.

When assessing an athlete's current participation level it is important to determine their athletic goals. Athletes may strive to achieve certain goals or reach

Case history 15.4

A 23-year-old semi-professional soccer player returned for treatment complaining of bilateral shin pain. Eighteen months previously he had been successfully treated for patellofemoral syndrome after being prescribed an exercise programme and orthoses for his football boots and AstroTurf training shoes. His shin pain had been present for 6 weeks and was gradually deteriorating. It was initially suspected that the shin pain was due to the orthoses becoming worn and less effective. Additional support was therefore added to the orthoses and the athlete was reviewed 2 weeks later. The pain was still present and it was at this stage that the athlete revealed that his training schedule had changed slightly. In addition to his normal soccer training, which consisted of 5 hours' practice and one game per week, he had started to attend a high-impact aerobics class. This was in a school hall with a non-sprung hardwood floor. For the 90-minute classes he wore an old pair of running shoes in which his orthoses did not fit.

He was advised to discontinue the aerobics class and the shin pain resolved within 10 days. High-impact aerobics on hard surfaces is associated with significant ground reaction forces and this had caused him to develop medial tibial stress syndrome. The lack of orthotic control and the poor shock absorption of his old running shoes had probably exacerbated the situation.

a specific level of performance, such as running a distance in a given time or becoming a regular first team player for a sports club. Although these goals may be achievable the athlete will often have unrealistic expectations of the time it will take to reach that level of skill or fitness. Part of the assessment of athletes and their injuries may involve the practitioner giving advice on whether an athlete's goals are achievable in the short term.

Injury history

As much information as possible should be gained about both previous lower-limb injuries and the current injury. Previous injuries are important as they can make the athlete more susceptible to injury and they may also cause structural or functional compensations. Information on this area can be gained easily by asking questions such as the following:

- Have you broken any bones within the lower limb?
- Have you ruptured or torn any ligaments or tendons in the lower limb?
- Is there a history of prolonged or intermittent swelling of any joints in the lower limb?
- Have you had any injuries, which have resulted in missing more than 2 weeks from sport?

With acute injuries there is often a history of a single traumatic event. The athlete may be able to describe how the injury occurred, making it easier for the practitioner to determine the mechanism or pattern of injury. This information can enable the practitioner to identify the injured structure and the likely level of force that caused the injury. Diagnosis of both the injured structure and the injury severity is therefore easier. Identifying the injury mechanism in chronic or overuse injuries is harder as these injuries are usually associated with multiple minor traumatic events and the injury may have led to functional compensation.

The location, duration and the type of pain can all assist the diagnosis of the injury. The location of pain may be diffuse and generalised or focal and specific to a single structure. This characteristic is important, as both generalised and focal pain can be typical of specific conditions. As an example, consider patellofemoral syndrome and patella tendinopathy, which are both causes of anterior knee pain. Patella tendinopathy will cause pain within the tendon or its sheath and is focal in nature. Patellofemoral syndrome is characterised by pain, medial, posterior or lateral to the patella and is generalised in nature. This is sometimes referred to as the 'grab' sign, as the patient will grab the whole of the front of the knee when asked to locate the area of pain.

The duration of pain will inform the practitioner both of how long the injury has been present and its severity. As a general rule, the longer the injury has been present the longer the recovery period will be from the initiation of treatment. This is usually because the injury has become more severe. Consider pathology of tendons as an example. Long-standing tendinopathy can be associated with the formation of adhesions, scar tissue and mucinous degeneration of the tendon itself. This is referred to as tendinosis and will require more intensive and prolonged treatment that may take many weeks or months to resolve. Injuries which are intermittent in nature may be less severe or specifically associated with a sporting activity.

Descriptions of the type of pain experienced are somewhat subjective (see Ch. 3). However, certain pain descriptions are characteristic of trauma to specific anatomical structures. Neurogenic symptoms usually involve paraesthesia, numbness or a burning sensation. A dull or intense aching sensation usually represents an injury to deep structures, especially muscle or bone. Sharp or throbbing pain may represent trauma to articular structures. The severity of the pain is especially subjective, as patients have differing tolerance and pain coping strategies. It is therefore best to assess the pain severity in conjunction with all other injury factors.

Other factors to note about the injury are previous conservative treatment and what exacerbates or improves the injury. The majority of sports patients have usually been treated by another healthcare practitioner or attempted self-treatment prior to attending the podiatrist. This information may be particularly useful in determining injury severity and appropriate treatment planning. Accurate information on treatment by other healthcare practitioners may require communication between practitioners, which can also assist in making an accurate diagnosis through case discussion. Factors which exacerbate injury are usually sport-related and may include any of the intrinsic and extrinsic risk factors discussed earlier. Factors outside the athlete's sport may also contribute, such as occupation, social activities and non-athletic footwear.

Many injuries have such characteristic histories that the injury diagnosis requires only minimal examination. A common example of this is exercise-induced leg pain, traditionally known as shin splints. The characteristics of the common causes of exercise-induced leg pain are shown in Table 15.3. The relationship of the pain to exercise is very diagnostic, as each condition significantly varies. In chronic compartment syndrome the pain is induced by exercise and the athlete must stop or reduce their exercise intensity. On cessation of exercise the pain disappears within minutes. In medial tibial stress syndrome pain is rarely present during exercise but occurs within hours following exercise and may last up to 2 days post exercise. The pain from stress fractures is exacerbated by exercise and usually becomes constant in nature unless the athlete completely rests.

Examining the injured structure

Following a thorough injury history, the practitioner may have formulated a provisional list of differential diagnoses. This process is assisted by observation of the injured site and adjacent structures. Marked swelling, bruising and erythema often accompany acute injuries, whereas in chronic injuries these signs may be subtle or absent. Observation of adjacent structures is useful to gauge the level of any swelling or to determine deformity. Unilateral injuries should always be visually compared with the asymptomatic side. This will require having the athlete prone when the injury is on the posterior surface such as with Achilles tendon injuries.

From the history and visual inspection the practitioner should be able to identify the potential injured anatomical structures. The next phase of the examination will be to individually isolate the structures and then apply stress to them in a controlled manner. The application of stress should be gradually increased until the athlete's symptoms are reproduced. Stress is initially applied by gentle and then firm palpation. The level of pressure required when palpating the area is determined by the tissue type and depth. Deep dense structures such as tendon or bone will require firmer pressure than more superficial structures or those that are less dense such as muscle or ligament.

Table 15.3 Characteristics of the common causes of exercise-induced leg pain

Pain characteristic syndrome	*Medial tibial stress syndrome*	*Tibial stress fracture*	*Chronic compartment*
Location	Tenoperiosteal junction	Bone	Muscle compartment
Nature	Diffuse	Focal	Diffuse
Description	Dull ache	Intense ache	Tightness, fullness, cramping
Relationship to exercise	Post-exercise, lasts <2 days	Constant, made worse by exercise	Induced by exercise, relieved by rest

Movement of the injured structure should also be performed. This should initially be passive, with the practitioner directing the movement. If this is pain-free, the patient should be directed to move the structure actively with no resistance applied. In the majority of sports injuries both of these types of movements are unlikely to cause pain. The next step is to apply active resistance to the movement. This should first be performed with concentric contraction and then eccentric if the first movement did not induce symptoms. These contractions should be held for between 10 and 20 seconds. In the majority of cases resisted eccentric or concentric contraction will induce symptoms.

The method of achieving the greatest stress is to have the athlete perform dynamic or functional exercises: examples of these movements are double or single knee squats to stress the patellofemoral joint and the single leg tiptoe test to stress the posterior tibial tendon or have the athlete go up and down on their forefoot with the heel over the edge of a stair to stress the Achilles tendon. A dynamic functional assessment should be included in any orthopaedic examination. For the athlete with a sports injury this may require the practitioner to observe the athlete's sporting technique in addition to normal static stance and gait analysis. Many of these sporting movements can be performed in a relatively small space or on a treadmill. Occasionally, a practitioner may have to go and observe the athlete in his natural sporting environment or ask the patient to video their sporting activity.

Specialist investigations

As with any investigation, specialist tests should only be performed if the results may change the treatment plan. Specialist investigations in sports medicine are primarily used to assist in diagnosing and grading the severity of an injury. Table 15.4 summarises the various tests and the common sports injuries they may be used to diagnose. X-ray remains the mainstay diagnostic test for osseous pathology and magnetic resonance imaging (MRI) or ultrasound for soft-tissue pathology. A number of conditions such as stress fractures, osteochondral defects and the osteochondritides may be diagnosed by several different modalities. In these cases the choice of modality will depend on the injury history, and the cost and access of the modalities.

Table 15.4 Specialist investigations used in sports injury assessment

Investigation	*Main uses*	*Common sports injuries diagnosed*
X-ray	Articular and osseous	Fractures, ligament ruptures or laxity, osteochondritides
Computed tomography (CT)	Osseous, especially cortical pathology	Stress fractures, cartilage tears, osteochondral defects
Magnetic resonance imaging (MRI)	Tendon, ligament, muscle, cartilage, bone marrow pathology	Tendinopathies, ligament injuries, muscle tears, cartilage tears, stress fractures, osteochondral defects
Nuclear bone scanning	Abnormal bone activity	Stress fractures, medial tibial stress syndrome, osteochondritises
Ultrasound	Tendon, ligament, muscle, fascial pathologies	Tendinopathies, plantar fasciitis
Intracompartmental pressure studies	Muscle/fascial pathology	Compartment syndromes
Nerve conduction studies	Nerve pathology	Exercise-related nerve entrapments
Arteriography/venography arterial	Arterial and venous pathology	Effort-induced deep vein thrombosis, entrapment syndromes

Table 15.5 Grading systems for ligament injuries and tendonitis

Grade	*Ligament injuries*	*Tendinopathy*	*Muscle tears*
1	Stretching of the ligament without macroscopic tears	Pain after exercise	Minimal tear with no loss of strength
2	Partial macroscopic tear	Pain pre- and post-exercise, pain reduced during exercise	Macroscopic tear with loss of strength
3	Complete rupture	Pain before, during and after exercise	Complete tear with no function
4		Constant pain and volume of exercise reducing	

Injury grading systems

As with many pathologies, sports injuries are often graded by their severity. These classification systems are primarily used to direct treatment protocols. As an example, grade 1 ankle sprains are treated differently from grade 3 sprains. Grading systems are also useful when communicating with other members of the sports medicine team about the patient. They can also be used to help explain the nature of the pathology to the athlete or coach. Grading systems may describe an injury to a tissue type such as ligament, bone or tendon, or be specific to a certain injury such as posterior tibial tendon dysfunction, osteochondral talar defects or Achilles tendon injuries. The grading systems for muscle and ligament injuries and tendinopathy are given in Table 15.5. The numerical grading system for Achilles tendon disorders has changed recently to peritendonitis, tendinosis, or a combination of both (Khan et al 2002), as this more accurately reflects the actual pathology.

Summary

The practitioner should involve the patient as much as possible in the assessment process. Athletes are often well educated in their area of sport and this can greatly assist the practitioner. Likewise, the practitioner must educate the patient, as this will play a crucial role in the success of the treatment. The majority of sports injury treatments require the athlete to follow specific advice or instructions. Compliance is intricately linked to understanding so the practitioner must educate the athlete about the injury and the purpose of any treatment.

A structured holistic approach is essential in the assessment of the sports patient. Practitioners should develop a logical assessment protocol that meets the patient's and their own needs in whatever assessment environment they are working in. The successful treatment of lower-limb sports injuries requires the practitioner to assimilate knowledge from areas as diverse as sports psychology, exercise physiology and sports biomechanics. This knowledge will assist in the diagnosis of the injury risk factors. Identification of these intrinsic and extrinsic risk factors should form the main focus of the assessment due to the multifactorial nature of most lower-limb sports injuries. Diagnosis of the injury itself requires detailed knowledge of the regional anatomy and common sports injuries that affect the lower limb. Athletes with chronic overuse injuries can be very difficult to treat. The assessment principles outlined in this chapter are designed to help the practitioner meet these management challenges.

References

Almeida S A, Trone D W, Leone D M et al 1999 Gender differences in musculoskeletal injury rates: a function of symptom reporting. Medicine and Science in Sport and Exercise 31(12):1807–1812

Amako M, Oda T, Masouka A et al 2003 Effect of static stretching on prevention of injuries in military recruits. Military Medicine 168(6):442–446

Anderson B, Burke E R 1994 Scientific, medical, and practical aspects of stretching. In: Delee J C, Drez D (eds) Orthopaedic sports medicine, vol 1. W B Saunders, Philadelphia

Beck B 1998 Tibial stress injuries: an aetiological review for the purposes of guiding management. Sports Medicine 26(4):265–279

Bennell K L, Malcolm S A, Thomas S A et al 1996 Risk factors for stress fractures in track and field athletes: a 12 month prospective study. American Journal of Sports Medicine 24:810–818

Bowers K D, Martin R B 1976 Turf toe: a shoe surface related football injury. Medicine and Science of Sports 8:81–83

Bradshaw C 2000 Exercise related lower leg pain: vascular. Medicine and Science in Sports and Exercise S34–36

Brukner P, Bennell K 2001 Stress fractures. In: O'Conner F, Wilder R (eds) Textbook of running medicine. McGraw-Hill, New York, pp 227–256

Brukner P, Bennell K, Matheson G 1999 Stress fractures. Blackwell Science, Oxford

Bruns W, Maffulli N 2000 Lower limb injuries in children in sports clinics. Sports Medicine 19:637–662

Cantu R, Micheli L (eds) 1991 American College of Sports Medicine guidelines for the team physician. Lea & Febiger, Philadelphia

Cavanagh P R, Kram R 1990 Stride length in distance running. Medicine and Science in Sports and Exercise 21(4):467–479

Cheung R, Ng T, Chen B 2006 Association of footwear with patellofemoral syndrome in runners. Sports Medicine 36(3):199–205

Colville M R 1998 Surgical treatment of the unstable ankle. Journal of the American Academy of Orthopaedic Surgeons 6:368–377

Conaghan P 2002 Update on osteoarthritis part 1: current concepts and the relation to exercise. British Journal of Sports Medicine 36(5):330–333

Cook S D, Kester M A, Brunet M E 1985 Shock absorbing characteristics of running shoes. American Journal of Sports Medicine 13:248–253

Dalton S E 1992 Overuse injuries in adolescent athletes. Sports Medicine 13(1):58–70

Dib M, Smith J, Bernhardt K 2005 Effect of environmental temperature on shock absorption properties of running shoes. Clinical Journal of Sports Medicine 15(3): 172–176

Ferran N, Maffulli N 2006 Epidemiology of sprains of the lateral ankle ligament complex. Foot and Ankle Clinics 11(3):659–662

Fradkin A, Gabbe B, Cameron P 2006 Does warming up prevent injury in sport? The evidence from randomised controlled trials. Journal of Science & Medicine in Sport 9(3):214–220

Friberg O 1982 Leg length asymmetry in stress fractures: a clinical and radiological study. Journal of Sports Medicine 22:485–488

Gardner L I, Dziados J E, Jones B H et al 1988 Prevention of lower extremity stress fractures: a controlled trial of a shock absorbent insole. American Journal of Public Health 78:1563–1567

Gerrard D F 1993 Overuse injury and growing bones: the young athlete at risk. British Journal of Sports Medicine 27(1):14–18

Gerson L, Stevens J 2004 Recreational injuries among older Americans. Journal of Injury Prevention 10(3):134–138

Goss D, Moore J, Slivka E et al 2006 Comparison of injury rates with limb length inequalities and matched controlled subjects over 1 year of military training and athletic participation. Military Medicine 171(6):522–555

Griffin L Y 1994 The female athlete. In: Delee J C, Drez D (eds) Orthopaedic sports medicine Vol 1. W B Saunders, Philadelphia

Hergenroeder A 1998 Prevention of sports injuries. Journal of Paediatrics 101:1057–1063

Herring K 1993 Injury prediction among runners. Preliminary report on limb dominance. Journal of American Podiatric Medical Association 83(9):523–528

Hootman J, Macera C, Ainsworth B et al 2002 Predictors of lower extremity injury among recreationally active adults. Clinical Journal of Sports Medicine 12(2):99–106

Hreljac A, Marshall R N, Hume P A 2000 Evaluation of lower extremity overuse injury potential in runners. Medicine and Science in Sports and Exercise 32:1635–1641

James S L, Bates B T, Osternig L R 1978 Injuries to runners. American Journal of Sports Medicine 6:40–50

Jarvinen T, Kannus P, Maffulli N et al 2005 Achilles tendon disorders: etiology and epidemiology. Foot and Ankle Clinics 10(2):255–266

Jones B H, Vogel J A, Manikowski R et al 1988 Incidence of and risk factors for injury and illness among male and female army basic trainees. US Army Research Institute of Environmental Medicine technical report T19–88

Kannus P 1997 Etiology and pathophysiology of chronic tendon disorders in sport. Scandinavian Journal of Sports Medicine 7(2):78–85

Kannus P, Jozsa L 1991 Histopathological changes preceding spontaneous rupture of a tendon. A controlled study of 891 patients. Journal of Bone and Joint Surgery 73:A1507–1525

Khan K, Cook J, Kannus P et al 2002 Time to abandon the 'tendinitis myth'. BMJ 324(7338):626–627

Knapik J J, Jones B H, Bauman C L et al 1992 Strength, flexibility and athletic injuries. Sports Medicine 14(5):277–288

Knowles S, Marshall S, Bowling J et al 2006 A prospective study of injury incidence among North Carolina high school athletes. American Journal of Epidemiology 164(12):1209–1221

McKenzie D C, Clement D B, Taunton J E 1985 Running shoes, orthotics and injuries. Sports Medicine 2:324–327

McQuillan R, Campbell H 2006 Gender differences in adolescent injury characteristics: a population based study of hospital A and E data. Journal of Public Health 120(8):732–741

Marks R M 1999 Achilles' tendonopathy. Foot and Ankle Clinics 4(4):789–809

Milgrom C, Finestone A, Segey S et al 2003 Are overground runners more likely to sustain a tibial stress fracture than treadmill runners? British Journal of Sports Medicine 37(2):160–163

Myburgh K H, Grobler N, Noakes T D 1988 Factors associated with shin soreness in athletes. Physician and Sports Medicine 16:129–134

Neely F 1998 Intrinsic risk factors for exercise-related lower limb injuries. Sports Medicine 26(4):253–263

Nicholl J P, Coleman B A, Williams B T 1991 Pilot study of the epidemiology of sports injuries and exercise related morbidity. British Journal of Sports Medicine 25(1):61–66

Nigg B M, Yeadon M R 1987 Biomechanical aspects of playing surfaces. Journal of Sports Science 5:117–145

Pope R P, Herbert R D, Kirwan J D 1998 Effects of flexibility and stretching on injury risk in army recruits. Australian Journal of Physiotherapy 44:165–172

Pope R P, Herbert R D, Kirwan J D et al 2000 A randomized trial of pre-exercise stretching for the prevention of lower limb injury. Medicine and Science in Sport and Exercise 32(2):271–277

Protzman R, Griffis C 1977 Stress fractures in men and women undergoing military training. American Journal of Bone and Joint Surgery 59(6):825

Rauh M, Macera C, Trone D 2006 Epidemiology of stress fracture and lower extremity overuse injury in female recruits. Medicine and Science in Sport and Exercise 38(9):1571–1577

Richie D, Devries H, Endo C 1993 Shin muscle activity and sports surfaces: an electromyographic study. Journal of American Podiatric Medical Association 83(4):181–189

Ross J, Woodward A 1994 Risk factors for injury during basic military training: is there a social element in injury pathogenesis. Journal of Occupational Medicine 36:1120–1126

Rossiter N, Galbraith K 1996 The incidence of hypermobility in a military population [abstract]. Meeting of the Combined Services Orthopaedic Society, Aldershot, UK, 165

Sassmannshausen G 2006 The older athlete. In: Johnson D, Mair S. Clinical sports medicine, Elsevier, Philadelphia pp 91–96

Strocchi R, DePasquale V, Guizzardi S et al 1991 Human Achilles tendon: morphological and morphometric variations as a function of age. Foot and Ankle 12:100–104

Tallay A, Kynsburg A, Toth S et al 2004 Prevalence of patellofemoral syndrome. Evaluation of the role biomechanics malalignments and the role of sports activity. Orvosi Hetilap 145(41):2093–2101

Taunton J, Ryan M, Clement D et al 2003 A prospective study of running injuries: the Vancouver sun run 'in training' clinics. British Journal of Sports Medicine 37(3):239–244

Thacker S, Gilchrist J, Stroup D et al 2004 The impact of stretching on sports injury risk: a systematic review of the literature. Medicine and Science in Sport and Exercise 36(3):371–378

Tomten S E, Falch J A, Birkeland K I et al 1998 Bone mineral densities and menstrual irregularities: a comparative study on cortical and trabecular bone structures in runners with alleged normal eating behavior. International Journal of Sports Medicine 19: 92–97

Walsh W M 1994 Patellofemoral joint. In: Delee J C, Drez D (eds) Orthopaedic sports medicine, Vol 2. W B Saunders, Philadelphia

Witvrouw E, Lysons R, Bellemans J et al 2000 Intrinsic risk factors for the development of anterior knee pain in an athletic population. American Journal of Sports Medicine 28:480–489

Witvrouw E, Danneels L, Asselman P et al 2003 Muscle flexibility as a risk factor for developing muscle injuries in male professional soccer players: a prospective study. American Journal of Sports Medicine 31(1):41–46

Wolf S 1998 Diabetes mellitus and predisposition to athletic pedal fracture. Journal of Foot and Ankle Surgery 37(1):16–22

Yates B, White S 2004 The incidence and risk factors in the development of medial tibial stress syndrome among naval recruits. American Journal of Sports Medicine 32(3):772–780

Further reading

Brukner P, Khan K 2006 Clinical sports medicine, 3rd edn. McGraw-Hill, Sydney

Brukner P, Bennell K, Matheson G 1999 Stress fractures. Blackwell Science, Victoria

Delee J C, Drez D Miller M (eds) 2003 Orthopaedic sports medicine, 2nd edn. Saunders, Philadelphia

Hartley A 1995 Practical joint assessment: lower quadrant, 2nd edn. Mosby, St Louis

Johnson D, Mair S 2006 Clinical sports medicine. Mosby, Philadelphia

O'Connor F, Wilder R 2001 Textbook of running medicine. McGraw-Hill, New York

CHAPTER

16

Assessment of the older person

H B Menz

Indicates figures on DVD, including colour

Chapter contents

Introduction

Ageing is associated with significant alterations in the cutaneous, vascular, neurological and musculoskeletal characteristics of the foot and ankle. As a consequence of these age-related changes, foot pain and deformity commonly accompany advancing age. Community-based studies indicate that foot problems are reported by approximately 30% of older people (Barr et al 2005, Dunn et al 2004, Gorter et al 2000) and are associated with reduced walking speed (Benvenuti et al 1995), impaired balance (Menz et al 2005, Menz & Lord 2001a), difficulty performing activities of daily living (Barr et al 2005, Benvenuti et al 1995, Leveille et al 1998) and an increased risk of falls (Menz et al 2006a). Due to the strong association between mobility and independence in older people, the maintenance of foot health can have a significant impact on an older person's quality of life (Fig. 16.1). Footcare specialists therefore have an important role in the assessment of the lower limb in older people, not only to provide diagnostic clues regarding foot disorders, but also to provide insights into broader issues of physical well-being associated with mobility impairment.

The general principles of lower-limb assessment in older people are essentially the same as for younger people. However, although the foot undergoes several characteristic age-related changes, the ageing process is highly variable and is affected by a multitude of factors, including the presence of co-morbidities, effects of previous surgery, medication use, level of physical activity and footwear. Subsequently, it is often difficult to delineate normal age-related changes and those related to an underlying disease process. Therefore lower-limb assessment in older people should be individualised and should not rely too heavily on strict interpretations of 'normal' reference values.

History taking

The initial assessment interview described in Chapter 2 is equally relevant for the assessment of the older person. However, because impairments in vision,

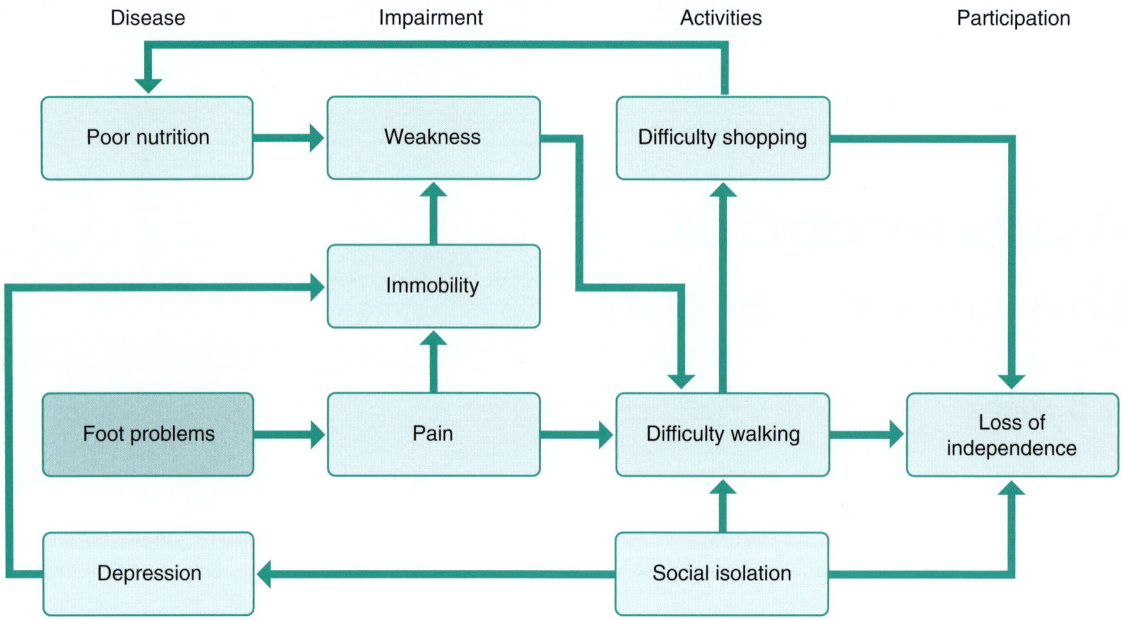

Figure 16.1 Conceptual map of the relationships between foot problems, impaired mobility and independence in older people.

hearing and cognition are common in older people, it is essential that the initial assessment interview is conducted in a quiet, well-lit and unhurried clinical environment. History taking in older people may also require the aggregation of information from multiple sources, including family members, friends and carers. This can be challenging, particularly when the information gathered is inconsistent. In some cases it may be necessary to obtain relevant information from each of these sources in isolation in order to develop a more accurate picture of the presenting complaint. This clearly requires striking a balance between patient confidentiality and family involvement (Tinetti 2003).

Documenting a thorough social history is essential to the management of foot problems in older people, as chronic foot conditions will often require ongoing self-management by the older person in their home environment. Inspection of foot lesions, use of appropriate footwear and regular changing of wound dressing are all aspects of care that may be compromised if the level of social support is inadequate. Thorough questioning of the older person's household situation may also highlight limitations in the awareness of supportive care services, such as community nursing, for which the older person may indeed be eligible.

Use of medications

Due to the age-related increase in prevalence of chronic conditions, the use of prescription and over-the-counter medications increases dramatically with advancing age, with over 80% of people over 65 taking at least one medication, and at least 20% taking five or more (Kaufman et al 2002). Prescribing medications for older people is inherently difficult due to age-related changes in drug absorption, distribution, metabolism and secretion. Furthermore, because most prescription drugs are trialled in younger people, their effects on older people are less predictable, and the likelihood of adverse reactions is not as well understood (McMurdo et al 2005). It is therefore not surprising that a large proportion of hospital admissions in older people are due to adverse drug reactions (Burgess et al 2005, Pirmohamed et al 2004).

Another issue that needs to be considered when documenting medication use in older people is the use of supplements and herbal medications. Use of these medications is highly prevalent among older people, however practitioners often do not document their use, and older patients may not report their use during the medical history interview. A study of 1539 older people found that, although 34% used some form of herbal medication, 70% of these had not informed their physician (Eisenberg et al 1993). This is problematic, as all medications, irrespective of their prescription status, have the potential to interact and contribute to adverse events. Common herbal medications that have been shown to have clinically important interactions with prescription medications include St John's wort, gingko biloba, echinacea, saw palmetto, garlic and ginseng (Izzo & Ernst 2001, Ernst 2002).

Although not all practitioners involved in the management of older people can prescribe and withdraw medications, all healthcare professionals should thoroughly document medication use at the initial assessment, undertake regular reviews of medication use, and be wary of potential adverse reactions. It is often necessary to request that older people bring their medications to their clinical appointments to ensure accuracy in documentation, and to ask specific questions regarding over-the-counter medications such as vitamin supplements, herbal medications, eye drops, creams and ointments. Regular communication with the patient's general practitioner is essential.

Pain assessment

The effect of ageing on pain is complex. The overall prevalence of pain complaints, with the exception of joint pain, seems to reduce with age (Gagliese & Melzack 1997). While changes in peripheral and central nervous system function that lead to increased pain thresholds in older people may partly explain this reduction (Gibson & Farrell 2004), other factors cannot be excluded, such as the reluctance of older people to report pain. Nevertheless, the degree of functional impairment and level of interference in daily activities associated with pain increases with age (Thomas et al 2004), and because of the key role that the foot has in mobility tasks, foot pain has a considerable impact on health-related quality of life (Chen et al 2003).

As outlined in Chapter 4, numerous multidimensional pain rating scales have been reported and validated in the literature, but they are generally too time-consuming for routine administration in the clinical setting. Visual analogue pain scales provide very limited insights into functional and psychosocial impairments associated with pain, but they are useful indicators of pain intensity, and are easily understood and simple and quick to administer. The use of visual aids, such as lower-limb diagrams or anatomical models, can be useful in determining the location of the pain, particularly if the older person has difficulty describing the location or is physically incapable of pointing to it. Direct questioning regarding pain in other body regions often provides useful diagnostic clues that may not have been otherwise volunteered.

Assessing pain in older people who are incapable of verbal communication is a considerable challenge, and requires observation of physical responses (such as guarding, fidgeting, or restricted movement of the painful body part) and facial expressions (such as frowning, grimacing, or excessive blinking) (Herr et al 2006). Never assume that those who are incapable of reporting pain do not experience it, and all attempts should be made to ensure that physical examination procedures are as pain-free as possible.

Assessment of cognitive status

Evaluation of cognitive status is an important aspect of lower-limb assessment in older people for two major reasons. First, obtaining informed consent to commence a clinical intervention requires that the older person is fully cognisant of the implications of the decision they are making. This is particularly important in relation to more invasive procedures such as foot surgery, where the advantages and disadvantages need to be carefully considered. Second, the success of many clinical management strategies depends on the ability of the older person to undertake activities after they leave the clinical environment. Failure to assess whether the older person is capable of undertaking these tasks may significantly reduce the likelihood of a good clinical outcome.

Although the astute practitioner may be able to detect moderate to severe levels of cognitive impairment from general observations and history taking, a structured approach using validated assessment tools will yield more valid findings. The most commonly used clinical screening tool for cognitive evaluation is the Mini-mental State Examination (MMSE), a clinician-administered questionnaire consisting of 30 questions addressing several components of cognitive function (Folstein & McHugh 1975). However, the MMSE it is generally not feasible to implement into routine clinical practice due to its length, and several shorter screening tools have been developed, which are highly correlated with the MMSE. The simplest and most widely used of these tests is the Clock Drawing Test (CDT) (Shulman 2000). Although there are several versions of this test, the most basic approach requires the patient to draw a clock face with all the numbers and hands placed correctly, and to then state the time they have drawn. The following

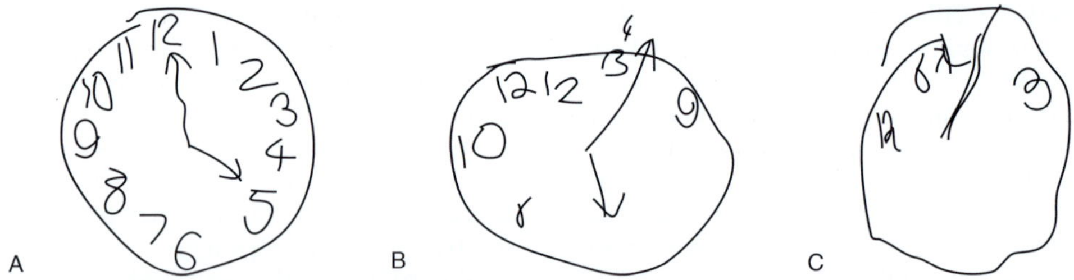

Figure 16.2 The clock-drawing test of cognitive impairment. **A** normal (score 6); **B** moderate cognitive impairment (score 4); **C** severe cognitive impairment (score 0).

scoring system is then applied:

1. The number 12 appears on top (3 points)
2. There are 12 numbers (1 point)
3. There are two clearly distinguishable hands (1 point)
4. The time is correctly stated (1 point).

Scores of <4 are indicative of moderate to severe cognitive impairment (Shua-Haim et al 1996), and warrant further diagnostic evaluation by a geriatrician. Examples of the CDT are shown in **Figure 16.2**.

Systems examination

The systems examination of the lower limb in older people should be essentially the same as that for younger people, with some particular issues requiring additional consideration. The most fundamental issue in relation to systems examination in the older patient is the tendency for some practitioners to undertake less thorough assessments, due to the incorrect assumption that many aspects of ageing cannot be effectively managed. This is by no means limited to footcare specialists – indeed, ageist assumptions have been demonstrated in most fields of medicine and often result in less detailed diagnostic approaches and the provision of less aggressive treatment approaches (Fraenkel et al 2006). Somewhat paradoxically, systems examination of the lower limb in older people is likely to have a far greater diagnostic yield, and older people may be more likely to benefit from thorough assessments than younger, relatively healthy patients.

The following section outlines the key age-related changes in the dermatological, vascular neurological and musculoskeletal systems and discusses the implications of these changes for the clinical assessment.

Dermatological assessment

Age-related changes

Advancing age is associated with several significant changes to the structure and function of the skin. The thickness of the epidermis does not change appreciably with age, however, the dermal-epidermal junction becomes flattened which may give the impression of atrophy (Gosain & DiPietro 2004). In the foot, there may be an increase in epidermal thickness due to thickening of the stratum corneum associated with plantar calluses (Thomas et al 1985). The shape and size of epidermal keratinocytes becomes more variable, and the rate of production and turnover of keratinocytes may reduce to only 50% of a young person (Smith 1989). Due to this delay in turnover time, the moisture content of keratinocytes is reduced, which, combined with the reduction in sweat gland density, contributes to the dry, scaly appearance of elderly skin (Balin & Pratt 1989). Older people exhibit a significant reduction in the number of capillary loops in the papillary dermis, increased porosity of endothelial cells and a thickened basement membrane, all of which contribute to a less efficient superficial blood supply (Ryan 2004). With advancing age, the rate of growth of the nails also decreases (Orentreich et al 1979), due to both a reduction in the turnover rate of keratinocytes and a reduction in size of the nail matrix itself.

The above changes have several implications for the assessment and treatment of elderly skin. The decreased water content of keratinocytes and decreased density of eccrine glands leads to an overall drying of the skin, which predisposes to hyperkeratosis and fissuring. The reduction in epidermal and dermal immune function increases the risk of infection (Albright & Albright 1994), and the reduced rate of epidermal turnover may increase the time required to successfully treat these infections

(Muehleman & Rahimi 1990). Wound healing is also significantly delayed in older people, due to both a reduction in wound contraction and reduced rate of epithelialisation and angiogenesis (Eaglstein 1986). Even if a wound successfully heals, the tensile strength at the wound site is diminished, which increases the likelihood of dehiscence. Subsequently, wounds in older people often require much longer periods of treatment and frequently recur. Bruising is also more likely to occur due to the decreased integrity of superficial blood vessels leading to leakage of red blood cells into the papillary dermis (Muehleman & Rahimi 1990). Due to the reduction in nail growth rate and subsequent thickening of the nail plate, treatment of onychomycosis with either oral or topical agents may take considerably longer in older people, and the possibility of reinfection is much higher (Tosti et al 2005).

Clinical assessment considerations

Dermatological assessment is primarily based on history taking and clinical observations, although as stated in Chapter 8, investigations such as mycology, bacterial and viral culture, histological assessment and patch testing may provide useful diagnostic information. Mycology is particularly important in relation to confirmation of suspected onychomycosis in older people, as dystrophic nails may test positive for a wide range of organisms, and no fungal organisms can be identified in approximately 20% of cases of suspected onychomycosis (Scherer et al 2001). In general, all foot lesions in older people should be investigated for evidence of underlying tissue breakdown and ulceration, and chronic lesions should be carefully documented for potential malignant changes. The ABCD mnemonic (A: asymmetry; B: border irregularity; C: change in colour, and; D: increase in diameter) is a useful general rule for routine assessment of suspect lesions. Practitioners should have a particularly high index of suspicion with regard to non-healing subungual lesions, as this is a relatively common site for the development of malignant melanomas (Lemon & Burns 1998).

Assessment of skin dryness in the clinical setting can be standardised using the xerosis scale developed by Rogers et al (1989). This scale consists of six images of feet with varying degrees of skin dryness, ranging from a mild, dusty appearance with some small skin flakes, to large scaly plates and deep fissuring (Fig. 16.3). Although the scale has not yet been validated against gold standard measurements of skin hydration (such as electrical capacitance; Lee & Maibach 2002), it has been shown to be a sensitive measurement of skin hydration in response to emollient application (Jennings et al 1998).

Vascular assessment

Age-related changes

Considerable changes take place in the intima of all vessels and the media of large arteries with advancing age. The size and shape of endothelial cells become more irregular, and the overall thickness of the intima and media increases due to collagen cross-linking and invasion of smooth muscle cells (Virmani et al 1991). Elastin fibres in the media of large arteries break down and stiffen, resulting in a reduction in elastic recoil, reduction in overall flow and an elevation in blood pressure (Ferrari et al 2003). At the capillary level, basement membrane thickening and collagen deposition result in a narrowing of the lumen and an overall reduction in blood flow, particularly in the lower limb (Richardson & Schwartz 1985). Relatively little is known about age-related changes in veins, however collagen cross-linking may have a role in the development of perforator vein incompetence (Delis 2004).

The end result of these changes is a generalised reduction in limb blood flow, which partly explains the approximate twofold increase in risk of developing peripheral arterial disease for every 10-year increase in age (Vogt et al 1993). Older people are also more likely to develop conditions associated with venous insufficiency, such as varicose veins and venous ulcers (Carpentier et al 2004).

Clinical assessment considerations

The vascular assessment approaches outlined in Chapter 6 are particularly important in older people, given that age is a major independent risk factor for the development of peripheral arterial disease (PAD). PAD affects approximately 15% of people aged 70 years and over (Selvin & Erlinger 2004), but often goes unrecognised in a large number of patients until the onset of symptoms (Kuller 2001). Given that many older people with asymptomatic PAD have evidence of subclinical cardiovascular disease, the ankle–brachial index has been described as one of the 'vital signs' of an older person's health status (Lawson 2005), and footcare specialists are well placed to detect early signs of vascular disease in asymptomatic older people.

Venous disorders are also common in older people (Carpentier et al 2004), therefore clinical evaluation

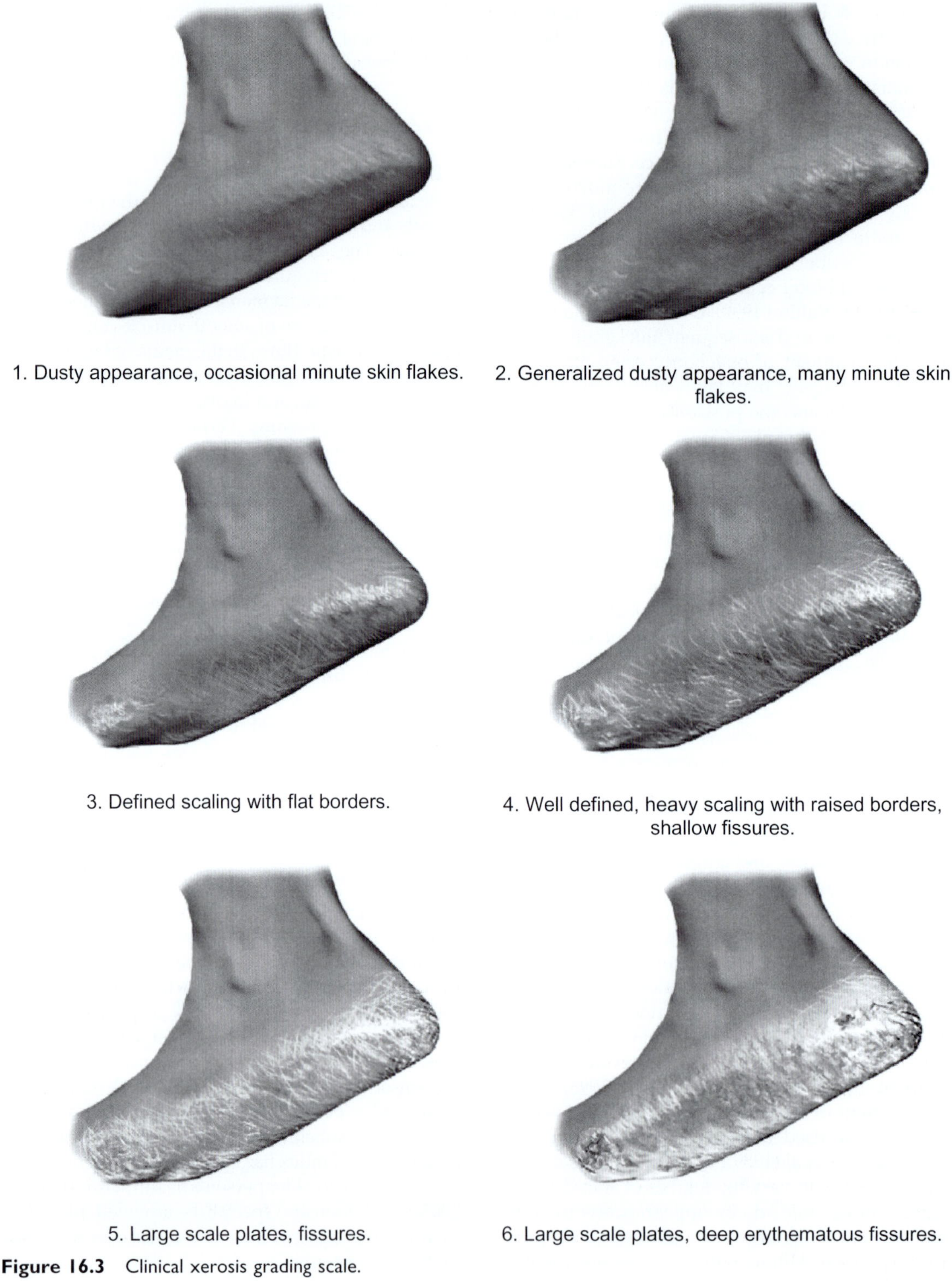

Figure 16.3 Clinical xerosis grading scale.

Table 16.1 Clinical prediction rule for the diagnosis of deep vein thrombosis (DVT)

	CLINICAL FEATURES
Major points	Active cancer Paralysis, paresis or recent plaster immobilisation of the lower limb Recently bedridden >3 days and/or major surgery within 4 weeks Localised tenderness along the distribution of the deep venous system Thigh and calf swollen Calf swelling 3 cm > asymptomatic side (measured 10 cm below tibial tuberosity) Strong family history of DVT (≥2 first-degree relatives with history of DVT)
Minor points	History of recent trauma (≥60 days) to the symptomatic leg Pitting oedema: symptomatic leg only Dilated superficial veins (non-varicose) in symptomatic leg only Hospitalisation within previous 6 months Erythema
	CLINICAL PROBABILITY
High	≥3 major points and no alternative diagnosis ≥2 major points and ≥2 minor points and no alternative diagnosis
Low	1 major point +≥2 minor points and has an alternative diagnosis 1 major point +≥1 minor point and no alternative diagnosis 0 major points +≥3 minor points and has an alternative diagnosis 0 major points +≥2 minor points and no alternative diagnosis
Moderate	All other combinations

of venous insufficiency, including observations of telangiectasis, varicosities, oedema and venous ulcers, should be a routine component of geriatric lower-limb assessment. The most serious and potentially life-threatening lower-limb venous disorder, deep vein thrombosis (DVT), should always be suspected in older people presenting with a hot, painful, swollen leg. However, because anticoagulant therapy has potentially serious side effects, it is important that DVT is also accurately ruled out when it is not present. To assist in this process, the clinical prediction rule (Table 16.1) of Wells et al (1995) is particularly useful. This consists of 12 medical history items and clinical observations which can easily be undertaken as part of a routine consultation. The classification of a patient as having a 'high clinical probability' of DVT on this scale has been shown to have 91% sensitivity and 100% specificity for the eventual imaging diagnosis of DVT.

Finally, it has recently been demonstrated that the assessment of foot veins provides a useful insight into the hydration status of an older person (Rosher & Robinson 2004). Given that dehydration is very common in older people (particularly those in institutional care), this simple assessment may help in the early detection of impaired fluid balance. To perform the assessment, the dorsal venous arch vein is occluded by finger pressure and the vein is emptied by stroking proximally. The finger is then released, and the rate and degree of venous return is observed, with a delay of >3 seconds being indicative of potential dehydration.

Neurological assessment

Age-related changes

With advancing age, there is a generalised decline in the size and number of axons, and the myelin sheaths surrounding the axons undergo significant deterioration, leading to a reduction in nerve conduction velocity (Verdu et al 2000). As a result of changes in receptor structure and function, ageing is associated with significant reductions in tactile sensitivity, spatial acuity, and vibration sense, and these changes are particularly pronounced in the lower limb compared with the upper limb. Proprioception (the ability to detect the position of body parts) and kinaesthesia (the ability to detect movement of body parts) rely partly on skin receptors and on Golgi tendon organs and receptors in muscle spindles. As with other mechanoreceptive abilities, ageing is associated with significant decline in proprioception and kinaesthesia in the sagittal plane of the knee (Petrella et al 1997) and the sagittal and frontal plane of the ankle (Gilsing et al 1995, Thelen et al 1998).

Clinical assessment considerations

Lower-limb neurological assessment in older people can be challenging, as it is often difficult to delineate between observations of normal age-related changes and those related to a neuropathic process. The initial assessment interview and history taking may provide useful insights into conditions commonly associated with neuropathy, such as diabetes, chronic alcoholism, vitamin B_{12} deficiency and the side effects of certain medications. However, self-reported 'numbness of the feet' has been shown to be a poor predictor of electrodiagnostically confirmed neuropathy in older people (Franse et al 2000). Furthermore, the use of ankle reflex testing or tuning forks alone to detect neurological problems is confounded by the fact that over a third of people aged over 70 years do not seem to have an ankle reflex (Bowditch et al 1996), and a similar proportion cannot detect vibratory stimuli at the ankle (Prakash & Stern 1973). Therefore, the clinical tests described in Chapter 7 may not provide the same level of diagnostic accuracy when applied to older people.

To address this issue, Richardson (2002) recently developed a clinical screening approach incorporating a range of clinical tests conducted in 100 older people, and correlated their findings with electrodiagnostic tests of peripheral polyneuropathy. The results indicated that all clinical tests differentiated between older people with and without electrodiagnostically confirmed neuropathy. The best prediction of neuropathy was made by using a combination of three tests: the Achilles reflex, vibration sense at the toe, and position sense at the toe. Having two or three abnormal signs demonstrated a sensitivity of 91% and specificity of 93% for neuropathy (Table 16.2). Interestingly, the diagnostic accuracy of this protocol was not greatly affected by whether or not the participants had diabetes, indicating that it may have broad application for the detection of neuropathy resulting from a range of conditions.

Musculoskeletal assessment

Age-related changes

There is now extensive literature demonstrating age-related changes in muscle, tendon, ligament and joint structure and function. Due to reductions in the size and number of muscle fibres, older people exhibit between 30% and 60% of the ankle strength of younger people (Doherty 2003), and two recent studies have indicated that older people demonstrate 30% less toe plantarflexor strength than younger people (Endo et al 2002, Menz et al 2006c). Changes in joint tissues may also be responsible for the reduction in range of motion of lower-extremity joints observed in older people. Several studies have shown that ankle dorsiflexion-plantarflexion range of motion reduces with age (James & Parker 1989, Nigg et al 1992, Nitz & Low-Choy 2004), and Nigg et al (1992)

Table 16.2 Clinical screening approach for the detection of neuropathy in older people

Test	*Description*	*Cut-off score*
Achilles reflex	Achilles tendon is struck with a reflex hammer	Absent plantarflexion response
Vibration sense	128 Hz tuning fork applied just proximal to the nail bed of the hallux, and time taken until patient reports that the vibration has disappeared is recorded in seconds	<8 s
Position sense	Dominant hallux grasped on medial and lateral surfaces by thumb and forefinger. Ten small amplitude up and down movements randomly administered, with patient asked to report direction of movement	<8/10 correct responses

have also noted a significant reduction in inversion-eversion and abduction-adduction motion of the ankle joint complex.

More recently, Scott et al (2007) showed that older people had significantly less range of motion at the ankle joint (36° versus 45°, using a weightbearing lunge test), and less passive range of motion of the first metatarsophalangeal joint (56° versus 82°, measured non-weightbearing) than younger controls. Assessment of foot posture also indicated that older people had significantly flatter feet, as indicated by a higher foot posture index and arch index, and a reduction in the height of the navicular tuberosity.

Clinical assessment considerations

Musculoskeletal assessment is clearly of considerable importance in older people, and each of the lower-limb orthopaedic assessments outlined in Chapter 10 are of direct relevance to the assessment of the older foot. However, due to age-related differences in foot structure and function and the higher prevalence of foot deformity, there are several clinical tests of foot deformity, posture, range of motion and strength that are of particular importance when assessing older people.

Foot deformity

The prevalence of foot deformity increases markedly with age, due to the combined effects of musculoskeletal changes and detrimental effects of footwear. The most common foot deformities in older people – hallux valgus and lesser toe deformities – are often associated with the development of hyperkeratosis and forefoot pain, and have a detrimental impact on balance and functional ability. Hallux valgus can be easily graded in the clinical environment using the Manchester scale (Garrow et al 2001), which consists of four standardised photographs covering the spectrum of the deformity (Fig. 16.4). A study by Menz & Munteanu (2005a) showed that gradings using this scale were significantly associated with hallux abductus and intermetatarsal angles obtained from foot radiographs. Lesser toe deformities (hammer toes, claw toes, mallet toes and retracted toes) can be simply evaluated by assessing the position and range of motion of the metatarsophalangeal, proximal, and distal interphalangeal joints. Thorough assessment of lesser toe function may have some prognostic value, as it has been demonstrated that mobilisation treatment is effective in reducing forefoot pain in people with limited metatarsophalangeal range of motion, but is not effective in people with severely retracted toes (Waldecker 2004).

Foot posture

Despite the proposed relationships between foot posture and the development of overuse conditions affecting the lower limb, there is still considerable disagreement regarding how best to assess and classify foot posture (Razeghi & Batt 2002). Furthermore, very few tests have been performed on the older foot. To address this issue, Menz & Munteanu (2005b) recently compared three clinical tests of foot posture (the arch index, navicular height and the Foot Posture Index) with arch-related measurements obtained from lateral foot X-rays in 95 older people. The results indicated that all three tests were significantly correlated with radiographic measurements, with the strongest associations found for navicular height and the arch index. A subsequent study involving plantar pressure measurements indicated that the arch index is a significant predictor of forces under the midfoot during walking (Menz & Morris 2006), suggesting that this technique may be a useful clinical assessment to perform in older patients.

To determine the arch index, a static footprint is obtained using a carbon-paper imprint system, and the area of the middle third of the footprint is divided by the total area of the footprint (ignoring the toes) (Fig. 16.5). A higher arch index represents a flatter foot. Because the calculation of the arch index can be time consuming, a simple classification of high, normal and flat based on a visual observation of the print may be more feasible for routine clinical use. **Figure 16.6** shows representative footprints obtained from a sample of 176 people aged between 65 and 96, along with their arch index ranges.

Range of motion

Assessing the available motion in all of the foot joints is a standard and necessary component of the lower-limb assessment. In older people, two joints are of particular importance – the first metatarsophalangeal joint and the ankle joint – as these joints provide the main sagittal plane pivots during propulsion, and both joints undergo significant reductions in motion with advancing age (Scott et al 2007). First metatarsophalangeal joint range of motion (assessed in a non-weightbearing position) is significantly correlated with the loading of the first ray during gait (Menz & Morris 2006), and restricted motion in this joint is associated with impaired forward leaning ability (Menz et al 2005). Although there are several methods of assessing the range of motion of the ankle joint, the weightbearing lunge test provides a functionally relevant indicator of available ankle dorsiflexion, and has been shown to

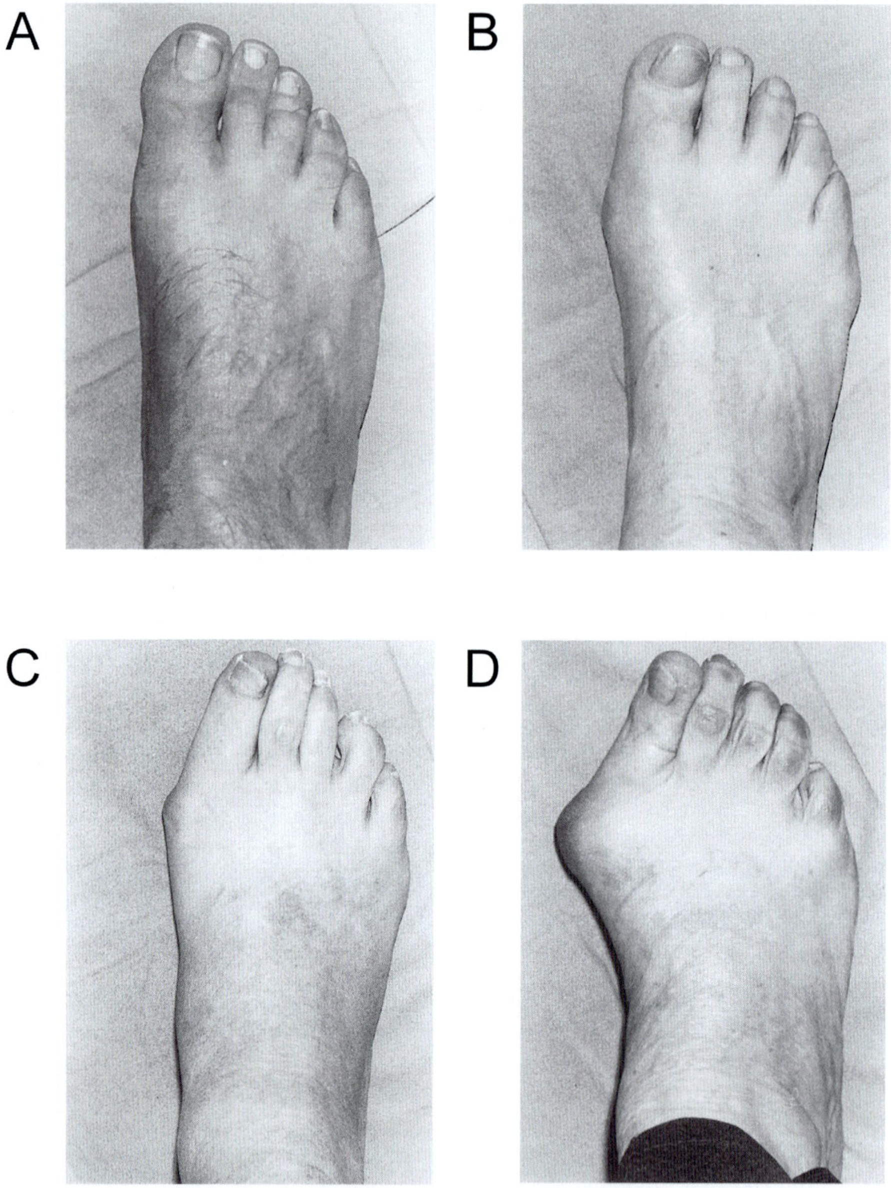

Figure 16.4 Manchester scale for grading hallux valgus severity.

be reliable and related to balance and functional ability in older people (Menz et al 2003, Menz et al 2005). To perform the test, the lateral malleolus and head of the fibula are located and marked in ink. The patient is then asked to stand with their foot placed alongside a vertically aligned clear acrylic plate inscribed with 2° protractor markings, and instructed to take a comfortable step forwards with the contralateral leg. In this position, the patient is requested to bend their knees to squat down as low as possible, without lifting the right heel from the ground and while keeping the trunk upright. The position of the fibular head is marked on the clear acrylic plate, and the angle formed between the lateral malleolus and the fibular head is measured (Fig. 16.7). The normal range of motion when performing this test is approximately 30–50°, with smaller values being associated with impaired

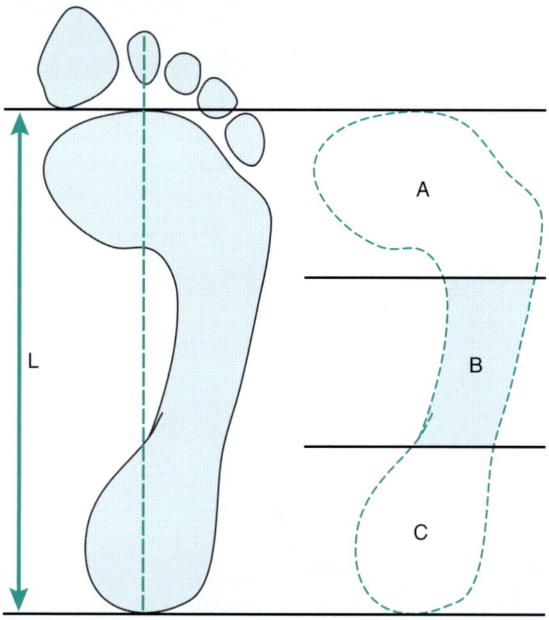

Figure 16.5 Calculation of the arch index. The length of the footprint excluding the toes (L) is divided into equal thirds. The arch index (AI) is then calculated as the area of the middle third of the footprint divided by the entire footprint area (AI = B/A+B+C).

balance and functional ability, and an increased risk of falls (Menz et al 2005, 2006a).

Strength testing

Although there are several instrumented techniques for the measurement of muscle strength (such as hand-held dynamometry), simple manual muscle testing of the foot and ankle can provide useful insights into strength deficits in older people (Perry et al 1986). The basic principle of manual muscle testing is to adequately stabilise the body part proximal to the muscle being tested, and to apply firm pressure directly opposite the line of pull of the muscle. Descriptions of hand placement and force application are shown in Table 16.3. The simple grading system initially proposed by Kendall & Kendall (1949) is then applied (Table 16.4). Although there is some subjectivity involved in this grading system (and care needs to be taken when comparing findings between practitioners), it has been demonstrated that foot and ankle muscle testing observations are related to the intensity of muscle activity during gait (Perry et al 1986).

Another useful clinical muscle test is the paper grip test, which was first developed to assess muscle paralysis in the feet of leprosy patients (deWin et al

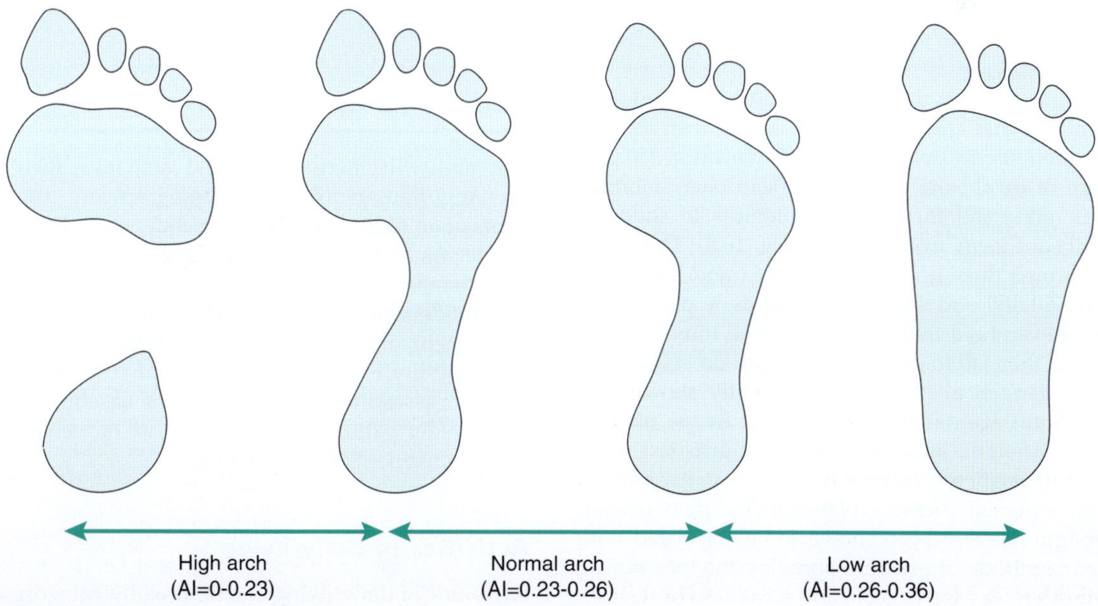

Figure 16.6 Simple visual categorisation of the arch index.

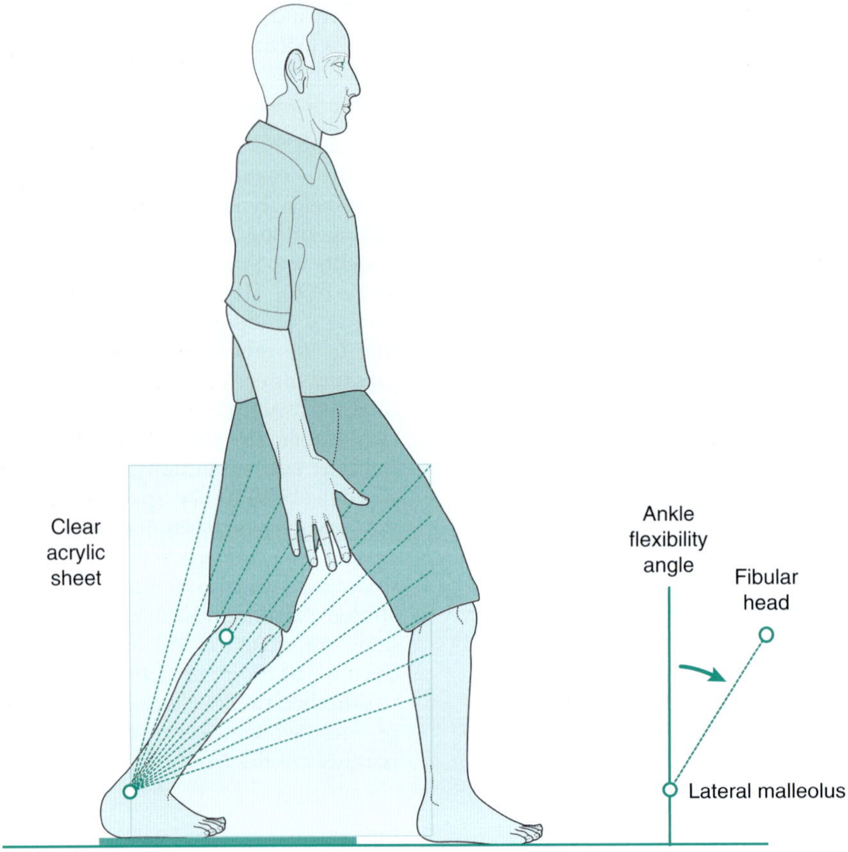

Figure 16.7 The ankle lunge test for assessing ankle range of motion.

2002). To perform the test, the patient is seated with their hip, knee and ankle at 90°, and are instructed to use their toe muscles to push down on a 280 gsm piece of cardboard while the practitioner stabilises their ankle and forefoot and attempts to slide the cardboard away from the toes (Fig. 16.8). The test is performed three times for the hallux and lesser toes individually, and is documented as a pass if the patient can hold the cardboard for all three trials or a fail if they fail to grip the cardboard on at least one trial. Menz et al (2006c) have recently shown that significant age-related changes exist in toe plantar-flexor strength, and that the paper grip test is an accurate predictor of strength measurements obtained from a plantar pressure platform. Toe plantarflexor strength has also been shown to be correlated with the magnitude of pressure borne by the toes during gait (Menz & Morris 2006) and weakness of the toes is associated with impaired balance and falls in older people (Menz et al 2005, 2006a).

Functional assessment

The ability to perform routine activities such as dressing, housework and shopping are key components of an older person's independence and quality of life. As stated in the introduction, there is now considerable evidence that foot problems have a significant detrimental impact on these abilities. Clinical assessment of an older person's functional ability and mobility is therefore an integral component of geriatric assessment to determine the baseline status of the older patient and also as a way of measuring the effectiveness of interventions.

Activities of daily living

Activities of daily living can be broadly categorized as: basic activities of daily living (BADLs); instrumental activities of daily living (IADLs) and advanced

Table 16.3 Manual muscle testing procedures

Motion	*Positioning of patient*	*Stabilising hand placement*	*Resistance hand placement*	*Instruction to patient*	*Muscles tested*
Ankle dorsiflexion	Seated, leg extended off table	Distal posterior tibia	Dorsomedial surface of the foot	Dorsiflex and invert the foot by bringing toe towards shin	Tibialis anterior
Ankle plantarflexion	Seated, foot and leg extended off table	Distal anterior tibia	Plantar surface of the foot	With knee extended (gastrocnemius) and flexed >45° (soleus) point foot against resistance	Gastrocnemius, soleus
Ankle plantarflexion	Standing on one leg using hand on table for balance	None	None	Raise heel 20 times, or until unable to complete full motion	Gastrocnemius, soleus
Inversion	Lying on side to be tested, foot slightly plantarflexed	Distal medial tibia	Medial aspect of foot	Raise medial border of foot toward ceiling	Tibialis posterior
Eversion	Lying on side not be tested, foot slightly plantarflexed	Distal lateral tibia	Lateral aspect of foot	Raise lateral border of foot toward ceiling	Peroneus longus and brevis
2nd–5th MTPJ and IPJ toe flexion	Supine, foot resting on table	MTPJ: metatarsal PIPJ: proximal phalanx DIPJ: middle phalanx	MTPJ: proximal phalanx PIPJ: middle phalanx DIPJ: distal phalanx	Flex or curl toes	PIPJ: flexor digitorum brevis DIPJ: Flexor digitorum longus MTPJ: Lumbricals and flexors above
2nd–5th MTPJ and IPJ toe extension	Supine, foot resting on table	Metatarsals	Distal phalanx	Extend toes	Extensor digitorum longus and brevis
Hallux flexion	Supine, foot resting on table	MTPJ: 1st metatarsal	MTPJ: Proximal phalanx	Flex big toe	MTPJ: Flexor hallucis brevis IPJ: Flexor hallucis longus
Hallux extension	Supine, foot resting on table	1st metatarsal	Proximal and distal phalanx	Extend big toe	Extensor hallucis brevis (MTPJ) and longus (IPJ)
Hallux abduction	Supine, foot resting on table	1st metatarsal	Medial aspect of proximal phalanx	Abduct the toe against resistance or place in abduction and say 'don't let me move you'	Abductor hallucis

MPTJ, metatarsophalangeal joint; IPJ, interphalangeal joint.

activities of daily living (AADLs). Table 16.5 shows examples of tasks in each of these categories. BADLs are considered necessary but not sufficient for maintaining independence, whereas IADLs are necessary to maintain an independent household environment and AADLs are complex tasks requiring high levels of physical and cognitive functioning (Katz et al 1970). Assessment of functional status is relatively straightforward and may simply require a brief checklist to be completed by the patient as part of the

Table 16.4 Manual muscle testing grades

Grade	*Interpretation*
4 (normal)	Resists strong pressure
3 (good)	Resists moderate pressure
2 (fair)	Resists gravity through full range of motion
1 (poor)	Resists gravity through partial range of motion
0 (none)	No muscle activity

Table 16.5 Activities of daily living

Basic	*Instrumental*	*Advanced*
Feeding	Paying bills	Paid employment
Maintaining continence	Taking medications	Attending religious services
Transferring	Shopping	Volunteering
Toileting	Doing housework	Undertaking hobbies
Dressing	Cooking meals	
Bathing		

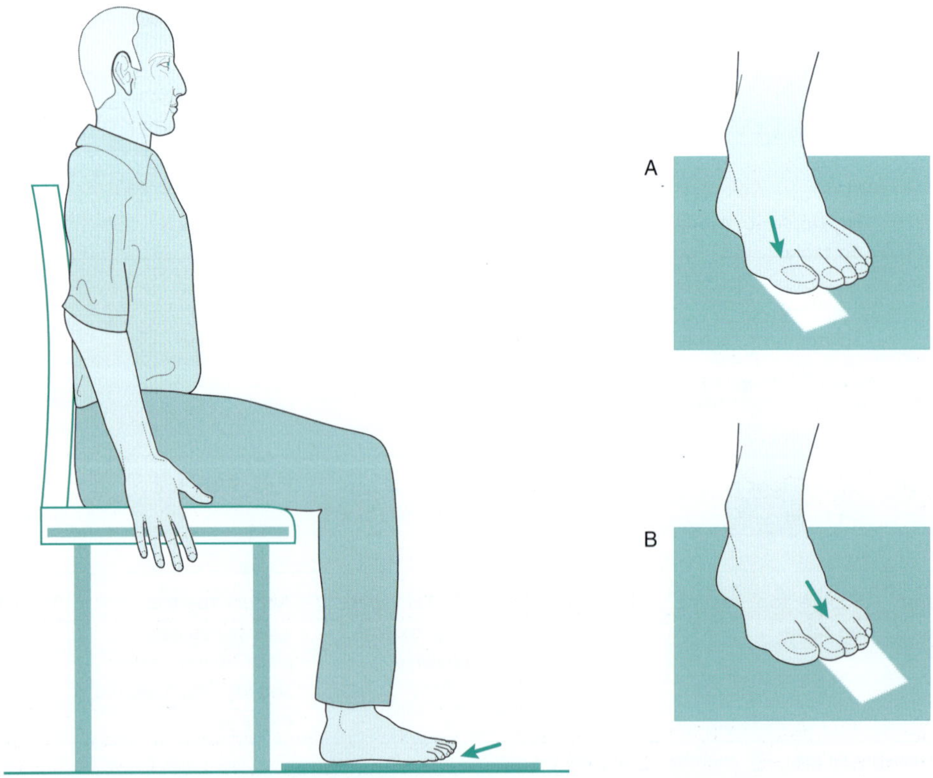

Figure 16.8 The paper grip test. **A** hallux; **B** lesser toes.

consultation. Several validated tools have also been developed, including the Barthel Index, which consists of 10 questions relating to bowel continence, bladder continence, grooming, toilet use, feeding, transfers, mobility, dressing, stair climbing and bathing (Mahoney & Barthel 1965). These scales are able to predict functional decline, institutionalisation and mortality in older people (Rozzini et al 2005). However, they are generally not sensitive enough to detect short-term changes in relatively highly functioning older people.

Objective measures of mobility

Objective measures of gait mobility, such as walking speed and rising from a chair, are also useful tools for assessing functional status and are sensitive enough to be used as clinical outcome measures. Walking speed, which can be simply measured with a stopwatch over a distance of 6 m, provides an indicator of not only lower limb muscle strength but also balance, reaction time and psychological status (Tiedemann et al 2005). Prospective studies have also shown that walking speed is a strong predictor of institutionalisation and mortality in older people (Woo et al 1999). Similarly, measuring the time taken to rise from a chair five times (the sit-to-stand test) provides an overall measure of physical ability, and can identify older people at risk of falling. Both walking speed and sit-to-stand have been shown to be impaired in older people with foot problems (Menz & Lord 2001a, Menz et al 2005). Some objective tests of mobility are also accurate predictors of falls (see section on falls risk assessment).

Evaluation of gait disorders

At least 20% of older people report difficulty walking or require assistance with gait-related tasks (Ostchega et al 2000). Although a small reduction in walking speed and step length seems to be a normal consequence of ageing (Oberg et al 1993), there is increasing evidence that most other gait changes frequently observed in older people are the result of underlying conditions that increase in prevalence with advancing age, such as osteoarthritis, stroke, peripheral neuropathy and dementia. In many older people with a gait problem, more than one potential contributing condition is present, which can make accurate diagnosis difficult.

Alexander & Goldberg (2005) have proposed a classification of gait disorders according to the level of the sensorimotor system they primarily affect. Low level gait disorders are those that influence structures distal to the central nervous system, including peripheral sensory impairments (such as peripheral neuropathy, vestibular disorders and visual problems) and peripheral motor impairments (such as arthritic and myopathic conditions). Middle level gait disorders include those resulting from spasticity (such as myelopathy, vitamin B_{12} deficiency and stroke), parkinsonism (idiopathic or drug-induced) and cerebellar ataxia (resulting from alcohol abuse). High level gait disorders include cautious gait (resulting from behavioural adaptations due to fear of falling) and those related to frontal lobe problems (such as stroke affecting the cortex or basal ganglia). See Table 16.6 for a summary of these disorders, including their characteristic gait changes and associated physical findings. Although this system provides a useful clinical summary of gait changes associated with specific conditions, there is often considerable overlap in their presentation.

The clinical assessment of gait disorders involves a thorough systems examination, in addition to the direct visual observation of movement patterns (see Ch. 10, section B). For the footcare specialist, visual observation of gait features (Table 16.6), including documentation of temporo-spatial parameters such as velocity, cadence and step length, is probably a sufficient basis for determining whether a referral is required for further diagnostic evaluation. In the clinical setting, all this requires is sufficient space to conduct a brief gait assessment (preferably at least 10 m) and a stop-watch. As a general rule, gait can be defined as impaired if the walking speed is less than 0.6 m/s (Studenski et al 2003).

When considering the contribution of gait patterns to foot disorders, more detailed lower-limb assessments may be required. The use of treadmills to observe frontal plane movements of the foot during gait is popular, however, the reliability of such visual observations is, at best, moderate (Keenan & Bach 1996) and walking patterns on a treadmill may differ from normal overground walking (Marsh et al 2006). Furthermore, some older people may find treadmill walking difficult due to balance problems. A recent study of healthy older people assessed the time required to become familiarised to treadmill walking, by comparing temporospatial characteristics and sagittal plane kinematics of the knee to overground walking. After 15 minutes of treadmill walking, two-thirds of the sample still required support of the handrails, and knee kinematics and cadence did not reflect overground walking values (Wass et al 2005). These findings suggest that gait

Table 16.6 Classification of common gait disorders in older people

Level	*Classification*	*Condition*	*Gait characteristics*	*Associated physical findings*
Low	Peripheral sensory	Sensory ataxia	Steppage gait	Loss of tactile sensitivity and proprioception
		Vestibular ataxia	Weaving from side to side; may fall to one side	Nystagmus
		Visual ataxia	Tentative, cautious	Visual impairment
	Peripheral motor	Arthritic	Shortened stance phase on affected side; Trendelenburg's sign	Avoidance of weightbearing on affected side; limited knee flexion; decreased lumbar lordosis; stooped posture; kyphosis
		Myopathic and neuropathic – proximal	Exaggerated lumbar lordosis; Trendelenburg's sign; waddling gait; foot slapping	Weakness of hip musculature
		Myopathic and neuropathic – distal	Foot drop; steppage gait	Weakness of ankle dorsiflexors
Middle	Spasticity	Hemiplegia/paresis	Leg circumduction; loss of arm swing; foot dragging	Leg weakness/spasticity; knee hyperextension; ankle equinovarus; arm weakness/spasticity
		Paraplegia/paresis	Bilateral leg circumduction; scissor gait	Leg weakness/spasticity
	Parkinsonism		Small shuffling steps; absent arm swing; freezing	Rigidity; bradykinesia; trunk flexion
	Cerebellar ataxia		Wide base of gait; increased trunk sway; staggering	Poor control of trunk; incoordination
High	Cautious gait		Wide base of gait; shortened stride; decreased velocity	Fear of falling
	Frontal-related gait disorders	Cerebrovascular	Wide base of gait; shortened stride; decreased velocity; difficulty initiating gait; freezing	Atherosclerotic disease; cognitive impairment; leg weakness/spasticity; incontinence

assessments using treadmills may be of limited value in older people.

Plantar pressure systems (either platform-based or in-shoe) are useful for identifying areas of high pressure that may predispose to plantar calluses and ulceration, and in-shoe systems may assist in optimising pressure redistribution with various insoles and orthoses (Orlin & McPoil 2000). When undertaking such assessments, however, bear in mind that the pressure distribution under the foot depends on a wide range of factors, including walking speed, step length, body weight, foot deformity, and the degree of peripheral sensory loss (Menz & Morris 2006). Because of this complexity, it is difficult to extrapolate foot motion characteristics (such as the degree of foot pronation) from plantar pressure recordings. While it seems that foot pronation does result in greater medial loading of the midfoot in older people, forefoot pressures are more closely correlated to the degree of hallux valgus deformity and the available range of motion in the first metatarsophalangeal joint (Menz & Morris 2006). Examples of foot pressure

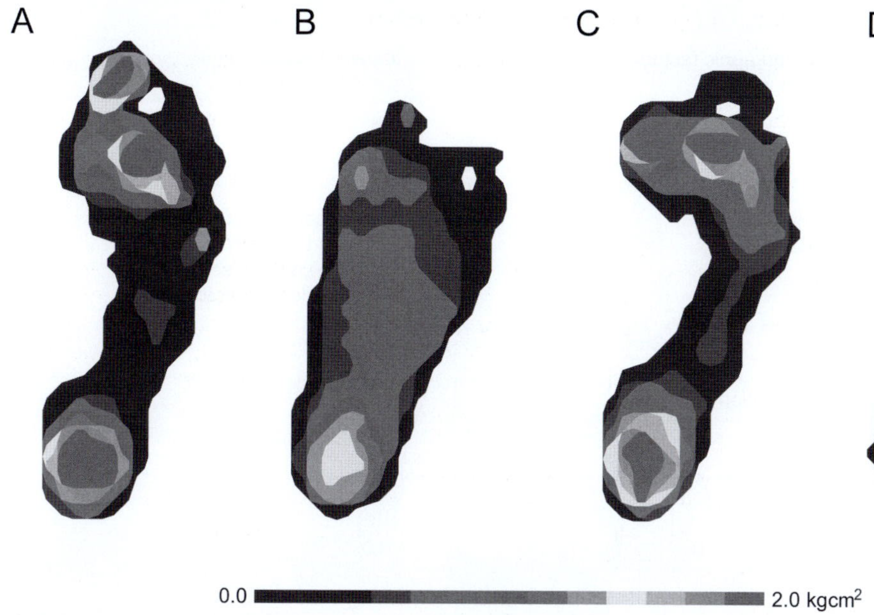

Figure 16.9 Examples of foot pressure recordings from older people. **A** hallux limitus; **B** tibialis posterior dysfunction; **C** severe hallux valgus deformity and associated plantar lesions; **D** pes cavus foot type.

recordings from older people are shown in Figure 16.9, and a summary of the strongest clinical predictors of plantar forces in older people is shown in Figure 16.10.

Falls risk assessment

Community-based studies indicate that 1 in 3 people aged over 65 years will fall in any given year. Falls frequently result in injury, and are the leading cause of injury-related death in older people (Lord et al 2001). The role and scope of podiatry in falls prevention is poorly defined, but is gaining considerable attention in response to recent studies indicating that foot problems (including foot pain, hallux valgus, decreased ankle flexibility, peripheral sensory loss and toe plantarflexor weakness) are independent risk factors for falling (Menz et al 2006a). Given these observations, it is likely that most older people attending footcare specialists have a higher risk of falling than the general elderly population. However, documenting medical conditions that are strong risk factors for falling, and undertaking some simple clinical tests will provide more accurate identification of very high risk older people who are most likely to benefit from falls prevention activities. Key demographic and medical risk factors for falling are shown in Figure 16.11, and Table 16.7 describes some

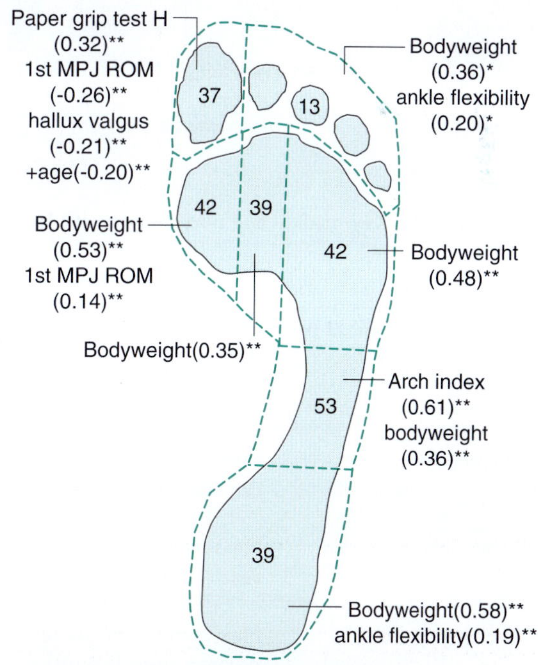

Figure 16.10 Determinants of plantar forces in older people. Values displayed in mask regions represent r^2 values, and values contained in brackets represent β-weights for each significant independent (predictor) variable. *$p < 0.05$, **$p < 0.01$. MPJ, metatarsophalangeal; ROM, range of motion.

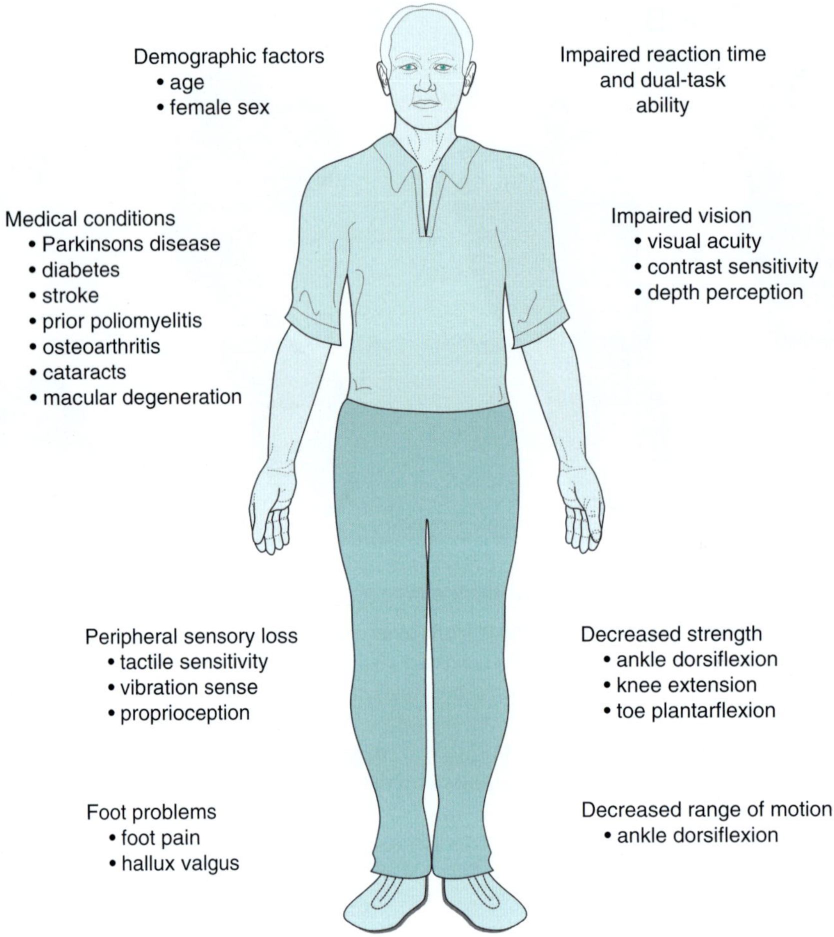

Figure 16.11 Key medical and physiological risk factors for falls in older people.

Table 16.7 Clinical mobility tests that can be used to predict risk of falling

Test	*Description*	*Cut-off score that indicates increased risk of falling*
Unipedal stance	Measurement of the time (in seconds) that an individual can stand on one leg unsupported	<30 s
Functional reach test	Measurement of the distance that an individual can reach forwards without moving their feet	<15 cm
Walking speed	Measurement of the time taken to walk a certain fixed distance (usually 6 m)	<0.56 m/s
Timed up and go test	Measurement of the time taken to stand from a chair, walk 3 m, turn around and again sit down	>14 s

simple tests that have been shown to be useful predictors of falls (Duncan et al 1992, Hurvitz et al 2000, Shumway-Cook et al 2000, VanSwearingen et al 1998). Footwear evaluation also has a role in falls risk assessment (see later section on footwear assessment).

Assessment of the ability to perform basic footcare

Many clinical interventions of foot problems require some level of self-management in the household environment. For this reason, foot specialists need to be aware of the ability of older patients to maintain adequate foot hygiene and undertake basic footcare tasks, such as cutting and filing nails, applying emollient creams, washing and drying feet, managing areas of dry skin and calluses, putting on shoes and hosiery, inspecting the foot for lesions and changing wound dressings. Failure to adequately assess an older person's competence to perform these tasks can have serious ramifications, particularly in older people with peripheral vascular disease or diabetes.

Basic footcare is inherently difficult for older people, as it requires not only adequate joint flexibility but also a high level of manual dexterity and visual acuity; all of which decline with advancing age. A particularly good example of the importance of assessing basic footcare competence was provided by Thomson & Masson (1992), who evaluated the ability of older people with and without diabetes to reach down to their feet to inspect a 'virtual lesion' (an adhesive red spot placed on the toes or on the plantar surface of the foot). The results indicated that 39% of those with diabetes could not reach their toes, and only 14% of all older participants could detect the plantar 'lesions'. It is therefore clear that advising older people about basic footcare tasks is not helpful unless they are actually capable of performing the task.

The ability for self-management can be evaluated during a routine consultation by simply observing whether the patient is capable of removing their footwear, and whether they have sufficient flexibility to reach and indicate the location of the foot problem. Assessing other aspects of self-management, such as using nail files, changing dressings and applying emollients, may require the clinician to specifically request that the patient demonstrate these skills. Assistive devices (such as long-handled shoe horns, nail files and devices to assist with footwear fixation) should also be available and demonstrations provided to patients who may benefit from them.

Footwear assessment

Evaluation of footwear is one of the most fundamental components of lower-limb assessment in older people. It has been demonstrated that between 50% and 80% of older people wear ill-fitting shoes (Burns et al 2002, Chung 1983), and there is evidence that the constriction associated with tightly fitting shoes predisposes to the development of common foot problems. Menz & Morris (2005) recently evaluated footwear fitting in 176 older people, and found that 80% wore shoes narrower than their feet. Those wearing shoes narrower than their feet were more likely to have corns on the toes, hallux valgus deformity and foot pain, whereas those wearing shoes shorter than their feet were more likely to have lesser toe deformity. Heel elevation in women's shoes was associated with both hallux valgus and plantar calluses.

Due to the strong association between ill-fitting footwear and foot problems, footwear evaluation is an essential first step in investigating the potential causes of foot problems. Indeed, changing footwear may be the only intervention necessary to successfully manage many common foot problems, particularly those related to toe deformities and associated hyperkeratotic lesions. Footwear also needs to be evaluated for suitability in relation to the provision of toe splints, in-shoe plantar padding and foot orthoses, as the efficacy of these interventions is highly dependent on the ability of the shoes to support and facilitate the function of these devices.

The first issue to consider when assessing footwear is whether the shoes that the older person is wearing at the time of the consultation are those that are worn most frequently – in many cases the shoes worn may be 'dress shoes' only worn for special occasions (such as attending medical appointments). It is also important to ensure that indoor footwear is also assessed, as some older people may spend more of their time indoors than outdoors. Although indoor shoes are generally wider fitting than outdoor shoes (Menz & Morris 2005), they also tend to be less supportive and are replaced far less frequently (Munro & Steele 1999). **Figure 16.12** summarises the key features of footwear that should be routinely assessed in older people.

Footwear and falls

An additional consideration when assessing footwear in older people is their potential contribution to impaired balance and falls. Certain footwear

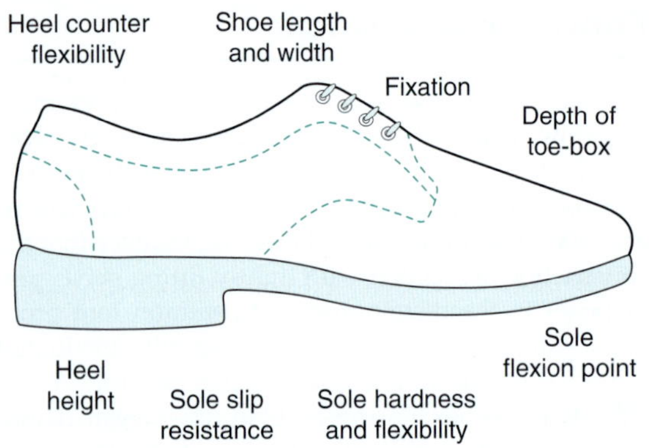

Figure 16.12 Key components of footwear evaluation in older people.

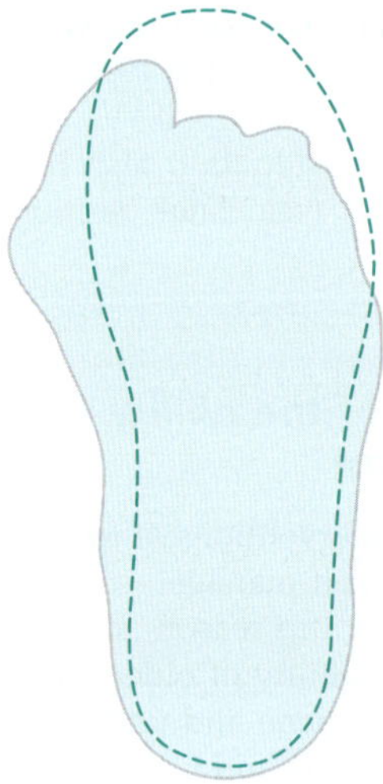

Figure 16.13 A typical shoe and foot tracing for an older woman.

characteristics, such as high heels, soles with poor grip and inadequate fixation, have been associated with impaired gait, balance, falls and hip fracture (Menz & Lord 1999, Sherrington & Menz 2003). Laboratory studies have shown that balance is maximised in shoes with low heels (Lord & Bashford 1996) and high heel collars (i.e. boot) (Lord et al 1999), and that the addition of a bevel to the rear section of a shoe can improve slip resistance (Menz & Lord 2001b). Older people should therefore generally be advised to wear appropriately fitting shoes with low heels, textured soles, laces, and if feasible, a high heel collar for additional ankle support. A standardised screening tool – the Footwear Assessment Form – has been developed for the purpose of assessing footwear in relation to balance and falls (Menz & Sherrington 2000). Patients with a history of falls whose footwear exhibits multiple potentially hazardous features should be advised to consider the purchase of more appropriate shoes.

Compliance issues

Fashion has a powerful influence over footwear selection, so compliance with footwear advice is often very low. The American podiatrist Bill Rossi (1980) stated that the provision of footwear advice is 'an exercise in eternal futility', and it is clear that this aspect of footcare is one of the most frustrating issues for foot specialists. Nevertheless, many aspects of behavioural change required to improve health are difficult to achieve (e.g. weight loss, exercise, smoking cessation), and it would be negligent to simply ignore these issues simply because they are difficult.

When providing footwear advice to older patients, it is worth considering the underlying concepts of the Health Belief Model (Janz & Becker 1984). This model suggests that a patient's decision to carry out a particular health protective behaviour (such as changing footwear) is influenced by how vulnerable they perceive themselves to be to the particular health problem, how serious they perceive the particular health condition to be, the benefits that they perceive the health protective behaviour will produce, and what barriers there are to carrying out the behaviour. Considering how these principles differentially affect individual patients may assist in the development of more effective strategies to enhance compliance with footwear recommendations. A useful first step in this process is to provide patients with a visual indication of the disparity between their foot size and their shoe size. This can be very simply and effectively demonstrated by making a tracing of the patient's bare foot on a piece of paper, and using the same piece of paper to trace around their shoe (Fig. 16.13).

Outcome measurement

Historically, determining the efficacy of a clinical intervention has been based primarily on subjective reports of pain relief, or objective measures considered important to the clinician (e.g. radiographic measurements of angular correction of hallux valgus following surgery). In recent times, a more patient-centred approach has been advocated, necessitating the development of questionnaires which reflect the broader construct of health-related quality of life. As outlined in Chapter 4, several such tools have been

Table 16.8 Manchester Foot Pain and Disability Index

Because of pain in my feet:	*Participant's response*	*Construct measured*
1. I avoid walking outside at all	None of the time On some days On most days/every day	Functional limitation
2. I avoid walking distances	None of the time On some days On most days/every day	Functional limitation
3. I don't walk in a normal way	None of the time On some days On most days/every day	Functional limitation
4. I walk slowly	None of the time On some days On most days/every day	Functional limitation
5. I have to stop and rest my feet	None of the time On some days On most days/every day	Functional limitation
6. I avoid hard or rough surfaces where possible	None of the time On some days On most days/every day	Functional limitation
7. I avoid standing for a long time	None of the time On some days On most days/every day	Functional limitation
8. I catch the bus or use the car more often	None of the time On some days On most days/every day	Functional limitation
9. I need help with housework/shopping	None of the time On some days On most days/every day	Functional limitation
10. I still do everything but with more pain or discomfort	None of the time On some days On most days/every day	Pain intensity
11. I get irritable when my feet hurt	None of the time On some days On most days/every day	Functional limitation
12. I feel self-conscious about my feet	None of the time On some days On most days/every day	Concern about appearance
13. I get self-conscious about the shoes I have to wear	None of the time On some days On most days/every day	Concern about appearance

Table 16.8 *Continued*

Because of pain in my feet:	*Participant's response*	*Construct measured*
14. I have constant pain in my feet	None of the time On some days On most days/every day	Pain intensity
15. My feet are worse in the morning	None of the time On some days On most days/every day	Pain intensity
16. My feet are more painful in the evening	None of the time On some days On most days/every day	Pain intensity
17. I get shooting pains in my feet	None of the time On some days On most days/every day	Pain intensity

developed for the foot and ankle, including the Foot Function Index (Budiman-Mak et al 1991), the Foot Health Status Questionnaire (Bennett et al 1998), a range of scales developed by the American Orthopaedic Foot and Ankle Society (Kitaoka et al 1994), the Manchester Foot Pain and Disability Index (Garrow et al 2000), and the Bristol Foot Score (Barnett et al 2005). Although each of these scales provides a quantitative measure of foot health status, they vary considerably in relation to the constructs measured, the level of psychometric validation undertaken, and their responsiveness to change.

The only scale to have been specifically validated in a large sample of older people is the Manchester Foot Pain and Disability Index (MFPDI). Menz et al (2006b) administered this scale to a random sample of 301 people aged 75 years and over, and reported a similarly high level of internal consistency to that found in the initial validation study by Garrow et al (2000). The MFPDI has also been used as an outcome measure in a clinical trial of a basic footcare self-management programme for older people (Waxman et al 2003). Table 16.8 outlines the MFPDI and its components.

Conclusion

The general principles of lower-limb assessment in older people are essentially the same as for younger people, and the clinical examination should be equally thorough and systematic. Key additional considerations when assessing older people include the variability of the ageing process, the multifactorial nature of foot disorders in older people, and the broader implications of mobility impairment. The clinical assessment techniques outlined in this chapter will hopefully assist practitioners in the accurate diagnosis of lower limb disorders, and contribute to the development of targeted and effective management strategies for older people.

References

Albright J W, Albright J F 1994 Ageing alters the competence of the immune system to control parasitic infection. Immunology Letters 40:279–285

Alexander N B, Goldberg A 2005 Gait disorders: search for multiple causes. Cleveland Clinic Journal of Medicine 72:586–600

Balin A K, Pratt L A 1989 Physiological consequences of human skin aging. Cutis 43:431–436

Barnett S, Campbell R, Harvey I 2005 The Bristol Foot Score: developing a patient-based foot-health measure. Journal of the American Podiatric Medical Association 95:264–272

Barr E L M, Browning C, Lord S R et al 2005 Foot and leg problems are important determinants of functional status in community dwelling older people. Disability and Rehabilitation 27:917–923

Bennett P, Patterson C, Wearing S et al 1998 Development and validation of a questionnaire designed to measure foot-health status. Journal of the American Podiatric Medical Association 88:419–428

Benvenuti F, Ferrucci L, Guralnik J M et al 1995 Foot pain and disability in older persons: an epidemiologic survey. Journal of the American Geriatrics Society 43:479–484

Bowditch M G, Sanderson P, Livesey J P 1996 The significance of an absent ankle reflex. Journal of Bone and Joint Surgery (Br) 78:276–279

Budiman-Mak E, Conrad K J, Roach K E 1991 The Foot Function Index: a measure of pain and disability. Journal of Clinical Epidemiology 44:561–570

Burgess C L, Holman C D, Satti A G 2005 Adverse drug reactions in older Australians, 1981–2002. Medical Journal of Australia 182:267–270

Burns S, Leese G, McMurdo M 2002 Older people and ill-fitting shoes. Postgraduate Medical Journal 78:344–346

Carpentier P H, Maricq H R, Biro C et al 2004 Prevalence, risk factors, and clinical patterns of chronic venous disorders of lower limbs: a population-based study in France. Journal of Vascular Surgery 40:650–659

Chen J, Devine A, Dick I M et al 2003 Prevalence of lower extremity pain and its association with functionality and quality of life in elderly women in Australia. Journal of Rheumatology 30:2689–2693

Chung S 1983 Foot care – a health care maintenance program. Journal of Gerontological Nursing 9:213–227

Delis K T 2004 Perforator vein incompetence in chronic venous disease: a multivariate regression analysis model. Journal of Vascular Surgery 40:626–633

deWin M, Theuvenet W, Roche P et al 2002 The paper grip test for screening of intrinsic muscle paralysis in the foot of leprosy patients. International Journal of Leprosy and other Mycobacterial Diseases 70:16–24

Doherty T J 2003 Aging and sarcopenia. Journal of Applied Physiology 95:1717–1727

Duncan P W, Studenski S, Chandler J et al 1992 Functional reach: predictive validity in a sample of elderly male veterans. Journal of Gerontology 47: M93–98

Dunn J E, Link C L, Felson D T et al 2004 Prevalence of foot and ankle conditions in a multiethnic community sample of older adults. American Journal of Epidemiology 159:491–498

Eaglstein W H 1986 Wound healing and aging. Dermatologic Clinics 4:481–484

Eisenberg D M, Kessler R C, Foster C et al 1993 Unconventional medicine in the United States: prevalence, costs, and patterns of use. New England Journal of Medicine 328:246–252

Endo M, Ashton-Miller J A, Alexander N B 2002 Effects of age and gender on toe flexor muscle strength. Journal of Gerontology 57A:M392–397

Ernst E 2002 The risk-benefit profile of commonly used herbal therapies: gingko, St. John's wort, ginseng, echinacea, saw palmetto, and kava. Annals of Internal Medicine 136:42–53

Ferrari A U, Radaelli A, Centola M 2003 Invited review: aging and the cardiovascular system. Journal of Applied Physiology 95:2591–2597

Folstein M F, McHugh P R 1975 Mini-mental state: a practical method for grading the state of patients for the clinician. Journal of Psychiatric Research 12:189–198

Fraenkel L, Rabidou N, Dhar R 2006 Are rheumatologists' treatment decisions influenced by patients' age? Rheumatology 45(12):1555–1557

Franse L V, Valk G D, Dekker J H et al 2000 'Numbness of the feet' is a poor indicator for polyneuropathy in type 2 diabetic patients. Diabetic Medicine 17:105–110

Gagliese L, Melzack R 1997 Chronic pain in elderly people. Pain 70:3–14

Garrow A P, Papageorgiou A, Silman A J et al 2001 The grading of hallux valgus: the Manchester Scale. Journal of the American Podiatric Medical Association 91:74–78

Garrow A P, Papageorgiou A C, Silman A J et al 2000 Development and validation of a questionnaire to assess disabling foot pain. Pain 85:107–113

Gibson S J, Farrell M 2004 A review of age differences in the neurophysiology of nociception and the perceptual experience of pain. Clinical Journal of Pain 2004:227–239

Gilsing M G, VandenBosch C G, Lee S G et al 1995 Association of age with the threshold for detecting ankle inversion and eversion in upright stance. Age and Ageing 24:58–66

Gorter K J, Kuyvenhoven M M, deMelker R A 2000 Nontraumatic foot complaints in older people: a population-based survey of risk factors, mobility, and well-being. Journal of the American Podiatric Medical Association 90:397–402

Gosain A, DiPietro L A 2004 Aging and wound healing. World Journal of Surgery 28:321–326

Herr K, Bjoro K, Decker S 2006 Tools for assessment of pain in nonverbal older adults with dementia: a state-of-the-science review. Journal of Pain and Symptom Management 31:170–192

Hurvitz E, Richardson J, Werner R et al 2000 Unipedal stance testing as an indicator of fall risk among older outpatients. Archives of Physical Medicine and Rehabilitation 81:587–591

Izzo A A, Ernst E 2001 Interactions between herbal medicines and prescribed drugs: a systematic review. Drugs 61:2163–2175

James B, Parker A W 1989 Active and passive mobility of lower limb joints in elderly men and women. American Journal of Physical Medicine and Rehabilitation 68:162–167

Janz N K, Becker M H 1984 The health belief model: a decade later. Health Education Quarterly 11:1–47

Jennings M B, Alfieri D, Ward K et al 1998 Comparison of salicylic acid and urea versus ammonium lactate for the treatment of foot xerosis: a randomized, double-blind, clinical study. Journal of the American Podiatric Medical Association 88:332–336

Katz S, Downs T D, Crash H et al 1970 Progress in development of the index of ADL. Gerontologist 10:20–30

Kaufman D W, Kelly J P, Rosenberg L et al 2002 Recent patterns of medication use in the ambulatory adult population of the United States: the Slone survey. Journal of the American Medical Association 287:337–344

Keenan A, Bach T 1996 Video assessment of rearfoot movements during walking: a reliability study. Archives of Physical Medicine and Rehabilitation 77:651–655

Kendall H O, Kendall F P 1949 Muscles: testing and function. Williams & Wilkins, Baltimore

Kitaoka H B, Alexander I J, Adelaar R S et al 1994 Clinical rating systems for the ankle-hindfoot, midfoot, hallux, and lesser toes. Foot and Ankle International 15:349–353

Kuller L H 2001 Is ankle-brachial blood pressure measurement of clinical utility for asymptomatic elderly? Journal of Clinical Epidemiology 54:971–972

Lawson G 2005 The importance of obtaining ankle-brachial indexes in older adults: the other vital sign. Journal of Vascular Nursing 23:46–51

Lee C M, Maibach H I 2002 Bioengineering analysis of water hydration: an overview. Exogenous Dermatology 1:269–275

Lemon B, Burns R 1998 Malignant melanoma: a literature review and case presentation. Journal of Foot and Ankle Surgery 37:48–54

Leveille S G, Guralnik J M, Ferrucci L et al 1998 Foot pain and disability in older women. American Journal of Epidemiology 148:657–665

Lord S R, Bashford G M 1996 Shoe characteristics and balance in older women. Journal of the American Geriatrics Society 44:429–433

Lord S R, Bashford G M, Howland A et al 1999 Effects of shoe collar height and sole hardness on balance in older women. Journal of the American Geriatrics Society 47:681–684

Lord S R, Sherrington C, Menz H B 2001 Falls in older people: risk factors and strategies for prevention. Cambridge University Press, Cambridge

Mahoney F I, Barthel D W 1965 Functional evaluation: the Barthel index. Maryland State Medical Journal 14:61–65

Marsh A P, Katula J A, Pacchia C F et al 2006 Effect of treadmill and overground walking on function and attitudes in older adults. Medicine and Science in Sports and Exercise 38:1157–1164

McMurdo M E, Witham M D, Gillespie N D 2005 Including older people in clinical research. BMJ 331:1036–1037

Menz H B, Lord S R 1999 Footwear and postural stability in older people. Journal of the American Podiatric Medical Association 89:346–357

Menz H B, Sherrington C 2000 The Footwear Assessment Form: a reliable clinical tool for the evaluation of footwear characteristics of relevance to postural stability in older adults. Clinical Rehabilitation 14:657–664

Menz H B, Lord S R 2001a The contribution of foot problems to mobility impairment and falls in older people. Journal of the American Geriatrics Society 49:1651–1656

Menz H B, Lord S R 2001b Slip resistance of casual footwear: implications for falls in older adults. Gerontology 47:145–149

Menz H B, Morris M E 2005 Footwear characteristics and foot problems in older people. Gerontology 51:346–351

Menz H B, Morris M E 2006 Clinical determinants of plantar forces and pressures during walking in older people. Gait and Posture 24(2):229–236

Menz H B, Munteanu S E 2005a Radiographic validation of the Manchester scale for the classification of hallux valgus deformity. Rheumatology 44:1061–1066

Menz H B, Munteanu S E 2005b Validity of 3 clinical techniques for the measurement of static foot posture in older people. Journal of Orthopaedic and Sports Physical Therapy 35:479–486

Menz H B, Tiedemann A, Kwan M M S et al 2003 Reliability of clinical tests of foot and ankle characteristics in older people. Journal of the American Podiatric Medical Association 93:380–387

Menz H B, Morris M E, Lord S R 2005 Foot and ankle characteristics associated with impaired balance and functional ability in older people. Journal of Gerontology 60:A1546–1552

Menz H B, Morris M E, Lord S R 2006a Foot and ankle risk factors for falls in older people: a prospective study. Journal of Gerontology 61A:M100–104

Menz H B, Tiedemann A, Kwan M M S et al 2006b Foot pain in community-dwelling older people: an evaluation of the Manchester Foot Pain and Disability Index. Rheumatology (Oxford) 45:863–867. Erratum in: Rheumatology (Oxford) 2007 46(2):375

Menz H B, Zammit G V, Munteanu S E et al 2006c Plantarflexion strength of the toes: age and gender differences and evaluation of a clinical screening test. Foot and Ankle International 27(12):1103–1108

Muehleman C, Rahimi F 1990 Aging integumentary system: podiatric review. Journal of the American Podiatric Medical Association 80:577–582

Munro B J, Steele J R 1999 Household-shoe wearing and purchasing habits – a survey of people aged 65 years and older. Journal of the American Podiatric Medical Association 89:506–514

Nigg B M, Fisher V, Allinger T L et al 1992 Range of motion of the foot as a function of age. Foot and Ankle 13:336–343

Nitz J C, Low-Choy N 2004 The relationship between ankle dorsiflexion range, falls and activity level in women aged 40 to 80 years. New Zealand Journal of Physiotherapy 32:121–125

Oberg T, Karsznia A, Oberg K 1993 Basic gait parameters: reference data for normal subjects, 10–79 years of age. Journal of Rehabilitation Research and Development 30:210–223

Orentreich N, Markovsky J, Vogelman J H 1979 The effect of aging on the rate of linear nail growth. Journal of Investigative Dermatology 73:126–130

Orlin M, McPoil T 2000 Plantar pressure assessment. Physical Therapy 80:399–409

Ostchega Y, Harris T B, Hirsch R et al 2000 The prevalence of functional limitations and disability in older persons in the US: data from the National Health and Nutrition Examination Survey III. Journal of the American Geriatrics Society 48:1132–1135

Perry J, Ireland M L, Gronley J et al 1986 Predictive value of manual muscle testing and gait analysis in normal ankles by dynamic electromyography. Foot and Ankle 6:254–259

Petrella R J, Lattanzio P J, Nelson M G 1997 Effect of age and activity on knee joint proprioception. American Journal of Physical Medicine and Rehabilitation 76:235–241

Pirmohamed M, James S, Meakin S et al 2004 Adverse drug reactions as a cause of admission to hospital: prospective analysis of 18820 patients. BMJ 329:15–19

Prakash C, Stern G 1973 Neurological signs in the elderly. Age and Ageing 2:24–27

Razeghi M, Batt M E 2002 Foot type classification: a critical review of current methods. Gait and Posture 15:282–291

Richardson D, Schwartz R 1985 Comparison of capillary blood flow in the nailfold circulations of young and elderly men. Age 8:70–75

Richardson J 2002 The clinical identification of peripheral neuropathy among older persons. Archives of Physical Medicine and Rehabilitation 83:1553–1558

Rogers R S, Callen J, Wehr R et al 1989 Comparative efficacy of 12% ammonium lactate lotion and 5% lactic acid lotion in the treatment of moderate to severe xerosis. Journal of the American Academy of Dermatology 21:714–716

Rosher R B, Robinson S B 2004 Use of foot veins to monitor hydration in the elderly. Journal of the American Geriatrics Society 52:322–324

Rossi W 1980 The frustration of 'sensible' shoes. Journal of the American Podiatry Association 70:257–258

Rozzini R, Sabatini T, Cassinadri A et al 2005 Relationship between functional loss before hospital admission and mortality in elderly persons with medical illness. Journal of Gerontology 60A:M1180–1183

Ryan T 2004 The ageing of the blood supply and the lymphatic drainage of the skin. Micron 35:161–171

Scherer W P, McCreary J P, Hayes W W 2001 The diagnosis of onychomycosis in a geriatric population: a study of 450 cases in South Florida. Journal of the American Podiatric Medical Association 91:456–464

Scott G, Menz H B, Newcombe L 2007 Age-related differences in foot structure and function. Gait and Posture 26(1):68–75

Selvin E, Erlinger T P 2004 Prevalence of and risk factors for peripheral arterial disease in the United States. Results from the National Health and Nutrition Examination Survey, 1999–2000. Circulation 110:738–743

Sherrington C, Menz H B 2003 An evaluation of footwear worn at the time of fall-related hip fracture. Age and Ageing 32:310–314

Shua-Haim J, Koppuzha G, Gross J 1996 A simple scoring system for clock drawing in patients with Alzheimer's disease. Journal of the American Geriatrics Society 44:335

Shulman K I 2000 Clock-drawing: is it the ideal cognitive screening test? International Journal of Geriatric Psychiatry 15:548–561

Shumway-Cook A, Brauer S, Woollacott M 2000 Predicting the probability for falls in community-dwelling older adults using the Timed Up & Go Test. Physical Therapy 80:896–903

Smith L 1989 Histopathologic characteristics and ultrastructure of aging skin. Cutis 43:414–424

Studenski S, Perera S, Wallace D et al 2003 Physical performance measures in the clinical setting. Journal of the American Geriatrics Society 51:314–322

Thelen D G, Brockmiller C, Ashton-Miller J A et al 1998 Thresholds for sensing foot dorsi- and plantarflexion during upright stance: effects of age and velocity. Journal of Gerontology 53:M33–38

Thomas E, Peat G, Harris L et al 2004 The prevalence of pain and pain interference in a general population of older adults: cross-sectional findings from the North Staffordshire Osteoarthritis Project (NorStop). Pain 110:361–368

Thomas S E, Dykes P J, Marks R 1985 Plantar hyperkeratosis: a study of callosities and normal plantar skin. Journal of Investigative Dermatology 85:394–397

Thomson F J, Masson E A 1992 Can elderly diabetic patients co-operate with routine foot care? Age and Ageing 21:333–337

Tiedemann A, Sherrington C, Lord S R 2005 Physiological and psychological predictors of walking speed in older community-dwelling people. Gerontology 51:390–395

Tinetti M E 2003 Approach to clinical care of the older patient. In: Hazzard W R, Blass J P, Halter J B et al (eds) Principles of geriatric medicine and gerontology, 5th edn. McGraw-Hill, New York, pp 95–110

Tosti A, Hay R, Arenas-Guzman R 2005 Patients at risk of onychomycosis – risk factor identification and active prevention. Journal of the European Academy of Dermatology and Venereology 19:13–16

VanSwearingen J M, Paschal K A, Bonino P et al 1998 Assessing recurrent fall risk of community-dwelling, frail older veterans using specific tests of mobility and the Physical Performance Test of function. Journal of Gerontology 53A:M457–464

Verdu E, Ceballos D, Vilches J J et al 2000 Influence of aging on peripheral nerve function and regeneration. Journal of the Peripheral Nervous System 5:191–208

Virmani R, Avolio A P, Mergner W J et al 1991 Effect of aging on aortic morphology in populations with high and low prevalence of hypertension and atherosclerosis. Comparison between occidental and Chinese communities. American Journal of Pathology 139:1119–1129

Vogt M T, Cauley J A, Kuller L H et al 1993 Prevalence and correlates of lower extremity arterial disease in elderly women. American Journal of Epidemiology 137:559–568

Waldecker U 2004 Limited range of motion of the lesser MTP joints – a cause of metatarsalgia. Foot and Ankle Surgery 10:149–154

Wass E, Taylor N F, Matsas A 2005 Familiarisation to treadmill walking in unimpaired older people. Gait and Posture 21:72–79

Waxman R, Woodburn H, Powell M et al 2003 Footstep: a randomized controlled trial investigating the clinical and cost effectiveness of a patient self-management program for basic foot care in the elderly. Journal of Clinical Epidemiology 56:1092–1099

Wells P S, Hirsh J, Anderson D R et al 1995 Accuracy of clinical assessment of deep-vein thrombosis. Lancet 345:1326–1330

Woo J, Ho S C, Lau J 1999 Walking speed and stride length predicts 36 months dependency, mortality, and institutionalization in Chinese aged 70 and older. Journal of the American Geriatrics Society 47:1257–1260

CHAPTER

17

The painful foot

B Yates

Indicates figures on DVD, including colour

Indicates video of assessment on DVD

Chapter contents

Introduction

The purpose of this chapter is not to cover the assessment of every possible cause of foot pain. To do so would be more than a complete text in its own right. What follows is a discussion on how pain within the foot may present itself and the findings on assessment for the common causes of foot pathology.

Pain is a subjective phenomenon – 'Pain is whatever the experiencing person says it is, existing whenever the experiencing person says it does' (McCaffery & Beeke 1989). We can assess pain in a variety of ways and it is essential for the practitioner to be aware of these assessment strategies when assessing foot pain (see Ch. 4). Assessment of the presenting complaint of the patient is covered in detail in Chapter 3.

There are many ways in which we can classify the pathologies that cause pain within the foot:

- Anatomical region – forefoot, midfoot, rearfoot
- Tissue type – articular, bone, tendon, etc.
- The cause – trauma, systemic disease, idiopathic, etc.

How common is foot pain?

Pain in the foot is a common complaint. Garrow et al (2004) in a survey of almost 5000 people found that 9.5% had disabling foot pain. Some studies have shown higher incidences: 14% in adolescents (Spahn et al 2004), rising to 36% in older patients (Menz et al 2006b). The incidence of foot pain increases with particular foot deformities or pathologies. Ribu et al (2006) found that 75% of patients with diabetic foot ulcers had foot pain from these ulcers, which may come as a surprise to many practitioners who believe that neuropathic ulcers are always painless.

Foot deformity is thought to be a common cause of foot pain. The evidence from the literature to support this hypothesis is variable. With certain deformities there is a strong correlation, such as pes cavus. A recent study found that 60% of subjects with this structural deformity had foot pain (Burns et al 2005). Hallux valgus and lesser toe deformities were not found to be a significant cause of foot pain in an elderly population (Badlissi et al 2005) but this is in contrast to the work of Benvenuti et al (1995) who found a significant relationship between pain and these and other foot pathologies such as plantar calluses and pes planus in a similarly aged population.

When considering foot deformity and its association with pain, one issue is the degree of deformity. It would be natural to assume that the bigger the deformity the more pain the patient would experience. However, this is not the case and has been demonstrated with several foot deformities, most recently hallux valgus. Thordarson et al (2005) found that the degree of pain experienced by patients waiting for hallux valgus surgery had no correlation with the degree of deformity measured clinically or radiologically. Such evidence reinforces the subjective nature of pain. However, this does not mean that foot deformity is not a major cause of morbidity. Even in those with foot deformity and no foot pain there is still the potential for significant other pathology and morbidity. Foot deformity, especially lesser toe deformities and hallux valgus, has been shown to increase the risk of falls in the elderly (Menz et al 2006a). Pes planus has been shown to increase the incidence of osteoarthritis in the knee and pes cavus has been shown to increase the incidence of osteoarthritis of the hip (Reilly et al 2006). Foot deformity is a known risk factor for foot ulceration in patients with diabetes and rheumatoid arthritis.

Examination of the patient with foot pain

You should first observe the patient, not the foot. It is useful to highlight those traits that have been discussed under medical history (Ch. 5) as the source of pain may be explained by general disease processes. Assess the patient's attitude. This may reveal psychological variations from normal and may influence your assessment strategy and the outcome of any treatment. Pointers concerning general health include the following:

- Does the patient look well?
- Is the patient well nourished (obese or thin and wasted)?
- Colour (pale and anaemic, jaundiced)?
- Look at the hands, are they misshapen (rheumatoid arthritis)?

The physical examination may reveal findings that raise concerns. For example, a manual worker who has thick calluses on his hands, and yet says he cannot work because of the pain in his foot, may be being less than fully honest.

Examination of the foot begins with watching the patient walk (see Ch. 10). An antalgic limp, where the patient will spend only a short period of time on the painful foot, is a clear positive sign. The limp may be linked with other problems associated with proximal joints or the back; these should be excluded. Look at shoe wear on the sole; this may indicate an abnormal gait pattern. Are the toes severely clawed, possibly suggesting a neurological problem? It is important to note any callosities, both dorsally and on the sole, as these indicate areas of high pressure and friction. Similarly, one must remember all the structures running under any area of tenderness.

The sources of pain are numerous and can be subdivided for convenience into problems affecting different tissues, different regions of the foot, generalised disorders and referred pain. Table 17.1 provides an overview of pathologies by tissue type which may cause foot pain. Tables 17.2–17.4 cover the common, less common and conditions not to be missed that can be the source of pain in the forefoot, midfoot and rearfoot respectively. In many cases the origins are not clear and assessment and further investigations are necessary to isolate the cause. The practitioner must always remember that multiple conditions may co-exist either in isolation or by association through compensation, for example a patient with a painful bunion may develop a Morton's neuroma through transfer metatarsalgia. It is important to identify these potential causal links as they can assist in the diagnosis and subsequent management of multiple conditions.

It is important to localise the current pain/symptoms to specific anatomical structures. Manikin diagrams or photographic pain maps (**Fig. 17.1**) are helpful in documenting this more quickly than is possible in words and provide a useful reference for future when the character or site of the pain changes over the course of treatment. The description of current pain/symptoms should be supplemented by an attempt to identify the precise structures affected and to reproduce the symptoms if appropriate either by direct palpation or by movement of the affected parts. The character of the symptoms (numbness, fatigue, pain), and, as appropriate, the pain characteristics (e.g. burning, bruised, achy) should be explored. Any influencing factors, for instance the effect of weightbearing/non-weightbearing activity, diurnal variation, footwear types will also help to

Table 17.1 Causes of foot pain by anatomical structure

Tissue type	*Condition*
Osseous	Fracture, accessory bones, bone tumour, metabolic bone disease, exostoses, traction apophysitis
Articular	Osteoarthritis, inflammatory arthritis, osteochondral defect, osteochondritis desiccans, tarsal coalition
Ligament	Sprain/tear/rupture
Muscle/tendon	Tear or rupture, tendinopathy, subluxing tendons, tibialis posterior dysfunction
Fascia	Plantar fasciitis, compartment syndrome, tumour, e.g. plantar fibroma
Nerves	Entrapments, peripheral neuropathy, referred pain (radiculopathy)
Skin/subcutaneous	Bursitis, soft tissue masses and tumours
Vascular	Peripheral vascular disease, vasculitis, deep vein thrombosis (DVT), venous insufficiency
All tissue types	Infection, complex regional pain syndrome

Table 17.2 Conditions that can cause forefoot pain

Common	*Less common*	*Not to be missed*
Corns/calluses	Plantar wart	Fractured sesamoid
Onychocryptosis/onychauxis	Subungual exostosis	Stress fracture (usually metatarsal)
Hallux valgus	Transverse plane deformity lesser MTPJ	Complex regional pain syndrome
Hallux rigidus	IPJ or lesser MTPJ arthritis	Charcot neuroarthropathy
Lesser toe deformity-Hammer/ claw toe	Lesser toe deformity – cross-over toe, clinodactyly, adductovarus toe	Glomus tumour
Morton's neuroma	Joplin's neuroma	Malignant melanoma
Inflammatory arthritis, e.g. Rh. A	Bursitis (usually MTPJ)	
Lesser MTPJ capsulitis (especially 2nd)	Sesamoiditis	
Gout	Soft tissue mass, e.g. ganglion, mucoid cyst Freiberg's Chilblains Tendinopathy (extensor or flexor)	

MPTJ, metatarsophalangeal joint; IPJ, interphalangeal joint.

Table 17.3 Conditions that can cause midfoot pain

Common	*Less common*	*Not to be missed*
Instep plantar fasciitis	Extensor/ tibialis anterior tendinopathy	Lisfranc dislocation
Plantar fibroma	Köhler's disease	Complex regional pain syndrome
Osteoarthritis 2nd/3rd TMT joints	Stress fracture – metatarsal base, navicular	Malignant melanoma
Soft tissue mass, e.g. ganglion	Lisfranc injury	
Charcot's neuroarthropathy	Osteoarthritis 1st TMT/ intercuneiform/ navicular-cuneiform joints	
Nerve entrapment (deep peroneal)	Nerve entrapment (superficial peroneal) Peripheral vascular disease, e.g. rest pain Gout	

TMT, tarsometatarsal.

Table 17.4 Conditions that can cause rearfoot pain

Common	*Less common*	*Not to be missed*
Plantar fasciitis	Plantar wart	Tarsal coalition
Nerve entrapment (lateral plantar nerve)	Tarsal tunnel syndrome	Bone tumour, e.g. osteoid osteoma
Tibialis posterior dysfunction	Peroneal tendinopathy/ subluxing tendons	Complex regional pain syndrome
Haglund's or retrocalcaneal exostosis	Accessory bone (os tibialis externum, os trigonum)	Charcot neuroarthropathy
Achilles tendinopathy	Osteochondral defect talus	Inflammatory arthropathies, e.g. ankylosing spondylitis, Reiter's disease
Osteoarthritis, subtalar joint	Osteoarthritis talonavicular joint	Fracture (traumatic or stress calcaneus or talus)
Sinus tarsi syndrome	Spring ligament injury	Malignant melanoma
Sever's disease	Retrocalcaneal bursitis Fat pad contusion Rheumatoid arthritis	

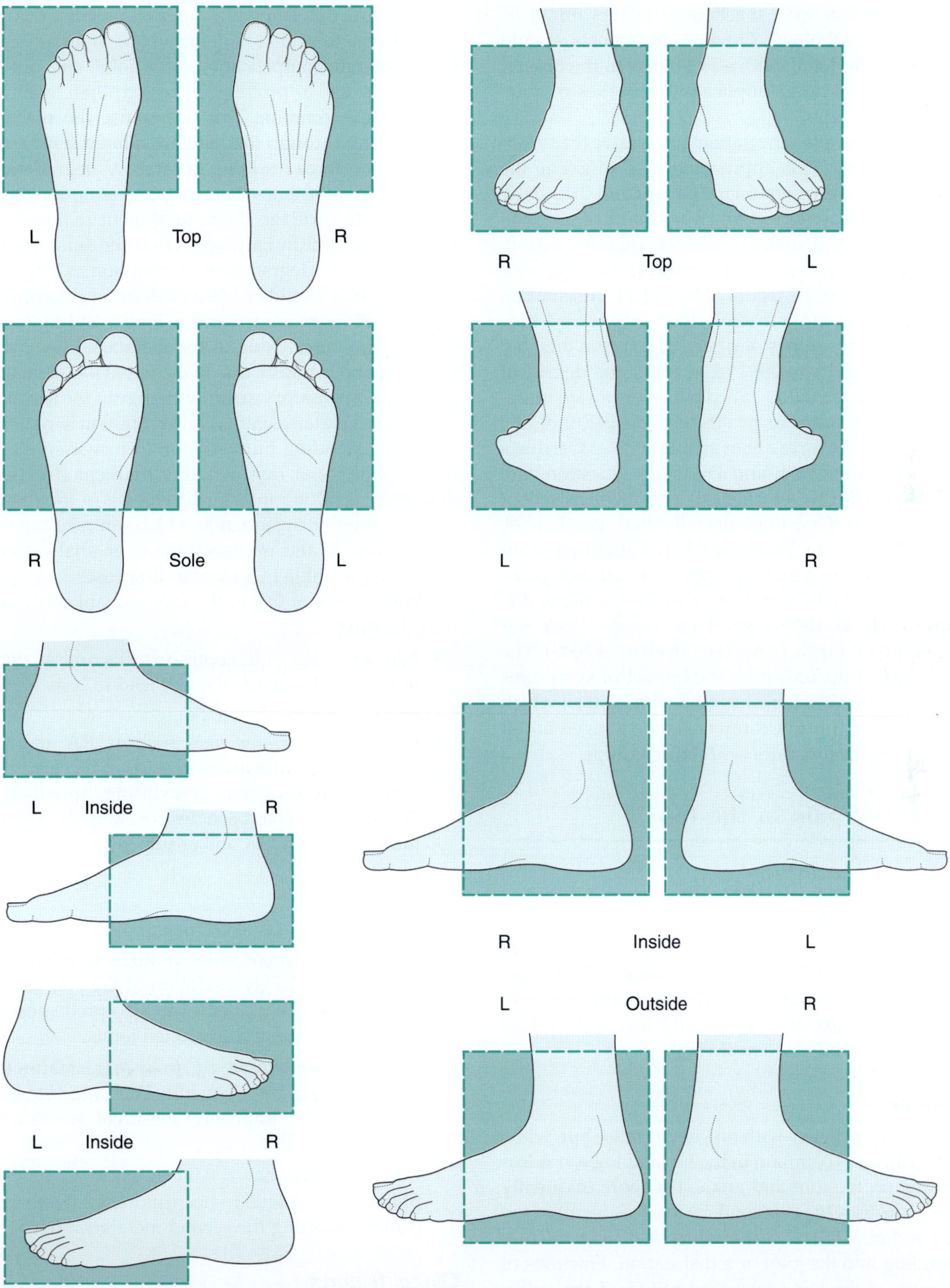

Figure 17.1 Pain map.

identify whether local mechanical factors might be driving the pathology. Previous treatments should be explored in detail, both as a pointer to the disease process and to avoid duplicating mistakes or ineffectual treatments.

Having prompted the patient to describe the symptoms themselves it is appropriate also to gauge the impact of the symptoms on the patient and their daily life. This can be done in several ways the most common being to use visual analogue scales to quantify simply pain or other aspects of impairment. It has long been common practice to record this sort of information empirically but more recently there has been a burgeoning of approaches designed to explore this in a more structured way and to quantify the degree of impact. These are the so-called patient reported measures of health status or health-related quality of life. A variety of measures are available such as Garrow's Manchester Foot Pain and Disability Questionnaire (MFPDQ) (Garrow et al 2000) and Bennett's Foot Health Status Questionnaire (Bennett et al 1998, Bennett & Patterson 1998) (see Ch. 4). Patient-reported measures can be generally applied to all foot problems such as the two above or may be specific to diseases (such as the Leeds Foot Impact Scale for rheumatoid arthritis (RA)) (Helliwell et al 2005). The advantage of documenting the impact of symptoms formally is that it establishes a baseline against which the success of future treatment can be gauged and it also acts as a comparator with other groups.

Causes of pain in the foot

Articular conditions

Osteoarthritis

Degenerative arthritis may affect any of the joints of the foot and ankle. The joints most commonly affected are the ankle, subtalar, talonavicular, and the first, second, and third tarsometatarsal joints, and the first metatarsophalangeal joint (MTPJ).

Aetiology

This may be primary with no known cause but, while such arthritis is common in the hip and knee, it is less common in the foot and ankle. Far more frequently osteoarthritis (OA) is secondary to some insult to the joint and may follow major injury, such as a fracture extending into the joint or a dislocation. Fractures of the neck of the talus may lead to OA of the ankle. Repetitive minor trauma is the most common feature for OA of the hip and knee but less common in the foot with the exception of the first MTPJ.

Structural deformity is a common precursor to OA either in the joint that is deformed or at an adjacent joint through compensation. If a joint sits out of alignment for a prolonged period then arthritic changes are common. This is because the reaction forces going through the joint are altered with areas of increased force resulting in cartilage degradation. It is also known that when cartilage is no longer in contact with cartilage the nourishment required for maintaining healthy cartilage is reduced again resulting in cartilage degradation. A common example of this in the foot would be hallux valgus where arthritic change within the joint is seen in long-standing cases, both on the medial side of the metatarsal head due to disuse and centrally due to increased joint reaction forces. Compensatory arthritic change in the second/third tarsometatarsal joints is also common in patients with long-standing bunions due to increased strain through the lesser rays. Another frequent structural deformity resulting in arthritic change in the foot is tibialis posterior dysfunction which can result in OA of the subtalar and midtarsal joints, medial column and even the ankle in long-standing cases.

Other causes of OA in the foot and ankle include the following:

- *Infection in the joint*. Septic arthritis, unless diagnosed and treated early, will lead to lysis of cartilage and secondary OA.
- *Inflammatory arthropathies* such as RA and the seronegative arthritides, e.g. psoriatic arthritis, Reiter's disease and ankylosing spondylitis. When the joint has been destroyed by the inflammatory process OA will ensue.
- *Metabolic disorders* such as gout and pseudogout.
- *Systemic diseases* such as diabetes mellitus, which can lead to Charcot's foot or ankle. Limited joint mobility due to glycosylation of the soft tissues in patients with diabetes can also predispose to arthritic change of the affected joints.
- *Proximal malalignment*, e.g. following a malunited fractured tibia, has frequently been stated to lead to arthritis by imposing abnormal stresses on distal joints.
- *Other miscellaneous conditions* such as haemophilia or avascular necrosis (e.g. Freiberg's disease affecting the second metatarsal head).

Clinical features

Generally these will be pain and stiffness in the area of the affected joint. Symptoms may start as aching after exercise and progress to pain after walking a distance. With time and progression of the arthritis the distance the patient can walk without pain gradually reduces. Pain may become constant and also present at night, disturbing sleep. How much pain the patient is experiencing is important to know but it is the impairment of function which probably influences us most when it comes to determining treatment. While one must be aware of the stoics who push themselves on regardless of the pain (and vice versa), how much a patient can do is often a good indicator of how severe the symptoms are. Stiffness may initially occur after the joint has been rested for a while, but with time the range of movement in the affected joint will decrease. Dorsiflexion is usually the first movement to be lost, and shoes with a slight heel raise may therefore be more comfortable. In severe OA the joint may completely lose movement and become virtually ankylosed. Patients may also complain of a limp, swelling or joint deformity.

The joint may appear enlarged or deformed or be held in an abnormal position. It may feel warm if the underlying cause is infection or an inflammatory arthropathy, but otherwise it does not feel warm in OA. An effusion may be present in ankle OA, but this is not usually clinically detectable in OA of other foot joints. Osteophytes may be felt in superficial joints as hard bony swellings and represent new bone formation around the periphery of affected joints. Localised tenderness may also be found. The range of movement of the joint will be reduced, the degree depending on how advanced the arthritis is, and movement will be painful, more so at the extremes. Often movement may feel 'dry', rather than smooth and easy. In advanced OA grating, crepitus or crunching may be felt by the examiner as the joint is moved.

Investigations

Plain X-rays, generally standing anteroposterior (AP for ankle, DP (dorsiplantar) for foot) and lateral, are essential (Ch. 12). The cardinal signs of OA are reduced joint space, sclerosis, cysts and osteophytes. Standing films are helpful as they may demonstrate deformity under load and the true loss of joint space due to cartilage erosion. Special views may be helpful to show particular structures more clearly such as Anthonsen's view, which shows the medial and posterior subtalar facets. If infection is suspected then any open wounds can be swabbed. Aspiration of the joint for bacterial cultures may be helpful. Results from blood tests will be normal and are unhelpful unless the OA is secondary to a systemic disease, infection or metabolic cause such as gout (Ch. 13). Further to the discussion on pain it should be noted that the degree of X-ray change does not always correlate in a linear fashion with the patient's symptoms or disability. It is always important to treat the patient and not the X-ray.

Differential diagnosis

In early OA, when X-rays are normal, a presumptive diagnosis may be made solely on information from the history, symptoms and signs. Other periarticular causes such as capsulitis should be considered however. In established OA, with X-ray changes, the differential diagnosis will usually lie in determining the underlying cause.

Osteochondroses

Osteochondral defects

A common articular injury is an osteochondral lesion or defect. These can be seen in any joint following a traumatic injury but are most often seen on the posteromedial or anterolateral aspects of the trochlear surface of the talus following an ankle sprain (Fig. 17.2). Other common sites include the first metatarsal head and the tibial plafond. Osteochondral lesions can be graded from I to IV (Table 17.5) and this helps dictate management. Classical symptoms are constant articular pain and stiffness with some swelling. Catching or locking can occur with grade III or IV lesions. Some residual pain and stiffness is often present and the patient should be counselled that early arthritis is likely to develop in the joint. Acute symptoms will be those of a sprained ankle, with the patient complaining of pain, swelling and difficulty walking. Chronic symptoms are more general, with patients complaining of discomfort, pain and perhaps stiffness during or after exercise. If an osteochondral fragment has become detached from the talar dome, then there may be locking and giving way in the ankle, suggestive of a loose body:

- Investigations (see Table 17.5)
  Plain X-rays should initially be requested but in the acute stage X-rays may appear normal, especially if the lesion is stage I, i.e. only the articular cartilage is damaged (Berndt & Harty 1959). Even in a chronic lesion it may be difficult to detect any changes on plain X-ray. Magnetic resonance imaging (MRI) is the most sensitive, as well as the most expensive way of demonstrating the osteochondral fractures. Blood tests are of no value in the investigation of this condition.

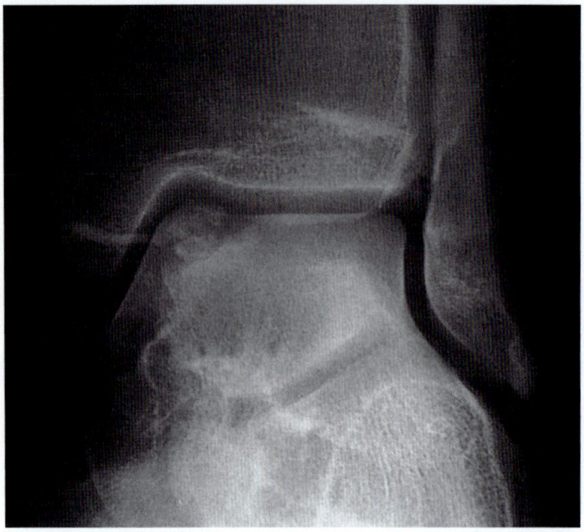

Figure 17.2 Osteochondral defect of the talus.

Table 17.5 Classification of osteochondral lesions

Grade of lesion	*Description*	*Imaging investigation required for diagnosis*
I	Subchondral cystic lesion with intact roof (also known as articular bone bruise)	Magnetic resonance imaging (MRI)
II	Subchondral cystic lesion with communication to joint surface	Computed tomography (CT)/MRI (may be visible on X-ray)
III	Separate non-displaced chondral lesion	CT/MRI/X-ray
IV	Displaced chondral lesion	CT/MRI/X-ray

- Differential diagnosis
  Acutely, this will be the co-existent trauma. Chronically, it will be other joint conditions such as capsulitis or synovitis. Around the ankle bony impingement, tendon or syndesmosis injuries should be suspected along with early OA.

Osteochondritis desiccans

Osteochondritis desiccans is triggered by avascular necrosis and is also termed osteonecrosis. It is most commonly seen in adolescents but can also occur in adults. It has been reported that trauma, either acute or chronic, is the cause in 50% of cases and the remainder is due to vascular compromise. There is still much we do not know about the aetiology of this condition. The bone most commonly affected is the lesser metatarsal (Freiberg's), followed by the navicular (Köhler's in children or Mueller–Weiss syndrome in adults), and then the cuneiforms (Bushke's disease).

Freiberg's

This is most commonly seen in the second metatarsal between 13 and 18 years of age and there is a female to male preponderance of 5:1. Symptoms include localised pain often with swelling of the affected MTPJ, and which is aggravated by weightbearing activities. Palpation of the joint and passive movement, especially plantarflexion, produce pain. Confirmation and staging of the condition can be confirmed on X-ray.

Köhler's or Mueller–Weiss syndrome

The paediatric form of this condition is most commonly seen in boys (6:1 male to female ratio) aged between 3 and 9 years. It is characterised by localised pain and swelling around the dorsal aspect of the navicular with warmth. The child often limps. In the adult form, the condition is usually more chronic in presentation with similar localisation of the pain and swelling but often with crepitus of the talonavicular joint and the development of a flatfoot posture. X-rays are used to confirm the presence of either form.

Buschke's disease

This rare condition can affect any of the cuneiforms. It occurs in children aged 5–13 years and is thought to be more prevalent in cavus feet. It is difficult to diagnose due to lack of localised swelling or erythema and initial X-rays are often negative.

Traction apophysitis

This condition is only seen in children either in the heel (Sever's disease) or at the base of the fifth metatarsal (Iselin's disease). It is caused by excessive traction of soft tissue on a secondary centre of growth before these centres have fused with the main body of the bone.

Sever's disease

This condition occurs usually between the ages of 10 and 15 years in athletic children. It used to be seen more commonly in boys but is now seen equally between sexes probably due to more girls playing sport. It is often associated with periods of rapid growth. The pain may be localised either posteriorly due to contracture of the Achilles or inferiorly due to contracture of the plantar fascia and intrinsic musculature. The presence of a tight Achilles and a flatfoot posture has also been highlighted as contributory factors. There is an absence of swelling but localised tenderness to palpation is the key to diagnosis. X-rays and other imaging modalities are not diagnostic.

Iselin's disease

This is not a commonly encountered condition. Pain is localised to the peroneus brevis insertion at the base of the fifth metatarsal, usually plantar-lateral, with minimal swelling. The epiphysis appears between the ages of 10 and 12 and fuses 2–3 years later. Stress testing of the peroneals can induce the symptoms. X-rays can be helpful to exclude fracture and are often characterised by fragmentation of the epiphysis.

Tarsal coalition

This is a congenital condition, inherited as an autosomal dominant trait, in which adjacent tarsal bones have a fibrous, cartilaginous or bone connection or bridge which progressively restricts normal movement. This may be termed syndesmosis, synchondrosis or synostosis, respectively, and occurs in less than 1% of the population (Lemley et al 2006). Generally, it begins as a fibrous union in infancy and progresses to cartilaginous and then bony union; however, it may remain fibrous. The most common coalition is the talocalcaneal, followed by calcaneonavicular (Lemley et al 2006), and these account for 95% of all coalitions. Although rare, most other possible combinations have been described.

Although these coalitions usually ossify between 8 and 16 years, symptoms may not develop until late childhood or into adulthood. Sometimes patients never develop symptoms and the diagnosis is made incidentally. When they do present, patients may complain of pain and stiffness around the hindfoot. The onset of initial symptoms is frequently after an ankle sprain and this often leads to inappropriate management. It is believed that the trauma of the ankle sprain triggers an inflammatory reaction around the coalition. Stiffness in the subtalar or midtarsal joint movements is usually the predominant sign. Patients may also have a valgus flatfoot with subtalar irritability, characterised by pain on forced plantarflexion of the ankle joint and some peroneal spasm. Tarsal coalition is the commonest cause of peroneal spastic flatfoot.

Appropriate plain X-rays may demonstrate a coalition; DP, lateral and medial oblique films should be taken. Medial oblique views show the calcaneonavicular coalition (**Fig. 17.3**). A Harris axial view may show a talocalcaneal coalition. Dorsal beaking on the head of the talus is a secondary change to abnormal movement, also suggesting this type of pathology (Case history 17.1). A long anterior calcaneal process may indicate a calcaneonavicular coalition on the lateral view. If X-rays are not diagnostic, a CT scan or MRI are the imaging modalities of choice to confirm the diagnosis.

Rheumatoid arthritis

RA is a systemic, inflammatory joint disease with an overall prevalence of about 0.8%. It is twice as common in females and usually presents in the fifth decade of life. The disease can lead to disabling pain with significant functional limitation associated with severe joint destruction and deformity. However, the

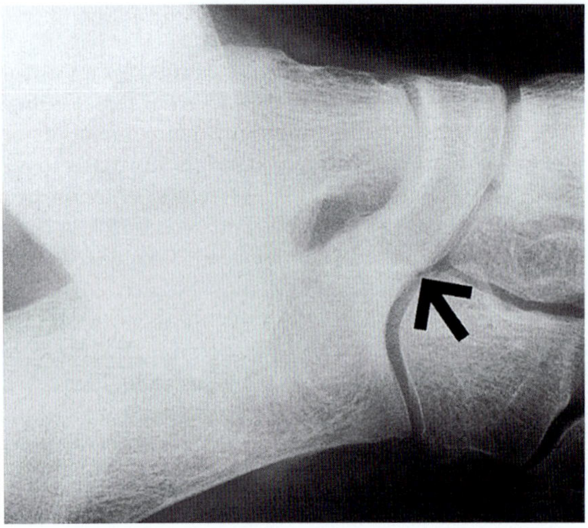

Figure 17.3 X-ray illustrating calcaneonavicular coalition (arrow) – medial oblique view.

Case history 17.1

A 25-year-old woman presented with a history of bilateral flat feet since childhood. She was now getting pain on walking after half a mile, which was interfering with her normal living. On examination, there was a normal range of movement in both ankle joints but both subtalar joints were rigid; there was slight decreased range of movement in the midtarsal joints bilaterally.

Plain X-rays showed talar beaking bilaterally. A CT scan showed bony left talocalcaneal fusion. On the right there was virtual talocalcaneal apposition but bony fusion could not be demonstrated and a fibrous coalition was diagnosed.

Diagnosis: Bilateral talocalcaneal tarsal coalition. The patient underwent subtalar fusion to achieve pain-free feet during walking.

course and severity of the disease varies widely and is often difficult to predict. The foot is affected in 90% of cases.

The diagnosis of RA is a clinical one based on observation of factors over a 6-week period (Table 17.6). The disease usually presents with morning stiffness, pain and swelling of the small joints of the hands and feet. It is estimated that RA first presents in the feet in 20% of cases. This is a key feature for podiatrists and other healthcare practitioners interested in the foot as many patients presenting with foot pain may have undiagnosed RA. This has led to the development of an early referral algorithm for RA (Emery et al 2002) which recommends immediate referral in the presence of:

- a positive forefoot squeeze test
- three swollen joints
- 30 minutes of morning stiffness.

Clinical features vary significantly depending on the severity of the disease, the location of symptoms, and whether the disease is early or established in duration. In the early stages of the disease the presenting symptoms are usually morning stiffness, pain and swollen joints. As the disease progresses foot deformity follows and this maybe the presenting feature in conjunction with painful swollen joints, calluses and ulceration. A pes planovalgus foot deformity is present in 50% of patients usually due to a combination of talonavicular or subtalar involvement often with tibialis posterior dysfunction. The ankle is less frequently affected.

Hallux valgus is present in up to 60% of established rheumatoid cases. The bunion deformity often pushes the lesser toes into either a hammered position, or more commonly causes lateral or 'fibula

Table 17.6 Components of an assessment

Component *Assessment interview*	*Presenting problem*
	Personal details
	Medical history
	Family history
	Social history
	Current health status
Observation and clinical examination	Vascular
	Neurological
	Locomotor
	Skin and nails
	Footwear
Laboratory and hospital tests	Urinalysis
	Microbiology
	Blood tests
	History
	Gait analysis
	X-ray
	Other imaging techniques
	ECG
	Nerve conduction

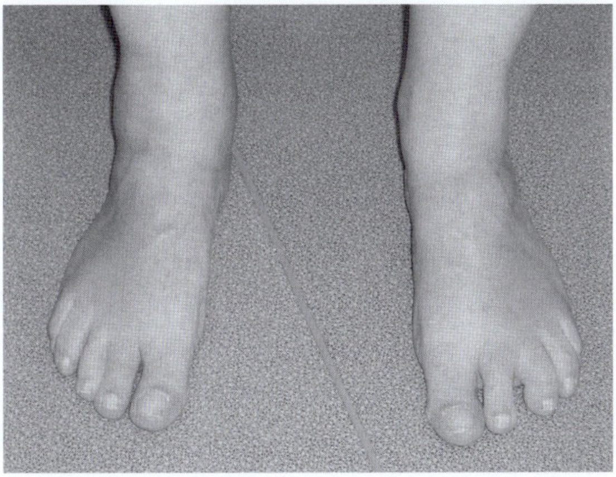

Figure 17.4 The Jacobs' daylight sign affecting the left second and third toes. Note the significant swelling of the contralateral ankle.

Case history 17.2

A 35-year-old woman was referred by her physiotherapist and podiatrist due to pain and swelling in her left forefoot and right ankle. The ankle pain had been present for a year following a mild ankle sprain and the left forefoot pain had been present for the past 6 months. On examination there was discomfort with ankle range of movement but no mechanical or functional instability. There was pain in the left forefoot with the squeeze test and compression of the second/third MTPJs and second intermetatarsal space. There was splaying between toes 2 and 3 (Fig 17.4).

An X-ray showed erosive changes in the lesser MTPJs of the left foot. The right ankle appeared normal. An MRI showed significant synovitis of the right ankle with small erosions. Blood tests revealed raised serum C-reactive protein (CRP) levels and positive rheumatoid factor.

Diagnosis: Rheumatoid arthritis.

deviation' of the toes in the transverse plane. Another common presenting symptom may be pain localised to two of the lesser toes associated with splaying of the digits termed Jacobs' daylight sign (Fig. 17.4). This is due to MTPJ synovitis in association with an intermetatarsal bursitis or other space-occupying mass such as a rheumatoid nodule. The localised inflammation often leads to neuroma symptoms due to irritation of the digital nerve and this may be the presenting complaint (see Case history 17.2).

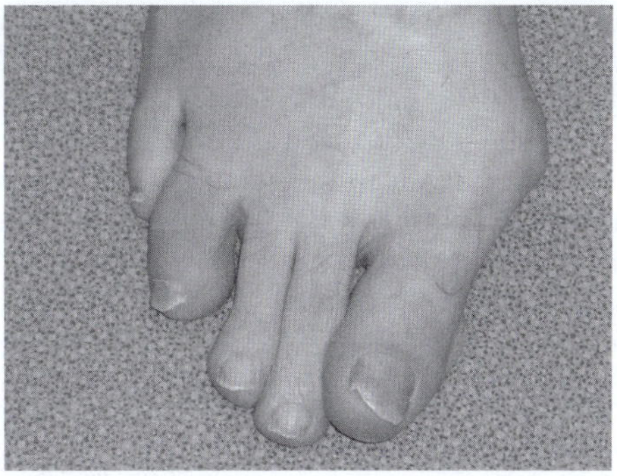

Figure 17.5 'Sausage fourth toe' due to psoriatic arthritis.

Psoriatic arthritis

Psoriatic arthritis (PA) is classically a seronegative enthesopathy with a small and large joint proliferative arthritis. It is estimated that between 1% and 2% of the population have psoriasis and approximately 10% of these will go on to develop PA. There are many forms of psoriasis but there does not appear to be any correlation with a particular form and the development of PA.

Oligoarticular (several joints) or monoarticular (single joint) arthritis is the classical presentation of this condition. The pattern of involvement usually affects the interphalangeal joints in an asymmetric manner. A chronically swollen toe or finger is a common feature (Fig. 17.5). This is called dactylitis or sausage toe. Contrary to historical teaching, the foot and ankle is the most common site for PA (Hammerschlag et al 1991). The patient usually presents with painful joint(s) in the forefoot often with heel pain due to enthesopathy and tendon involvement such as tibialis posterior tendinopathy.

X-rays will demonstrate small marginal erosions of the affected joints, and this is an early feature with peri-articular bony proliferation and periostitis at tendon attachments. There is a strong association with the HLA-B27 allele.

Reiter's syndrome

Reiter's syndrome is now considered a type of reactive arthritis. Both conditions occur in individuals with HLA-B27 following some form of infection. Reiter's syndrome usually presents as lower limb oligoarticular arthritis associated with a genitourinary or gastrointestinal infection. Eye complaints or cutaneous lesions such as keratoderma blennorrhagica on the soles of the feet are not uncommon associated complaints.

The arthritis usually affects the knees, ankles or forefoot with heel pain, and a fluffy periosteal reaction on X-ray is a classical feature. The arthritis is often additive with new joint involvement occurring within days of the first joint. Constitutional symptoms such as fever and weight loss are also common in the early stages.

Ankylosing spondylitis

Ankylosing spondylitis is a seronegative spondylitis that causes low back pain due to sacroiliitis and enthesopathy, which eventually can lead to ankylosis of the spine. The condition is associated with the HLA-B27 allele and also certain infections such as with *Klebsiella*. Enthesopathy of both the plantar fascia and Achilles tendon is a relatively common clinical feature.

Gout

Gout is associated with the deposition of uric acid crystals within joints and monosodium urate deposits within soft tissues following high uric acid serum levels. It usually occurs in middle age with 95% of cases being in males. There is a strong genetic link in primary gout. Secondary gout maybe triggered by hypertension, hypercholesteraemia, polycystic kidneys, obesity and high alcohol consumption.

The first MTPJ is affected in 50–75% of gout in a monoarticular pattern. It is associated with severe pain, swelling, heat and redness. The pain is often worse at night. The swelling and pain are often so severe that they cause desquamation of the skin resembling a cellulitis. With time other joints become affected and tophaceous deposits in the soft tissues are common. These usually occur in periarticular or subcutaneous tissue or tendons. The subcutaneous tophi appear as small white bumps under the skin, and may ulcerate (Fig. 17.6).

X-ray changes demonstrate large periarticular erosions. As the disease progresses osteoarthritis develops. Other radiographic features of gout include large periarticular cysts and intraosseous tophi which can calcify. Blood tests may show a hyperuricaemia but this has often passed in long-standing cases. A mildly raised CRP or erythrocyte sedimentation rate (ESR) is common. The only truly sensitive test for gout is the presence of sodium urate crystals in joint aspirant as seen by light microscopy.

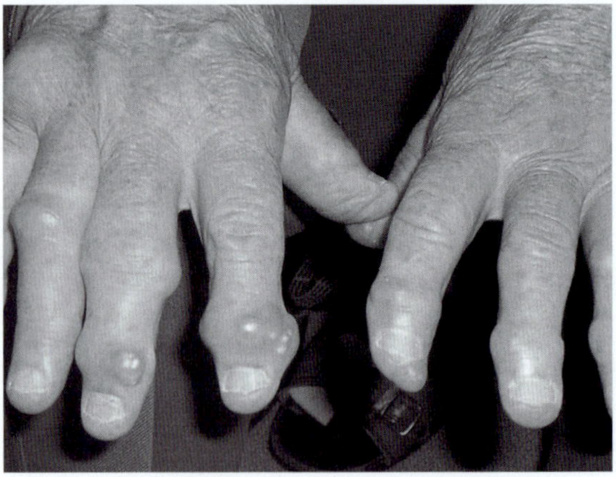

Figure 17.6 Subcutaneous gouty tophi of the fingers.

IMAGES

Bone conditions

Fracture

All bones within the foot are capable of being fractured. The commonest bones to be fractured are the phalanges of the toes, the metatarsals, and the calcaneum. Most acute fractures will not present themselves to the podiatrist but will be seen in accident and emergency departments. However, all practitioners with an interest in the foot and ankle should be aware of the common clinical findings associated with fracture of significant swelling and bruising with or without malalignment. The degree of malalignment will depend on the fracture type and the bone affected, for example long bone fractures are associated with more significant deformity.

Radiological assessment is crucial in the assessment of fracture as an aid to diagnosis, its management and the prognosis. X-ray is the standard assessment technique and two views should be taken to help identify the degree and location of fracture fragments (Ch. 12). In more complex fractures CT scanning is usually the modality of choice especially in relation to surgical planning.

Stress fracture

Stress fractures are the commonest bone pathology among athletes but they can also occur in the non-athletic populations. Repetitive loading of bone causes osseous micro-damage and results in the bone remodelling itself to become stronger. Stress fractures occur when these repetitive loads exceed a bone's ability to adapt. The incidence of stress fractures varies between different athletic, non-athletic and military populations. The incidence among track and field athletes has been shown to be as high as 21% (Bennell et al 1996) while among military recruits it can be as high as 27% (Finestone et al 1999). Lower rates have been shown in other sports and other military populations. No incidence figures are available for non-athletic/military populations.

Numerous risk factors have been proposed for the development of stress fractures with considerable variation in the level of supporting evidence. People with smaller bone geometry are more prone to stress fractures probably due to a reduced ability to resist osseous bending forces (Beck et al 2000). Reduced bone density has long been suggested as a cause of stress fractures, although only one well-controlled study demonstrated a significant reduction in bone density between those with and without a stress fracture (Bennell et al 1996). Menstrual irregularities increases the risk for stress fracture between two and four times compared with eumenorrhoeic females (Brukner & Bennell 2001). Muscle helps attenuate force and therefore reduces the stress applied to bone. This has been demonstrated in stress fracture populations where the muscle mass has been proportionally smaller than asymptomatic controls (Beck et al 2000) and the maximal muscle strength has also been less (Hoffman et al 1999). Physical fitness also has a role as reduced fitness can increase the ground reaction forces applying greater strain to the bone.

Poor biomechanics has long been thought to be a crucial risk factor. A cavus foot type has been shown to be associated with tibial and femoral stress fractures (Brosh & Arcan 1994, Giladi et al 1985) and also for repetitive stress fractures (Korpelainen et al 2001). A low arched foot type has been associated with pedal stress fractures (Simkin et al 1989). Limb-length discrepancy of greater than 5 mm has also been linked to the development of stress fractures in both military and athletic populations (Bennell et al 1996, Brunet et al 1990, Friberg 1982).

The location of stress fractures can vary depending on the activity, but the vast majority occur below the knee. In the four largest series of over 1100 stress fractures 38–54% occurred in the tibia, 7–13% the fibula, 9–23% the metatarsals, and 2–10% the navicular (Cameron et al 1992, Hulkko & Orava 1987, Matheson et al 1987, Orava 1980). The presenting features of a stress fracture are different from an acute fracture as there is usually no history of trauma, malalignment and bruising, and swelling is subtle, not significant. The diagnosis is also complicated by the fact that X-ray is often negative for 2–3 weeks in

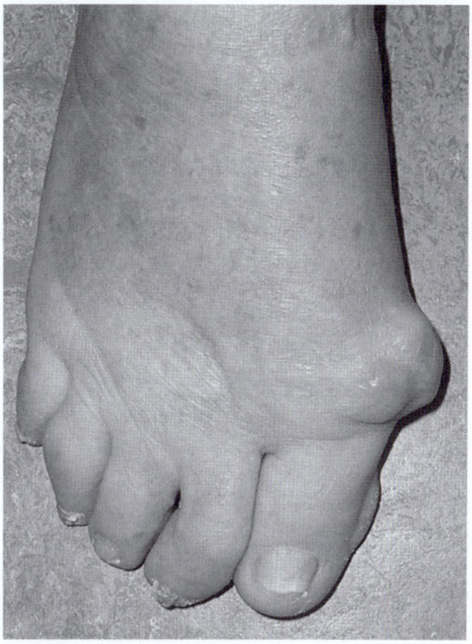

Figure 17.7 Dorsal and medial exostoses of arthritic hallux valgus.

IMAGES

long-bone stress fractures and 5 weeks in cancellous bones. Diagnosis is based on the location of symptoms and exclusion of the other differential diagnoses. The practitioner should have a high index of suspicion in athletic or military patients and the clinical picture, relation to activity and local tenderness should point towards the correct diagnosis. One should be aware of metatarsal 'stress fractures' in the diabetic patient, as they may be the precursor of Charcot's foot.

Exostoses

A bony outgrowth is termed an exostosis and the location within the foot and ankle varies. Most exostoses are associated with joints and can be related to osteoarthritis (termed an osteophyte). Common locations for these are the dorsal aspect of the first MTPJ in hallux rigidus, and the dorsal aspect of the second and third tarsometatarsal joints. Exostoses can also occur at joints without arthritis and the obvious site in the foot is the medial exostosis of the first metatarsal in hallux valgus. In cases of arthritic hallux valgus deformity exostoses will be found both on the medial and dorsal aspects (Fig. 17.7).

Exostoses can also develop away from joints and the two commonest sites in the foot are the posterior aspect of the calcaneum (termed retrocalcaneal exostosis) and under a toenail (termed subungual exostosis). The latter is technically an osteochondroma and is usually congenital rather than traumatic in origin like the other exostoses. The aetiology of true exostoses is likely to be due to repetitive microtrauma resulting in bony proliferation. This causes localised tenderness of the soft tissues and can result in the development of an adventitious bursa which often becomes inflamed, exacerbating the symptoms.

Accessory bones

Accessory bones are anatomical variants found within tendons. Some are always present, such as the patella or hallucal sesamoids where they are present to increase the mechanical advantage of the attached muscle by acting as a pulley. Numerous other accessory bones have been documented within the lower limb. The vast majority are asymptomatic but some have been associated with pathology. These include:

- os tibialis externum or accessory navicular with posterior tibialis tendinopathy
- os peroneum in peroneus longus tendon (often following an ankle sprain)
- os trigonum causing posterior ankle impingement.

The os trigonum causes symptoms with activities in repeated plantarflexion, affecting football players and dancers standing 'en pointe'. Patients complain of posterolateral ankle pain when the ankle is plantarflexed and impingement occurs. An accessory navicular may cause rubbing in a shoe, because of local pressure, or may become symptomatic following a twisting injury to the foot. It is associated with a flatfoot posture and often first presents in sporty adolescents. The accessory navicular is easily palpated within the tibialis posterior tendon and usually can be mobilised with gentle pressure which causes pain. Pain on resisted inversion is common. With a symptomatic os trigonum tenderness may be felt behind the lateral malleolus and peroneal tendons and forced passive plantarflexion of the ankle will be painful. Pain around an os peroneum usually occurs following an inversion ankle sprain with localised tenderness and pain up resisted eversion.

Plain X-rays will demonstrate the presence of accessory bones (Fig. 17.8) but their presence is not proof of their guilt. A bone scan may help to demonstrate a symptomatic accessory bone. MRI or ultrasound can pick up localised inflammation. A diagnostic local anaesthetic injection can also be used.

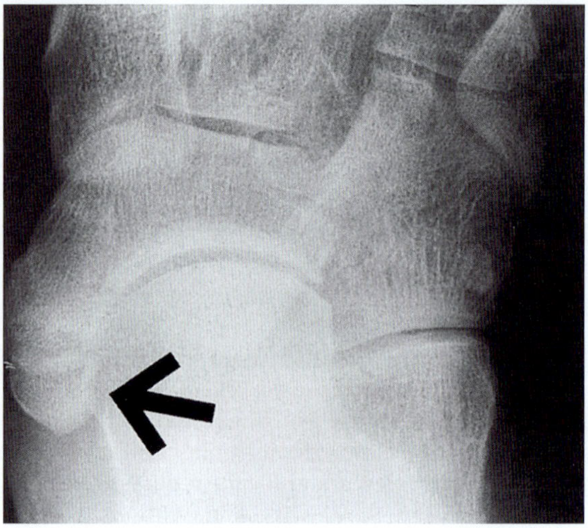

Figure 17.8 X-ray showing accessory navicular (arrow) – dorsiplantar view.

Sesamoiditis

Flexor hallucis brevis inserts into the base of the proximal phalanx of the hallux and within its tendons two sesamoid bones lie under the first metatarsal head. Sesamoids can be a source of pain for a variety of reasons:

- If they become arthritic (often with hallux rigidus or long-standing hallux valgus)
- Stress fracture or complete fracture
- Hypertrophy of a sesamoid can lead to a painful plantar callosity
- Inflammatory arthropathy or gout can affect the sesamoids
- Chondromalacia-type changes have also been reported.

The presenting symptom is primarily pain localised to either bone. Inflammation of the plantar structures of the first MTPJ including bursitis may also be present along with a plantar callosity. A high arch or cavus foot type with a plantarflexed first ray is usually a contributory factor. Resisted extension at the first MTPJ may be limited and painful. A standing DP and axial X-rays depicting the sesamoids should be requested. Careful examination of the sesamoids is required as they may frequently appear fractured when in fact the sesamoid is naturally separated into two or more pieces (bipartite or tripartite). In cases of true fracture the fragments are irregular and do not have a complete cortical rim. If X-rays are normal, a bone scan or MRI may be helpful.

Bone tumours

Bony or cartilaginous tumours are fortunately rare in the foot. Nevertheless, a number have been reported, both benign and malignant. Among the most common benign ones are osteoid osteoma, enchondroma and osteochondroma. Osteoid osteomas may occur in the tarsus in the foot, enchondromas in metatarsals or phalanges and osteochondromas normally only occur as subungual exostoses. Malignant tumours reported include osteosarcoma, chondrosarcoma and Ewing's tumour. Osteosarcomas and chondrosarcomas have been reported in the tarsus and metatarsals, and Ewing's in the tarsus. Although a secondary deposit is the most common bony tumour in the body as a whole, secondaries are rare in the foot but may occur: if they do, the most likely primary is a bronchial carcinoma. For a fuller discussion of bone tumours see Chapter 12.

Metabolic bone disease

Metabolic bone disease is an umbrella term that covers a number of disorders related to the weakening of the bone or impaired systems function caused by an imbalance in vitamin D_3, calcium and phosphorus. This imbalance may be caused by a lack, or too much of one of these three essential elements or the failure to provide one or more of them in a bioavailable form. The common causes of metabolic bone disease include osteoporosis, osteogenesis imperfecta, osteopetrosis, Paget's disease, rickets, osteomalacia, hyperparathyroidism, and vitamin D intoxication. Abnormalities of bone metabolism can cause a variety of symptoms primarily associated with bone pain and pathological fractures affecting any part of the body. The radiological features of these conditions are given in Chapter 12.

Ligaments injuries

Grading of ligament injuries

Ligament injuries are very common in the lower limb. The lateral collateral ligament injury to the ankle is the commonest acute ligament injury. Other common sites include the anterior cruciate and medial collateral ligaments of the knee, interosseous ligament of the sinus tarsi and occasionally the deltoid ligament, spring ligament, bifurcate ligament, and medial collateral ligament of the first metatarsophalangeal joint. Ligament injuries are graded from 1 to 3 depending on the severity of the injury:

- Grade 1: stretching of the ligament without macroscopic tears or joint laxity
- Grade 2: partial macroscopic tear with joint laxity
- Grade 3: complete rupture with excessive joint laxity.

Injuries to ligaments are invariably acute in nature and occur when the mechanical strength of the ligament is exceeded by the applied force. Joint pathology such as arthritis can follow ligament trauma due to the reduced mechanical stability of the joint.

Although ligaments are primarily avascular, ligament injuries involve significant swelling due to trauma to the adjacent soft tissues. The degree of swelling is often commensurate with the degree of damage to the ligament. Therefore, grade 3 injuries are associated with more swelling than grade 1 injuries.

Ankle ligament sprains

The majority of ankle sprains involve grade 1 injuries to the anterior talofibular ligament that heal without complication. However, up to 40% of ankle sprains are associated with persistent pain that may be due to mechanical or functional instability of the ankle, subtle fractures, osteochondral defects of the talus, or additional soft-tissue injuries to adjacent structures (Fallat et al 1998, Gerber et al 1998). Diagnosis of these additional injuries starts with the practitioner having a high level of suspicion that additional pathology can and often does occur with an ankle sprain. Attention to detail of the injury mechanism and location of symptoms is essential in identifying the additional injured structure. Finally specific tests or imaging techniques can confirm the diagnosis.

Mechanical instability occurs with grade 2 or 3 sprains and is associated with the ankle repeatedly giving way. This mechanical instability can affect both the ankle and subtalar joints (Clanton & Berson 1999, Hertel et al 1999). It may be associated with a cavus foot type, weak or dysfunctional peroneal muscles, or an ineffective treatment plan following the initial ankle sprain. Examination may reveal these associated factors along with laxity of the anterior talofibular ligament with tenderness and minor swelling. Functional instability occurs due to impaired proprioception following an ankle sprain. This loss of the protective action of the peroneals greatly increases the susceptibility of the ankle to further spraining. Both forms of instability can, and frequently do, co-exist.

Syndesmosis injuries to the anterior inferior tibiofibular ligament are relatively common with lateral ankle sprains. They occur in 15% of ankle sprains and are the commonest cause of persistent pain following

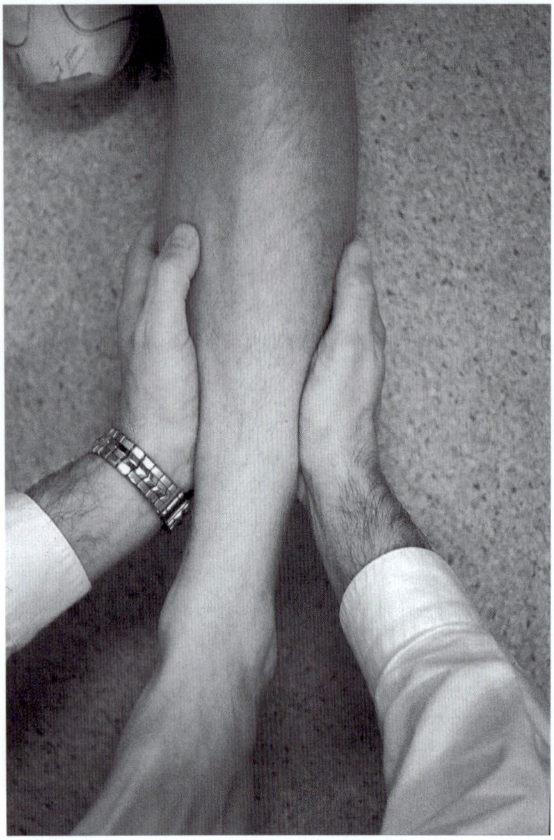

Figure 17.9 Squeeze test for syndesmosis injury.

an ankle sprain (Gerber et al 1998). They can be diagnosed clinically by combined dorsiflexion and external rotation of the foot which pushes the talus against the fibula stretching the ligament and causing pain. This can also be achieved by squeezing the fibula against the tibia at the mid-shaft level. This is called the squeeze test (Fig. 17.9). Diagnosis can be confirmed by weightbearing X-rays or MRI.

Lisfranc injuries

Lisfranc injuries are fortunately not common, accounting for only 1% of all joint dislocations. However, when they do occur, they are associated with a high level of morbidity particularly if a fracture dislocation has occurred, if the diagnosis is missed, or reduction incomplete. The mechanism of injury is usually a forced plantarflexion of the forefoot on a stable rearfoot. The commonest cause for this injury is following a motor vehicle accident or following more innocuous trauma such as stepping in a hole or slipping down the stairs. Patients are

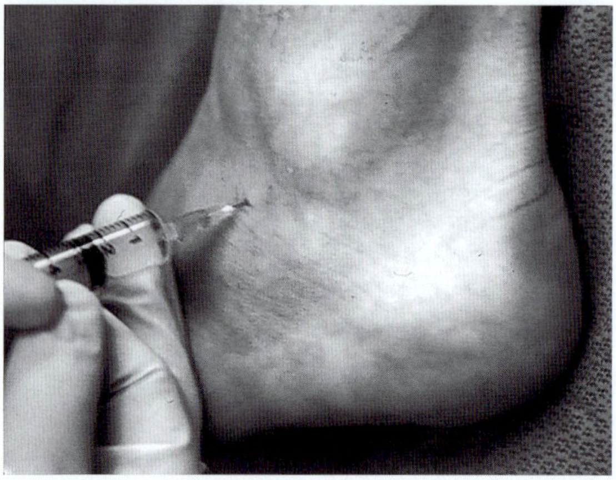

Figure 17.10 Injection into the sinus tarsi.

often aware of a snapping or popping sound at the time of the injury.

As with all ligament injuries complete rupture of the ligaments is associated with significant swelling and usually malalignment due to fracture dislocation. The more subtle injuries with little swelling are harder to diagnose. The practitioner should have a high index of suspicion based on the location of symptoms and injury history. There are several classification systems which have been recommended for Lisfranc injuries such as the classifications of Hardcastle and Wilson. All of these classifications are wholly or partly based on radiographic findings. X-rays remain the cornerstone of diagnosis of these complex injuries, although CT scanning is now commonly used especially to aid surgical planning.

Sinus tarsi syndrome

This syndrome was first described in 1958 by O'Connor. It involves inflammation and fibrosis of the contents of the sinus tarsi following a sprain of the coronary and talocalcaneal ligaments. This usually occurs as part of an ankle sprain but may also be due to compression of the lateral aspect of the subtalar joint in severe pronation. The patient will complain of localised pain with minimal swelling that is exacerbated by subtalar motion. Firm palpation of the sinus tarsi also reproduces the pain. Diagnosis should be confirmed by injection of local anaesthetic into the sinus tarsi. Frequently this is mixed with corticosteroid to reduce symptoms (Fig. 17.10).

Flexor plate tears

Tears in the joint capsule are usually caused by an acute injury such as hyperextension of a toe causing a tear in the plantar joint capsule of the metatarsophalangeal joint. This is often caused by a stubbing injury. They are often misdiagnosed in the acute form as the symptoms of pain and swelling without deformity or abnormal movement are similar to many soft-tissue injuries. Often it is not until the pain becomes constant and a deformity develops that the diagnosis is made. The localised swelling and inflammation often irritates the plantar digital nerve mimicking neuroma symptoms, which further complicates diagnosis. The situation is compounded by the inability of MRI or ultrasound to pick up tears in the joint capsule, as these tests are the standard for soft-tissue pathology. Tears can really only be seen by injecting a dye into the joint and then imaging the joint using X-ray, MRI or CT. It is also possible to assess the degree of laxity of the joint by firmly grasping the base of the second proximal phalanx and mobilising it in the sagittal plane on the metatarsal head. Excessive movement indicates plantar disruption of the joint capsule.

Tendon pathology

Tear or rupture

The diagnosis of acute tendon rupture is generally straightforward due to the level of pain, swelling, and lack of function of the torn tendon. However, in cases of long-standing tendinosis that progress to rupture, the diagnosis often requires imaging for confirmation as these signs and symptoms are already present from the tendinosis. A tear will result in a reduction of the physiological strength of the tendon and if it is significant then this can be determined clinically by stress testing of the tendon and by comparing strengths to the unaffected side. Stress testing should be progressively harder to determine which tendon is affected and to assess the degree of pathology. Initially testing is by concentric contraction, progressing to eccentric contraction and finally functional stress testing if painful symptoms are not induced by the first two.

The commonest tendons affected in the foot and ankle are the Achilles tendon, tibialis posterior, the peroneals, tibialis anterior, and the flexor hallucis longus tendon.

Tendinopathy

Tendon pathologies usually occur at specific well-recognised sites along the tendon path. Certain factors are usually present which predispose that specific part of the tendon to injury. These factors are:

- reduced blood supply (hypovascular or water-shed area)
- section of the tendon adjacent to a bony prominence
- section of the tendon which changes direction
- section of the tendon with re-orientation of its fibres.

One or several of these factors are usually present in tendinopathy. Consider tibialis posterior tendinopathy which characteristically occurs inferior to the medial malleolus, about 4 cm proximal to the insertion. This section of the tendon is associated with a change in direction, it lies close to a bony prominence, and has the least blood supply. Awareness of these principles can assist the practitioner in diagnosis of tendinopathies. Many factors exist which can predispose tendon injury including; muscle inflexibility/weakness, joint stiffness, malalignment, increased age, obesity, systemic disease, oral or injectable corticosteroids, and fluoroquinolone antibiotics.

Tendinosis

The exact pathological process that causes the pain in tendinopathy is not fully known. Inflammation of the tendon itself does not occur and therefore the term tendonitis should not be used. Inflammation of the tendon sheath or paratenon (tenosynovitis or paratenonitis) can occur and results in obvious swelling with occasional crepitus and formation of nodules. Fibrous thickening of the tendon sheath can occur in long-standing cases (Fig. 17.11). The patient will often complain of localised stiffness and discomfort after resting. Pain is often felt with strenuous exercise and the patient may recall instances of sharp pain during exercise which may represent partial tears. It is important to note that both tenosynovitis/paratenonitis and tendinosis can co-exist, giving mixed symptoms. Ultrasound (US) or MRI are the imaging modalities of choice in the assessment of tendon pathologies.

Subluxing tendons

The commonest site for subluxing tendons in the foot and ankle are the peroneal tendons around the lateral malleolus. The tendons normally run posterior to the malleolus and are held in place by the peroneal groove on the posterior aspect of the fibula and the peroneal retinacula. Disruption of the retinacula causes the tendons to sublux anteriorly which usually causes pain with resultant tendinopathy in long-standing cases. The subluxation often causes an

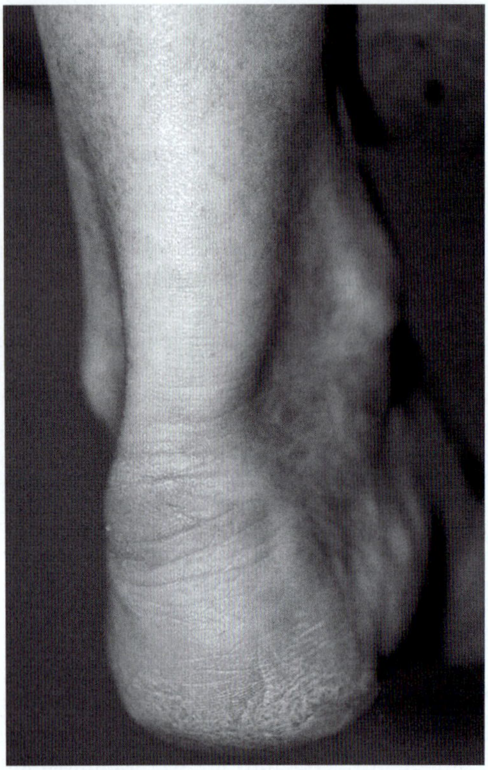

Figure 17.11 Achilles tendinopathy.

audible snap or popping sound and can be reproduced by resisted eversion with the ankle dorsiflexed.

Tibialis posterior tendon dysfunction

Tibialis posterior tendon dysfunction requires special mention as tendinopathy is often accompanied by significant structural changes affecting the midtarsal, then subtalar and finally the ankle joints. Tendon changes have been classified based on MRI appearance by Conti et al (1992):

- Grade 1 – accumulation of fluid and longitudinal micro-tears
- Grade 2 – attenuation with frank tears and intramural degeneration
- Grade 3 – partial or complete rupture of the tendon, marked swelling and scar tissue.

As the tendon changes progress the foot becomes more pronated with lowering of the medial longitudinal arch, inversion and abduction of the forefoot, and eversion of the rearfoot. These changes are due to the loss of supinatory power of the tibialis posterior and exacerbated by ankle equinus which is invariably present. In long-standing cases the rearfoot joints become fixed in this position and significant arthritis develops. Besides Conti's classification, other classifications have been proposed to take into account these structural changes and the Myerson classification is more meaningful as it can help in the management of the condition (Table 17.7).

Table 17.7 Classification of tibialis posterior dysfunction

Classification	*Clinical features*
I	Tenosynovitis without significant flatfoot deformity and no tendon tear
II	Partial rupture with flexible flatfoot deformity. Can be further subclassified into IIB with flexible forefoot supination and IIC fixed forefoot supination
III	Complete rupture with rigid hindfoot valgus, rigid forefoot supination due to arthritis
IV	Complete rupture with ankle valgus associated with deltoid ligament rupture. The ankle valgus deformity is either flexible (rare) or fixed

The patient will present with localised pain around the medial aspect of the ankle in the early stages of the condition. As it progresses and the heel moves into valgus pain may also occur laterally due to sinus tarsi syndrome or peroneal impingement. As the foot becomes progressively flatter arthritis will develop in the midtarsal, subtalar and medial column joints with localised pain and stiffness present. Eventually ankle malalignment and arthritis will develop and stress fracture of the fibula can occur. Severe flatfoot will be present with gross malalignment (Fig. 17.12).

The cornerstone of clinical diagnosis is stress testing of the tibialis posterior to assess its strength and function. This is achieved by asking the patient to invert their foot against resistance, and usually invokes pain along the course of the tendon below the medial malleolus. For functional testing of the tendon ask the patient to stand on tiptoe. This is called the tiptoe test and in the normal individual the

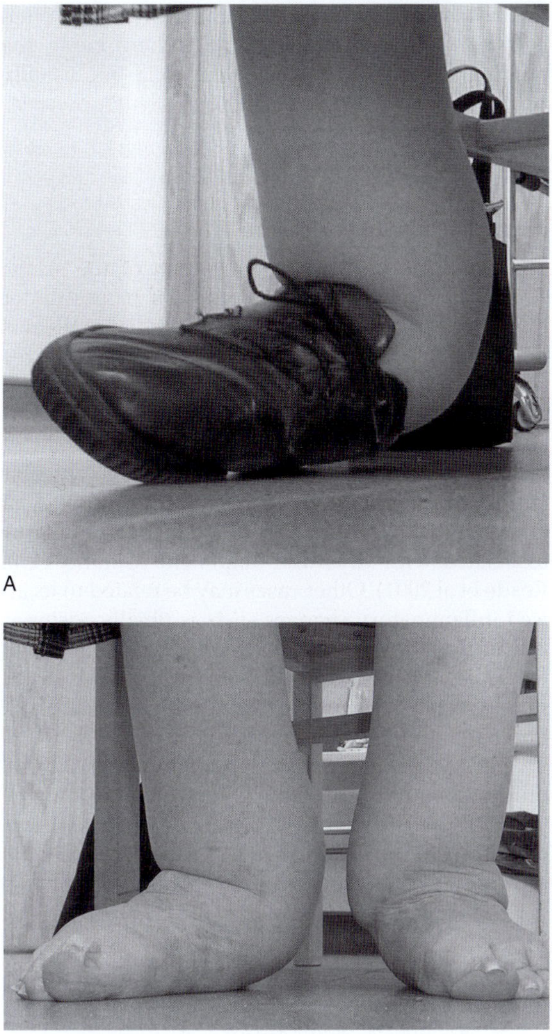

A

B

Figure 17.12 Gross flatfoot deformity with stage IV tibialis posterior dysfunction. **A** With shoe on. **B** Bare feet.

heel will invert under the action of the tibialis posterior as the heel lifts from the ground. In patients with stage I tibialis posterior dysfunction the heel may invert but not to the same extent as the unaffected side. Also asking the patient to repeat the test 10 times with the contralateral knee flexed will often induce pain in the tendon. In stage II tibialis posterior dysfunction, the heel will not invert and in stages III or IV the patient often cannot lift their heel at all.

Imaging of the tendon via ultrasound or MRI will show the degree of pathology not only to the tendon but also to the surrounding soft tissues and can help dictate management.

Fascia

Plantar fasciitis

Plantar fasciitis is undoubtedly one of the commonest causes of foot pain. It has been estimated to affect two million people a year in the USA (Pfeffer et al 1999) and is thought to affect 15% of all adults at some stage of their life. In the vast majority of cases the cause of the condition is mechanical overload of the fascia resulting in localised inflammation. The aetiology is multifactorial and includes:

- overuse (e.g. occupations involving prolonged standing, runners)
- obesity (most studies report average body mass index >30)
- biomechanical dysfunction (pronated foot type, hallux rigidus)
- age (highest incidence is in middle age)
- muscle inflexibility (ankle equinus)
- inflammatory arthropathy.

The evidence to support these causes is often lacking but one or more are usually present clinically.

Plantar fasciitis usually presents with an insidious onset of pain. Occasionally patients may recall an instance of a sharp stabbing pain that then became chronic in nature. This is usually due to a small tear in the plantar fascia. Post-static dyskinesia or 'first step' pain is invariably present with patients reporting pain following standing or walking after a period of rest/sleep. This is thought to be due to stiffening of the soft tissues with the initial stages of scar tissue formation during the period of rest. Then when the person walks the scar tissue breaks down and stiffened structures are stretched, causing pain.

The pain is localised to the medical calcaneal tubercle or more distally along the central or medial bands of the fascia. The best way to reproduce the symptoms is to first dorsiflex the ankle and toes to stretch the plantar fascia and then with the other hand run the thumb down the length of the plantar fascial bands from distal to proximal to see if this produces pain in the instep. Then examine the heel by firm palpation again with the plantar fascia on stretch. Firm palpation is required as the plantar fat pad is approximately 15 mm thick and the fascia lies directly deep to this structure. Localised pressure should be applied to the central, medial and lateral aspects of the underside of the heel to locate the area of inflammation. Pain on the medial/inferior border of the heel is usually due to localised nerve entrapment and not plantar fasciitis, although the two conditions often co-exist. In acute cases the patient often limps or walks without putting pressure on the heel. With time this will cause compensatory symptoms such as Achilles tendinopathy, metatarsalgia, and occasionally medial or lateral ankle pain.

Imaging may demonstrate a thickened plantar fascia, calcaneal marrow oedema or spur. The presence of a spur is not diagnostic, although spurs are more frequently present in patients with plantar fasciitis than those without the condition. US is now the modality of choice for diagnosing plantar fasciitis.

Chronic compartment syndrome

Chronic compartment syndrome (CCS) occurs when the intracompartmental pressure within a myofascial compartment is abnormally high. During exercise muscle volume increases by up to 20%. The muscles within the lower leg and foot are surrounded by inelastic fascial boundaries. If these boundaries cannot accommodate the increase in muscle volume then the intracompartmental pressure rises and interstitial fluid accumulates. The exact cause of the pain that ensues is not known at present. It may be that the increased pressure inhibits muscle blood flow causing ischaemic pain. It may also be that there is increased pressure on the pacinian corpuscles (pressure receptors) within the fascia causing pain.

CCS most commonly occurs in the lower leg. CCS of the foot has been reported more frequently in the recent literature but it still remains a rare condition. When present it usually occurs in the medial compartment. Patients complain of a cramping aching pain that is induced by exercise. The patient will have to reduce the intensity of exercise or stop exercising before the pain disappears. Pain usually resolves within 5 minutes to an hour of stopping exercise. Occasionally the patient will complain of numbness distal to the affected compartment due to the elevated pressure inhibiting sensory nerve function. It is possible to measure the increased intracompartmental pressure to confirm the diagnosis.

Plantar fibroma

Plantar fibroma is one of the commonest benign tumours of the foot and ankle and occurs within the plantar fascia. They are genetically linked to palmer fibromatoses, also known as Dupuytren's contracture of the hand. They are more common in males with a peak incidence in the third to fifth decades. They are slow growing and usually only present when the patient becomes aware that there is a lump on the sole of the foot. As the lump grows it will often become tender. It can occur anywhere along the medial or central bands of the fascia but usually occurs in the instep.

Nerves

Tarsal tunnel syndrome

The posterior tibial nerve, a branch of the sciatic nerve, may become compressed as it passes under the flexor retinaculum behind the medial malleolus (Fig. 17.13). The condition is analogous to carpal tunnel syndrome in the wrist, but it is not as common as the latter. The compression may cause direct pressure, leading to motor and sensory symptoms. Most commonly the compression affects the vascular supply causing sensory symptoms only. Aetiology of tarsal tunnel syndrome is idiopathic, traumatic or associated with structural alignment (Cimino 1990, Reade et al 2001). Other cases may be related to localised inflammatory changes such as tibialis posterior dysfunction or systemic disease such as RA or diabetes. Compression within the tunnel can also occur due to a space-occupying lesion such as a ganglion, lipoma or venous varicosities.

The patient is likely to complain of a diffuse, burning, tingling or numbness type of pain along the path of the affected nerve. With time symptoms may become more localised. Often pain is worse on activity and better at rest. A proportion of patients get night-time pain and about 30% have proximal

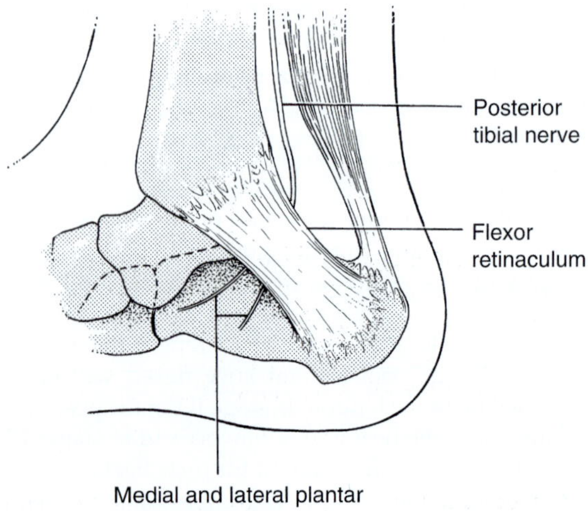

Figure 17.13 Gross anatomy of the tarsal tunnel – lateral view.

radiation of pain to the midcalf region, known as the Valleix phenomenon (Mann 2006). Sensory deficit or motor weakness is rare but should be carefully looked for. The commonest sign of motor weakness is weak toe flexion. Most diagnostic is a positive Tinel's sign, obtained by starting proximally and percussing along the course of the nerve. At the site of entrapment percussion will cause radiation of pain along the course of the nerve.

Plain X-rays may demonstrate any post-traumatic bony spurs causing compression but do not in themselves constitute a diagnosis. MRI or US may show a space-occupying lesion or localised inflammation. Electrodiagnostic tests can confirm the diagnosis via nerve conduction studies looking at sensory conduction velocities and the amplitude and duration of motor-evoked potentials (Ch. 7). Tests should be performed bilaterally and peripheral neuropathy should be excluded. Nerve conduction studies often fail to identify localised nerve entrapments such as to the medial calcaneal nerve or branch of the lateral plantar nerve to abductor digiti quinti.

Because of the diffuse nature of the symptoms the differential diagnosis is quite wide, but two possibilities should be particularly looked for. A peripheral neuropathy, for example from diabetes, may cause burning pains in the foot, but is usually bilateral where as tarsal tunnel syndrome is rarely bilateral. Sciatica with nerve root irritation causing distal pain also needs to be excluded. Straight leg raising will be restricted and painful.

Other entrapments

Other entrapments which have been described include the deep peroneal nerve under the inferior extensor retinaculum, the superficial peroneal nerve as it exits the deep fascia about 10 cm above the lateral malleolus, the medial plantar nerve at the master knot of Henry, the first branch of the lateral plantar nerve between abductor hallucis and quadratus plantae muscles at the inferior-medial border of the heel, and the dorsomedial nerve at the first MTPJ. The aetiology is due to localised compression from acute or chronic trauma to the nerve and may be due to:

- repetitive compression from sports (e.g. runners) – often the medial plantar nerve
- obesity – usually the branch of the lateral plantar nerve
- foot deformity – pronated foot posture with plantar nerves, supinated foot posture with deep peroneal nerve, Joplin's neuroma with hallux valgus
- arthritis – usually the deep peroneal nerve with second tarsometatarsal OA, Joplin's neuroma with hallux rigidus
- acute trauma –superficial peroneal nerve with an ankle sprain.

Symptoms and signs

Deep peroneal nerve

Patients complain of pain over the dorsum of the foot and sometimes numbness and paraesthesia in the first webspace. There may be altered sensation in the first webspace and a positive Tinel's sign. A common finding is arthritic change at the second tarsometatarsal joint or pes cavus foot type with dorsal prominence of the midfoot.

Superficial peroneal nerve

Symptoms include pain over the dorsum of the foot and ankle and inferior lateral border of the calf. Symptoms can be induced by inversion and plantarflexion of the foot which puts the nerve on stretch. As a sensory nerve there are no motor signs but there may be a positive Tinel's sign. Look for a fascial defect or muscle herniation where the nerve exits the deep fascia.

Medial plantar nerve

Patients complain of an aching pain over the medial aspect of the arch, often radiating into the medial three toes, becoming worse on running. Again, Tinel's sign may be positive and there may also be tenderness under the medial arch (Case history 17.3).

First branch of lateral plantar nerve

Patients complain of chronic pain, often increased with prolonged weightbearing or waking. On examination there will be tenderness over the nerve deep to abductor hallucis and firm localised pressure reproduces the patient's symptoms. Plantar fasciitis is the main differential diagnosis and the conditions often co-exist.

Joplin's neuroma

Repetitive compression of the dorsomedial nerve to the first MTPJ against a bony prominence either due to hallux valgus or rigidus can cause this neuroma. Numbness or paraesthesia radiating up the medial aspect of the hallux will be present and the symptoms can be reproduced by firm compression over the nerve.

Case history 17.3

A 48-year-old keen runner, and squash and badminton player presented with an 18-month history of bilateral paraesthesia affecting the medial aspect of the soles of both feet, in the distribution of the medial plantar nerve, when running. Symptoms initially settled after exercise but over the next 6 months the patient developed shooting pains without any pattern of onset with increasing numbness in both feet. On examination, Tinel's sign was positive above both medial malleoli. Some loss of sharp and blunt sensory discrimination on the medial aspect of the sole was identified.

Nerve conduction studies showed conduction blocks bilaterally at the level of the tarsal tunnel. Medial plantar responses were absent on the right and delayed on the left.

Diagnosis: Bilateral tarsal tunnel syndrome. Operative findings included high division of the posterior tibial nerve into medial and lateral plantar branches on both sides. A sharp edge to abductor hallucis was compressing the medial plantar nerve bilaterally. In addition there was a large vascular pedicle crossing the medial plantar nerve and compressing it more proximally. Pain settled following surgery.

Nerve conduction studies are rarely helpful as they cannot consistently detect sensory dysfunction in these small nerves.

Peripheral neuropathy

Peripheral neuropathies may be due to a variety of causes. In the West the leading cause is diabetes and in developing countries the leading cause is leprosy. Other common causes are spina bifida, pernicious anaemia, drugs and alcoholism (Ch. 7). The different patterns of peripheral neuropathy may vary but in diabetes the most common is a symmetrical distal polyneuropathy, encompassing motor, sensory and autonomic components.

Peripheral neuropathy is often painless. The first inkling of a problem may be when a patient presents with a complication such as ulceration or infection. In the patient with diabetes who usually has a painless foot with no sensation the presence of pain is important and may indicate deep infection, such as an abscess or osteomyelitis or the development of Charcot's neuroarthropathy. If the presentation is of a painful neuropathy the patient may complain of a burning sensation in the legs and feet, commonly worse at night and usually bilateral.

Morton's neuroma

This condition is a type of entrapment neuropathy affecting a plantar digital nerve. It most commonly affects the common digital nerve to the third/fourth interspace, but may also occur in the second/third interspace. The diagnosis probably does not exist in the first or fourth webspaces, probably due to the wider space between these metatarsals, although in truth any nerve is capable of developing a neuroma. The incidence of a second neuroma in the same foot is 4% (Thompson & Deland 1993). Women are affected at least four times more often than men and the condition can affect adults of any age. The nerve develops a fusiform swelling, just proximal to its bifurcation, at the level of the intermetatarsal bursa (Fig. 17.14). Although frequently termed a neuroma, technically it is not as the histology shows a degenerative process rather than a proliferative one.

The patient complains of a burning pain on the sole of the foot, just distal to the metatarsal heads and commonly radiating into one or two toes. It may feel

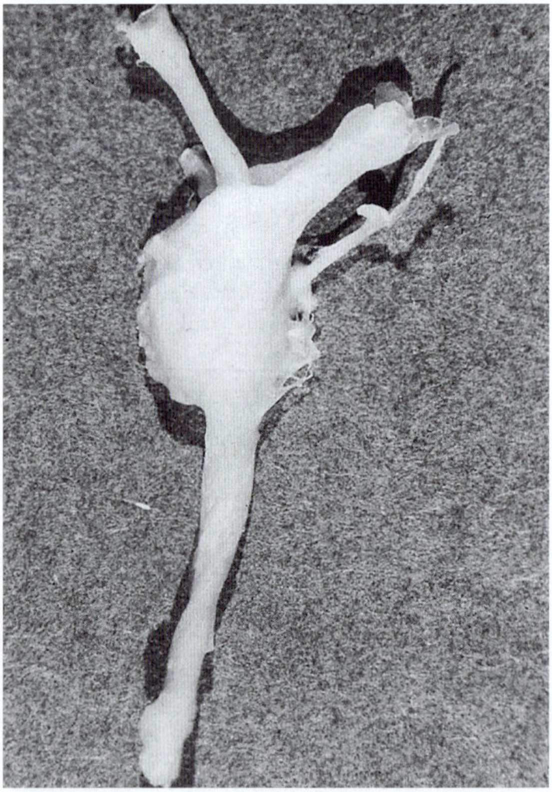

Figure 17.14 Resected Morton's neuroma showing terminal digital branches following operation.

to the patient like walking on a sharp pebble or is often described as an electric shock to the area. Occasionally, pain will radiate proximally. Pain is often worse on walking and may be particularly exacerbated by tight-fitting shoes, as these will compress the metatarsal heads together, thus 'trapping' the nerve. Resting or removing tight shoes may settle the pain. Only 25% of patients complain of numbness in the toes. The condition is usually insidious in onset, although occasionally it may be triggered by a particular activity. A common finding in patients with Morton's neuroma is forefoot deformity. Hallux valgus increases pressure and shear across the lesser MTPJs as does digital deformity such as hammer and claw toes. Inflammation of the intermetatarsal bursa or other space-occupying mass will also compress the nerve leading to a neuroma in long-standing cases.

Firm compression of the relevant interspace will usually reproduce the patient's pain. This is best achieved by splaying the affected digits with one hand and then using the thumb and index finger of the other hand to compress the intermetatarsal space initially distal to the MTPJs and then between the metatarsal heads. In the second clinical test, squeezing the forefoot just behind the first and fifth metatarsal heads closes the distance between the metatarsal heads. A painful click may be obtained, which is known as Mulder's click and is only helpful if it reproduces pain (Mulder 1951). Then the thumb of the other hand is used to push the soft tissues against the second/third metatarsal heads and then the third/fourth. This affectively traps the neuroma and reproduces the symptoms. It is important to demonstrate the test on an unaffected area first so that the patient can experience what is normal before the painful area is examined.

The use of a diagnostic local anaesthetic injection is possible but the practitioner must be very accurate in the placement of the injection especially if a differential diagnosis of capsulitis is present. US is more sensitive in the diagnosis of Morton's neuroma than MRI but neither give 100% reliability. In the author's experience they are only useful if bilateral neuromas are suspected or with mixed symptoms in the second intermetatarsal space where capsulitis of the second MTPJ is a common pathology.

Referred pain (radiculopathy)

The main source of referred pain in the lower limb is sciatica due to nerve root compression in the back. Most commonly this is due to a prolapsed intervertebral disc and over 90% of these occur at the L4/5 or L5/S1 levels.

Patients will usually complain of low back pain radiating into a buttock and down the leg. They may have little back pain and mainly leg pain. A careful history may indicate the nerve root involved. Pain radiating down the back of the leg into the sole of the foot or heel is generally S1 and this is a differential diagnosis in patients with inferior heel pain. Pain down the lateral border of the leg and into the hallux is generally L5 in origin.

In an acute disc prolapse the patient experiences considerable pain and cannot move easily. They may have a scoliotic tilt to the spine when viewed from behind, paraspinal muscle spasm and tenderness in the buttock. The clinical diagnosis can be confirmed with a straight leg raise test. The patient should lie supine with the arms at their sides and the examiner then slowly raises the limb with the knee fully extended and ankle in neutral. If the test is positive hip flexion is limited and the pain reproduced in the distribution of the nerve root. Sensory changes and muscle weakness appropriate to that nerve root may be found but are not common unless the condition is longstanding. Reflexes may be diminished; the knee jerk is L3/4 and the ankle jerk is L5/S1.

A positive straight leg raise test does not mean that all foot pain is referred and the practitioner should continue to assess the lower limb for other potential causes of the foot pain as conditions may co-exist (see Case history 17.4).

Skin and subcutaneous tissues

Bursitis

There are many anatomical bursae within the foot and ankle. Any of these can become inflamed, as can adventitious bursae which develop at sites of increased friction. The common sites for bursitis in the foot and ankle are the first MTPJ, second or third intermetatarsal space, and the posterior aspect of the calcaneum at the Achilles insertion.

Retrocalcaneal bursitis

There are two bursae at the heel: one is deep to the tendo Achilles and the other lies superficial to its insertion. The deep bursa is infrequently affected but, as it has a synovial lining, symptoms may be early indicators of an inflammatory arthropathy such as rheumatoid arthritis. Another cause for inflammation of this deep bursa is Haglund's prominence. Men are affected more often than women. Inflammation of the superficial bursa often occurs with

Case history 17.4

A 58-year-old man was referred by his general practitioner for a surgical opinion. He had a 2-year history of recalcitrant inferior heel pain. Previous treatments for the heel pain had involved orthoses, stretching exercises, ice, physiotherapy, non-steroidal anti-inflammatory drugs (NSAIDs) and two steroid injections. There was a history of long-standing lower back pain 4 years ago and two spinal operations (laminectomy) at the L4/5 and L5/S1 discs 18 months ago. Sciatic symptoms had resolved following the last operation but the foot pain remained. On examination, palpation of the heel could not reproduce the pain in the heel which was diffuse in nature. Straight leg raise reproduced the symptoms in the heel with hip flexion at 60°.

US scan confirmed no inflammation of the plantar fascia. MRI of the spine demonstrated a small bulge at the S1 nerve root.

Diagnosis: Radiculopathy. Patient was referred back to the spinal team.

insertional calcific Achilles tendinopathy or a retrocalcaneal exostosis on the posterolateral aspect of the heel (Fig. 17.15).

Patients commonly complain of a tender prominence at the heel when wearing shoes. This led to the eponym of 'heel or pump bump'. Palpation of the area will induce symptoms with the bony prominence or calcification of the tendon feeling hard with an overlying soft bursitis that appears red due to the localised inflammation. A functional or structural heel varus often with ankle equinus is a common finding.

Inflammation of the deep bursa will produce tenderness deep to the tendo Achilles. A lateral weight-bearing X-ray should be taken. With deep bursitis calcaneal erosions or Haglund's deformity should be looked for. In heel bumps the X-ray is usually normal but will show calcification of the Achilles insertion if this is present.

First metatarsophalangeal joint bursitis

Bursitis can occur plantar to the first MTPJ or on the medial or dorsomedial aspects of the joint. The latter two are associated with hallux valgus. Dorsomedial bursitis can also be present with hallux rigidus or an arthritic hallux valgus deformity. A similar bursitis may occur over the fifth MTP with a tailors bunion. All forms of these bursae are adventitious. Plantar bursitis of the first MTPJ is often associated with a

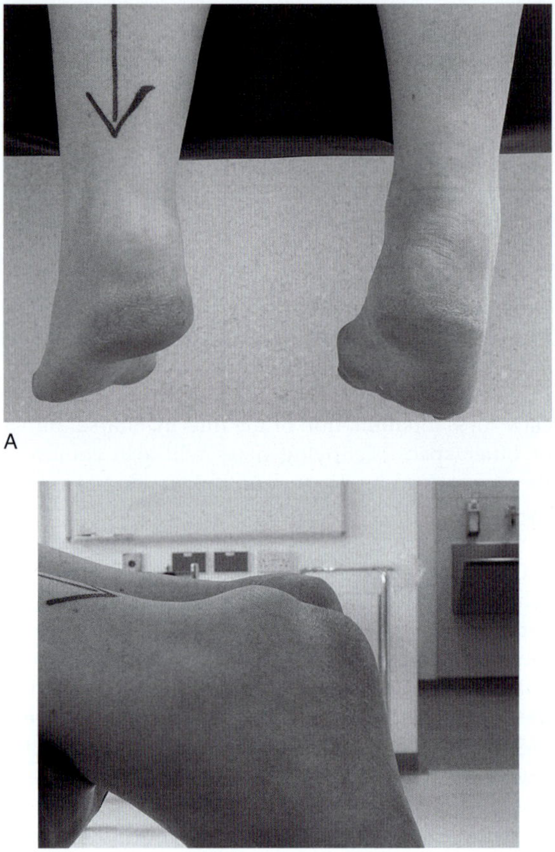

A

B

Figure 17.15 Bilateral retrocalcaneal exostosis with overlying bursitis. **A** Posterior view. **B** Lateral view.

IMAGES

plantarflexed first ray or previous injury to the plantar capsuloligamentous structures including the sesamoids. Plantar bursitis is always more fibrous than the dorsal or medial bursitis. Any may become infected which obviously greatly increases the degree of swelling and pain. The bursa will feel motile and soft. Localised erythema is present on the medial or dorsomedial bursitis but not plantar.

An ultrasound scan is useful in the diagnosis of plantar bursitis and to exclude other causes of plantar first MTP pain such as sesamoiditis or joint effusion.

Soft-tissue masses or tumours

The foot and ankle is the second most common site for soft-tissue masses or tumours after the hand and wrist. The most common benign soft-tissue mass of the foot and ankle is a ganglion. A ganglion is a mucoid cyst which usually arises from an underlying

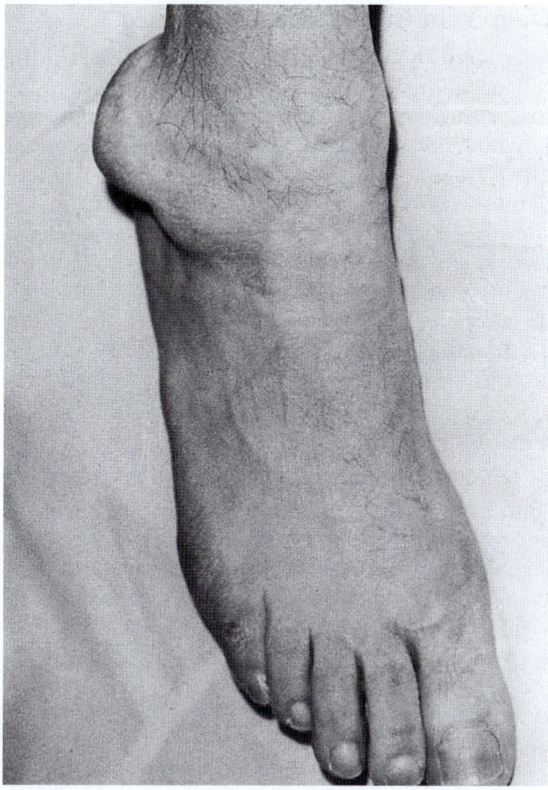

Figure 17.16 Large ganglion on lateral aspect of the ankle.

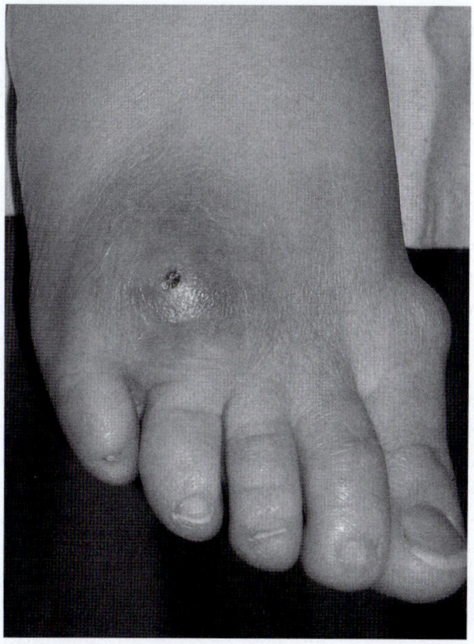

Figure 17.17 Large ganglion on the dorsal aspect of the forefoot with overlying sinus.

IMAGES

joint or occasionally from a tendon sheath. In the foot and ankle they most commonly occur around the ankle (Fig. 17.16) or the dorsum of the foot (Fig. 17.17). Other common soft-tissue tumours or masses of the foot and ankle are:

- giant cell tumour of tendon sheath – usually in an intermetatarsal space or dorsal midfoot
- lipoma – most commonly around the ankle
- angioleiomyoma – usually in the digits
- mucoid cyst – dorsal aspect of an interphalangeal joint
- plantar fibroma – within the plantar fascia
- epidermal cyst – superficial to the skin usually plantar
- glomus tumour – usually subungual or on the apex of the toe
- rheumatoid nodule – usually around a joint and most often in the forefoot.

The commonest presenting feature of a soft-tissue mass or tumour is localised pain. However, many patients may only be concerned about a diagnosis to ensure that the lump that has appeared is not cancer. Fortunately, soft-tissue tumours of the foot and ankle are rarely malignant but the clinician should be cognisant of the patient's concerns and refer them if there is any doubt about the diagnosis. When assessing these lumps the size, sponginess, motility, growth rate, and medical history can all help in the diagnosis.

Exact diagnosis can usually only be made by histological examination following excision or aspiration of the mass. US or MRI can be useful in surgical planning to delineate the morphology of the mass but cannot fully differentiate between the different types of soft-tissue tumours.

Vascular

Vascular pathology rarely presents itself just in the foot. There are usually significant signs of arterial or venous disease more proximally in the lower limb such as intermittent claudication of the calf in peripheral vascular disease or varicose veins in the calf or thigh due to venous incompetence. This reinforces the concept of a holistic approach to assessing the patient's foot pain, considering systemic causes of a distal localised complaint. Vascular assessment is covered in detail in Chapter 6.

Peripheral vascular disease

The common presenting features of peripheral vascular disease (PVD) may be intermittent claudication, usually of the calf, rest pain, or an ulcer. Rest pain and ischaemic ulceration affecting the foot and ankle are usually preceded by a history of intermittent claudication. However, if the patient cannot walk a reasonable distance due to other co-morbidities, intermittent claudication is often absent.

Rest pain usually occurs in the heel or arch most commonly at night as the feet are elevated. Patients often report that symptoms are relieved by hanging the feet down over the side of the bed. The pain is usually described as a cramping or burning sensation due to a lack of oxygenated blood to the affected tissues.

Ischaemic ulceration usually occurs around bony prominences such as the malleoli or fifth MTPJ and in the absence of neuropathy is exquisitely painful. Clinical signs of PVD will be present in the foot such as thin waxy skin, absence of hairs, thickened brittle nails, cold feet and a brick red discoloration to the plantar surface which is a sign of critical ischaemia.

Vasculitis

The symptoms of vasculitis depend on the particular blood vessels that are involved by the inflammatory process. Different types of vasculitis involve blood vessels in characteristic locations throughout the body. For example, giant cell arteritis typically involves the medium- to large-sized blood vessels supplying the head and neck. Other common sites include the blood vessels to the kidneys, the lungs, the upper respiratory tract, the skin and the small vessels of the fingers and toes. Gangrene can result from a profound lack of blood flow.

Patients with vasculitis often have fever, weight loss, fatigue, a rapid pulse, and diffuse aches and pains that are difficult to pinpoint. It has been said that vasculitis is a 'hurting disease', because it is so commonly associated with pain of one type or another: pain from a nerve infarction, pain from insufficient blood to the gastrointestinal tract, pain from skin ulcers. Joint pain is another common feature usually associated with swelling. The ankle is a common site. Abnormal sensations in the limbs including paraesthesia is common with nerve involvement.

Accurate diagnosis of vasculitis is often difficult as true diagnosis requires histopathological examination of an inflamed blood vessel. However, careful history taking and assessment will often lead to a provisional diagnosis of the condition.

Deep vein thrombosis

Deep vein thrombosis (DVT) usually occurs in the calf, occasionally in the thigh, and hardly ever in the foot. However, symptoms can occur in the foot with proximal occlusion leading to venous incompetence. The common symptoms of a DVT are localised tenderness, swelling, and sometimes erythema at the site of the occlusion. This will rarely cause pain in the foot. In the post-phlebitic syndrome foot symptoms can occur and usually involve pain, redness, thickening, and glossy appearance of the skin. An ulcer can occur months to years after the blood clot, most often around the medial malleolus.

Venous insufficiency

In venous insufficiency states, venous blood escapes from its normal antegrade path of flow and refluxes backwards down the veins into an already congested leg. Venous insufficiency syndromes are caused by valvular incompetence in the high-pressure deep venous system, low-pressure superficial venous system, or both. Untreated venous insufficiency in the deep or superficial system causes a progressive syndrome involving pain, swelling, skin changes and eventual tissue breakdown.

Patients present with a wide variety of symptoms within the leg and foot. The symptoms are most commonly described as burning, throbbing, aching and heaviness in the leg and foot. These symptoms are usually accompanied by swelling. Restless legs and leg fatigue are also common symptoms. The most common physical signs of venous insufficiency are those of the progressive syndromes of chronic venous stasis and chronic venous hypertension, and include: oedema, hyperpigmentation (haemosiderosis, see Ch. 6, Fig. 6.26), venous dermatitis (varicose eczema, see Ch. 6, Fig. 6.26), chronic cellulites, cutaneous infarction (atrophie blanche, see Ch. 6, Fig. 6.25), and venous ulceration (see Ch. 6, Fig. 6.28). The location of the varicose eczema, atrophie blanche, haemosiderosis and potential ulceration is always close to the superficial veins themselves so common sites include the dorsal aspect of the midfoot and around the ankle.

Global foot pain

Many conditions can cause pain all over the foot. The majority are systemic conditions such as severe RA, autoimmune conditions (e.g. vasculitis) and painful diabetic neuropathy. Significant trauma to multiple joints can also result in global foot pain initially in the acute phase and also in chronic states. Trauma is also the cause of complex regional pain syndrome (CRPS), which is a significant cause of globalised foot pain. Another potential cause of total foot pain is extensive infection. Both CRPS and infection are discussed below.

Infection

Infection may occur as cellulitis in the soft tissues, as osteomyelitis in the bone or as septic arthritis in a joint. The cause may be direct inoculation following an open wound, either traumatic or surgically created, or via haematogenous spread. Traumatic or surgical infection may occur at any time but septic arthritis is more likely to occur in the very young, the elderly or immunocompromised patient. *Staphylococcus aureus* is the commonest pathogen to cause cellulitis, septic arthritis and osteomyelitis and is responsible for between 50% and 75% of all of these types of infection. Other common pathogens are the streptococci.

The degree of swelling and pain will vary according to the tissue involved and degree of infection. Cellulitis will present with intense pain, swelling and erythema of the involved area. Sleep is often disturbed due to the degree of pain. Because the bones are very superficial in the foot, osteomyelitis should always be suspected under any area of cellulitis. Septic arthritis is likely to present with exquisite pain on moving a joint, usually the ankle, and with overlying swelling and erythema. However, in the elderly, ischaemic or immunocompromised patient, symptoms may be strikingly muted, reducing suspicion of an underlying infection. In acute septic arthritis, extensive cellulitis or osteomyelitis the patient is likely to have systemic signs of being unwell with a high temperature and nausea being common symptoms.

The cause of the infection should obviously be sought and investigations to determine the extent of infection carried out. These will include X-rays to exclude osteomyelitis or gas in the tissues. MRI and bone scintigraphy are both more sensitive for bone infection than X-ray, and MRI will also demonstrate soft-tissue infection. In septic arthritis a diminution in joint space or adjacent osteomyelitis may be seen. Aspiration of fluid from a joint and Gram stain and culture can provide a diagnosis. Blood cultures should also be done, and a full blood count will show a raised white cell count and ESR or CRP. CRP has now become the mainstay blood test in the assessment of acute infection and its response to treatment. Obviously, if there is an open discharge with pus then swabs should be taken, although direct samples of the infected tissue are more reliable for demonstrating the true infective organisms.

Complex regional pain syndrome

CRPS is a chronic pain condition that is believed to be the result of dysfunction in the central or peripheral nervous systems. Typical features include dramatic changes in the colour and temperature of the skin over the affected body part, accompanied by intense burning pain, skin sensitivity, sweating and swelling. CRPS I is frequently triggered by tissue injury; the term describes all patients with the above symptoms but with no underlying nerve injury. Patients with CRPS II experience the same symptoms but their symptoms are clearly associated with a nerve injury. Older terms used to describe CRPS are 'reflex sympathetic dystrophy syndrome' and 'causalgia'. CRPS can strike at any age and affects both men and women, although it is more common in young women and smokers. The key symptom of CRPS is continuous, intense pain out of proportion to the severity of the injury, which gets worse rather than better over time. CRPS usually follows a traumatic event such as a fracture or following surgery. However, it may also be triggered by an innocuous injury such as tripping on a kerb, falling down a few stairs. CRPS most often affects one of the extremities (arms, legs, hands, or feet) and common symptoms include:

- 'burning' pain
- increased skin sensitivity changes in skin temperature: warmer or cooler compared to the opposite extremity
- changes in skin colour: often blotchy, purple, pale, or red
- changes in skin texture: shiny and thin, and sometimes excessively sweaty
- changes in nail and hair growth patterns
- swelling and stiffness in affected joints
- motor disability, with decreased ability to move the affected body part.

Often the pain spreads to include the entire limb, even though the initiating injury might have been only to a toe. Pain can sometimes even travel to the opposite extremity. It may be heightened by emotional stress (see Case history 17.5). The symptoms of CRPS vary in severity and length. Some experts believe there are three stages associated with CRPS, marked by progressive changes in the skin, muscles, joints, ligaments, and bones of the affected area,

Case history 17.5

A 13-year-old schoolgirl presented following nail surgery (phenolisation) with positive subungual exostosis over the left hallux. This was confirmed by X-ray. Following an exostectomy to remove the bone, intractable pain developed in a pattern unusual for postoperative events at 6 weeks. Stabbing and crushing pain was described, with extreme sensitivity over the foot. On examination, the foot was swollen and blue. Analgesics were of minimal help. The patient had a tendency to hysterical fits. Over an 18-month period the contralateral side became affected.

Infection was excluded. Surgery was performed on two further occasions by different surgeons in case an exostosis was still present. Amitriptyline 10 mg at night provided minimal help in reducing vasomotor activity. A lumbar sympathectomy (guanethidine) only gave temporary relief. Psychiatric assessment was considered.

Diagnosis: CRPS with hysteria.

although this progression has not yet been validated by clinical research studies.

Case history 17.5 highlights the ease with which inappropriate management and additional physical insult can elevate the patient's problem. CRPS is a difficult problem to manage and non-invasive techniques should be emphasised, with total pain-blocking control and maintenance of mobility if the pain syndrome is diagnosed (Tollafield 1991).

Stage 1 is thought to last from 1 to 3 months and is characterised by severe, burning pain, along with muscle spasm, joint stiffness, rapid hair growth and alterations in the blood vessels that cause the skin to change color and temperature. Stage 2 lasts from 3 to 6 months and is characterized by intensifying pain, swelling, decreased hair growth, cracked, brittle, grooved, or spotty nails, softened bones, stiff joints and weak muscle tone. In stage 3 the syndrome progresses to the point where changes in the skin and bone are no longer reversible. Pain becomes unyielding and may involve the entire limb or affected area. There may be marked muscle loss (atrophy), severely limited mobility, and involuntary contractions of the muscles and tendons that flex the joints. The limbs may become contorted.

CRPS is diagnosed through observation of the signs and symptoms. The practitioner should have a high index of suspicion in patients presenting with any of the above symptoms especially following a traumatic episode. Early diagnosis and treatment usually improves the prognosis of CRPS. Plain X-rays may show osteopenia within a few weeks and subperiosteal bone resorption. A bone scan will show generalised increased uptake in the affected area. Patients have a characteristic delayed bone scan pattern of diffuse increased tracer throughout the foot, with juxta-articular uptake accentuation (Holder et al 1992). Temporary pain relief from a lumbar sympathetic block is also a useful test, although a negative test does not exclude CRPS.

Summary

There are many causes of foot pain. Knowledge of the common causes of foot pain both by region and tissue type will aid the practitioner in formulating an accurate list of differential diagnoses. Pain is subjective and is a very personal experience, and the pain associated with certain foot conditions can manifest at various levels. Practitioners must undertake a careful history, examination and relevant investigations to assess a patient with foot pain if an accurate diagnosis is to be made. Only then can effective treatment plans be implemented.

References

Badlissi F, Dunn J, Link C et al 2005 Foot musculoskeletal disorders, pain, and foot related functional limitation in older persons. Journal of the American Geriatric Society 53(6):1029–1033

Beck T, Ruff C, Shaffer R 2000 Stress fracture in military recruits: gender differences in muscle and bone susceptibility factors. Bone 27(3):437–444

Bennell K, Malcolm S, Thomas S et al 1996 The incidence and distribution of stress fractures in competitive track and field athletes. American Journal of Sports Medicine 24(2):211–217

Bennett P J, Patterson C 1998 The Foot Health Questionnaire (FHSQ): a new instrument for measuring outcomes of foot care. Australian Journal of Podiatric Medicine 32(3):87–92

Bennett P J, Patterson C, Wearing S et al 1998 Development and validation of a questionnaire designed to measure foot-health status. Journal of the American Podiatric Medical Association 88(9):419–428

Benvenuti F, Ferrucci L, Guralnik M et al 1995 Foot pain and disability in older persons: an epidemiologic study. Journal of the American Geriatrics Society 43(5):479–484

Berndt A, Harty M 1959 Transchondral fractures (osteochondritis dissecans) of the talus. Journal of Bone and Joint Surgery (Am) 41:988–1020

Brosh T, Arcan M 1994 Toward early detection of the tendency to stress fractures. Clinical Biomechanics 9:111–116

Brukner P, Bennell K 2001 Stress fractures. In: O'Connor FG, Wilder RP (eds) Textbook of running medicine. McGraw Hill, New York, pp 227–256

Brunet M, Cook S, Brinker M et al 1990 A survey of running injuries in 1505 competitive and recreational runners. Journal of Sports Medicine and Physical Fitness 30:307–315

Burns J, Crosbie J, Hunt A et al 2005 The effect of pes cavus on foot pain and plantar pressure. Clinical Biomechanics 20(9):877–882

Cameron K, Wark J, Telford R 1992 Stress fractures and bone loss: the skeletal cost of intense athleticism. Excel 8:39–55

Cimino W R 1990 Tarsal tunnel syndrome: a review of the literature. Foot and Ankle 11:47–52

Clanton T, Berson L 1999 Subtalar joint athletic injuries. Foot Ankle Clinics 4(4):729–743

Conti S, Michelson J, Jhass M 1992 Clinical significance of MRI in pre-operative planning for reconstruction of posterior tibial tendon ruptures. Foot and Ankle 13:208–214

Emery P, Breedveld F, Dougados M et al 2002 Early referral recommendation for newly diagnosed rheumatoid arthritis: evidence based development of a clinical guide. Annals of the Rheumatic Diseases 61:290–297

Fallat L, Grimm D, Saracco J 1998 Sprained ankle syndrome: prevalence and analysis of 639 acute injuries. Journal of Foot Ankle Surgery 37(4):280–285

Finestone A, Giladi M, Elad H et al 1999 Prevention of stress fractures using custom biomechanical shoe orthoses. Clinical Orthopaedics 164(2):153–156

Friberg O 1982 Leg length asymmetry in stress fractures: a clinical and radiological study. Journal of Sports Medicine 22:485–488

Garrow A, Papageorgiou A, Silman A J et al 2000 Development and validation of a questionnaire to assess disabling foot pain. Pain 85(1–2):107–113

Garrow A, Spilman A, Macfarlane G 2004 The Cheshire foot pain and disability survey: a population survey assessing prevalence and associations. Pain 110:378–384

Gerber J, Williams G, Scoville C et al 1998 Persistent disability associated with ankle sprains: a prospective examination of an athletic population. Foot and Ankle International 19(10):653–660

Giladi M, Milgrom C, Stein M et al 1985 The low arch, a protective factor in stress fractures: a prospective study of 295 military recruits. Orthopaedic Review 14:709–714

Hammerschlag W, Rice J, Caldwell D et al 1991 Psoriatic arthritis of the foot and ankle: analysis of joint involvement and diagnostic error. Foot and Ankle 12:35–39

Helliwell P, Reay N, Gilworth G et al 2005 Development of a foot impact scale for rheumatoid arthritis. Arthritis Care and Research 53(3):418–422

Hertel J, Denegar C, Monroe M et al 1999 Talocrural and subtalar joint instability after lateral ankle sprain. Medicine and Science in Sports and Exercise 31(11):1501–1508

Hoffman J, Chapnik L, Shamis A 1999 The effect of leg strength on the incidence of lower extremity overuse injuries during military training. Military Medicine 164(2):153–156

Holder L E, Cole L A, Myerson M S 1992 Reflex sympathetic dystrophy in the foot: clinical and scintigraphic criteria. Radiology 184(2):531–535

Hulkko A, Orava S 1987 Stress fractures in athletes. International Journal of Sports Medicine 8:221–226

Korpelainen R, Orava S, Karpakka J et al 2001 Risk factors for recurrent stress fractures in athletes. American Journal of Sports Medicine 29(3):304–310

Lemley F, Berlet G, Hill K et al 2006 Current concepts review: tarsal coalitions. Foot and Ankle International 27(12):1163–1169

McCaffery M, Beeke A 1989 Pain: clinical manual for nursing practice. C V Mosby, Toronto

Mann R A 2006 Diseases of the nerves. In: Coughlin M, Mann R, Saltzmann C (eds) Surgery of the foot and ankle, 8th edn. C V Mosby, St Louis

Matheson G, Clement D, McKenzie D et al 1987 Stress fractures in athletes: a study of 320 cases. American Journal of Sports Medicine 15:46–58

Menz H, Morris M, Lord S 2006a Foot and ankle risk factors for falls in older people: a prospective study. Journal of Gerontology and Biological and Medical Sciences 61(8):866–870

Menz H, Tiedemann A, Kwan M et al 2006b Foot pain in community dwelling older people: an evaluation of the Manchester foot pain and disability index. Rheumatology (Oxford) 45(7):863–867

Mulder J D 1951 The causative mechanism in Morton's. Journal of Bone and Joint Surgery (Br) 33:94–95

O'Connor D 1958 Sinus tarsi syndrome: a clinical entity. Journal of Bone and Joint Surgery (Am) 40:720

Orava S 1980 Stress fractures. British Journal Sports Medicine 14:40–44

Pfeffer G, Bacchetti P, Deland J et al 1999 Comparison of custom and prefabricated orthoses in the initial treatment of proximal plantar fasciitis. Foot and Ankle International 20(4):214–221

Reade B, Longo D, Keller M 2001 Tarsal tunnel syndrome. Clinics in Podiatric Medicine and Surgery 18(3):395–408

Reilly K, Barker K, Shamley D et al 2006 Influence of foot characteristics on the site of lower limb osteoarthritis. Foot and Ankle International 27(3):206–211

Ribu L, Rusteon T, Birkeland K et al 2006 The prevalence and occurrence of diabetic foot ulcer pain and its impact on health related quality of life. Journal of Pain 7(4):290–299

Simkin A, Leichter I, Giladi M et al 1989 Combined effect of foot arch structure and an orthotic device on stress fractures. Foot and Ankle 10:25–29

Spahn G, Schiele R, Hell A et al 2004 The prevalence of pain and deformities in the feet of adolescents: results of a cross sectional study. Zeitschrift fur Orthopaedia und Ihre Grenzgebeite 142(4):389–396

Thompson F M, Deland J T 1993 Occurrence of two interdigital neuromas in one foot. Foot and Ankle 14:15–17

Thordarson D, Ebramzadeh E, Rudicel S et al 2005 Age adjusted baseline data for women with hallux valgus undergoing corrective surgery. Journal of Bone and Joint Surgery (Am) 87(1):66–75

Tollafield 1991 Reflex sympathetic dystrophy in day case foot surgery. British Journal of Podiatric Medicine 3(1):2–6

CHAPTER

18

Assessment of the at-risk foot

A McInnes

Indicates figures on DVD, including colour

Indicates video of assessment on DVD

Chapter contents

Introduction

Life expectancy is increasing steadily throughout the Western world as a result of improvements in public health, advances achieved by the pharmaceutical industry and advances in health technologies. However, this good news is tempered by the fact that as a result of modern lifestyles, new public health challenges have emerged. The new epidemics are cancer, diabetes, chronic heart disease, mental distress and illness (Hewitt 2006). The World Health Organization has estimated that if we could eliminate the major risk factors of smoking, obesity and physical inactivity, the great majority of heart disease, strokes and type 2 diabetes would be prevented. The prevalence of diabetes in the UK is estimated to be around 2.5 million adults today and is expected to rise to around 3 million by the year 2010 (Diabetes UK 2004). The International Diabetes Federation Diabetes Atlas, which provides data for 215 countries, estimates that in 2007 approximately 246 million people had diabetes worldwide. The worldwide estimate is expected to rise to 380 million by 2025.

For disability, which is a major concern for later life, research has shown that while the level of severity of disability has diminished overall, the additional years of life gained are not free from disability. Chronic diseases that affect the ageing population include disorders of the musculoskeletal system such as the inflammatory arthropathies (e.g. rheumatoid arthritis and gout). According to Michelson et al (1994) foot pain has been reported in up to 94% of people suffering from rheumatoid arthritis. With due consideration of the health problems now and in the future, it is timely to focus on the concept of the 'at-risk' foot and the associated complications. The aim of this chapter is to inform the lower-limb practitioner in the identification, assessment and evaluation of the patient at risk of the pedal complications of ulceration, structural deformity, infection and gangrene.

Normal homeostasis of the lower limb is dependent on structurally sound and physiologically normal function of hormonal, circulatory, neurological, musculoskeletal and dermatological systems. Tissue vitality may be affected by any disruption of these systems and is most reliant on the integrity and physiology of the skin. Maintenance of tissue viability of the skin is vital to prevent the unwanted aforementioned adverse events that result from a break in the integrity of the skin. The key protective functions of the complex organ that is the skin are covered in detail in Chapter 8.

The at-risk foot

The term 'at-risk foot' is used to describe the foot that is at risk of ulceration and loss of tissue viability. Many risk factors have been identified and it is the combination of intrinsic risk factors together with extrinsic factors in the form of mechanical stress that leads to a break in the continuity of epithelial tissue and subsequent complications. The associated morbidity and mortality is significant, particularly in those affected with diabetes mellitus and the prognosis for many is poor (Laing et al 2003). The threat of amputation looms over many of the at-risk group with resultant reduction in mobility, poor quality of life and decrease in life expectancy (Frykberg et al 2007). It has been estimated that every 30 seconds, worldwide, a lower limb or part of a lower limb is amputated as a consequence of diabetes.

The role of the healthcare practitioner when managing the patient 'at risk' includes:

- adopting a holistic, biopsychosocial approach to assessment
- identifying those at risk
- appropriately assessing and evaluating risk factors
- developing effective preventive and education strategies
- appropriately negotiating care planning and risk factor management
- recording and charting assessment findings
- developing an integrated care pathways and acting on them
- appropriate and timely referrals when dealing with emergency situations
- instituting appropriate rehabilitation programmes.

This list of skills suggests 'appropriate' action. It may be useful to deconstruct the term 'appropriate' and suggest that the above skill set requires underpinning knowledge of medical sciences, evidence-based practice, clinical reasoning, interpersonal and communication skills and reflective practice. This will be explored later in the chapter.

Tissue viability

A number of factors are essential to maintain the viability of tissues. The integrity of skin is dependent on its ability to withstand the everyday mechanical stresses and hazards of the environment including ultraviolet radiation, extremes of temperature, chemical trauma, opportunistic bacterial, viral and fungal pathogens and dehydration.

Trauma

Skin and the underlying soft tissues have a great capacity to withstand the mechanical stresses from everyday activities and the integral strength and elastomeric properties of skin is provided by the unique properties of collagen and elastin (Tzaphlidou 2004). However, depending on the degree of sustained trauma to the skin, the body's response to inflammation will initiate the repair process in a complex series of biochemical events (Williamson & Harding 2000).

Trauma may occur in many forms including burns, lacerations, incisions and compression injuries. More minor trauma that occurs more frequently include friction, shear, pressure and ultraviolet radiation. In the healthy individual, the minor stresses will be attenuated or dissipated with no noticeable damage to the tissues. In the 'at-risk' population, these minor stresses may result in a cascade of events that leads to significant tissue loss. Once the skin has been breached, the potential for infection is enhanced in those who are susceptible and healing will be delayed. It is important at this point to emphasise the requirement to identify the source of extrinsic trauma that leads to the development of ulceration and infection. This provides important information to evaluate the wound and to adopt preventive strategies. For example, with the neuroischaemic diabetic foot, which is at great risk of ulceration, there is usually a source of extrinsic pressure that initiates a breakdown in the skin with subsequent ulceration. It is important for the practitioner to appreciate the fact that through the minor trauma of ill-fitting footwear, a limb may require amputation and a life may be threatened as a consequence (Adler et al 1999).

Assessing the extrinsic factors and developing preventive strategies is a key component of management and it is not always possible to eradicate all of

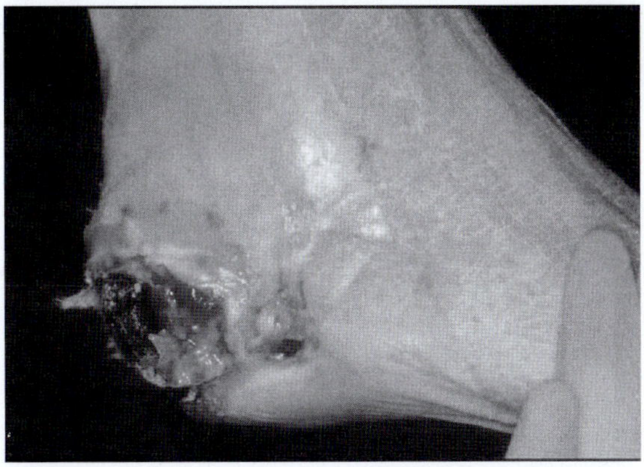

Figure 18.1 Heel pressure ulcer in neuro-ischaemic foot.

the various sources of trauma. One potential source of excessive pressure is, ironically, generated by lying supine in a hospital bed. In a study by Boulton (1996) heel to bed pressures were measured to be between 50 mmHg and 94 mmHg. If this exceeds normal capillary pressure, then as a result of the ischaemia and reperfusion cycle, pressure necrosis can occur (Fig. 18.1) (Tsuji et al 2005).

IMAGES

Other reported sources of trauma precipitating foot ulceration include rubbing from footwear and as a consequence of surgery. Macfarlane & Jeffcoate (1997) reported that rubbing from footwear was the most common precipitant (20.6%) in a prospective study of 669 ulcers seen in a multidisciplinary foot clinic. Trips and falls have also been identified as contributors to foot ulceration and the *National service framework for older people* has stated the aim is to reduce the number of falls which result in serious injury (Department of Health 2001). This initiative may help in the reduction of foot wounds in the at-risk population.

There is a substantial body of evidence that has identified the risks of ulceration in the diabetic population. Whilst there are other at-risk groups, people with diabetes are considered to have the greatest risk of ulceration. Approximately 2–3% of individuals with diabetes develop one or more foot ulcers each year and an estimated 15% will develop a foot ulcer during their lifetime (Frykberg et al 1998). Foot ulceration impacts on the individual's functional ability and quality of life (Price & Harding 2000). Pecoraro et al (1990) demonstrated that in more than 80% of cases, amputation was preceded by a foot ulcer. The economic burden is high with an estimated £244 million spent in 2001 on foot ulcers and amputations in the UK (Gordois et al 2003).

Risk factors in diabetic foot ulceration

It is important to be able to identify the most significant risk factors that predispose the diabetic person to foot ulceration. Similarly it is imperative to identify and evaluate the risk factors that may affect the prognosis and outcomes of such wounds. This process will aid the healthcare practitioner to develop a care pathway with appropriate referral criteria to other healthcare agencies. Many researchers have identified causal pathways and risk factors for ulceration. Targeting modifiable risk factors can reduce the incidence of foot ulcers or amputations (Malone et al 1989, Uccioli et al 1995).

The risk factors that are most commonly found in the causal pathway to a foot ulcer are:

- neuropathy
- peripheral arterial disease
- deformity (Reiber et al 1999).

A pivotal prospective study in a North American Indian population (Rith-Najarian et al 1992) identified risk factors that were predictive for foot ulceration. These included:

- structural foot deformity (hallux valgus or varus, claw and hammer toes, bony prominence or Charcot foot)
- peripheral neuropathy
- history of previous ulcer or amputation.

In this study, the researchers found that an ulcer was about five times more likely to occur in a patient with a history of disease or lack of sensation than in a patient without these factors. In another prospective study, Boyko et al (2006) followed 1285 diabetic subjects without foot ulcer (mostly male) over 3 years (mean 3.38). Significant predictors of foot ulcers included: impaired vision, prior foot ulcer, prior amputation, monofilament insensitivity, tinea pedis and onychomycosis. Merza & Tesfaye (2003) in a review of risk factors for diabetic foot ulceration describe other identified risk factors (Box 18.1).

Screening

Screening for risk factors for ulceration is recommended by various national and international guidelines (Scottish Intercollegiate Guidelines Network 2001, National Institute for Clinical Excellence 2004) and is an important part of a primary prevention programme. However, it may not be a cost-effective activity if the whole diabetic population has to be

Box 18.1 Risk factors for diabetic foot ulceration

- Diabetic neuropathy
- Peripheral vascular disease
- Biomechanical factors
- Previous foot ulceration
- Poor glycaemic control
- Long duration of diabetes mellitus
- Race
- Smoking
- Retinopathy and nephropathy
- Insulin use and poor vision
- Age and male sex
- Other factors

Other identified risk factors

- Old age
- Oedema
- Renal disease
- Psychosocial factors
- Obesity
- Previous history of ulceration
- Ill-fitting footwear
- Limited joint mobility
- Presence of skin callus
- Self-treatment
- Social isolation
- Social deprivation

screened in order to identify the 'at-risk' group of patients. Any screening programme has to be carefully considered and the resources have to be identified. The implications and consequences of screening programmes are far-reaching and will impose a significant burden of the health economy. Identification of risk factors may be important, however, it may be considered even more important that prevention programmes can achieve their aims.

International guidelines suggest that people with diabetes should be examined for potential foot problems at least once a year (Apelqvist et al 2007). The Consensus on the Diabetic Foot suggests a risk categorisation system should be adopted with a recommended check-up frequency (see Table 18.1).

There is evidence that the identification of the risk category can predict an episode of ulceration (Leese et al 2006). This may help to target resources to the appropriate patient groups. Numerous guidelines have suggested reliable tools to use in the identification of peripheral neuropathy and the presence of

Table 18.1 Risk categorisation system

Category	*Risk profile*	*Check-up frequency*
1	No sensory neuropathy	Once a year
2	Sensory neuropathy	Once every 6 months
3	Sensory neuropathy, signs of peripheral arterial disease and/or foot deformities	Once every 3 months
4	Previous ulcer	Once every 1–3 months

arterial disease (Best practice pathway 2007). However, there remains debate about the number of test sites required to ascertain loss of protective sensation. Table 18.2 gives the clinical tests used to identify risk based on best available evidence. In addition, a medical history to assess other risk factors, e.g. history of ulceration, will be required. There are other methods to determine extent of neuropathy, e.g. the Neuropathy Disability Score (Boulton 2005), but for a simple screening tool, the above tests are recommended.

Having a history of a previous ulcer is a significant risk factor for a recurrence (Abbott et al 2002, Boyko et al 1999, Peters et al 2001). In an important publication by Frykberg et al (1998) of the 251 patients studied, 99 patients had a current or prior history of ulceration, and 33 with active ulcers. Recurrence rates have been reported to range from 28% at 12 months (Chantelau et al 1990) to 100% at 40 months (Uccioli et al 1995). Apelqvist et al (1993) reported a recurrence rate of 34% and 70% after 2 and 5 years, respectively. Clearly having had a history of ulceration is the most important risk factor for further ulceration.

Renal failure

Identification of risk factors does not only inform the practitioner who is at risk, but also informs treatment options and likely prognosis. For example the diabetic patient with end-stage renal failure and peripheral arterial disease who presents with a foot ulcer

Table 18.2 Simple identification of risk factors

	Sites
DEGREE OF SENSORY NEUROPATHY	
Loss of protective sensation (10 g nylon monofilament)	Pressure sites of plantar aspect of the hallux, 1st and 5th metatarsal heads of both feet
Loss of vibration perception (128 Hz tuning fork) **or** vibration perception threshold (neurosthesiometer)	Distal end of hallux and medial and lateral malleolus Same sites above >25 V
PERIPHERAL ARTERIAL DISEASE	
Absence of two or more pedal pulses	Dorsalis pedis and tibialis posterior pulses
Ankle–brachial pressure index	Both dorsalis pedis and posterior tibial pulses
OBSERVATION OF FOOT DEFORMITY	Hallux abductovalgus, hallux rigidus, pes cavus pes planus and Charcot's foot deformity
Limited joint mobility syndrome	Positive prayer sign (see Fig. 18.2)
Observation of plantar callus	Pressure points of hallux, all metatarsophalangeal joints, apices of digits and heels of both feet

IMAGES

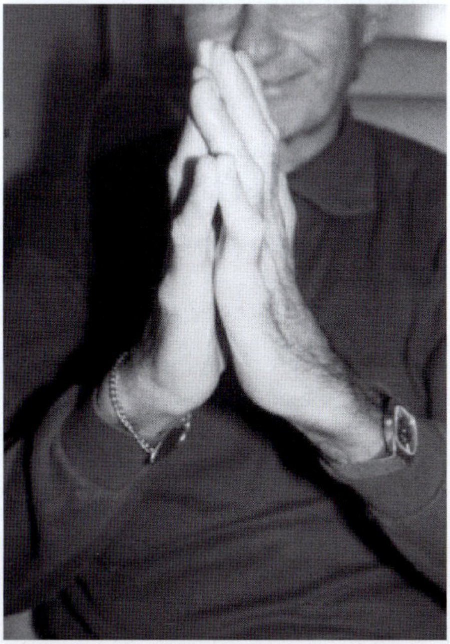

Figure 18.2 Limited joint mobility as demonstrated by the prayer sign.

has a high risk of infection and a poor prognosis (Boufi et al 2006).

Established renal failure in diabetes is associated with a high incidence of foot ulcers and gangrene. This problem may be particularly associated with the onset of renal replacement therapy. There is evidence that haemodialysis causes hypoxaemia and this can be reflected in the subsequent decrease in lower limb transcutaneous oxygen tension ($TcPO_2$) (Hinchcliffe et al 2006). These patients are liable to be prescribed immunosuppressant drugs and are therefore at great risk of infection. This patient group will have underlying advanced diabetic microangiopathy and often have concomitant peripheral arterial disease and are hypertensive. Clearly, a holistic assessment of all of the risk factors is needed to evaluate risk factor status for possible future ulceration.

Practice point

Chronic renal insufficiency can be identified by the following criteria: creatinine >4.0 mg/dl, current dialysis or a history of renal transplantation (Savage et al 1996).

Biopsychosocial approach

Following a primary screening programme, patients may be referred to a podiatrist for further assessment, education and treatment if required. Many of the at-risk patients may be over 50 years of age and suffer from other co-morbidities. A comprehensive assessment is needed to have a full appreciation of the patient's life, their heath beliefs and behaviours, risk of developing a wound and likely prognosis. In addition any negotiated care plan will have been informed by a full assessment. It may be helpful to consider the following factors.

Psychosocial factors

Recognition of the importance of both psychological and social factors in the care of people with diabetes is required to assess and facilitate optimum management. Neuropathy, pain, foot ulceration and amputation can have a devastating effect on the person with diabetes. This may lead to social isolation, depression and failure to maintain healthy behaviours. As a consequence there may be a downward spiral of poor health, further complications and early death (Vilekyte et al 2003).

The quality of life can be severely affected by the complications of neuropathy and foot ulceration. The psychosocial assessment of patients suffering from these complications is vital to determine further risk of the complications and improve care. A seminal research study by Vilekyte and colleagues (2003) led to the development of a validated quality-of-life instrument (NeuroQoL) that can reliably capture the key physical and psychosocial effects. Psychosocial factors that are measured include disruption of daily living and interpersonal-emotional burden. Healthcare practitioners should consider the use of this assessment tool to inform any behavioural strategy and evaluate effectiveness of quality of care.

The podiatrist and other healthcare providers have to develop the skills and knowledge in order to embrace a biopsychosocial approach to caring for the at-risk diabetic person (Kinmond et al 2003). Psychological and emotional wellbeing is the foundation on which all other aspects of the treatment regimen rest and failure to consider these aspects in management of the diabetic foot can lead to poor outcomes (Clark 2006).

The psychological and social barriers to diabetes self-management and quality of life are given below.

Psychological factors

- Low levels of self-efficacy
- Personal illness models and health beliefs
- Depression.

Social factors

- Stress
- Low levels of support from family and close friends.

Albert Bandura first described self-efficacy in 1977 and recognised that it is a key psychological factor that influences a wide range of health behaviours. In essence, self-efficacy is a belief in one's own ability that by carrying out a set of actions, one will achieve the desired goals. In the context of the high-risk diabetic patient, if he or she strongly believes that by carrying out certain foot health preventive practices, foot ulceration will be prevented, then they are more likely to adhere to those healthy behaviours. Conversely, if the high-risk patient has low self-efficacy, and does not hold those aforementioned health beliefs, then it is unlikely that they will adopt healthy footcare practices.

Motivational interviewing

Assessment of psychosocial factors requires good communication skills that lead to developing a rapport with patients. Once a relationship has been established, the patient's self-efficacy can be explored. It is not the purpose of this chapter to expand on the psychology of diabetes. However, the assessment of health beliefs, attitudes and self-efficacy do need to be explored.

Hampson and colleagues (1996) have shown that personal models of diabetes, e.g. beliefs about the consequences of having diabetes and the effectiveness of treatment can predict self-care behaviour. It is therefore important to explore with the person with diabetes or other chronic illness about their perceptions of how their illness affects them. This holistic approach to assessment needs to include an exploration of the patient's perceived susceptibility to their illness and foot complications. It is only by adopting an empathetic approach and willingness on behalf of the patient to disclose such information that valuable insights may be gained to facilitate change in self-management.

Practice point

Consider the following assessment strategy: use of open ended questions, e.g. 'How are you today, Mrs Smith?' or 'How have you been getting on with your insoles?'. This approach needs to be accompanied by affirmation, e.g. 'Well done for making your appointment today and well done for trying out the insoles.' It is important to be sincere and genuine with questioning and praise. If not, the practitioner may be perceived as patronising and this will result in failure to establish a rapport. It is vital that active listening is adopted. The patient may be trying to disclose other information.

At this stage, some summarising can be very helpful. This demonstrates that the practitioner has been listening and gives the patient an opportunity to reflect on what has been said. The patient-centred approach is best practice and will enhance the assessment process.

Self-efficacy can be explored by a skilled practitioner. Consider the following: 'How important is it for you Mrs Smith to get the ulcer healed on your foot? On a scale of 1–10, 1 representing not at all important and 10 being very important?'. Many patients will consider it to be very important and score highly.

This can lead to the practitioner asking the following: 'On a scale of 1–10, how confident are you that by sticking to your treatment plan, the ulcer will heal?' The response may shed some light into the self-efficacy of Mrs Smith. She may score a 2. This provides the practitioner the opportunity to praise the 2 scored, and enquire why Mrs Smith did not score a zero. The dialogue that follows allows the patient to reflect on her beliefs about her confidence and consider what it might take to move along the scale.

These are simple tools that practitioners may consider to enhance the assessment process. This patient-centred approach has been recommended (Lincoln et al 2007) and is a key part of the assessment process. In addition many of the at-risk patients may well have depression, which will affect their health behaviours and communication. All practitioners should consider that diabetes doubles the risk of depression (Anderson et al 2000).

Assessment of foot health knowledge and behaviour is often overlooked as part of the assessment process and yet it is often the health behaviours that lead to an episode of ulceration and further recurrence. One new assessment tool that has been validated is the Nottingham Assessment of functional Footcare (NAFF). This questionnaire explores both knowledge and behaviour and could be used to test the effectiveness of education and identify specific areas of poor protective behaviour that individuals may have (Lincoln et al 2007).

Other useful health-related quality of life and diabetic foot ulcer assessments include:

- The Diabetic Foot Ulcer Scale (DFS): a quality of life instrument for use in clinical trials (Abetz et al 2002).
- The Diabetic Foot Ulcer Scale – short form (DFS-SF) (Bann et al 2003).

Socioeconomic factors

Many of the leading causes of mortality and morbidity are related to low socioeconomic status. Individuals with low socioeconomic status suffer from more diseases and their consequences than from those who enjoy higher socioeconomic status (Alder et al 1993). Studies have shown that low socioeconomic status is associated with obesity, depression and diabetes (Everson et al 2002). The relationship is complex and there is evidence that those with low socioeconomic status have a greater prevalence of smoking, higher alcohol consumption, poorer diets and more sedentary lifestyles. These health behaviours are more likely to put the person at greater risk of developing the chronic disorders stated.

Socioeconomic factors are not routinely assessed in clinical practice and are more likely to be explored in research studies. However, it may be useful to consider these socioeconomic factors as they may impact on your assessment and management of the at-risk foot:

- Education
- Income
- Housing tenure
- Area (deprived)
- Race
- Social class (occupation).

Although it has been acknowledged that poor socioeconomic status is a risk factor for diabetic foot complications (Apelqvist 2000), the evidence is fairly sparse. The at-risk population tend to be older, and there are some difficulties in measuring socioeconomic factors with this group. As an example, social class measured by occupation is not possible with a retired population. The lower-limb practitioner should take into account the socioeconomic status of the patient as this may inform the assessment and prognosis. In addition, the practitioner may be able to refer the patients to other agencies, for example social services, voluntary support for further assistance.

Age

The ageing population in the UK and other developing countries is well acknowledged and statistics from Help Age International suggest there are 550 million older people worldwide, which will increase to 1.2 billion by 2025 (Help Age International 2005). With this demographic background and an expected increase in the prevalence of diabetes, the proportion of at-risk patients will increase substantially. In the context of the at-risk foot, tissue viability may be compromised by the ageing process. The ageing process is a complex process and can be divided into intrinsic and extrinsic ageing.

Intrinsic ageing is mostly genetically determined and extrinsic ageing, more commonly referred to as photoaging, is caused by environmental exposure in the form of ultraviolet radiation (Fisher et al 2002). These aging processes have both qualitative and quantitative effects on collagen and elastic fibres in the skin (El-Domyati et al 2002). Although the pathomechanisms of collagen deficiency differ between intrinsic and extrinsic ageing, the cumulative effects result in dermal atrophy and decrease in the elasticity of the skin (Tzaphlidou 2004).

Wound healing and repair processes decline with age and the inflammatory response, proliferative phase and maturation have all been shown to alter with age (Hardy 1989). Growth factors and their receptors which regulate the wound healing process are also affected by the ageing process (Ashcroft et al 1997). The aged skin is at greater risk of damage and wound dehiscence occurs more frequently in people over the age of 60 (Falanga & Eaglstein 1988).

The main contributing risk factors that can lead to the development of ulceration, infection and gangrene have been identified. However, a number of both local and systemic factors may affect wound healing and facilitate infection (Table 18.3).

Table 18.3 Conditions which may affect healing

Category	*Examples*
Cardiovascular	Peripheral arterial disease, venous insufficiency, lymphatic obstruction
Endocrine	Diabetes, malnutrition, deficiency syndromes, obesity
Immunological	DiGeorge syndrome, hypogammaglobulinaemia, human immunodeficiency virus infection, rheumatoid arthritis and hypersensitivity
Immunosuppressive agents	Long-term steroids, immunosuppressive drugs, radiation, cytotoxic drugs
Infectious	Cytomegalovirus, infectious mononucleosis, bacterial and fungal agents
Haematological	Luekaemia, anaemias, haemophilia, sickle-cell anaemia
Musculoskeletal	Deformities, hypermobility
Neoplasia	Carcinoma, lymphomas, sarcomas
Respiratory	Chronic obstructive airways disease
Renal	Chronic nephropathy
Traumatic	Burns, foreign bodies, repeated minor trauma, tight hosiery
Exogenous factors	Inappropriate dressings, antiseptics, harsh environment, caustics and irritants

Practice point

It is important to consider a biopsychosocial approach to assessment not only to determine the contributing risk factors but also to gain valuable information that may inform treatment, management and prognosis.

Wound assessment

Despite the widespread use of preventive and intervention strategies, many patients receiving footcare may go on to develop a foot ulcer. An ulcer by definition is a break in the continuity of epithelial tissue, which may range from the loss of superficial tissues of the epidermis to a full-thickness wound involving the dermis and deeper underlying tissues. This may include fascia, fat, muscle, tendon and bone. Accurate wound assessment is a prerequisite for care planning. Assessment skills must be accompanied by an understanding of the normal physiology of wound healing and an appreciation of factors that may affect wound healing.

The process of wound assessment is important for:

- determining the aetiology, extent and severity of the wound and the risks posed to the patient
- determining the health and nutritional status of the patient and their ability to heal normally without complications
- designing and justifying a management plan and documenting the improvement/deterioration accordingly
- classifying the wound for clinical management, audit and research purposes
- providing a complete, concise documentation including wound size, appearance and perfusion as a written record of a pattern of treatment. This needs to be consistent with agreed standards of care and best practice.

The requirement for complete documentation is vital, considering that litigation is an increasing problem. The first and most essential aspect of wound assessment is to carry out a thorough risk assessment of the patient (see holistic assessment) with the wound to determine what action needs to be considered. A relevant medical and drug history should be taken along with the history of the wound. The key aspects of history taking for the at-risk foot are given in Box 18.2.

The purpose of the history taking is to help determine the health status of the patient and to identify the factors that may have contributed to the development of the wound. Most foot wounds are a result of a combination of intrinsic and extrinsic factors. For example, people with diabetes are often at risk of developing an ulcer due to the common complication of peripheral neuropathy. Peripheral neuropathy may be a contributing factor but has to be accompanied by some form of direct trauma for ulceration to occur. The trauma may be in the form of intermittent high pressure on a weightbearing part of the foot. Common sites for ulceration include metatarsal heads, plantar aspect of the hallux and heel areas.

Box 18.2 Factors to be covered in the patient history

- Name
- Address
- Date of birth
- Medical history
- Drug history
- Surgical history
- Social history (smoking, alcohol intake, exercise)
- Nutrition status
- Wound history
- Identifiable cause
- Duration
- Colour changes
- Size
- Location

The patient with rheumatoid arthritis who is receiving treatment with corticosteroid drugs as part of a treatment regimen may also have a wound that has resulted from a foot deformity. Deformity is common in rheumatoid arthritis and may contribute to a foot wound. In addition the complication of vasculitis may accompany the inflammatory arthropathy which also may contribute to the formation of the wound.

Chronic diseases such as diabetes mellitus and the inflammatory arthropathies are not only risk factors for foot wounds but also affect the healing process. In addition, certain drugs may impair the normal healing processes – for example, in the cancer patient who is receiving chemotherapy, in the arthritic patient on high doses of corticosteroids, and in the diabetic patient who is receiving dialysis treatment, all of these treatments can lead to wound-healing complications.

Wound size

Wound size is one of the most useful parameters to evaluate. The size of the wound can be monitored to evaluate the effectiveness of treatment, can act as a visual record to provide the patient with evidence of improvement and can be an important measure for clinical research. There are a number of techniques that can be considered for clinical practice. Methods that are usually reserved for clinical research will also be discussed here.

Wound size involves both surface area and depth. The surface area is easier to determine, whereas the depth of the wound is more problematic to measure. Wound depth is assessed in most ulcer classification systems by a description of the tissues involved as opposed to an actual measurement (see section on classification systems).

Practice point

In a pivotal study by Oyibo et al (2001), ulcer area significantly predicted the outcome of foot ulcers ($p = 0.04$).

Linear measurement

Perpendicular linear measurements of wounds are often made in clinical practice. The measurements can be taken by a ruler or tape measure. There are limitations with this practice as wounds are not a uniform size. Common practice involves measuring two dimensions which assumes a simple shape, i.e. a circle (diameter and diameter), an ellipse (major and minor diameter) or a rectangle (length and width). The most representative linear method is the measurement of an ellipse. This can be calculated based on the formula for an ellipse (length × width × 0.785).

Wound tracing

Wound outlines can be traced by the use of a marker pen and acetate paper. A second sheet of paper can be placed directly against the wound and discarded after measurement, so that the first sheet can be kept clean for the patient notes and prevent cross-infection. Wound tracings can be kept in a sequential format to help monitor the progress and shown to the patient as evidence of improvement. The reliability of this technique is improved if the practitioner remains constant throughout the management of the wound.

Area measurement

Wound area can be measured by the use of a wound mapping chart in the form of an acetate sheet with a grid to measure the wound in square centimetres. This has similar limitations to the linear measurements, depending on calculation of the squares. However, if an elliptical shape is assumed, then the margin of error is reduced. This method is useful for clinical research and compares well with computerised planimetry.

Digital planimetry

This method has been described as having excellent intra-rater and inter-rater reliability and validity. This involves a computerised programe using two area calculations of the same tracings (Goldman & Salcido 2002). However, this process takes time and is usually reserved for clinical research.

Visitrak

Visitrak (Smith & Nephew, Hull, UK) is a portable digital device that provides a standardised approach to wound measurement. The Visitrak grid film and Visitrak depth indicator allow for surface area and depth measurements respectively.

Volume measurement

Volume measurement in foot wounds (especially those on the plantar surface) is difficult and not widely used either in clinical practice or research. Techniques include the use of calcium alginate to form a mould of the wound space which is then weighed and used as a baseline measurement for monitoring over time. This technique is an attempt to measure depth of the wound. Other techniques include the use of a sterile probe. Care has to be taken to avoid further trauma to the wound.

Kundin device

This is a disposable plastic gauge, which is a three-dimensional ruler. Length, width and depth are multiplied with a constant factor (0.327) which calculates a volume about 60% of a spheroid. Good validity and inter-rater and intra-rater reliability has been demonstrated (Goldman & Salcido 2002).

Colour

Colour of the wound has been used as a basis for an ulcer classification system and as a guideline for treatment options. Visual assessment of colour can aid the practitioner in the assessment process but with obvious limitations. Foot wounds may be red (granulating), yellow (infected/sloughy), green (infected), black (necrotic) or pink (epithelialising). wound may have a mixture of the colours, in which case a percentage estimate can be used for documentation purposes.

Digital photography is far superior; however, this requires personnel to take the photographs, analyse the images and organise the files. Computerised stereophotogrammetry is the most accurate method of wound assessment and includes objective information on size, outline, shape, area, colour and surrounding tissue changes. However, it is a costly and complex method which is reserved for research only.

Perfusion

A vital part of assessment of the at-risk patient with a wound is the measure of vascular perfusion of the tissues. Vascular assessment is described in detail in Chapter 6. Assessment of the underlying vasculature provides much needed information. Clearly there will be treatment options that may be contraindicated, for example the use of total-contact casting with a neuro-ischaemic ulcer. It has been suggested that a wound with an ankle–brachial pressure index (ABPI) of less than 0.4 is unlikely to progress to healing. The use of toe pressures and transcutaneous oxygen levels may also provide useful information for prognosis of healing.

Infection

Infection is the major complication that threatens the at-risk population who develop foot ulcers. Many at-risk patients have chronic diseases that result in an immunocompromised state. This may be a direct result of the disorder, e.g. diabetes or as a result of drug therapy such as corticosteroids for those with rheumatoid arthritis. For the majority of diabetic patients, infection is a pivotal event that complicates ulceration causing substantial morbidity, amputation and death (Lipsky et al 2005).

Several studies have suggested that amputations can be reduced in the at-risk population by providing a multidisciplinary team approach to facilitate preventive strategies (Apelqvist et al 1994, Edmonds 1987). It is extremely important that the presence of infection is detected early in order to prevent further tissue loss and failure of the wound to heal. This section considers criteria for severity of infection, methods of assessment, evaluation and diagnosis.

Assessment of the patient with an infected ulcer

Assessment of the at-risk patient with an infected foot ulcer should ideally be carried out by multidisciplinary specialist healthcare team. However, the patient may first be seen by a healthcare auxiliary or other care worker in the community and it is vital that they have the necessary training to identify the severity of the condition and refer to the appropriate services. Any delay without medical intervention will affect the duration of therapy required and affect the prognosis.

The diagnosis of infection is a clinical decision and is based on the signs and symptoms of inflammation. Laboratory investigations may help to confirm the presence of pathogenic bacteria and in the detection of soft tissue and bone infection (osteomyelitis) (Lipsky et al 2005).

Practice point

It is important to remember that the signs and symptoms may be absent or diminished in the diabetic neuro-ischaemic foot. There may be absence of pain, diminished inflammation, and reduced swelling. If in doubt, refer immediately to a specialist podiatrist or other member of the footcare protection team. Delay can only result in prolonged treatment and further tissue damage.

Lipsky et al (2005) described the clinical manifestations of infection in the diabetic foot (see Table 18.4). **Figures 18.3–18.5** provide clinical pictures of mild, moderate and severe infection. The PEDIS system of grading the ulcer is discussed later in this chapter (see ulcer classification). The 'PREPSOCS' acronym has been used (Turner & McLeod-Roberts 2002) to aid in the clinical identification of a foot infection (see Box 18.3). IMAGES

The implications of the severity of the infection will dictate the management of the patient. While it is important to detect the pathogenic bacteria that are involved, the severity of the infection must be ascertained in order to facilitate appropriate management. The patient with a severe foot infection using the criteria above, clearly requires immediate hospital admission in order to save life and limb.

Delayed healing and increasing pain may indicate that the wound may progress to overt infection. Critical colonisation may represent the transition from colonisation to overt infection, or the transition to

Table 18.4 Clinical classification of a diabetic foot infection

Clinical manifestations of infection	*Infection severity*	*PEDIS grade*
Wound lacking purulence or any manifestations of inflammation	Uninfected	1
Presence of ≥2 manifestations of inflammation (purulence, or erythema, pain, tenderness, warmth or induration), but any cellulitis/erythema extends ≥2 cm around the ulcer, and infection is limited to the skin or superficial subcutaneous tissues; no other local complications or systemic illness	Mild	2
Infection (as above) in a patient who is systemically well and metabolically stable but who has ≥1 of the following characteristics: cellulitis extending >2 cm, lymphangitic streaking, spread beneath the superficial fascia, deep tissue abscess, gangrene, and involvement of muscle, tendon, joint or bone	Moderate	3
Infection in a patient with systemic toxicity or metabolic instability (e.g. fever, chills, tachycardia, hypotension, confusion, vomiting, leucocytosis, acidosis, severe hyperglycaemia or azotaemia)	Severe	4

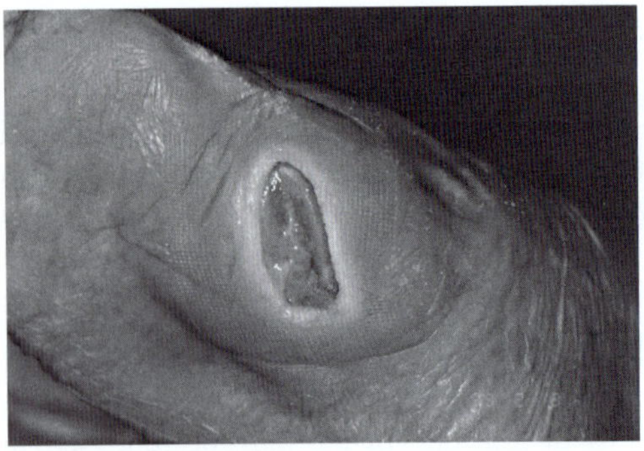

Figure 18.3 Mild infection.

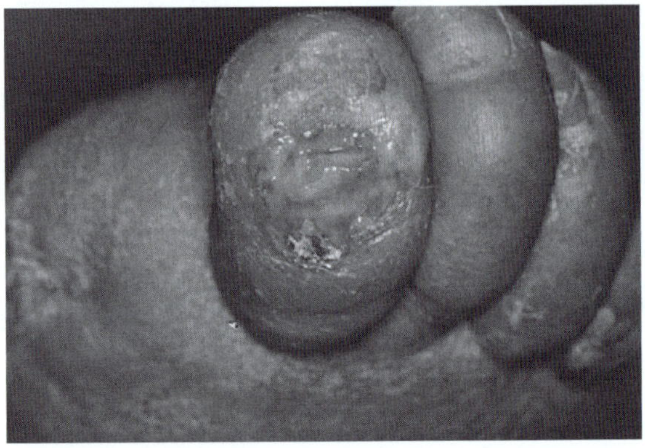

Figure 18.4 Moderate infection.

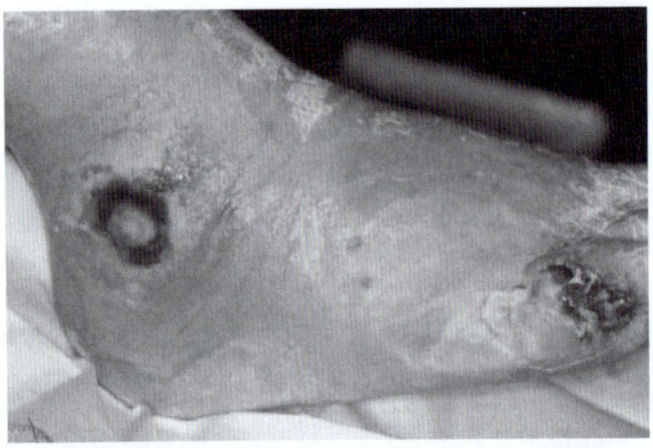

Figure 18.5 Severe infection.

persistence and chronic inflammation (Cooper 2005). There is a possibility that in some polymicrobial communities formation of biofilms can occur. Their presence in chronic wounds may be linked with failure to heal (Cooper 2005).

Practice point

With elevation of the limb, the redness of ischaemia will rapidly disappear, while the redness of cellulitis as a result of infection will remain. This may be helpful in identifying the presence of infection.

The items in Table 18.4 and Box 18.3 may not capture all of the signs and symptoms of the presence of infection. Other observations and assessments include:

- the presence of dorsal foot phlegmon (spreading inflammatory reaction visible on the dorsum of the foot)
- 'sausage toe' – in the absence of inflammatory arthropathy, this is invariably an indicator of infection usually osteomyelitis

Box 18.3 'PREPSOCS' indicators of foot infection

- **P**ain – may be diminished with sensory neuropathy. However, in the neuropathic diabetic foot, a new episode of pain may be indicative of infection. The pain may be throbbing, pulsatile and persistent. There may be tenderness in the lymph glands.
- **R**edness – cellulitis may radiate from the ulcer site and colour may vary in intensity, depending on arterial perfusion and invading pathogens. Spread of cellulitis indicates severity of infection.
- **E**xudation – the amount, colour and consistency of exudates can inform assessment and management. There is an increase in the volume of exudate with infection present. Thick, creamy pus may indicate staphylococcal infection, whereas thin watery exudate may indicate the presence of anaerobes. Green exudate may be indicative of the presence of *Pseudomonas* species.
- **P**yrexia – temperature increase may not always be present, depending on the vascular status of the patient. Temperature awareness may be absent in the neuropathic foot. Diabetic patients may not have a rise in systemic temperature even when dealing with limb-threatening infection. Causes of increased temperature, e.g. Charcot's arthropathy, need to be excluded.
- **S**low healing – infection will slow down the healing process. Slow healing may occur when critical colonisation is suspected or a state of chronic inflammation has been achieved.
- **O**edema – unilateral swelling of the foot may be a sign of infection. Need to consider other causes of oedema/swelling.
- **C**olour – change in colour of the base of the ulcer. Greyish/yellowish discoloration may indicate infection.
- **S**mell – malodorous wounds may signify the presence of anaerobic bacteria. Foul smelling ulcers are often infected.

- crepitus in the joint – this may be felt on joint palpation as a cracking or grating sensation suggestive of gas-producing bacteria
- fluctuance – this is felt by palpation of the area and may denote the presence of pus and breakdown of the involved tissues
- blue-black discoloration and haemorrhage halo – associated with septic vasculitis (Fig. 18.6)

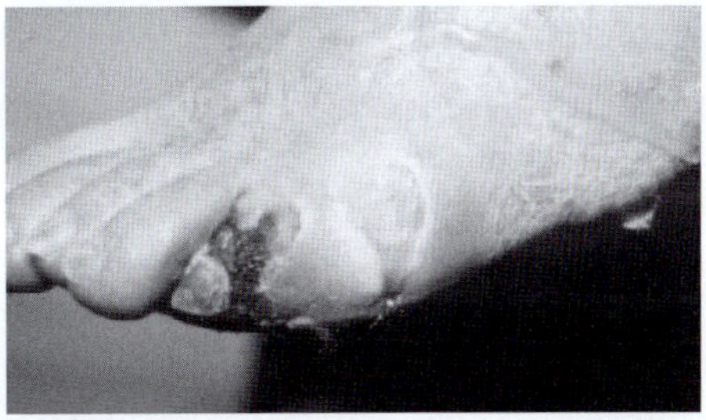

Figure 18.6 Septic vasculitis.

- friable granulation tissue that bleeds easily
- the presence of a sinus
- general increase in moisture of the wound
- the presence of sloughy devitalised tissue.

Clinical investigations and laboratory tests

While the diagnosis of soft-tissue infection is a clinical one, microbiological investigations are very useful to diagnose osteomyelitis, identify pathogens and direct antimicrobial drug management. In addition, laboratory advice may be required when:

- confirmation of infection is needed
- when an antimicrobial intervention has failed
- when healing is delayed
- when a patient requires screening for a specific organism (Vowden & Cooper 2006).

Superficial swab specimens yield a greater range of organisms and may fail to identify deeper pathogenic organisms. In addition, anaerobic bacteria may be missed, unless appropriate means of transportation have been used.

Procedure

For best results, clean and debride the wound before a swab is taken from the floor of the ulcer. Debridement includes the removal of slough and the surrounding callus. This helps to remove colonising bacteria. Care must be taken with the interpretation of results and generally superficial swabs are regarded as less than helpful.

For more accurate results, tissue specimens curettaged from the ulcer base yield more accurate results. This can be done by scraping with a scalpel blade. Use a swab designed for culturing aerobic and anaerobic organisms and ensure early transportation to the laboratory. Needle aspiration of pus can be useful. The specimen type and location must be identified

IMAGES

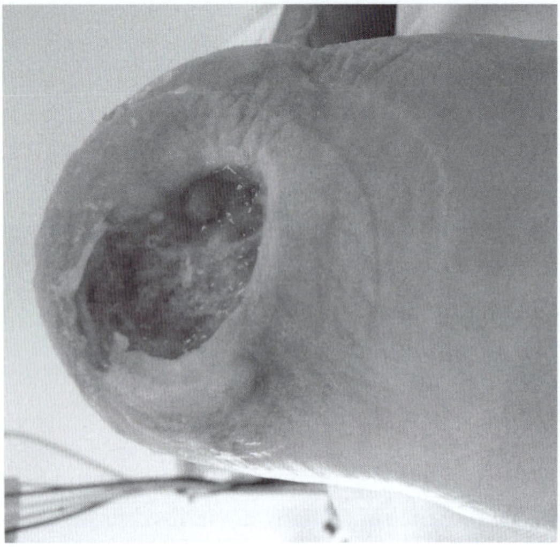

Figure 18.7 Osteomyelitis of the heel.

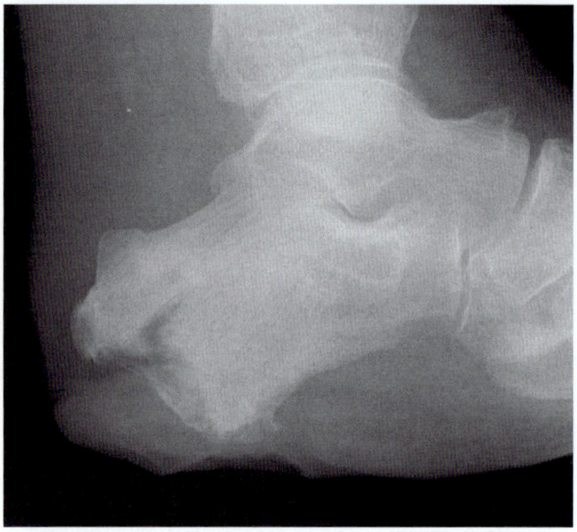

Figure 18.8 X-ray of osteomyelitis of the heel.

along with any current antimicrobial therapy (Lipsky et al 2005). See Chapter 13 for more details.

Osteomyelitis

The detection of osteomyelitis can be complex. This is particularly the case when dealing with the diabetic patient who has peripheral neuropathy and may have neuropathic bone changes. Clinical assessment of the infected wound includes probing of the tissues to determine depth and to detect bone infection. There remains some controversy about the validity of the 'probe to bone' test. However, it may be useful to remember that not being able to probe to bone does not necessarily eliminate the presence of osteomyelitis. A sterile metal probe is best for this purpose. Confirmation of the presence of osteomyelitis by bone biopsy is the gold standard test for bone infection.

US and CT scanning may detect deep abscess or sinus tracks (Lipsky et al 2005). However, X-rays, bone scintigraphy and MRI (see Ch. 12) are best in the detection of bone infection (Lipsky et al 2005). MRI has greater sensitivity and specificity than plain X-ray and standard scintigraphy. **Figures 18.7** and **18.8** demonstrate the clinical and X-ray appearance in a patient with osteomyelitis of the heel.

Blood tests

It is important that blood tests are performed when systemic involvement is suspected in the at-risk patient. Diabetic subjects may also experience metabolic derangement which needs to be urgently addressed. In order to monitor the effects of any antimicrobial intervention, it may be useful to measure the serum level of C-reactive protein (CRP) and the erythrocyte sedimentation rate (ESR) as indicators of inflammation and infection (see Ch. 13). CRP is a highly sensitive inflammatory marker and is commonly used in the management of infection. HbA_{1C}, electrolytes and other tests for renal status should be considered as routine investigations in the patient with suspected infection.

Implications for management

The assessment of the patient with an infected ulcer has to be accompanied by an interpretation of all of the clinical findings (see Box 18.4). Clinical reasoning needs to be as accurate as possible and decision-making is based on objective and subjective findings. The patient's symptoms and complaint may not necessarily reflect the severity of the condition, for example the patient with peripheral neuropathy may not experience much pain. However, spreading cellulitis of >2 cm^2 indicates the requirement for hospitalisation and intravenous antibiotic treatment. The patient with an apparently small wound but a critically ischaemic foot has to be treated as a clinical emergency and immediately referred on to the specialist team.

There is no substitute for clinical experience. However, reflection on all thoughts, hypothetico-deductions and actions should enable the practitioner to make the right decision. If in doubt, refer to a member of the specialist team.

Box 18.4 Factors to consider when assessing patients with a suspected infected ulcer

- Assess general well-being of the patient
- Assess full medical history
- Pain/symptom history
- History of wound
- Previous antibiotic treatment
- Systemic infection evidence
- Critical limb ischaemia
- Full wound assessment
- Extent of tissue involvement
- Spreading cellulitis
- Psychosocial status

Practice point

If the patient has had a puncture wound, the wound may not have the characteristics of infection. In the at-risk patient, the wound will inevitably be deeply infected and will require antibiotic therapy. The use of prophylactic antibiotics remains controversial, particularly in light of the emergence of multi-resistant strains of bacteria. However, in the diabetic patient with significant co-morbidities of nephropathy and ischaemia, there is a strong case for their use.

Pain

In the at-risk patient, the complaint of pain has to be fully investigated. A pain history includes onset, duration, type, location, identified exacerbations and identified means of relief. The history of pain in the critically ischaemic foot, particularly rest pain (ischaemic neuritis) which is usually felt in the dorsal aspect of the forefoot requires speedy referral to the vascular services team. It is a sign of impending tissue loss.

New pain felt in an otherwise neuropathic foot ulcer may herald the arrival of infection and the wise practitioner will look out for subtle signs of infection and ensure that the patient receives appropriate antibiotic treatment as required.

Ulcer classification

Wound assessment involves extensive documentation including assessment of all of the characteristics of the wound and results of laboratory tests and clinical investigations. The tests required will be determined by the underlying presenting pathologies and other aetiological factors. Further classification of the ulcer is an all too often neglected aspect of wound care. Failure to utilise a valid, reliable and repeatable classification system has resulted in difficulty in identifying best practice and evaluating any intervention. Sound clinical evidence should be based on a classification that is selected by as many healthcare practitioners as possible. Current diabetic foot ulcer classification systems include: Wagner's, University of Texas San Antonio Diabetic Wound Classification System, the Frykberg, Coleman, and Knighton S(AD) SAD system, and the newly proposed PEDIS system. This is by no means an exhaustive list, and is perhaps one reason why practitioners are reluctant to use a system, as there are too many to select from.

Table 18.5 Wagner's ulcer classification system

Grade	*Lesion*
0	No open lesions; may have deformity or cellulitis
1	Superficial diabetic ulcer (partial or full thickness)
2	Ulcer extension to ligament, tendon, joint capsule or deep fascia without abscess or osteomyelitis
3	Deep ulcer with abscess, osteomyelitis or joint sepsis
4	Gangrene localised to portion of forefoot or heel
5	Extensive gangrenous involvement of the entire foot

Aim and purpose

Clearly, before selection of a classification system, the practitioner needs to consider the role of the selected system. The most widely used classification in recent times has been Wagner's system (Table 8.5). This was designed to describe the dysvascular foot, even though evidence of it validity and reliability are lacking (Smith 2003).

While the Wagner classification has been the 'gold' standard for several years, the factors that have not been adequately addressed in this classification are

Table 18.6 San Antonio wound classification system

	0	*I*	*II*	*III*
A	Pre- or post-ulcerative lesion completely epithelialised	Superficial wound, not involving tendon, capsule or bone	Wound penetrating to tendon or capsule	Wound penetrating to bone or joint
B	Pre- or post-ulcerative lesion completely epithelialised with infection	Superficial wound, not involving tendon, capsule or bone, with infection	Wound penetrating to tendon or capsule with infection	Wound penetrating to bone or joint with infection
C	Pre- or post-ulcerative lesion completely epithelialised with ischaemia	Superficial wound, not involving tendon, capsule or bone with ischaemia	Wound penetrating to tendon or capsule with ischaemia	Wound penetrating to bone or joint with ischaemia
D	Pre- or post-ulcerative lesion completely epithelialised with infection and ischaemia	Superficial wound, not involving tendon, capsule or bone with infection and ischaemia	Wound penetrating to tendon or capsule with infection and ischaemia	Wound penetrating to bone or joint with infection and ischaemia

The San Antonio system uses four grades of ulcer (0–III) and four stages of infection and ischaemia (A–D). This system can help to predict outcome and help in the appropriate management, which may include referral for vascular services.

those of ischaemia and infection. The purpose of a classification system for the practitioner is to be able to identify the grade of ulcer and to aid in the logical approach to management. This may also help predict the prognosis and predict the outcome. In addition, the use of a classification system will enable the process of clinical audit and to compare practice with national and international data. Without the use of a classification system, clinical research in this much needed area will be hampered accordingly. The development of the San Antonio Diabetic Wound Classification System (Armstrong et al 1998) (Table 18.6) helped to address the parameters of ischaemia and infection and its use has been increasingly apparent in the research literature.

Another important development in ulcer classification system is the S(AD) SAD System devised by Treece et al (2004) (Table 18.7). The authors have identified the problems that arise in the development of classification systems and have reproduced a model that is valid and easy to use. The problems that they identified included:

- multiple factors involved in the healing and non-healing of wounds
- difficulty in deciding which aetiological factors predominates in any one case
- the lack of simple and reproducible methods of determining the extent and severity of factors, e.g. neuropathy and infection.

These authors, unlike the San Antonio group, have considered the inclusion of neuropathy in their system which is useful for audit and research purposes. The S(AD) SAD system has also included degrees of ischaemia which may be useful for both the practitioner and the researcher. It is important to consider that this system has been designed as an aid to audit and research.

Systems approach to risk assessment

The at-risk foot is generally considered to describe the potential of the patient to develop foot ulceration, infection and gangrene. The threat to tissue viability may arise from a number of systemic diseases. Diabetes mellitus is probably the most prevalent disease that contributes to the risk status. However, other diseases can threaten tissue viability and the ability of the subsequent wounds to heal appropriately. The following systems are considered with regard to risk status and response.

Cardiovascular system

A functioning cardiovascular system is necessary to maintain homeostasis and delivery of oxygen and other nutrients to all of the tissues including skin and

Table 18.7 The S(AD) SAD classification

Grade	*Area*	*Depth*	*Sepsis*	*Arteriopathy*	*Denervation*
0	Skin intact	No infection	No infection	Pedal pulses palpable	Pinprick sensation/VPT normal
1	<10 mm^2	Skin and subcutaneous tissues	Superficial: slough or exudate	Diminution of both pulses or absence of both	Reduced or absent pinprick sensation/VPT raised
2	10–30 mm^2	Tendon, joint capsule, periosteum	Cellulitis	Absence of both pedal pulses	Neuropathy dominant: absent pinprick palpable pedal pulses
3	>30 mm^2	Bone and/or joint spaces	Osteomyelitis	Gangrene	Charcot's foot

VPT, vibration perception threshold.

soft tissues of the lower limb and foot. There are many circulatory disorders that affect the foot and lower limb. The main group of peripheral arterial disorders that affect the lower limb are occlusive arterial disease in the form of atherosclerosis, vasospastic disease in the form of Raynaud's disease, and vasculitis often associated with connective tissue disorders.

It is important to consider that any circulatory disease that affects delivery of nutrients and removal of waste products can be detrimental to tissue viability. Assessment of medical history and drug treatment may reveal additional conditions that can affect tissue perfusion. An increasingly important aspect of care for the podiatrist is their role in heath promotion. It is useful to consider the risk factors for the development of cardiovascular disease. Preventive action taken at an early stage to reduce the risk factors (see Table 18.8) can dramatically reduce the incidence of the disease. It is important to consider risk factor reduction as an important aspect of practice and record any such reduction appropriately.

The risk factors for coronary heart disease are similar to those for peripheral arterial disease. Hyperlipidaemia and hypertension have a strong association with coronary heart disease. Additional key factors for peripheral arterial disease include diabetes mellitus, smoking and advanced age. The prevalence of peripheral arterial disease increases by up to twofold per decade of life and diabetes and smoking increase the risk fourfold (Case history 18.1). One worrying statistic is that cigarette smoking can result in symptoms of peripheral arterial disease much earlier and the likelihood of peripheral arterial disease increases by 40% for every 10 cigarettes smoked (Almahameed 2006).

Table 18.8 Cardiovascular disease risk factors for the development of foot ulceration

Systemic	*Local*
Heart failure	Peripheral arterial disease
Ischaemic heart disease	Peripheral venous disease
Valvular disease	
Cardiac arrhythmias	
Congenital heart disease	
Pulmonary heart disease	
Infective endocarditis	
Myocardial, pericardial and endocardial disease	
Hypertension	
Marfan's syndrome	

Many podiatry patients present with type 2 diabetes. These patients are at risk for the development of cardiovascular disease, especially atherosclerosis via

Case history 18.1

A 65-year-old man with type 2 diabetes comes to the clinic complaining of fatigue in both legs, pain at night and had an ulcer on the medial side of his left first metatarsophalangeal joint. He is a life-long smoker, smoking 20 cigarettes per day. Foot pulses are absent.

Clinical reasoning:

- The extent and severity of his peripheral vascular disease may be masked as a result of any co-existing sensory neuropathy. He does not complain of intermittent claudication.
- Remember that only 10–30% of all patients with peripheral arterial disease present with classical symptoms of claudication. Patients may complain of fatigue or heaviness in the legs. In addition, patients who may have co-existing coronary artery disease, may not exert themselves sufficiently to bring on the pain of claudication.
- It is important to assess vascular status. With an ABPI of <0.4 it is unlikely that healing of the ulcer will occur and the patient should be referred to vascular services.
- Take a careful pain history. Night pain may be either of neuropathic or ischaemic origin.
- APBIs can be misleading in the presence of calcified arteries (falsely elevated).

the complications of insulin resistance. They often have hypertension and hyperlipidaemia. It is important that the podiatrist recognises the complications and is able to communicate with other members of the multidisciplinary team if there are any concerns regarding management.

Practice point

Remember values of cholesterol to identify risk (Table 18.9).

Table 18.9 Values of cholesterol in identifying risk

Cholesterol	*Risk*	*Treatment*
<5.2 mmol/l	Low	Lifestyle + diet
5.2–6.5 mmol/l	Intermediate	Lifestyle + diet
6.6–8 mmol/l	High	Lifestyle + drugs + diet
>8 mmol/l	Very high	As above + other treatments

Assessment of the critically ischaemic limb

Chronic limb-threatening ischaemia is indicated by rest pain (ischaemic neuritis) which tends to affect the dorsal aspect of the forefoot and is characterised by burning, shooting pain. The presence of ischaemic ulcers or gangrene is also associated with critical ischaemia. These patients are often forced to sleep in a chair as elevation of the limbs is too painful. Unfortunately this can lead to dependent oedema which may further compromise the limb.

Practice points

Elevate the limb and observe elevation pallor. Assessment using the hand-held Doppler can provide further information. Place the probe over the artery for insonation and if the Doppler sounds disappear while gently elevating the limb, then the degree of ischaemia warrants referral to vascular services. It is imperative not to delay in the face of critical ischaemia, especially if infection is suspected. If foot pulses are not palpable and the ABPI is >1, reduced Doppler arterial waveform indicates ischaemia (Edmonds & Foster 2006).

This chapter does not consider treatment options. However, in the Heart Protection Study (Heart Protection Study Collaborative Group 2002), patients with peripheral arterial disease who took statins had a lower incidence of cardiovascular ischaemic events than those who did not take them. The use of statins to reduce risk of ischaemic events, and improves leg function is now becoming a common preventive measure in patients with diabetes.

Skin

Dermatological assessment of the skin and appendages is covered in depth in Chapter 8. The consequences for the at-risk patient involve a breach of the skin and therefore any co-existing skin condition that threatens the integrity of the skin needs to be identified. There are risks factors that significantly affect the skin.

The majority of the at-risk patients have systemic disease and the resultant complications predispose the foot to develop ulceration (Case history 18.2).

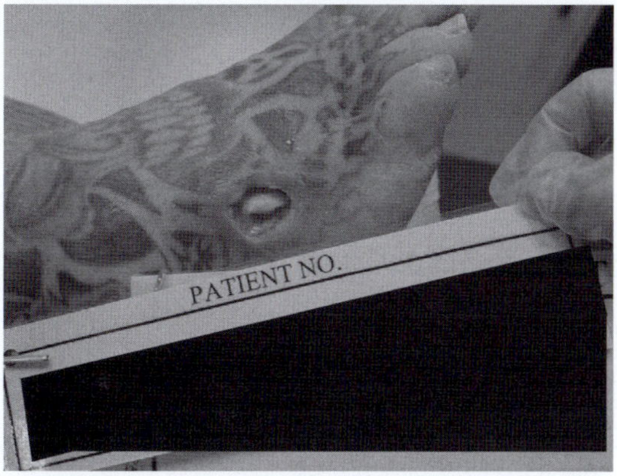

Figure 18.9 Critical ischaemic foot ulcer.

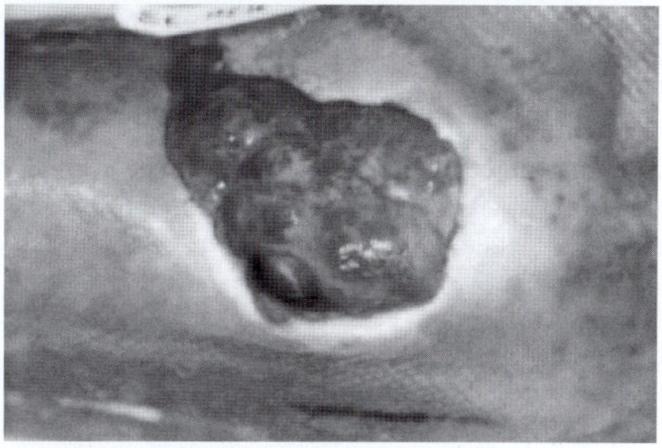

Figure 18.10 Exuberant hypergranulation.

Case history 18.2

A 53-year-old man with type 2 diabetes visits the clinic with a foot ulcer. He has peripheral arterial disease, peripheral neuropathy and a history of poor diabetes control. He also has many tattoos. The ulceration is at the site of the most recent tattoos (Fig. 18.9).

Clinical reasoning:

- Prolonged hyperglycaemia leads to tissue complications. Full assessment needs to be carried out.
- Most foot ulceration results from a combination of peripheral neuropathy, peripheral arterial disease and external pressure.
- Determine the presence of infection.
- Consider relationship of recent tattoo and ulceration.

Many of the patients are elderly and often present with other co-morbidities that can complicate the wounds and impair healing.

There are few published data on decorative tattoo-induced diabetic foot ulceration. In general, complications are relatively rare. However, the introduction of substances from tattoo ink can cause toxic or immunologic responses. These reactions include acute inflammatory reaction, allergic hypersensitivity and granulomatous, lichenoid and pseudolymphomatous types of histopathologic reactions (Tanzi 2007). In addition there are risks of developing the blood-borne viral infection, hepatitis B, and the possibility of acquiring hepatitis C and human immunodeficiency virus infection.

The patient in Case history 18.2 rapidly developed an infection which may have been directly derived from the repeated puncture of tattoo ink into the dermis. Further complication may have resulted from a reaction to the components of the red ink. Despite the use of intravenous antimicrobial treatment, he proceeded to partial amputation.

Practice point

Whilst the decision to have a tattoo or body piercing is entirely the decision of the patient, they need to be informed of the risks, especially if they are an at-risk patient. It is best to avoid having a tattoo on a diabetic neuropathic foot.

Malignancy

Foot ulceration tends to be either predominantly neuropathic or neuro-ischaemic in nature. However, more rarely the diagnosed foot ulcer may mask undetected malignancy. It is vital to detect any abnormality early on in order to refer on for an expert opinion. In a retrospective study of 60 patients with foot/ankle melanoma, the most common location was on the plantar aspect of the foot (Fortin et al 1995). Common misdiagnosis includes plantar warts, fungal disorders, non-healing diabetic ulcers and hyperkeratotic lesions.

Practice point

Atypical hypergranulation (Fig. 18.10) or surrounding warty appearance must alert the clinician to seek further opinion, preferably from a consultant dermatologist. Similarly, while delayed healing of an ulcer may suggest chronic inflammation or critical colonisation, there is also the possibility of malignancy. If in doubt, seek further opinion. IMAGES

Primary melanoma of the foot has a poorer prognosis and early biopsy is indicated. Practitioners need to have a high index of suspicion when attempting to differentiate malignant melanoma from other common skin conditions (Kong et al 2005). Although melanoma accounts for only 4% of all skin cancers, it remains the leading cause of skin cancer-related deaths worldwide (Fernando et al 2006).

There have also been reports about metastatic squamous cell carcinoma resembling osteomyelitis affecting the digits. Metastasis of tumours to the phalanges most commonly causes the signs and symptoms of infection. Peripheral metastasis is associated with a poor prognosis. The survival time for a patient with a pedal lesion is 3–9 months (Libson et al 1987).

Periulcer area and dry skin

Diabetic patients and other at-risk patients can develop dry skin on their legs and feet and the use of emollients is often advised. In addition, the use of an emollient may be advocated for the periulcer area to protect the skin from the adverse effects of the wound exudates. Aqueous cream has often been suggested for this use. However, there have been several reports that irritant reactions can occur (Highet 2002). Also, cutaneous reactions have been associated with formulations of aqueous creams containing phenoxyethanol but not those containing chlorocresol (Cork et al 2003). Aqueous cream was originally designed as a wash product and not to be left on as an emollient.

Practice point

Aqueous cream should not be advised to use as an emollient. Other types of emollients should be advocated.

Endocrine system

Assessment and evaluation of the at-risk patient includes a full medical and drug history. Many of the at-risk patients are older and may have other disorders and treatment that contribute to the development of an ulcer and delay healing. It is not the intention in this section to describe every endocrine disorder, but rather to highlight the common endocrine disorders and consider key aspects that may contribute to the at-risk status and affect prognosis. The endocrine system controls development and growth, energy regulation, internal homeostasis and reproduction. The effects of diabetes mellitus have previously been discussed. The metabolic rate of many tissues is controlled by the thyroid hormones and underactivity and overactivity of the thyroid gland are the most common of all of the endocrine disorders (Table 18.10).

Table 18.10 Signs and symptoms of thyroid dysfunction that may complicate the at-risk foot

Underactive thyroid	*Overactive thyroid*
Weight gain	Muscle weakness
Dry, coarse skin	Onycholysis
Muscle weakness/ stiffness	Proximal muscle wasting
Muscular hypertrophy	Sweating
Proximal myopathy	Grave's dermopathy (rare)
Cold peripheries	Proximal myopathy
Oedema	

Complications of hypocalcaemia (most commonly deficiency of parathyroid hormone) can lead to bone resorption, rickets or osteomalacia, with a tendency for fracture. This would increase the risk of Charcot's arthropathy in patients with diabetes. The post-menopausal syndrome may lead to osteoporosis and the potential for crush fractures affecting the spine and wrist.

Neurological system

Any neurological condition that affects the sensory system would clearly contribute to the at-risk status of the patient. Many neurological disorders affect sensory, motor and autonomic nerves and all can affect the at-risk status (Table 18.11). Whilst diabetes is the most common disease that affects the peripheral nervous system, some other conditions can result in a deficit in all nerve fibres.

Charcot's neuroarthropathy

Ulceration of the foot may well occur in any of the above conditions, especially where there is a

Table 18.11 Conditions that may lead to lower-limb neuropathies

Condition	*Effect*
Diabetes mellitus	Sensorimotor neuropathy mononeuropathies and radiculopathies
Cerebrovascular disease (stroke)	Motor neuropathy
Cerebral palsy	Motor neuropathy
Friedreich's ataxia	Sensory and motor involvement
Motor neurone disease	Motor neuropathy
Vitamin B_{12} deficiency (very low levels)	Polyneuropathy
Multiple sclerosis	Spastic paraparesis
Syringomyelia	Spastic paraparesis and neuropathic joints
Parkinson's disease	Motor neuropathy
Chronic alcoholism	Sensorimotor and neuropathic joints
Poliomyelitis	Motor neuropathy
Malignancy	Mostly sensory
Hansen's disease	Sensory neuropathy
Guillain–Barré syndrome	Mostly sensory involvement
Certain drugs/toxins	Polyneuropathies
HIV/AIDS	Distal symmetrical polyneuropathy
Rheumatoid arthritis	Sensory and mononeuropathies

significant sensory loss. One neurological complication that affects the at-risk foot is the development of the Charcot's foot or Charcot's neuroarthropathy. While diabetes is the most common condition associated with this complication, other diseases can cause this destructive joint disorder (Box 18.5).

The aetiology of Charcot's neuroarthropathy remains elusive and the condition can be difficult to diagnose especially in the presence of osteomyelitis. Jeffcoate et al (2005) has suggested a hypothesis for this disabling condition which may well help to

Box 18.5 Conditions associated with Charcot's foot

- Diabetes mellitus
- Spinal cord injury
- Syphilis
- Syringomyelia
- Chronic alcoholism
- Renal dialysis
- Leprosy
- Congenital insensitivity to pain
- Meningomyelocele

develop treatment strategies for the future. Charcot's foot is characterised by pathologic fractures, joint dislocation and deformity (Armstrong & Peters 2002) and ulceration can complicate the condition. Infection can further complicate Charcot's joint, leading to prolonged treatment and poorer prognosis.

Jeffcoate et al (2005) has proposed a role for pro-inflammatory cytokines in the cause of the Charcot's foot. It is interesting to note that similar pathological mechanisms may be responsible for the altered inflammation associated with the non-healing chronic ulcer. Early detection is important, as therapeutic intervention at this stage is considered to help prevent gross deformity and subsequent ulceration. The practitioner should consider the risk factors that can lead to Charcot's arthropathy (Box 18.6) and have a high index of suspicion in the presence of a warm swollen foot in patients with neuropathy (Fig. 18.11). The differential diagnoses include gout, pseudogout, severe sprain, rheumatoid arthritis, septic arthritis and osteomyelitis. There is often a history of trauma reported by patients with Charcot's joint, but this finding may not always be present. Of all the potential alternative diagnoses osteomyelitis is by far the most common and hardest to differentiate. The use of an indium-labelled white blood cell bone scan or MRI scan is helpful to distinguish infective from neuropathic causes but even the most sophisticated technique cannot provide 100% sensitivity. It is also important to consider that the two conditions can, and frequently do, co-exist. This is most frequently seen in long-standing Charcot's in which ulceration and subsequent bone infection has developed due to the severe bony prominences and joint deformity (Fig. 18.12).

Box 18.6 Risk factors associated with Charcot arthropathy

- Diabetic peripheral neuropathy
- History of trauma
- Elevation in skin temperature of 3–7°
- Excessive alcohol
- Osteopenia
- Poor diabetic control
- Long duration of diabetes
- Retinopathy
- Nephropathy
- History of previous ulceration
- Obesity

Practice point

Where there is an absence of a break in the skin and a history of trauma, assume a diagnosis of Charcot's joint until confirmation with interpretive radiology. It is important to request blood tests and X-ray early on. With the patient supine, elevate the leg for 5–10 minutes. If the swelling and redness dissipates, the

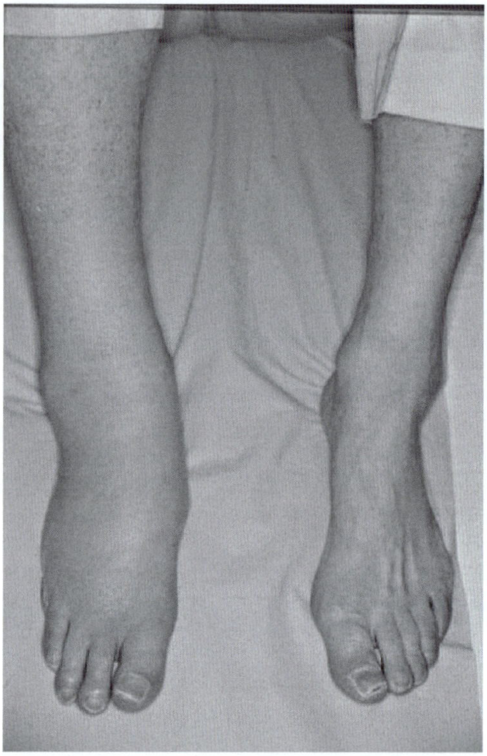

Figure 18.11 Acute Charcot's foot.

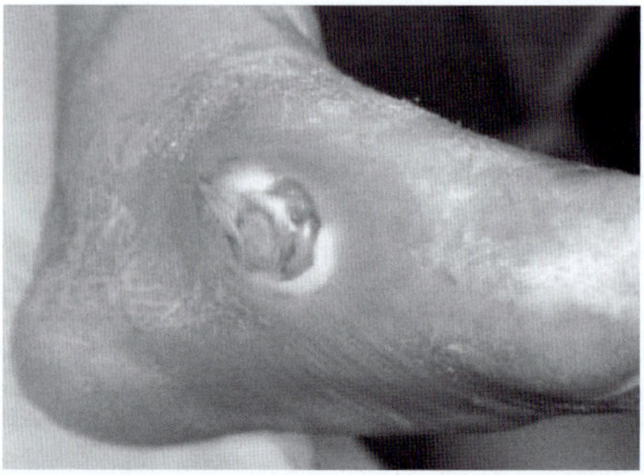

Figure 18.12 Longstanding Charcot's arthropathy with ulcer and osteomyelitis.

diagnosis of Charcot's joint is supported. If swelling and redness persists, then infection is more likely (Brodsky 1993a,b).

Blood tests can be very helpful in the diagnosis of Charcot's arthropathy and include:

- CRP
- ESR
- full blood count
- HbA_{1C}
- serum uric acid
- alkaline phosphatase
- parathyroid hormone.

Care must be taken in interpretation of serologic results. CRP is a reliable marker for the detection of infection (sensitivity 88% and specificity of 96%). However, diabetic patients may have elevated CRP as a result of vascular insult and other conditions so that interpretation of a raised result should be undertaken by appropriate specialists. It has been reported that the CRP is not raised as a result of the inflammatory flare that is characteristic of the acute phase of Charcot's joint. This may be useful in the differential diagnosis of the condition (Judge 2007).

Classification of Charcot's neuroarthropathy has been proposed by Eichenholz (1999) (Table 18.12) and by Sella & Barette (Table 18.13). The classification systems are useful as they help in the diagnosis, staging and treatment of the condition.

Table 18.12 Classification of Eichenholz

Phase	*Description*
Development	Bone fragmentation
Coalescence	Absorption of small bone fragments, fusion of joints (ankylosis)
Remodelling	Healing and new bone formation

Table 18.13 Classification of Sella and Barette

Stage	*Description*
0	Localised heat and swelling. Bone scan may be positive. Minimal radiological changes
1	Localised osteopenia, subchondral cysts, erosions and possible diastasis
2	Joint subluxations
3	Joint dislocations and joint collapse
4	Healing: sclerosis and fusion with trabecular patterns

Musculoskeletal system

Tissue viability can be affected by a number of musculoskeletal or connective tissue disorders. In addition the prolonged use of steroid drug therapy can lead to atrophic changes in the skin. Foot deformity is a common complication of some inflammatory arthropathies and ulceration is a frequent complication.

Rheumatoid arthritis

Rheumatoid arthritis is a chronic inflammatory disease that often involves the foot being affected by pain, oedema, deformity, callus and ulceration (Wiener-Ogilvie 1999). Tissue viability can be further threatened by the presence of nodules which can ulcerate. Vasculitis can add further complications by delaying wound healing. The theoretical mechanism for forefoot deformity in rheumatoid arthritis is shown in **Figure 18.13**.

Foot pain has been reported in up to 94% of patients with long-standing rheumatoid arthritis. The Manchester Foot Pain and Disability Questionnaire is a valid tool to assess disabling foot pain and is easy to use for evaluation (Garrow et al 2000). To assess the risk status of the patient in terms of impending ulceration it may be useful to consider the use of this questionnaire in tandem with the Disease Activity Score (Van der Heijde et al 1990). Tissue viability may be compromised by the effect of vasculitis which ranges from inflammation of the venules and small arteries to a necrotising arteritis that can affect small- and medium-sized arteries (Firth 2005). This may manifest as purpura, erythematous nodules or ulceration and necrosis in the lower limb and foot (Ehrlich 1993).

Differential diagnosis

The vasculitic ulcer may occur on the lower leg and dorsal aspect of the foot. It can manifest suddenly, often preceded by palpable purpura and ecchymosis.

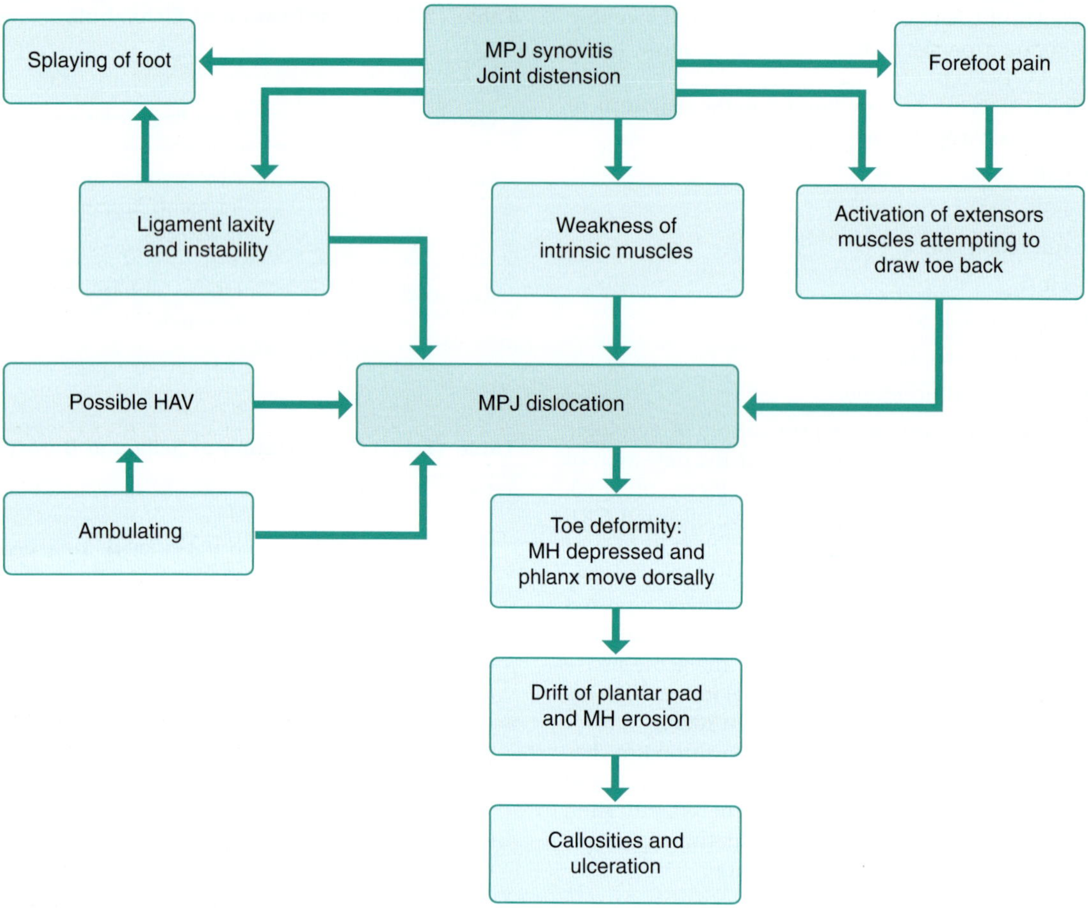

Figure 18.13 Mechanism of deformity in the forefoot. (After Wiener-Ogilvie 1999.) MPTJ, metatarsophalangeal joint; MH, metatarsal head; HAV, hallux abductovalgus.

The ulcers may be well demarcated and are often painful and slow healing. The risk factors for foot ulcers associated with rheumatoid arthritis are shown in Table 18.14. Crucial in the development of ulceration is foot deformity and there is strong evidence to suggest that prevention of foot deformity greatly reduces the risk of foot ulceration and disabling foot pain (Woodburn et al 2002, 2003).

Practice point

Consider the drug regimen of patients with rheumatoid arthritis in the assessment process. Anti-tumour necrosis factor (TNF) alpha agents are indicated for treatment in those who have progressive clinically active rheumatoid arthritis that has not responded to at least two disease-modifying anti-rheumatic drugs, including methotrexate. These agents should not be started if there is an active source of infection. TNF alpha is a key regulator of innate immunity (Otter et al 2005).

Gout

Gout is an inflammatory condition which occurs when monosodium urate crystals are deposited in body tissue. These crystal deposits are referred to as tophi and can be found in synovial membranes, bones, tendons, ligaments and skin. The most common site in the foot involves the first metatarsal phalangeal joint. The interphalangeal joint can also be affected. Bone can be destroyed as the tophus grows, the bone cortex becomes thin and is replaced by urates (Larmon 1970).

Differential diagnosis

The diagnosis of gout is usually a clinical one, after careful history taking and examination. The

Table 18.14 Risk factors for foot ulcers associated with rheumatoid arthritis

Factor	*Effect*
Reduced mobility	Increase in pressure sites; difficulty with self-care
Poor nutrition	Depressed appetite, delayed healing
Medication	Atrophy of skin, delayed/ impaired healing
Extra-articular effects	Vasculitis, peripheral neuropathy, nodules
Foot deformity	Increased plantar pressure, shear stress from shoes
Peripheral arterial disease	Dry, atrophic skin, delayed healing
Use of inappropriate footcare products	Tissue breakdown and infection

differential diagnosis includes septic arthritis, osteomyelitis, rheumatoid arthritis and Charcot's neuroarthropathy. A request for a blood test will reveal a raised serum uric acid level (normal 2–6 mg/100 ml).

Practice point

CRP and ESR are usually higher in those patients with septic arthritis than those with gout. Gout has often been described as 'exquisitely painful' and often is worst at night.

Haematological system

Several blood disorders can affect tissue viability and healing of foot wounds. Essential thrombocythemia and secondary thrombocythemia results in the overproduction of platelets, which may lead to clotting of small vessels. The secondary form of the disease can be due to iron deficiency anaemia, leukaemia, lymphoma, polycythemia vera, rheumatoid arthritis and cancer that has metastasised. Hydroxyurea is a common cancer chemotherapy agent and is considered the drug of choice for the treatment of chronic myelogenous leukaemia and essential thrombocythemia. Leg ulcers have been identified in 8.5% of patients receiving continuous treatment with hydroxyurea, although the cause is unknown (Velez et al 1999).

Sickle cell anaemia is caused by an abnormal type of haemoglobin called haemoglobin S. This type reduces the amount of oxygen inside the red blood cells, distorting their shape (sickle). This can lead to blocked blood vessels and organs. Sickle cell disease affects 1:500 African Americans. A child who inherits haemoglobin S from one parent and normal from the other parent (type A), will have sickle cell trait. Someone who inherits type S and another abnormal type of haemoglobin will have another form of sickle cell disease called thalassaemia. In both thalassaemia and sickle cell disease tissue viability can be compromised by the onset of leg ulcers, susceptibility to infections and bone pain.

Hydroxyurea is also used to treat this condition and there have been some concerns about the possibility of the drug causing leukaemia.

Practice point

Patients with sickle cell disease are more likely to develop infections in any leg wound or ulcer.

Clinical decision making

With the shift in demographics to an older population and the increase in chronic disease, especially diabetes, there is an anticipated increase in patients with at-risk feet. From the newly qualified to the advanced practitioner, there is a requirement for the skills of clinical reasoning and critical reflective practice.

Clinical reasoning

Clinical reasoning is a process of reflective inquiry, involving the patient, which seeks to promote a deep and contextually relevant understanding of the clinical problem in order to provide a sound basis for clinical intervention. It is much more than the diagnostic process.

Schon (1988) contends that clinical reasoning is far-reaching and goes beyond 'the professional activity of instrumental problem solving made rigorous by the application of scientific theory and technique'. Technical problem solving needs to be considered in a much broader context of reflective enquiry and 'link the practice of uncertainty and uniqueness to the scientist's art of research.' Clinical reasoning consists of three core elements:

- knowledge
- cognition
- metacognition.

Knowledge

The acquisition of knowledge by the student is a staged process which includes the development of concepts from the basic sciences and the biomedical sciences. Problem-solving skills develop alongside the knowledge gained as the concepts are developed (Boshuizen & Schmidt 1992). Previously detailed pathophysiological/biomedical knowledge becomes encapsulated into broader clinical concepts. Students do not have to activate all possible biomedical knowledge to understand what is occurring.

Example

The patient with rheumatoid arthritis may present with ulnar deviation of both hands, primarily affecting the metacarpal joints. The biomedical knowledge of the development of pannus formation and other pathological changes is not required to recognise the presence of inflammatory arthritis.

Cognition

The development of cognitive skills will manifest in methods of data analysis and synthesis of inquiry strategies. The student develops problem forming which is an ability to construct an abstract concept from a collection of factual information. This will lead to a form of pattern recognition. This is referred to as inductive reasoning.

Example

The patient with symmetrical involvement of the synovial joints of the hands and feet, and who complains of stiffness in the morning. This is typical of the pattern of rheumatoid arthritis. Recognition of this pattern is inductive reasoning. This skill develops with experience and exposure to such patterns. The student who has little experience and has not developed the knowledge concepts will engage in deductive reasoning by the generation of several hypothesis, in an attempt to identify the problem.

The experienced clinician when solving a clinical problem activates one or a few illness scripts. The enabling conditions of the patient are matched to the elements of the script. Illness scripts also generate expectations about other signs and symptoms the patient may have. Activated scripts provide an opportunity to seek clinical findings/values that are expected by the presentation of the patient. If the scripts fail to match they are deactivated. The activated script provides a differential diagnosis, when a few competing scripts remain active.

Example

The diabetic patient presents with a hot swollen, red foot. There is little pain and a history of trauma. The expert clinician recognises a pattern of signs and symptoms and activates an illness script via a series of questions. Depending on the responses of the patient, a working differential diagnosis of Charcot's foot, cellulitis, severe soft-tissue injury or gout may be made. Further tests and investigations will be requested to determine a definite diagnosis.

This is a difficult skill for the student to develop. Illness scripting requires experience with patients. The difficulties in scripting for the students include the lack of information available and the inability to recognise information that may be relevant. Overlooked information occurs as a lack of knowledge concepts and experience.

Example

A diabetic patient with an infected neuro-ischaemic ulcer who suffers from renal failure. The experienced clinician will recognise the risks that infection poses in this patient, whilst the student may not realise the implications of co-existing renal failure. This vital information is overlooked.

Metacognition

This is rather an esoteric term, but it is an essential component of clinical reasoning. This is the integrative element between cognition and knowledge. Throughout the reasoning process, the core elements of knowledge, cognition and metacognition interact. Clinical data are processed against the practitioner's knowledge and experience. Metacognition is the process of thinking about one's thinking. It has been described as thinking in action, or reflection in action (Higgs & Jones 1995). Metacognition is about thinking at a higher level.

Example

The Charcot patient – practitioner's metacognition:

- Have I considered everything?
- What about the possibility of osteomyelitis?
- Have I addressed the patient's concerns?
- Have I requested the correct tests?
- Should the patient be admitted today?

Metacognition, in a sense is about professional responsibility and discipline. This thinking discipline may be considered as the core elements of reflective practice.

Reflective practice

'Reflective practice is the form of practice which seeks to problematise many situations of professional performance so that they can become potential learning situations and so the practitioners can continue to learn, grow and develop in and through practice' (Jarvis 1992).

The three domains that the clinician is required to reflect on include:

- cognitive (thinking)
- affective (feelings)
- behavioural (actions).

These domains fit with the identified learning styles by Honey & Mumford (1992) of the activists, reflectors, theorists and pragmatists. The skill of critical reflection requires the learning style of the reflector.

Without reflective practice, the practitioner will fail to develop and will not learn from mistakes and more importantly will not be providing the best care they can to their patients. Clinical practice is never completely perfect, but with reflective practice, care can continually improve.

Critical incident analysis

Despite the best care systems, working with the at-risk patients can result in amputation. This may be a devastating consequence of the combination of peripheral neuropathy, peripheral arterial disease and infection. The multidisciplinary footcare team can analyse these events with a view to identify the reasons for the amputation and learn from the event in an attempt to prevent similar future events. Amputation may be unavoidable at times, but it is important to scrutinise team practice to ensure that any system faults are eradicated.

An example of a model of reflection is Gibb's (1988) cycle of reflection which can be used to analyse a situation as described above (Fig. 18.14).

Using a simple model of reflection, the event of an amputation can be closely scrutinised and lessons learned from the event. It is important to carry out this reflection in an environment that is blame-free and aimed at better organisational performances. This will lead to better results rather than focusing on individuals. The emphasis is on improving care and preventing future adverse outcomes (Chadwick & Young 2006). Reflective practice makes a useful

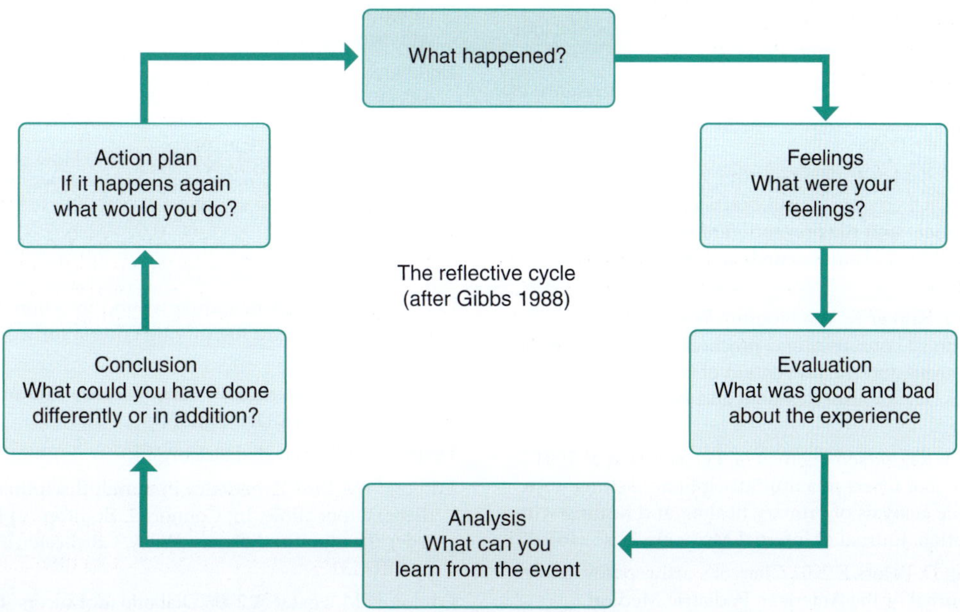

Figure 18.14 Gibb's model of reflection.

contribution to the development of knowledge and improved practice (Wilkinson 1999).

Summary

Assessment of the at-risk foot is one of the most important and difficult aspects of clinical practice that the practitioner will ever engage in. While the rewards may be profound in assessing and healing the 'at-risk' foot, conversely the failures can have tragic and devastating consequences. A sound knowledge base, clinical reasoning and reflective practice skills are the essential components for the successful practitioner. Perfect practice may not be an achievable goal, but to continually strive to improve practice is the hallmark of the professional practitioner.

References

Abbott C A, Carrington A L, Ashe H et al 2002 The North-West Diabetes Foot Care Study: incidence of, and risk factors for, new diabetic foot ulceration in a community-based patient cohort. Diabetic Medicine 19(5):377–384

Adler A, Boyko E, Ahroni E et al 1999 Lower-extremity amputation in diabetes: the independent effects of peripheral vascular disease, sensory neuropathy and foot ulcers. Diabetes Care 22(7):1029–1035

Alder N, Boyce W, Chesney M et al 1993 Socioeconomic inequalities in health: no easy solution. Journal of the American Medical Association 269:3140–3145

Almahameed A 2006 Peripheral arterial disease: recognition and medical management. Cleveland Clinic Journal of Medicine 73(7):621–638

Anderson R, Lustman P, Clouse R et al 2000 Prevalence of depression in adults with diabetes: a systematic review. Diabetes. 49(1):A64

Apelqvist J, Bakker K, Van Houtum W et al 1993 International consensus and practical guidelines on the management and the prevention of the diabetic foot. Diabetes Metabolism Research and Reviews 16(1): S84–92

Apelqvist J, Bakker K, Van Houtum W H 2000 International consensus and practical guidelines on the management and the prevention of the diabetic foot, Diabetes/Metabolism Research and Reviews 16(suppl 1):S84–S92

Apelqvist J, Ragnarson-Tennval G, Persson U et al 1994 Diabetic foot ulcers in a multidisciplinary setting – An economic analysis of primary healing and healing with amputation. Journal of Internal Medicine 235(5):463–471

Armstrong D, Peters E 2002 Charcot's arthropathy of the foot. Journal of the American Podiatric Medical Association 92(7):390–394

Ashcroft G, Horan M, Ferguson M 1997 The effects of ageing on wound healing: immunolocalisation of growth factors and their receptors in a murine incisional model. Journal of Anatomy 190(3):351–365

Bandura A 1977 Self-efficacy: toward a unifying theory of behaviour change. Psychological Review 84:191–215

Bann C M, Fehnel S, Gagnon D D 2003 Development and validation of the diabetic foot ulcer scale-short form (DFS-SF). Pharmacoeconomics 21(17):1277–1290

Best practice pathway of care for people with diabetic foot problems 2007 The Diabetic Foot Journal 10(1)

Boshuizen H, Schmidt H 1992 On the role of biomedical knowledge in clinical reasoning by experts, intermediates and novices. Cognitive Sciences 16:153–184

Boufi M, Ghaffari P, Allaire E et al 2006 Foot gangrene in patients with end-stage renal disease: a case control study. Angiology 57:355–361

Boulton A J 1996 The pathogenesis of diabetic foot problems: an overview. Diabetic Medicine 13 Suppl 1: S12–S16

Boulton A J M 2005 Management of diabetic peripheral neuropathy. Clinical Diabetes 23:9–15

Boyko E J, Ahroni J H, Stensel V et al 1999 A prospective study of risk factors for diabetic foot ulcer: the Seattle Diabetic Foot Study. Diabetes Care 22:1036–1042

Boyko E, Ahroni J, Cohen V et al 2006 Prediction of diabetic foot ulcer occurrence using commonly available clinical information. Diabetes Care 29:1202–1207

Brodsky J W 1993a Outpatient diagnosis and care of the diabetic foot. Instructive Course Lectures 42:121–39

Brodsky J W 1993b The diabetic foot. In: Mann RA, Coughlin MJ (eds). Surgery of the foot and ankle, 6th edn. Mosby, St Louis

Chadwick P, Young R 2006 Critical event analysis: reflecting on major amputations. Diabetic Foot 9(2):66–74

Chantelau E, Kushner T, Spraul M 1990 How effective is cushioned therapeutic footwear in protecting diabetic feet? Diabetic Medicine 7:355

Clark M 2006 The long and winding road. Practical Diabetes International 23(2):69–74

Cooper R 2005 Understanding wound infection: EWMA position document. Identifying criteria for wound infection.

Department of Health 2001 National service framework for older people. DH, London

Diabetes UK (www.diabetes.org.uk)

Edmonds M 1987 Experience in a multidisciplinary diabetic foot clinic. In: Connor H, Boulton A J M et al (eds). The foot in diabetes. Wiley, Chichester, pp 121–131

Edmonds M, Foster A 2006 Diabetic foot ulcers. BMJ 332(7538):407–410

Ehrlich M 1993 Vasculitic ulcers: a complication of collagen-vascular disorders. Wound Management 39(1):12–25

El-Domyati M, Attia S, Saleh F et al 2002 Intrinsic aging vs. photoaging: a comparative histopathological, immunohistochemical, and ultrastructural study of skin. Experimental Dermatology 11:398–405

Everson S, Maty S, Lynch J et al 2002 Epidemiologic evidence for the relation between socioeconomic status and depression, obesity, and diabetes. Journal of Psychosomatic Research 53(4):891–895

Falanga V, Eaglstein W 1988 Wound healing: practical aspects. Progress in Dermatology 22(3):1–12

Fernando D, Rajendra J, Emmerson E 2006 A non-healing foot ulcer in a patient with type 2 diabetes mellitus. European Journal of Internal Medicine 17(6):452

Firth J 2005 Tissue viability in rheumatoid arthritis. Tissue Viability Society 15(3):12–18

Fisher G, Kang S, Varani J et al 2002 Mechanisms of photoaging and chronological skin aging. Archives of Dermatology 138:1462–1470

Fortin P, Freiberg A, Rees R et al 1995 Malignant melanoma of the foot and ankle. Journal of Bone and Joint Surgery (Am) 77:1396–1403

Frykberg R, Abraham S, Tierney E et al 2007 Syme amputation for limb salvage: early experience with 26 cases. Journal of Foot and Ankle Surgery 46(2):93–100

Frykberg R, Lavery L, Pham H et al 1998 Role of neuropathy and high foot pressure in diabetic foot ulceration. Diabetes Care 21(10):1714–1719

Garrow A, Papageorgiou A, Silman A et al 2000 Development and validation of a questionnaire to assess disabling foot pain. Pain 85:107–113

Gibbs G 1988 Learning by doing: a guide to teaching and learning methods. Further Education Unit, Oxford Polytechnic, Oxford

Goldman R, Salcido R 2002 More than one way to measure a wound: an overview of tools and techniques. Advances in Skin and Wound Care 15(5):236–243

Gordois A, Scuffham P, Shearer A et al 2003 The healthcare costs of diabetic neuropathy in the UK. Diabetic Foot 6:62–73

Hampson S, McKay H, Glasgow R 1996 Patient–physician interactions in diabetes management: consistencies and variations in the structure and content of two consultations. Patient Education and Counselling 29(1):49–58

Hardy M 1989 The biology of scar formation. Physical Therapy 69:1014–1024

Heart Protection Study Collaborative Group 2002 MRC/BHF Heart Protection Study of cholesterol lowering with simvastatin in 20,536 high risk individuals: a randomised placebo-controlled trial. Lancet 360:17–22

Help Age International 2005 www.helpage.org

Hewitt Rt Hon Patricia Secretary of State for Health 2006 A vision for public health in the 21st century. Public Health 120(12):1098–1101

Higgs J, Jones M 1995 Clinical reasoning. Clinical Reasoning in the Health Professions 1:3–19

Highet A 2002 Using emollients effectively. Dermatological Practice 10:12–15

Hinchcliffe R, Kirk B, Bhattacharjee D et al 2006 The effect of haemodialysis on transcutaneous oxygen tension in patients with diabetes. Nephrology and Dialysis Transplant 21:1981–1983

Honey P, Mumford A 1992 The manual of learning styles, 3rd edn. Maidenhead, Maidenhead: Peter Honey Publications

Jarvis P 1992 Reflective practice and nursing. Nurse Education Today 12:174–181

Jeffcoate W, Game F, Cavanagh P 2005 The role of inflammatory cytokines in the cause of neuropathic osteoarthropathy (acute Charcot foot) in diabetes. Lancet 366(9502):2058–2061

Judge M 2007 Continuing Education: using serologic screening to identify and monitor at-risk Charcot patients. Podiatry Today 17(8)

Kinmond K, McGee P, Gough S et al 2003 'Loss of self': a psychosocial study of the quality of life of adults with diabetic foot ulceration. Journal of Tissue Viability 13(1):6–16

Kong M, Jogia R, Jackson S et al 2005 Malignant melanoma presenting as a foot ulcer. Lancet 366(9498):1740

Laing S, Swerdlow A, Slater S et al 2003 Mortality from heart disease in a cohort of 23,000 patients with insulin-treated diabetes. Diabetologia 46(6):760–765

Larmon W 1970 Surgical management of tophaceous gout. Clinical Orthopaedics 71:56–69

Libson E, Bloom R, Husband J et al 1987 Metastatic tumors of bones of the hand and foot a comparative review and report of 43 additional cases. Skeletal Radiology 16:387–392

Lincoln N B, Jeffcoate W J, Ince P et al 2007 Validation of a new measure of protective footcare behaviour: the Nottingham Assessment of Functional Footcare (NAFF). Practical Diabetes International 24: 207

Lipsky B, Berendt A, Deery H et al 2005 Diagnosis and treatment of diabetic foot infections. Journal of the American Podiatric Medical Association 95(2): 183–210

Macfarlane R, Jeffcoate W 1997 Factors contributing to the presentation of diabetic foot ulcers. Diabetic Medicine 14(10):867–70

Malone J, Snyder M, Anderson G et al 1989 Prevention of amputation by diabetic education. American Journal of Surgery 158(6):520–524

Merza Z, Tesfaye S 2003 The risk factors for diabetic foot ulceration. The Foot 13(3):125–129

Michelson J, Easley M, Wigley F M et al 1994 Foot and ankle problems in rheumatoid arthritis. Foot and Ankle International 15 (11):608–13

National Institute for Clinical Excellence 2004 Type 2 diabetes: prevention and management of foot problems. Clinical guidance 10. NICE, London

Otter S, Robinson C, Berry H 2005 Rheumatoid arthritis, foot infection and tumour necrosis factor alpha inhibition – a case history. The Foot 15(2):117–119

Oyibo S, Jude E, Tarawneh I et al 2001 The effects of ulcer size and site, patient's age, sex and type and duration of diabetes on the outcome of diabetic foot ulcers. Diabetic Medicine 18:133–138

Pecoraro R, Reiber G, Burgess E 1990 Pathways to amputation: basis for prevention. Diabetes Care 13(5):13–521

Peters E J, Lavery L A; International Working Group on the Diabetic Foot 2001 Effectiveness of the diabetic foot risk classification system of the International Working Group on the Diabetic Foot. Diabetes Care 24(8):1442–1447

Price P, Harding K 2004 Cardiff wound impact schedule: the development of a condition-specific questionnaire to assess health-related quality of life in patients with chronic wounds of the lower limb. International Wound Journal 1(1):10

Reiber G, Vileikyte L, Boyko E et al 1999 Causal pathways for incident lower-extremity ulcers in patients with diabetes from two settings. Diabetes Care 22(1):157–162

Rith-Najarian S, Stolusky T, Gohdes D 1992 Identifying diabetic patients at high risk for lower extremity amputation in a primary care health care setting: a prospective evaluation of simple screening criteria. Diabetes Care 15:1386–1389

Savage S, Estacio R, Jeffers B et al 1996 Urinary albumin excretion as a predictor of diabetic retinopathy, neuropathy, and cardiovascular disease in NIDDM. Diabetes Care 19(11):1243–1248

Schon D 1988 From technical rationality to reflection-in-action. In: Dowie J, Elstein A (eds) Professional judgement. Cambridge University Press, Cambridge, pp 60–77

Scottish Intercollegiate Guidelines Network 2001 The management of diabetes. SIGN guideline 55. Royal College of Physicians, SIGN, Edinburgh

Sella E J, Barette C 1999 Staging of Charcot neuroarthropathy along the medial column of the foot in the diabetic patient. Journal of Foot and Ankle Surgery 38:34–40

Shinsaku T, Shigeru I, Naomi S, et al 2005 Analysis of ischemia-reperfusion injury in a microcirculatory model of pressure ulcers. Wound Repair and Regeneration 13(2): 209–215

Smith L A 2003 Clinical experience using silver antimicrobial dressings on venous stasis ulcers. Ostomy Wound Management 2 February (Suppl):10–12

Stuart L, Gambling T, McInnes A 2004 Patient-centred education: time to reflect? The Diabetic Foot Journal. Winter edition.

Tanzi E 2007 Tattoo reactions. Available at: www.emedicine.com/derm/topic512.htm (accessed 3 January 2008)

Treece K A, Macfarlane R M, Pound N 2004 Validation of a system of foot ulcer classification in diabetes mellitus. Diabetic Medicine 21(9):987–991

Turner W, McLeod-Roberts J 2002 The at-risk foot. In: Merriman L M, Turner W (eds) Assessment of the lower limb, 2nd edn. Churchill Livingstone, Edinburgh, pp 427–449

Tzaphlidou M 2004 The role of collagen and elastin in aged skin: an image processing approach. Micron 35(3):173–177

Uccioli L, Faglia E, Monticone G et al 1995 Manufactured shoes in the prevention of diabetic foot ulcers. Diabetes Care 18(10):1376–1378

Van der Heijde D, van't Hof M, van Riel P et al 1990 Judging disease activity in clinical practice in rheumatoid arthritis: first step in the development of a disease activity score. Annals of Rheumatological Disease 49:916–920

Velez A, Garcia-Aranda J, Moreno J 1999 Hydroxyurea-induced leg ulcers: is macroerythrocytosis a pathogenic factor? Journal of the European Academy of Dermatology and Venereology 12:243–244

Vilekyte L, Peyrot M, Bundy C et al 2003 The development and validation of a neuropathy- and foot ulcer-specific quality of life instrument. Diabetes Care 26:2549–2555

Vowden P, Cooper R 2006 An integrated approach to managing wound infection. EWMA Position Document.

Wiener-Ogilvie S 1999 The foot in rheumatoid arthritis. The Foot 9:169–174

Wilkinson J 1999 Implementing reflective practice. Nursing Standard 13(21):36–40

Williamson D, Harding K 2000 Wound healing medicine 28:11 3–6

Woodburn J, Barker S, Helliwell P 2002 A randomised controlled trial of foot orthoses in rheumatoid arthritis. Journal of Rheumatology 29(7):1377–1383

Woodburn J, Helliwell P, Barker S 2003 Changes in 3d joint kinematics support the continuous use of foot orthoses in the management of painful rearfoot deformity in rheumatoid arthritis. Journal of Rheumatology 30(11):2356–2364

CHAPTER

19

Assessment of the surgical patient

I Reilly

Chapter contents

Introduction

The process of surgery can be broken down into three distinct phases: the pre-operative, intra-operative and post-operative phases. These phases are collectively known as the peri-operative period and may overlap and vary in relative importance, depending on the individual patient and the nature of the planned surgical procedure. The overall results of surgery depend on the effective assessment and management of each phase. Box 19.1 lists the key issues in the assessment process. Corrective surgery can help resolve many chronic foot conditions that have traditionally been treated with conservative or palliative care. For example, the treatment of ingrown toe nails in the UK has been transformed by the phenol-alcohol nail surgery technique. Hammer toes and hallux abductovalgus are other common forefoot complaints that can be corrected with surgery.

Pre-surgical assessment should be tailored to the individual patient with regard to their medical history, their expectations and their choice of anaesthesia. The majority of surgical procedures on the foot performed by podiatrists and podiatric surgeons in the UK are undertaken on an elective day-case basis under local or regional anaesthesia. Procedures on the hindfoot and the ankle and other operations that require prolonged periods of anaesthesia or immobility are more likely to be performed under general anaesthesia (GA). The option to perform regional anaesthesia was traditionally reserved for the medically compromised patient, but now it has become the first choice for many consultant anaesthetists. Published studies have demonstrated safer practice, reduced costs and high patient satisfaction to validate its place in modern anaesthesia. The most important advances in anaesthetic techniques include the development of new general anaesthetic agents of short duration and advanced techniques in the administration of spinal, epidural and regional nerve blockade. It is predicted that the number, variety and complexity of surgical procedures performed in an outpatient setting will continue to expand.

Box 19.1 The pre-operative assessment process

Information from the primary patient assessment

- What is the diagnosis?
- What are the important facets of the history?
- Is surgery indicated?
- What further investigations are required?

Health status and fitness for surgery

- Is the patient fit for the planned surgery?
- Are there any concomitant diseases that increase the peri-operative risk?
- Is the patient on any drugs that could influence the surgical outcome?
- What medical management is required?

The anaesthetic

- Local, regional or general anaesthetic?
- If local – which technique will be used – field, digital, ankle, popliteal, other?

The operation

- What is the aim of surgery?
- What is the surgical plan?
- Does the surgery itself pose any special problems?
- Has informed consent been obtained?

After the operation

- Can any problems be anticipated?
- What home support is required/available?
- Have re-dressing appointments been arranged?
- What other factors will affect the post-operative recovery?
- Is the patient able to use crutches?

Pre-operative assessment

It is the responsibility of the practitioner to determine the most likely diagnosis of the presenting problem based on a detailed history taking and physical examination. Appropriate laboratory investigations and diagnostic imaging support and confirm the provisional diagnosis. Clear communication between the practitioner and the patient is vital and forms the basis of informed consent, which is a prerequisite to any invasive procedure. The decision to recommend surgery to the patient is taken in light of the presenting problem and usually after non-surgical treatment options have been tried (or at least considered) and when the potential risks and benefits of invasive techniques have been calculated in the surgeon's mind and discussed with the patient as part of the consent process.

Purpose of the pre-operative assessment

The purpose of the pre-operative assessment is to:

- review the history of the presenting illness or complaint
- review the major systems of the body and ascertain whether these systems are functioning within normal limits and, if not, to facilitate the management of this
- arrive at an informed position regarding the medical appropriateness of the planned surgical procedure
- identify any factors that may contraindicate surgery or place the patient 'at risk'.

At the end of the assessment the practitioner will have formed an opinion as to whether the patient is fit for surgery and thus will be able to proceed with the management with the knowledge that the risk of encountering an intra-operative or post-operative complication has been reduced to a minimum. An inadequate assessment of the patient's health status may have serious consequences for the surgical patient:

1. The patient is placed at risk – inappropriate or unsafe surgery is performed because of an inadequate surgical assessment. Surgery carried out on patients with certain systemic pathologies carries an increased risk of post-operative morbidity. Medical disorders can complicate surgical practice in various ways, e.g. a patient with rheumatoid arthritis on steroid therapy is prone to impaired healing and infection. Invasive treatment in a patient with haemophilia or a patient taking anticoagulants requires special consideration because of the likelihood of very slow blood clotting and haemorrhage. The use of post-operative analgesia, especially if obtained on patient group directions, requires that the practitioner is familiar with the indications, contraindications, interactions and side effects of the analgesic medication.
2. The surgeon is placed at risk – the practitioner will inevitably encounter blood and tissue fluids. Inadequate history taking with regard to identifying known or potential blood-borne diseases such as hepatitis B places the practitioner and their assistant(s) at risk.

3. An increased risk of clinical emergencies – a number of intra-operative emergencies, such as hypertensive crises, can arise. A detailed pre-operative assessment should identify those at greatest risk. An occult condition may manifest under the stress of surgery, e.g. a cerebrovascular insult may occur intra-operatively or post-operatively in patients with undiagnosed or uncontrolled hypertension.
4. Poor treatment outcomes – a combination of any of the above factors can lead to a poor treatment outcome. Without a thorough assessment and a judicious use of laboratory investigations, certain disease states can be overlooked. Assessment of pre-operative radiographs is often essential if the practitioner is to effectively plan the appropriate surgical procedure.

   N.B. These factors have implications for the litigation risk and overall cost if not adequately discussed.

A systematic approach to the assessment process will ensure that the practitioner covers all relevant areas in the enquiry process. The use of questionnaires give the patient time to consider their answers, reduces the amount of time spent during the consultation and ensures that the patient's answers relate to their current and past health status (see Ch. 5). Health status can be classified using the American Society of Anesthesiologists (ASA) classification (Table 19.1). Patients who fall into either class 1 or 2 are the most suitable for elective procedures.

As already noted in the introduction it is assumed that the practitioner has undertaken a full medical and social history as detailed in Chapter 5. However, there are specific issues that need to be taken into consideration when assessing a patient for elective surgery under local anaesthesia. These are considered below.

Determining surgical need

American podiatrists favour the NLDOCAT system for primary patient evaluation (see Box 19.2). The key component in determining the need for surgery is the treatment received to date and its outcome. Before recommending surgery to a patient, due consideration must be given to non-surgical treatment options. Surgery is indicated either when non-surgical options have been tried but have been unsuccessful, or when conservative treatment is not indicated.

An operation causes physiological stress to the patient. The magnitude of the stress increases with the invasiveness of the procedure. The National Institute of Health and Clinical Excellence (NICE) has suggested a simple grading system for surgery-related stress in the absence of an accepted validated system:

- Grade 1 (minor) – e.g. nail surgery
- Grade 2 (intermediate) – e.g. knee arthroscopy
- Grade 3 (major) – e.g. hysterectomy
- Grade 4 (major +) – e.g. total hip replacement

Table 19.1 American Society of Anesthesiologists (ASA) surgical risk classification

Class	*Symptoms*
P1	The patient has no organic, physiological, biochemical or psychiatric disturbance. The pathological process for which the operation is to be performed is localised and does not entail systemic disturbance
P2	Mild to moderate systemic disturbance caused either by the condition to be treated surgically or by other pathophysiological processes
P3	Severe systemic disturbance or disease from whatever cause, even though it may not be possible to define the degree of disability with finality
P4	Severe systemic disorders that are already life-threatening, not always correctable by operation
P5	The moribund patient who has little chance of survival but is submitted to operation in desperation
P6	A declared brain-dead patient whose organs are being removed for donor purposes

Box 19.2 NLDOCAT system for primary patient evaluation

- N – Nature of the presenting problem
- L – Location
- D – Duration
- O – Onset
- C – Cause of the problem
- A – Aggravating and alleviating factors
- T – Treatment used and its effect

The author would classify most forefoot surgery as grade 2 and most rearfoot surgery as grade 3.

Current health status

General health

In general, patients who are unwell are not good candidates for elective surgical procedures or treatments which are likely to demand close compliance.

Nutrition

Obesity is a condition that may be more complicated than simple overeating. Obesity is associated with various endocrine diseases, such as type 2 diabetes mellitus, peripheral vascular disease, hypertension and cardiac disease, anaemia, deep vein thrombosis (DVT), cholecystitis and nutritional imbalances. Obese patients have an increased risk of post-operative DVT and wound complications such as infection and dehiscence.

It is commonly assumed that malnutrition is rare in Western societies. However, the malnutrition status among elderly people is alarmingly high. A percentage weight loss of 20% or greater is associated with a 10-fold increase in operative mortality following major surgery, and a threefold increase in post-operative infection. Vitamin B_1 (thiamine) and B_{12} deficiencies are associated with peripheral neuropathy. Vitamin C and serum zinc deficiencies may impair wound healing. Seriously underweight patients may be suffering from a range of systemic conditions or they could be poorly nourished due to alcoholism, drug misuse or anorexia nervosa. Fatigue and weight changes are symptoms of many systemic illnesses and are always worthy of note, especially if weight change appears to be rapid.

Pregnancy

Elective surgery is rarely indicated in a pregnant woman. An exception might be for an infected ingrown toe nail not responsive to conservative care. The practitioner should weigh up the relative risk of a small dose of anaesthetic to treat an ingrown toenail versus a protracted period of antibiotic therapy.

Past and current medication

Information about the patient's past and current drug therapy can provide useful information about the patient's health status. Patients should be asked if they are currently taking, or have taken in the past, any medicines or used any ointments or creams that have been prescribed by their doctor or bought over the counter. The practitioner should refer to the *British National Formulary* (BNF) or other pharmacological text if they unfamiliar with any drug the patient is taking. In particular, details of adverse reactions, either by the patient or any member of the patient's family, to previous local anaesthetic injections and other drugs (e.g. antibiotics, analgesics, etc.) should be sought.

Steroids such as prednisolone are commonly used in the treatment of asthma, obstructive airway disease and rheumatoid arthritis. They have three main effects, which can be of importance during the peri-operative period:

- suppression of the hypothalamus–pituitary–adrenal (HPA) axis
- poor wound healing
- predisposition to infection.

There will be a suppression of the HPA axis if the patient has taken more than 7.5 mg/day of prednisolone for more than 1 week. In such instances, consideration must be given to the administration of exogenous steroids to prevent hypotension or cardiovascular collapse. For minor procedures, no supplementary therapy is usually required; for more extensive (grade 3) procedures a typical regimen would be 15 mg PO (by mouth) at 6 a.m. on the day of surgery; and the same dose 12 hours and 24 hours later.

Anticoagulants are used in ischaemic heart disease, mitral stenosis, atrial fibrillation and in the prevention of post-operative thrombosis formation. Heparin inhibits the intrinsic clotting pathway and is used in the short-term prophylaxis of DVT. Warfarin inhibits the extrinsic clotting pathway and is used in long-term therapy. The use of an oral anticoagulant has obvious implications if surgical treatment is planned (Case history 19.1). Adjustment of the dosing regimen can be undertaken to allow surgery to proceed with relative safety. Current NICE guidelines recommend that with warfarin the international normalised ratio (INR) should be below 1.5 for elective surgical procedures. Drugs that alter platelet function include aspirin, non-steroidal anti-inflammatory drugs (NSAIDs), steroids and antihistamines. In patients regularly taking aspirin it may be necessary to stop its use because of delayed clotting after surgery. This should be done 1 week before surgery – with the consent of the patient's GP or drug prescriber. Women taking oral contraception have a slightly increased risk of post-operative DVT and consideration must be given to stopping contraceptive use during the peri-operative period, depending on the grade of surgery and post-operative immobility.

Case history 19.1

A 54-year-old woman presented with an interdigital corn that failed to respond to many years of palliative treatment. The history and physical examination revealed that she had atrial fibrillation for which she took warfarin (to prevent ventricular thrombosis).

Outcome: Surgery was indicated. At first assessment the patient's INR was 4.1. In consultation with her GP and in accordance with current NICE guidelines, her dosage was adjusted to reduce the INR to below 1.5. Surgery was carried out with INR 1.4 on the day. The post-operative course was unremarkable and the patient was discharged after the 12-week follow-up visit.

Case history 19.2

A 32-year-old woman presented with a hammered second toe on her right foot. After pre-surgical assessment she was listed for a proximal interphalangeal joint arthrodesis with percutaneous Kirschner (K) wire. It was planned that the wire would remain in situ for 4–6 weeks, until osseous fusion had been achieved. At the first post-operative visit she presented with a painful, swollen toe and mentioned (for the first time) that she could not wear cheap jewellery.

Diagnosis: Nickel allergy, a component of stainless steel K wires. The wire was removed 2 weeks after the surgery. The toe went on to form a painful pseudo-arthrosis that required revision surgery with a titanium K wire.

Case history 19.3

A 59-year-old widow was referred for treatment for a tailor's bunion. Palliative treatment did not control the symptoms. A pre-operative assessment was undertaken with a view to performing an osteotomy of the fifth metatarsal head. The typical post-operative course involves complete rest for 2 days and performing 'light duties' for between 2 and 4 weeks. Patients are asked not to perform any household duties and to have someone stay with them for the first 2 days in case of an emergency.

The present patient lived alone and had no children. The only home support she was able to organise was from neighbours. This support was not very reliable as the neighbours were out at work all day.

Outcome: In view of the lack of home support, surgery was not offered to the patient.

Counselling must therefore also be given on alternative forms of contraception.

The use of all recreational drugs should be recorded. Patients who use injectable drugs are at a higher risk of hepatitis and human immunodeficiency virus (HIV). Long-term or heavy use of tobacco can affect wound and bone healing due to the immediate vasoconstrictive effect of nicotine as well as the long-term effect of increased platelet adhesiveness and atherosclerosis. Tobacco smokers are also at greater risk of bronchitis, asthma and lung cancer. Heavy alcohol consumption can affect peripheral sensation, immune response, post-operative healing and the metabolism of local anaesthetics, as well as having implications for treatment compliance.

Past medical history

The past medical history consists of information about previous lower-limb problems and the treatment received, as well as details about any problems that have affected the patient's general health. The nature of previous treatment, the name of the practitioner, details of relevant investigations such as X-rays and the patient's view of the treatment success should be recorded. This information may prevent the repetition of tests or treatments which have previously been ineffective (Case history 19.2). Of particular interest is the operative history of the patient. In an audit of the author's National Health Service (NHS) surgical caseload, 10% of patients were referred for revision surgery.

Home circumstances

It is important to assess the patient's home situation. In the case of surgical treatment, the practitioner must establish who is going to transport the patient to and from surgery and who is going to assist them through the immediate post-operative recovery period. Lack of home support may rule out surgical intervention (Case history 19.3). Stairs, either outside or within the house are also important factors to be aware of and can have implications for post-operative recovery.

Occupation

A patient's occupation may be contributing to the lower-limb problem and may influence the decision as to whether surgery could or should be offered. Some patients may have difficulty taking time off work to attend for treatment and need to be aware of

Case history 19.4

A 47-year-old publican attended for a surgical opinion for a complex digital deformity. The pre-operative assessment indicated that he required extensive digital and soft-tissue reconstruction. While discussing his occupation as a landlord, the patient expressed his intention to return to bar work the evening following surgery. He equated the surgery he was to receive with tooth extraction under local anaesthesia. Clear (and written) advice was given regarding the need to rest in the post-operative period.

Outcome: The patient did not comply with the advice given. He presented at his first re-dressing appointment with marked forefoot swelling and pain – more than was expected from the procedure performed. The final result was a less than satisfactory 'sausage toe' because of failure to take appropriate advice. This example highlights the need to document the advice given to patients during the peri-operative period to protect the surgeon from litigious action.

the variable amount of time needed to recuperate from surgery (Case history 19.4). The patient who cannot commit to devoting the time required for healing after surgery is not a good surgical candidate.

Sports and hobbies

Details of any sporting hobby should be sought. As indicated in Case history 19.3, the patient needs to devote time to post-operative healing, and therefore cessation of sporting activity must be emphasised to the patient.

Foreign travel

Details of foreign travel should be recorded in case the patient has acquired an unusual foot infection. In particular, travel to tropical countries and any foot injuries sustained while walking barefoot should be recorded. Many countries have a higher incidence of human immunodeficiency virus (HIV) infection than the UK. A history of blood product transfusion abroad could, therefore, be important.

The systems enquiry

Cardiovascular system

Cardiovascular assessment is covered in detail in Chapter 6. What follows is a discussion of cardiovascular pathologies as they relate to planned elective surgical procedures of the foot. A history of cardiovascular disease should be taken with respect to systemic, peripheral and haematological disease states, followed up by a review of symptomatology.

Patients with ischaemic heart disease (IHD) may present with a history of previous myocardial infarction (MI), stable or unstable angina or a history of previous coronary artery bypass graft (CABG). A detailed history must be taken of all patients who have suffered previous cardiac problems or have high-risk factors such as obesity, hypertension, shortness of breath on exercise, smoking or a family history of cardiac problems. Ten per cent of patients over 50 presenting for non-cardiac surgery had previously had an MI. This is significant because there is a known risk of re-infarction in the peri-operative period. The relative significance of that risk depends on the time elapsed since the first MI. A quarter of patients presenting for non-cardiac surgery are likely to have another MI if less than 3 months has passed since their first attack. However, if more than 6 months is allowed to elapse, the incidence of repeat MI falls to less than 5 in 100 patients.

Angina may be classified as stable or unstable. Stable angina takes the form of chronic, predictable, exertional chest pain. In these circumstances, when there is no history of a previous MI, and other risk factors are absent, the risk of peri-operative MI is low, provided that the patient is not exposed to any excessive stress. The patient's anti-anginal medication should be continued peri-operatively. An assessment needs to be done of how the patient will respond to anaesthesia, local or general. Some patients may find being awake for an operation stressful and, therefore, would be considered unsuitable for local anaesthesia. For other patients a general anaesthetic may be deemed too stressful. Unstable angina is characterised by increased frequency, severity and duration of painful attacks that is not easily controlled by their medication. Angina of recent onset, angina at rest or with minimal exertion or angina awakening the patient from sleep should also be considered unstable. Such unstable angina symptoms carry the same peri-operative risk as having had an MI in the previous 6 months. Surgery is contraindicated until the angina has been stabilised by medical or surgical means. A history of CABG should also be taken into consideration. In essence, these patients have had their symptoms controlled by surgery but they may still have limited cardiac reserve and may not be able to respond well to the additional stress of surgery.

Patients with congestive heart failure (CHF) have diminished cardiac reserve and do not respond well to peri-operative stress. CHF carries a high peri-operative risk of MI in patients given a general anaesthetic, and therefore elective surgery must be avoided in patients presenting with third heart sounds, an elevated jugular venous pulse or pulmonary oedema. As patients undergoing procedures under local anaesthesia frequently experience considerable stress from fear and apprehension, those in cardiac failure represent a high risk of an adverse peri-operative cardiac event. Conduction defects represent a low risk in elective foot surgery under local anaesthesia; however, the opinion of the GP and anaesthetist is useful.

Patients with a history of fainting attacks may require specific assessment before any elective surgery under local or general anaesthesia. Patients will often offer a history of palpitations, 'missed heart beats' or fainting attacks. Any patient who gives a history suggestive of an arrhythmia should have an electrocardiogram (ECG) that can then be carefully assessed by a cardiologist prior to local anaesthesia.

Major heart valve disease is becoming rarer but a heart murmur is still a regular finding in routine medical examinations. Most murmurs are related to turbulent flow of blood in the heart and are not significant and do not represent heart valve damage. A history of valvular heart disease is of concern because it carries a risk of bacterial endocarditis, CHF and MI. The American Heart Association recommendation for cases of mitral valve prolapse and a detectable murmur is that antibiotic prophylaxis should be prescribed in all procedures where a transient bacteraemia is created. In the main, bone surgery on the foot is clean and prophylaxis is not required. Antibiotic prophylaxis is, however, required in nail surgery where there is paronychia or in any incision and drainage procedures of infected tissue.

Well-managed, mild-to-moderate hypertension poses no increased peri-operative risk, although in all cases hypertensive medication should be continued peri-operatively. Treated hypertension is associated with ischaemic heart disease and stroke. In cases of uncontrolled hypertension, the patient may present with a variety of symptoms, including headaches, transient visual impairment, anorexia or even nausea. Two significant findings are impaired renal function manifesting clinically as proteinuria and/or retinopathy. All patients with blood pressure above 160/95 mmHg on more than one occasion should be investigated and treated prior to surgery. Diastolic pressure greater than 120 mmHg is of grave concern and contraindicate any surgical intervention; such patients require urgent medical referral. Table 19.2 summarises the findings of a comprehensive literature review (Kilmartin et al 2001 – Trent Region Podiatric Forum) regarding peri-operative considerations of the patient with cardiovascular disease.

Anaemia represents a reduction in the oxygen-carrying capacity of the blood. Since there are

Table 19.2 Surgical recommendations for the cardiovascular patient (Kilmartin et al)

Myocardial infarctions (MI)	Surgery should be avoided in patients who have had an MI within the previous 6 months
Angina	In stable angina, where there is no history of an MI or other risk factors, the per-operative risk of an MI is low. In unstable angina, surgery is contraindicated until the angina has been controlled by medical or surgical means
Coronary artery bypass graft (CABG)	History of a CABG should be considered a low peri-operative risk
Congestive heart failure (CHF)	Patients with CHF represent a high risk of adverse cardiac events from the stress of surgery
Conduction disturbances	Conduction defects represent a low peri-operative risk
Arrhythmia	Any patient with a history suggestive of arrhythmia should have an ECG
Valvular heart disease	Antibiotic prophylaxis is not required in clean podiatric surgery to prevent bacterial endocarditis. It is, however, required in nail surgery

Box 19.3 Common clotting abnormalities

- von Willebrand's disease
- Haemophilia
  - Type A – classical haemophilia
  - Type B – Christmas' disease
  - Type C – PTA (plasma thromboplastin antecedent) deficiency
- Vitamin K deficiency

multiple causes and types of anaemia, pre-operative consultation is appropriate. Both cardiopulmonary integrity and wound healing depend on tissue oxygen levels. Anaemia is rarely a contraindication to surgery unless it is of severe magnitude. Haematocrit values below 30 are considered insufficient for elective foot surgery.

Patients with haemophilia or other clotting abnormalities (see Box 19.3) require thorough history taking. Enquire about bruising, nose bleeds and any previous surgical problems. Further studies that will be indicated include a platelet count and bleeding time.

Sickle cell disease affects those of African or West Indian descent. It is an autosomally inherited haemoglobinopathy resulting in the formation of haemoglobin S (HbS) instead of HbA. Small changes in oxygen tension cause HbS to polymerise and form pseudocrystalline structures, which distort red blood cells into the characteristic sickle shapes. Sickle cells increase blood viscosity and obstruct microvascular blood flow, leading to thrombosis and infarction. A comprehensive literature review regarding the use of tourniquets in this condition has been undertaken by a member of the Trent Region Podiatric Forum (Fig. 19.1).

Respiratory system

Post-operative morbidity and mortality from atelectasis and infection, following local or general anaesthesia, are significantly increased in individuals with pulmonary disease. These effects are most often noted in those individuals with known pulmonary risk factors, such as a history of heavy smoking and pre-existing pulmonary disease, and obesity and in elderly people. The pre-operative goal is to identify pulmonary risk factors and request an expert opinion as indicated. Smoking should be stopped at least 1 week prior to surgery and for at least 2 weeks following surgery, to promote healing.

Alimentary system

Gastrointestinal disorders are common and have many implications for the lower limb and its treatment. Patients with severe liver damage may be metabolically unstable and may not withstand the stress and the demands of surgery. Liver cirrhosis is not uncommon and should be identified in the history. Chronic alcoholism may cause osteoporosis, complicate anaesthesia (the metabolism of the anaesthetic), increase bleeding risk, decrease wound healing, increase the risk of infection and diminish adrenocortical responses to stress, and affect compliance with the post-operative regimen. Serious co-existing nutritional imbalances are often noted.

Genitourinary system

The kidneys regulate the body's electrolyte and fluid balance; this has implications for lower limb circulation and oedema, and it can delay wound healing. The presence of any renal symptoms such as haematuria, dysuria, polyuria, oliguria or flank pain mandates specific evaluation. Although the peri-operative risks for patients with renal disease are primarily related to fluid and electrolyte disturbances, hypertension and oedema may be related to renal dysfunction. Confirmation of kidney disease requires specific investigation. Screening urinalysis remains the classic measurement of renal performance (Ch. 13). Abnormal findings include the presence of glucose, protein, ketones, bilirubin, more than four red or white blood cells per field, bacteria, casts and crystals. Surgery should be postponed until renal function is stabilised.

Central and peripheral nervous system

Diseases of the nervous system may cause pain in the lower limb, deformity or gait abnormalities. The significance of some symptoms in the neurological enquiry will be difficult to interpret because the enquiry relies on the patient's subjective account. However, inadequate assessment of the neurological basis of foot pathology can lead to inappropriate surgical intervention through a missed diagnosis. A detailed assessment of the peripheral nervous system is given in Chapter 7.

Endocrine system

Diabetes, thyroid disease, growth disorders, obesity and problems associated with the menopause are particularly relevant. Diabetes mellitus is a complex systemic disease that may manifest as vascular, neurological, dermatological and structural changes in the foot and lower leg. The peri-operative goal is to

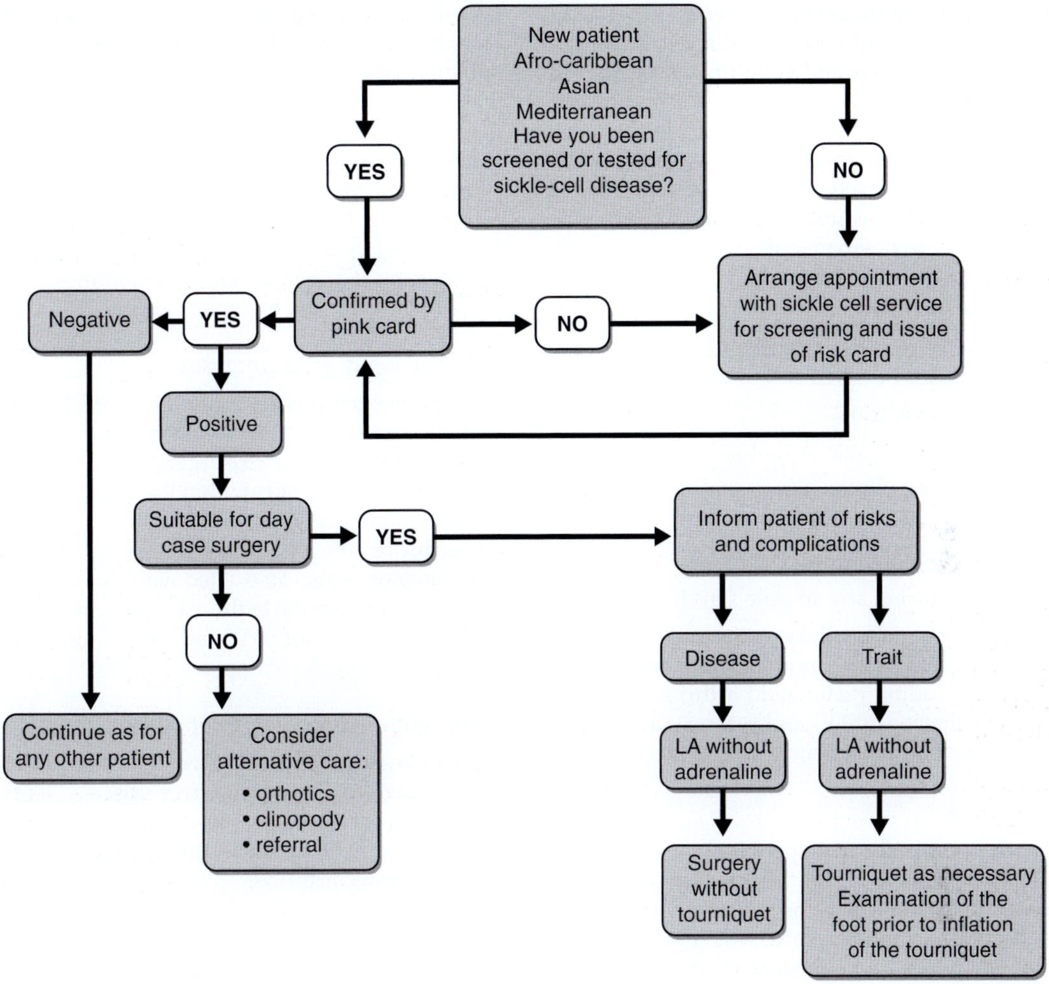

Figure 19.1 Decision-making algorithm for patients with sickle-cell anaemia. (With thanks to Mr C Bicknell of the Trent Forum.)

reduce hypoglycaemia or hyperglycaemia. Normally hyperglycaemia activates insulin production, but in the diabetic patient this feedback control loop is defective. Surgical stress causes a catabolic reaction, resulting in glucagon, adrenaline (epinephrine) and cortisol secretion. Blood glucose levels rise and other fuel pathways are mobilised.

The practitioner should ensure that a good metabolic balance is obtained pre-operatively. Avoidance of the extremes of hypoglycaemia or hyperglycaemia will help optimise wound healing and host defence function. Hyperglycaemia impairs wound healing by retarding wound closure, delaying wound contraction, slowing collagen synthesis, impairing granulocytes and reducing red blood cell viscosity. Elective surgery should be avoided in diabetic patients with blood sugar values greater than 11 mmol/l (200 mg/dl). Chronic hyperglycaemia greatly increases the risk of post-operative infection. The use of haemoglobin A_{1C}, an index of hyperglycaemia, is helpful in evaluating trends in diabetic control. Inadequate nutrition and reduced total plasma albumin have been shown to deter wound healing in patients with diabetes and should be normalised pre-operatively when possible. Patients with diabetes and a propensity towards ketosis require intra-operative intravenous insulin and monitoring. Wide blood sugar variations are associated with unpredictable healing ability and an increased surgical risk. A patient who is taking multiple medications is more prone to drug interactions, which may also affect diabetes management.

General anaesthesia creates a greater peri-operative risk because of increased insulin demands, the risk of silent MI, nausea and vomiting, and delays in food and oral medication intake. Early-morning surgery allows the optimal equilibrium between insulin dose and caloric intake, with immediate oral nutrition post-operatively. A sliding insulin scale is used to maintain this equilibrium in patients having surgery under a general anaesthetic.

Locomotor system

To determine the presence of musculoskeletal disease the patient should be asked if they have ever had:

- any form of arthritis
- back, hip, knee, ankle or foot pain
- fractured bones in the legs or feet
- torn or injured muscles in the legs
- joint swelling or stiffness
- limb pain during any specific activity.

Arthritic patients include those with single-joint osteoarthrosis and those with more complex multiorgan arthritides, including rheumatoid arthritis, systemic lupus erythematosus (SLE) and seronegative arthritis. Also review of the patient is able to use crutches.

Osteoarthrosis

There are no specific peri-operative considerations for the management of the osteoarthritic patient. However, the patient may be taking analgesic and anti-inflammatory preparations, which must be considered in the overall assessment of the patient. NSAIDs alter bleeding times and may inhibit bone healing and some authors recommend stopping their use before surgery.

Rheumatoid arthritis

Many patients coming to surgery have been on long-term steroids. These drugs suppress the HPA axis, and patients may require corticosteroid coverage during the peri-operative period. This should be given even if it has been a year since the patient has received medication (it is not necessary to treat a patient with steroids if they have only received intra-articular injections of cortisone). Disease-modifying drugs (e.g. methotrexate) and the newer biological agents such as the anti-tumour necrosis factor (TNF) or interleukin (IL)-1 agents suppress the bone marrow and can cause leucopenia and thrombocytopenia, increasing the likelihood of infection. Anti-TNF agents should be stopped 1 week prior to surgery and not reinstated until wound healing is complete (usually 2 weeks following surgery). This is to minimise the risk of infection and is undertaken in consultation with the prescribing doctor (Mohan et al 2003, Olsen & Stein 2004). With methotrexate the risk is less clear and two studies have shown no increase in the risk of infection if patients remain on methotrexate during the post-operative period and stopping the drug leads to a 5% risk of a rheumatoid flare (Grennan et al 2001, Sany et al 1993). Despite these findings most rheumatologists recommend similar guidelines as for the biological agents.

Systemic lupus erythematosus

Since systemic lupus erythematosus (SLE) is a multisystem disease, a careful history and assessment should be done prior to surgery. If the patient has received corticosteroids within the past year, consideration should be given to stress-coverage replacement during the peri-operative period. Raynaud's phenomenon is also associated with this disease, and it is a contraindication to the use of adrenaline (epinephrine) in foot surgery and may affect wound healing.

Seronegative spondyloarthropathies

If possible, elective foot surgery should be performed during periods between active disease flare-ups. Otherwise, there are no specific peri-operative considerations for Reiter's syndrome, psoriatic arthritis or enteropathic arthritis.

Gout

Any patient with a history of gout is at a substantially increased risk of a post-operative gouty attack. This may be due to local surgical trauma, dehydration and the temporary interruption of uricosuric medication. Those who have had an attack within the past year or those who are on hyperuricaemic medication are at highest risk.

Septic arthritis

Septic arthritis is a serious condition. The patient is likely to be generally unwell and should not undergo surgery if there is any chance that the joint is infected. Synovial fluid analysis should be considered where there is a recent history of infection.

Physical examination

The format of the physical examination is summarised in Box 19.4. The aim of the physical examination is to identify abnormality and delineate those patients who are fit for surgery. Opinions vary as to

Box 19.4 Physical examination

Cardiovascular system

- Blood pressure
- Ankle brachial pressure index (ABPI)
- Temperature and gradient
- Palpation of pulses
- Capillary refilling time (CRT)
- Oedema

Respiratory system

- Shortness of breath (SOB)
- Clubbing of fingers

Alimentary system

Rarely examined.

Genitourinary system

- Mid-stream urine reagent testing

Central nervous system

- Gait
- Motor system
- Sensory system

Endocrine system

- Blood glucose monitoring for diabetic patients

Locomotor system

- Joint range and quality of motion
- Neutral and relaxed calcaneal stance position
- Arch profile
- Digital position/deformity

the level of the examination required for the patient undergoing elective surgery under local anaesthesia. The practitioner is expected to have undertaken a detailed physical assessment of the systems (Ch. 5), vascular status (Ch. 6), neurological status (Ch. 7) and musculoskeletal status (Ch. 10), and a dermatological assessment (Ch. 8). As the physical examination has been considered in these chapters, it will not be dealt with in this chapter. For those patients having surgery under a general anaesthetic, NICE has produced standard national pre-operative test guidelines based on the level of surgery (minor to major +) and the anaesthetic surgical risk classification (NICE 2003).

Factors affecting operative risk

Use of local anaesthetics

Local anaesthetic agents can be defined as drugs which are used clinically to produce a reversible loss of sensation in a circumscribed area of the body. Because surgical techniques require their use, any contraindication to local anaesthetics must be identified. Contraindications that should be considered are given below.

Unstable epilepsy

High blood levels of local anaesthetic agents are known to cause convulsions in some epileptic patients through their action on brain tissue. Their use is therefore best avoided in such individuals.

Methaemoglobinaemia

Methaemoglobin is a form of haemoglobin consisting of globin with an oxidised haem-containing ferric iron. Methaemoglobin cannot transport oxygen and therefore compromises cardiovascular function. When prilocaine is metabolised by the liver, small amounts of a chemical called O-toluidine are produced which inhibits the enzyme involved in the conversion of methaemoglobin to haemoglobin. In patients with known methaemoglobinaemia, an alternative local anaesthetic agent to prilocaine should be used.

Pregnancy and breastfeeding

The British Medical Association suggests that drugs should only be used during pregnancy where the potential benefit outweighs the risk of harm to the fetus, particularly during the first trimester where all drugs should be avoided if possible. There is no specific guidance on the risks associated with the low doses of local anaesthesia used for foot surgery in pregnant women. However, because of the ability of local anaesthetics to cross the placental barrier, they are probably best avoided whenever possible during pregnancy. If a local anaesthetic was to be given during pregnancy it would seem prudent to avoid prilocaine hydrochloride, as fetal haemoglobin is more susceptible to the development of methaemoglobinaemia. Both lidocaine (lignocaine) and bupivacaine are considered safe for use in breastfeeding mothers, as only small quantities are secreted into breast milk.

Porphyrias

The porphyrias are a group of metabolic disorders, and drugs contraindicated for use in patients with porphyria include some local anaesthetics. These agents must therefore be avoided in known carriers of the porphyrogenic gene to avoid precipitating an acute attack. Where surgery is still indicated, the use of a general anaesthetic should be considered and the patient referred as necessary.

Psychiatric status

Patients approach surgery with an understandable amount of fear and anxiety. They know that they will be in an environment that is unfamiliar to which they are unaccustomed. Some fear that they will experience pain during the operation. Most of their anxiety is because of insufficient knowledge based on hearsay and rumour. During the pre-operative assessment it is important that the practitioner recognises the nervous patient and provides appropriate information and counselling to allay any concerns. However, it is important that the practitioner recognises when a patient is unsuitable for surgery under local anaesthesia and either refers the patient or organises for the patient to have their surgery under a general anaesthetic.

Significant psychiatric illness is a contraindication for most elective surgical procedures primarily due to compliance issues with post-operative care regimens.

Age

An increasing percentage of the population is over 65 years of age, a trend that is expected to continue well into the twenty-first century. Independent ambulation is an important component of wellness, although a majority of patients over the age of 65 complain of foot pain limiting their activity. In geriatric patients who have foot conditions which can be surgically corrected, and where the physical condition is satisfactory, surgery can safely be performed. The chronological age of the patient is less important, as long as the physiological age of the patient is adequate for the planned surgical procedure. Problems associated with surgery on the older patient include:

- adverse physiological status
- impact of surgery on the patient's lifestyle
- the use of a tourniquet – ankle tourniquet is tolerated for a shorter period in patients over the age of 70 (<40 minutes is recommended (Rudkin et al 2004))
- selection of the operative procedure – simple procedures versus complex procedures – even though the latter would give a better result.

Generally, in the older patient, destructive rather than functionally reconstructive procedures are often more appropriate. For example, amputation of a dislocated hammer second toe in the presence of asymptomatic hallux valgus, rather than reconstructive surgery of both the first and second toes.

With regard to surgical treatment in children, it is important to bear in mind child psychology, patient–parent relationships, stress levels, and parental presence during the operation should be considered.

Infection

In general, the elective procedure is performed when the patient is free from all systemic infection. A patient with established infection that does not respond to oral antibiotics and appropriate wound care demands a thorough pre-operative evaluation and specialist consultation.

Antibiotic prophylaxis

The spread of multi-resistant organisms, exacerbated by the over-use of antibiotics, is a major concern across all surgical disciplines. The difficulty is making a clinical judgement as to when the antibiotic is truly indicated and when their use is considered because of tradition and dogma. Recent studies suggest that an antibiotic should be used to supplement the body's natural defences with the ultimate aim of preventing a post-operative infection. Antibiotics are therefore indicated when there is a high probability that a bacterial invasion will overcome host defences. Four factors are key to this decision making:

1. timing
2. the at-risk patient
3. the procedure
4. the choice of antibiotic.

Antibiotics should be given in such as manner that they reach peak tissue concentrations during the procedure. To facilitate this, the intravenous (i.v.) route is preferred – the drug given 1 hour prior to the procedure. Consideration must then be given as to how long to continue treatment.

Systemic conditions that decrease host resistance and place the patient at an increased risk of infection include:

- diabetes mellitus
- rheumatoid arthritis
- peripheral vascular disease
- hepatic pathology
- corticosteroid therapy
- rheumatic valvular heart disease.

Case history 19.5

A 62-year-old diabetic patient had an involuted nail on the right hallux. Her diabetes was poorly controlled and she had a total knee replacement 4 years ago. The knee replacement was uneventful but her diabetic control has deteriorated since then. Will you request antibiotic cover in this patient?

Outcome: Although some authors feel that nail surgery is 'dirty' surgery because of the bacterial load beneath the nail plate, there is no evidence for routine use of antibiotic prophylaxis for nail surgery in patients with a prosthetic joint. However, with this patient's poor diabetic control you should consider performing the procedure under antibiotic cover.

The appropriate use of antibiotics in such patients remains controversial. The procedure itself must be considered. Surgery that involves prolonged operative times and/or extensive dissection increases the infection risk. The use of implants, such as screw fixation, affects the normal wound mechanics (Case history 19.5). Antibiotic prophylaxis is recommended for surgery in the presence of contaminated wounds or trauma. Finally, the practitioner must consider the likely infecting organism to decide the choice, route and dosage of an antibiotic. Cephalosporins are often prescribed because of their low toxicity, spectrum of activity and clinical efficiency.

Laboratory investigations and imaging modalities

The National Institute for Health and Clinical Excellence (NICE 2003) states that the main purpose of preoperative investigations is to provide additional diagnostic and prognostic information to supplement the clinical history of a patient with the aim of:

1. providing information that may confirm or question the correctness of the current course of clinical management
2. using this information to reduce the possible harm or increase the benefit to patients by altering their clinical management if necessary
3. using this information to help assess the risk to the patient and opening up the possibility of discussing potential increases of risk with the patient
4. predicting post-operative complications
5. establishing a baseline measurement for later reference (to refer back to post-operatively)
6. opportunistic screening that is unrelated to the surgery.

Urine testing

Urinalysis is an aid in the diagnosis of renal disease, hepatic disease and diabetes mellitus (see Ch. 13). Diabetes mellitus can have widespread consequences for the lower limb and is of particular interest to the surgeon. Renal and hepatic diseases may have serious systemic repercussions and, when identified, require further investigation before it is safe to proceed with surgery. Screening for a urinary-tract infection (UTI) or the presence of bacteria in urine can also identify those patients at increased risk of developing post-operative wound infections. Testing is non-invasive and cost-effective, and urine specimens are easily obtained. Urinalysis is therefore useful in the pre-operative assessment of patients to screen for illnesses that may complicate or contraindicate elective procedures.

Blood analysis

The use of blood analysis in the pre-operative assessment of the surgical patient is a matter for debate. Routine screening prior to surgery is only likely to reveal a small percentage with abnormalities, most of which are insignificant for anaesthetic or surgical management. Therefore, the general rule for the use of confirmatory diagnostic testing applies: their use is indicated from the initial patient assessment. In cases where systemic pathology is known or suspected, e.g. in anaemia to ascertain haemoglobin levels or blood glucose levels/HbA_{1C} in patients with diabetes, blood sampling is certainly indicated.

The patient on anticoagulant therapy has already been discussed. Similarly, patients who have clotting abnormalities also require further investigation (see Box 19.3).

Radiographs

Radiographs are vital for a number of reasons:

- Identification of rheumatological, metabolic, endocrine and infective disease
- Monitoring the progression of disease/deformity
- Showing the precise relationship between osseous anatomical structures that are of particular interest to the surgeon
- Implications for the intra-operative fixation of osteotomies

- Demonstration of the position of retained internal fixation
- Confirmation of bone healing in the post-operative phase.

Osteoporosis typically begins in middle life and is predominantly a disease of post-menopausal women. Histologically, bone formation is normal, but bone resorption is increased. If pre-operative radiographs suggest significant osteoporosis, systemic disease is likely and multiple contributing factors, including dietary deficiencies, endocrine imbalances, sedentary lifestyles and genetic predisposition, may be implicated. Apart from the surgical implications of systemic disease, radiographs of, for example, osteoarthritis are key if surgery is being considered. Identification and use of angular relationships, or charting, between the foot bones has become a key skill of the foot surgeon. Surgical planning is heavily influenced by charting and helps the surgeon select the most appropriate surgical technique.

Radiographic assessment is covered in Chapter 12.

Post-operative assessment

The post-operative phase is said to begin when the patient leaves the operating theatre. However, wound healing commences with the initial surgical incision. Wounds progress through the phases of inflammation to establish environmental homeostasis amenable to tissue repair. Careful pre-operative assessment and meticulous surgical technique assist the wound through this process and minimise post-operative complications.

A surgical complication is an unexpected set of circumstances that occur during the peri-operative setting and directly or indirectly prolong the patient's functional recovery period. Complications are inherent to all types of surgical procedures and foot surgery is no exception. If appropriately anticipated, some complications are preventable, whereas other complications can be minimised with early diagnosis. There must, therefore, be an awareness of the signs of impending complications to trigger prompt and decisive action appropriate to the situation.

Management is aimed at avoiding haematoma formation, excess oedema and infection, while attempting to keep the patient comfortable and protect the surgical site. The format of the post-operative assessment includes evaluation of:

- the wound dressing
- the wound
- pain.

Evaluation of the wound dressing

A wound dressing has several functions but the main goal is to provide an optimum environment for healing. The dressing must first protect the wound from contamination and prevent the overgrowth or penetration of pathogens. It must be absorptive and draw the fluids away from the wound and prevent their accumulation – this reduces tissue maceration. Different materials can be used to provide temporary immobilisation, with or without compression. This places a wound at rest and allows healing without undue mechanical forces impeding the physiological processes. Clots and newly formed capillaries are thus not disturbed and pain levels are decreased. Gentle compression will aid haemostasis and prevent the formation of haematoma. Immobilisation is particularly important in reconstructive surgery, to maintain the foot or a digit in its corrected position during the healing process.

The post-operative dressing regimen typically includes a dressing change and/or removal of sutures at 7–14 days after surgery. The inspection of the dressing is part of the overall assessment of the wound. Ensure that there are no overt signs of slippage, which may predispose exposure of the wound to contamination. If compression has been applied, has it been effective? Examine the inside of the dressing to gauge both the amount of blood loss and the nature of any exudate. A purulent, offensive exudate indicates bacterial infection and requires prompt antimicrobial therapy and/or drainage. It is important to record normal and abnormal findings throughout the healing period.

Evaluation of the wound

A classification of wounds is given in Box 19.5.

The majority of elective procedures on the foot are classified as clean, with the exception of nail surgery, where it is impossible to disinfect the invaginated nail sulci to the same standard as unbroken skin.

When examining the wound post-operatively, the surgeon should expect to see:

- an intact wound that shows no sign of dehiscence
- a 'normal' amount of inflammation
- no sign of excessive bleeding, oedema or haematoma formation
- the position maintained if any reconstructive technique has been performed.

Meticulous suturing technique combined with anatomical dissection, adequate haemostasis and careful

Box 19.5 Wound classification

Wounds can be classified as:

- Clean: surgical incisions are made with no break in aseptic technique; no known contamination and no inflammation is encountered
- Clean-contaminated: a minor break is made in aseptic technique
- Contaminated: a major break is made in aseptic technique, or in a fresh traumatic wound (less than 4 hours)
- Dirty: acute bacterial infection encountered with or without pus. A traumatic wound with delayed treatment (greater than 4 hours). A retained foreign body or infected surgery

skin handling are important to reduce the incidence of these complications. When the sutures are removed it is important to check the healing of the wound edges by gently applying tensile force across the area. Dehiscence will require further support of the wound until the area has regained its mechanical strength.

Evaluation of pain

The assessment and management of pain requires an understanding of both physiology and pharmacology. The degree and severity of pain in the post-operative period depends on:

- the site and nature of the operation
- the amount of surgical trauma
- the physiological and psychological make-up of the patient and their tolerance of pain.

Pain is a reflection of tissue injury, but it also represents the psychological dimension of the patient's suffering. Much unnecessary suffering may be avoided by the reduction of pre-operative anxiety. Simple, clear and honest communication with the patient should include an explanation of what will happen and when it will happen; this can have a positive influence on post-operative pain levels. Certain patients may benefit from prescription of an anxiolytic, used alone, or with analgesic medications to raise pain thresholds following surgery.

A long-acting local anaesthetic is usually injected at the time of surgery and will delay the onset of post-operative pain for some time. A combination of opioid analgesics and NSAIDs, however, provides the mainstay of post-operative pain management. Paracetamol may be combined with opioid analgesics such as codeine to gain enhanced analgesia, while NSAIDs may be added to an opioid regimen to provide additional anti-inflammatory and intrinsic analgesic effects.

During the post-operative period, a patient should be asked about pain and their response should be recorded. There are several tools available to assess pain, including visual analogue scoring and complex questionnaires such as the McGill Pain Questionnaire (Ch. 3). The use of (or lack of) prescribed analgesic medication should also be discussed. The most common causes of excessive post-operative pain in the first week after surgery are excessive swelling within a restrictive dressing and cast and haematoma formation. Pain is usually greatest within the first 48 hours following surgery. If pain increases following this initial peak, this 'returning pain' is suggestive of infection and usually occurs 4–10 days after surgery. Suspicion of haematoma formation or infection requires prompt intervention and management.

Summary

Surgical procedures of the foot vary enormously in their complexity. However, the continuum of surgical care encompassing the pre-operative, intra-operative and post-operative phases should remain the same. Careful attention to detail during each phase is essential for the achievement of a successful surgical outcome. Following the approach outlined in this chapter will ensure that a broad range of factors are taken into consideration when assessing the surgical patient.

References

Grennan D M, Gray J, Loudon J et al 2001 Methotrexate and early postoperative complications in patients with rheumatoid arthritis undergoing elective orthopaedic surgery. Annals of Rheumatic Diseases 60(3):214–217

Kilmartin T E, McInnes B, Wilkinson D J 2001 Peri-operative considerations for the podiatric patient with cardiovascular disease. British Journal of Podiatry 4:20–24

Mohan A K, Cote T R, Siegel J N et al 2003 Infectious complications of biological treatments of rheumatoid arthritis. Current Opinion in Rheumatology 15:179–184

National Institute of Clinical Excellence 2003 Preoperative tests. Clinical guideline no 3. NICE, London

Olsen N J, Stein M 2004 New drugs for rheumatoid arthritis. New England Journal of Medicine 350:2567–2579

Rudkin A k, Rudkin G E, Dracopoulos G C 2004 Acceptability of ankle tourniquet use in midfoot and forefoot surgery: an audit of 1000 cases. Foot & Ankle International 25(11):788–794

Sany J, Anaya J M, Canovas F et al 1993 Influence of methotrexate on the frequency of postoperative infections and complications in patients with rheumatoid arthritis. Journal of Rheumatology 20:1129–1132

Further reading

British National Formulary (BNF) [Updated twice yearly] British Medical Association and Royal Pharmaceutical Society of Great Britain, London

James Garden O, Bradbury A W, Forsythe J L R et al 2007 Principles and practice of surgery, 5th edn. Churchill Livingstone, Edinburgh

Greenberger N, Hinthorn D 1993 History taking and physical examination: essentials and clinical correlates. Mosby Year-Book, St Louis

Levy L A, Hetherington V J 2006 Principles and practice of podiatric medicine. Data Trace Publishing Company, Maryland, USA

McGlamry E D 2001 A comprehensive textbook of foot surgery, 3rd edn. Lippincott, Williams & Wilkins, Baltimore

National Institute of Clinical Excellence 2003 Preoperative tests. Clinical guideline no 3. NICE, London

O'Higgins N J, Chisholm G D, Williamson R C N 1991 Surgical management, 2nd edn. Butterworth-Heinemann, Oxford

Pinnock C et al 1999 Fundamentals of anaesthesia. Greenwich Medical Media, London

RCN 1999 Orthopaedic pre-admission assessment clinics. RCN Publishing Company Ltd

Seymour C, Siklos P 2004 Clinical clerking: a short introduction to clinical skills, 2nd edn. Press Syndicate of the University of Cambridge

Tally N, O'Connor S 1989 Clinical examination. Blackwell Scientific, Oxford

Turner R, Blackwood R 1991 Lecture notes on history taking and examination, 2nd edn. Blackwell Science, Oxford

Zier B 1990 Essentials of internal medicine in clinical podiatry. W B Saunders, Philadelphia

Index

Note: Page numbers in *italics* refer to figures and page numbers in **bold** refer to tables.

B

C

D

E

G

H

I

J

K

M

N

O

P

S

T